BARRON'S

DAT®
DENTAL ADMISSIONS
TEST

Joseph DiRienzo, Ph.D.
Professor of Microbiology and
Assistant Dean for Student Research
Department of Microbiology
School of Dental Medicine
University of Pennsylvania

Edwin H. Hines, DDS
Professor and Chairman
Department of Pediatric
Dentistry
Meharry Medical
College, School of
Dentistry

John J. Ference, DMD
Director of Undergraduate Prosthodontics
University of Pittsburg
School of Dental Medicine

John Swartwood, C.Phil.
Head Instructor at Swartwood Testing,
Admissions, and Review

Nicole D. Cornell, M.S.
Boise State University

J. Shield Wallace, Ph.D.
Professor of Chemistry
Central New Mexico Community College

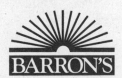

BARRON'S

ONLINE PRACTICE TESTS

Access the Diagnostic Test and a full-length online
practice test at *barronsbooks.com/tp/dat/*
or by scanning the QR Code below.*

*Be sure to have your copy of *Barron's DAT* handy
to complete the registration process.

All inquiries should be addressed to:
Barron's Educational Series, Inc.
250 Wireless Boulevard
Hauppauge, NY 11788
www.barronseduc.com

ISBN: 978 -1-4380-0634-5

Library of Congress Control Number: 2018934052

PRINTED IN THE UNITED STATES OF AMERICA
9 8 7 6 5 4 3 2 1

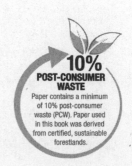

10%
POST-CONSUMER
WASTE
Paper contains a minimum
of 10% post-consumer
waste (PCW). Paper used
in this book was derived
from certified, sustainable
forestlands.

Contents

PART THREE: ORGANIC CHEMISTRY

PART FOUR: READING COMPREHENSION TEST

PART FIVE: QUANTITATIVE REASONING TEST

Introduction

ABOUT THE DAT

The American Dental Association (ADA) Department of Testing Services annually reports on the *appropriateness* of the DAT. It has been proved through statistical analysis that the test battery is a significant indicator of success in dental school as well as a valuable indicator of performance on Part I of the National Board Dental Examinations. The DAT is also used as a method of standardizing and quantifying the undergraduate preparation received at various academic institutions. The Dental Admission Testing Program is administered by the ADA Department of Testing Services. It consists of four timed sections:

- Survey of the Natural Sciences Test (SNST)
- Perceptual Ability Test (PAT)
- Reading Comprehension Test (RCT)
- Quantitative Reasoning Test (QRT)

Although there are only four timed sections, there are six scored sections. Notice in the list below that the Survey of the Natural Sciences has three scored sections that are administered in one timed section. You will receive the following **eight** score reports.

- **BIOLOGY** (Questions 1–40 of the Survey of the Natural Sciences Test)
- **GENERAL CHEMISTRY** (Questions 41–70 of the Survey of the Natural Sciences Test)
- **ORGANIC CHEMISTRY** (Questions 71–100 of the Survey of the Natural Sciences Test)
- **QUANTITATIVE REASONING**
- **READING COMPREHENSION**
- **TOTAL SCIENCE** (a combination of the biology, general chemistry, and organic chemistry raw scores)
- **ACADEMIC AVERAGE** (a composite score that is an average of the quantitative reasoning, reading comprehension, biology, general chemistry, and organic chemistry scores)
- **PERCEPTUAL ABILITY** (a score that is not incorporated in the other composite/combination score reports; it is always reported separately)

The specifics regarding the number of questions and the time allotted for each section are as follows for the Dental Admission Testing Program:

Section	Number of Questions	Time Average	Average Time Per Item
Survey of the Natural Sciences Test	100 questions (40 Biology, 30 General Chemistry, 30 Organic Chemistry)	90 minutes	54 seconds/question
Perceptual Ability Test	90 questions (composed of 6 different sections)	60 minutes	40 seconds/question (see section for specific timing)
Break		15 minutes	
Reading Comprehension Test	50 questions (3 passages, with 16–17 questions following each passage)	60 minutes	20 minutes/passage
Quantitative Reasoning Test	40 questions	45 minutes	1 minute, 7 seconds/question
TOTAL	280 questions	4 hours, 30 minutes (start to finish)	

SCORING

The DAT is scored on a 30-point scale, with 30 being the highest mark and 1 being the lowest mark. *There is no penalty for wrong answers.* The total number of correct answers on each section is the raw score.

Each section is scored separately. A total science score and an academic average are also given. The most important score is the academic average. The academic average is calculated by averaging the Biology, General Chemistry, Organic Chemistry, Reading Comprehension, and Quantitative scores (everything but the PAT). One of the first things that dental schools look at is the academic average (AA).

What you need to know is that a score of 17 (AA) is about the national average on most sections of the DAT. You should aim to get above this national average on all sections.

While every institution is different and every committee has its own standards, many find 19+ to be in the competitive range. Of course, some applicants with lower scores are admitted to top schools, and some applicants with higher scores are not.

A rough guideline that we use for many of our students is the following:

Academic Average:

19+ Competitive
20+ Strong
21+ Very Strong

PREPARING FOR THE TEST

In order to take the DAT, you need only pay the required fee, register, show up at the testing site, and spend several hours answering the battery of test questions. Alternatively, you have chosen to do more than just take the test. By purchasing this book, you have begun a commitment to something much greater. Your decision to engage in test preparation is a sign that you seek to take control of the test, and that you believe that performance is largely a result of preparation. Hopefully, the following comments regarding test preparation for the DAT will prove useful.

Studying and Preparation Strategies

Study What You Don't Know

After a few weeks of studying for the DAT, you will find that much of the material looks familiar. Concentrate on learning the information you don't know rather than focusing on the information that you've read before. This tip seems obvious, but failure to follow it will waste much of your time and will hurt your score.

Utilize All Your Senses

Read, write, and speak aloud the material to maximize the experience of learning. If you enhance the learning experience, you will enhance your ability to recall that experience.

Use Repetition

Read, write, and speak aloud the information for 6 weeks, and you will be able to recall important facts with greater ease.

Don't Study Just the Sciences

Any single low score on any section could be reason to *not* accept you, whereas a single high score will *not* greatly help your application. High scores across *all* sections is what is desired.

Create and Use Mnemonics

For an easier way to remember unfamiliar or unrelated science information, make up mnemonics. Make up phrases and words that stand for difficult to remember items of information in biology, chemistry, and organic chemistry.

Allow Sufficient Time

Do not schedule your exam before you can realistically be prepared to take it. Only you will know how much time you will need to spend reviewing. Use the model exams in this book and online to gauge your proficiency with the subject matter. Schedule a date that will permit you to thoroughly review all the material for the exam. Usually 6 weeks is sufficient for the average student; but, depending on how much time you will dedicate to studying each day, you may require only 4 weeks, or as many as 8 weeks, to fully cover all the material.

Be Disciplined

This is the common strategy of all test takers who score in the top percentiles. It is through hard work that high marks are achieved. Discipline yourself to a regimented schedule of studying for the DAT. Do not let anything come between you and the scores you desire. Between now and your test date, many things will try to distract your attention from your studies, but *be disciplined*!

Test-Taking Strategies

Answer Every Question

On the DAT, you are *not* penalized for wrong answers. You will have a 20% chance of guessing the correct answer if you respond randomly.

Beware of ALL and NONE Questions

The ADA Department of Testing Services does not want to have to rescore examinations and answer inquiries regarding ambiguous questions. Therefore, "gentle" words, such as *usually*, *often*, and *rarely*, are preferred in answer choices. "Harsh" words, such as *always, never, all*, and *none*, can prove disastrous if any one exception can be argued. If you are really baffled on a question, steer clear of choosing an answer containing a "harsh" word.

Be Knowledgeable About Distracters

The wrong answer choices to a question are termed distracters because their purpose is to distract you from the obvious correct answer. The ADA Department of Testing Services does not really want to confuse you; rather, it wants the correct answer to blend in with the wrong answers. The distracters lure you from the correct answer by presenting possible answers that may be partially correct. On any given question, the distracters will be similar in their "degree of distraction." The following example will illustrate how to identify and eliminate distracters.

Supplemental information must be used to eliminate the wrong answers. Do not get caught in the trap of choosing the most familiar and comfortable answer. On a difficult organic chemistry question involving an obscure reaction that you are not familiar with, undoubtedly at least two familiar reactions will appear in the answer choices as distracters. You will want to choose one of these as the correct response because we all like to feel comfortable with our answers. Use any knowledge you possess about any answer choices to identify distracters.

Draw It

You will almost always be able to more clearly understand what is being asked if you can sketch a chart, a figure, or some other graphical representation of the question you are asked. You will be given an erasable scratch board and marker upon request; use them to your advantage.

Know the PAT Directions

Before the test date, be sure that you know exactly what you will be asked to do in each section of the PAT. For the other tests, the directions are rather straightforward; for the PAT, however, they are not as clear-cut. A sufficient review of the material presented in this book should clear up any confusion as to what will be required of you on the PAT's six sections.

Be Sensible About Sleep, Eating, and Exercise

To give a peak performance on the day of the test, you will need to take care of yourself in the days prior. Eat right, get plenty of sleep, and exercise the week before the test. Getting adequate sleep the night before will not compensate for a series of late nights.

Prepare the Night Before

The night before the test, you should have everything accounted for so that no last-minute stresses will distract you on test day. Be sure that everything you need is in order and that plans are set for your timely arrival at the test site. Again, your focus on the test is reinforced by a general sense of control over the situation. Have clear plans for the test day that include what you will eat, wear, and take to the center.

Anxiety

By viewing your future goals as intimately connected to your actions in the present, you will undoubtedly acknowledge the value of engaging in preparative measures to ensure future success. You will possess a sense of control over your performance. Control will help you to stay focused, to remain in the present, and to use the mental tools that you have worked hard to refine. When you possess a high level of self-control, anxiety can serve you positively in two ways: It can help to keep you motivated as you actively prepare, and it can even help boost performance on the day of the test.

It is normal to be anxious about the DAT. The fact that you possess a degree of anxiety suggests that you respect the difficulty of the test and the value of a high score. Anxiety will be your mentor, reminding you to actively prepare for this test. Anxiety will help to ensure that you have taken care of important details, such as verifying that you have the proper identification and familiarizing yourself with the best way to get to the test site. On the day of the test, if you maintain a sense of being in control of your own destiny, you will walk into the testing center confident that your hours of preparation will pay off. During the test, your slightly rapid heart rate will serve to keep you working at a productive pace. You will remain alert, and you will perform to your best ability.

Become Comfortable with the Computerized Format

Because the test will be administered on computer, you should be certain to clear up any concerns about the computer format prior to your test date. It is strongly suggested that you order the computer tutorial from the ADA Department of Testing Services. This will help you know what the test will look like on the computer screen and how you can register your answers appropriately. You should also consider ahead of time how you will use your erasable boards and markers.

PRACTICE, PRACTICE, PRACTICE: ONLINE PRACTICE TEST

Now that you know the strategies that will help you do well on the DAT, be sure to use them whenever you take the model tests in this book and, of course, when you take your actual DAT. In addition to the tests in this book, you can get even more practice online at *barronsbooks. com/tp/dat/* with a downloadable Diagnostic Test and an additional online practice test. You will need your copy of *Barron's DAT* handy to complete your online registration.

ONLINE PRACTICE TESTS

Access a downloadable PDF Diagnostic Test and a full-length online practice test at *barronsbooks.com/tp/dat/* or scan the QR Code below.*

*Be sure to have your copy of *Barron's DAT* handy to complete the registration process.

PART ONE

Biology

BIOLOGY

Introduction

As detailed in the DAT 2018 Program Guide found at *www.ada.org/en/education-careers/ dental-admissions-test/dat-guide*, the Biology component of the Survey of the Natural Sciences section contains 40 multiple-choice questions. Biology makes up the largest percent (40%) of the Natural Sciences test, which also includes General Chemistry (30%) and Organic Chemistry (30%).

This section of the preparatory guide will cover the Biology portion of the Survey of the Natural Sciences test. As recently as in 2017, the Biology questions that appeared on past exams were selected from the following six general topics. These are very broad topics covered in most General Biology courses and textbooks.

1. **CELL AND MOLECULAR BIOLOGY.** This topic has included questions on theories of the origin of life, structure and function of cells and their organelles, cell metabolism and energy generating processes, basic principles of thermodynamics, cell replication/division including mitosis and meiosis, and experimental cell biology.

2. **DIVERSITY OF LIFE** questions about the biological organization and relationship of major taxa. Questions about the organization of living organisms into the three domains and six kingdoms that represent current classification schemes have been asked.

3. **STRUCTURE AND FUNCTION OF SYSTEMS.** Additional questions about organ systems of vertebrate animals, including integumentary, skeletal, muscular, circulatory, immunological, digestive, respiratory, urinary, nervous, endocrine, and reproductive, have also appeared on exams.

4. **DEVELOPMENTAL BIOLOGY.** The process of fertilization, descriptive and experimental embryology, and developmental mechanisms have been covered.

5. **GENETICS.** There have been questions on molecular biology and recombinant DNA technology as well as Mendelian (classical) and population genetics. There have also been questions specifically about human genetics.

6. **EVOLUTION, ECOLOGY, AND BEHAVIOR.** Lastly, the exam has included questions in the areas of phylogenetics, natural selection and ecology of populations, and social behavior.

The emphasis of this section will be to summarize the principles and concepts for these broad topics that formed the basis of questions on prior DAT exams. However, the study material will be supplemented with background information that is required for a thorough understanding of these subjects. The study material will be organized in a logical progression of information in which basic information will be presented in order to provide the background for more complex principles and concepts. In addition, the sequence of information will be summarized in flow charts to supply a convenient overview. Study material will be integrated, where possible, using a comparative approach to facilitate learning. The organization of the review is shown in the following flow chart (Figure 1.1).

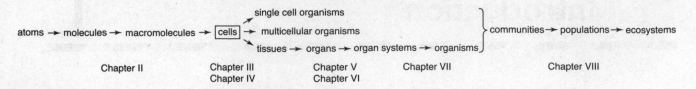

Chapter II   Chapter III   Chapter V   Chapter VII   Chapter VIII
                          Chapter IV   Chapter VI

Figure 1.1. Flow chart illustrating how the Biology review material
is organized. The cell is the central theme of the review material.

Basic Principles 2

Biology is defined as the scientific field that examines the organization, structures, functions, interactions, and relationships of living organisms. The foundation of the study of biology is the cell. The primary material used to build the cell includes **organic** compounds (carbon-containing compounds from living material), such as nucleotides, amino acids, sugars, and fatty acids (Figure 2.1). These molecules are typically composed of carbon [C], oxygen [O], and hydrogen [H] in various ratios. Some of these basic molecules also contain nitrogen [N], phosphorus [P], and/or sulfur [S]. Notice that C, O, N, P, and S are clustered on the Periodic Table of the Elements, and that all of these elements, plus H and selenium [Se], make up the nonmetals group (see Figure A.1 in the Appendix).

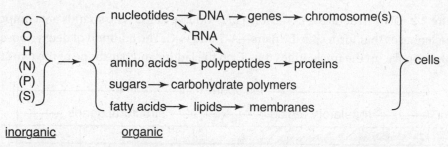

Figure 2.1. Flow chart of the approach used to organize the review topics in Chapter 2. The parentheses indicate that nitrogen, phosphorus, and sulfur are not present in all of the basic building blocks of cells.

COMPOSITION OF THE UNIT CELL

Nucleotides are molecules composed of a purine (adenine [A] or quanine [G]) or pyrimidine (cytosine [C], thymine [T], or uracil [U]), a 5-carbon sugar (ribose or deoxyribose), and phosphate. **Nucleic acids**, such as DNA (**deoxyribonucleic acid**) and RNA (**ribonucleic acid**), are comprised of nucleotides. U is substituted for T in RNA. DNA is organized in a coiled or twisted double-strand of paired nucleotides (Figure 2.2). Adenine always pairs with thymine, and guanine always pairs with cytosine. Notice that the additional hydrogen bond in a G-C pair makes G-C-rich DNA more stable than A-T-rich sequences. One strand extends from the 5′ to 3′ direction and the complementary strand extends from 3′ to 5′. **Genes** are composed of unique sequences of DNA. In some cases, genes that have related functions, such as coding for enzymes involved in the metabolism of a sugar, may be arranged in clusters or **operons** (Figure 2.3). The genes in an operon are usually under a common regulatory mechanism. The linear sequence of genes (either independent or in operons) makes up the **chromosome**.

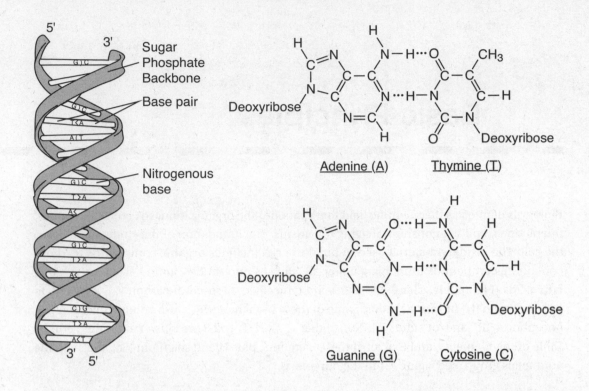

Figure 2.2. DNA structure is in the form of a "double helix." The strands are composed of nucleobases that form specific pairs—A-T and G-C. The addition of deoxyribose and phosphate make up the nucleotides that form the ladder and backbone of the two strands.

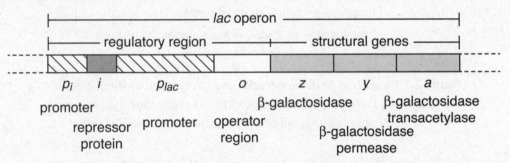

Figure 2.3. Typical genetic organization of an operon. Genes in the *lac* operon help the cell metabolize the sugar lactose.

The information contained in the DNA sequence of a gene is converted to an RNA species [ribosomal (r)RNA, transfer (t)RNA, or messenger (m)RNA] by a process known as **transcription**. In order for a specific gene to be expressed in a cell, a protein known as a sigma factor must bind to RNA polymerase. This creates a complex that binds to a sequence of DNA known as a promoter (initiation phase) (Figure 2.4). All genes have an assigned promoter that resides immediately before the gene or group of genes in an operon. The promoter-bound RNA polymerase separates the two stands of the DNA helix and catalyzes the addition of matching complementary RNA nucleotides (A, G, C, or U), in a 5′ to 3′ direction, by moving along one of the separated DNA strands in a 3′ to 5′ direction (elongation phase). A sugar-phosphate backbone is added to the growing chain of newly added nucleotides producing an mRNA strand that is complementary to the DNA sequence of the gene (DNA template). In the termination phase in prokaryotic cells, RNA transcription stops when a G-C enriched hairpin loop is formed. In eukaryotic cells, the addition of a series of adenines (A) at the 3′ end of the mRNA stops transcription. See Chapter 3 for definitions of prokaryotic and eukaryotic cells. The mRNA leaves its site of synthesis in the nucleus and enters the cytoplasm.

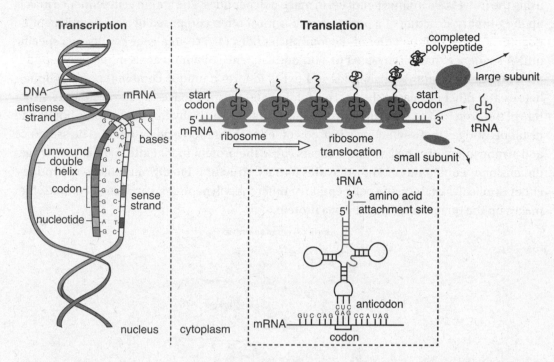

Figure 2.4. Transcription and translation. Inset shows how the tRNAs recognize each codon on the mRNA template adding specific amino acids to the growing polypeptide chain.

The RNA species are then used to make **polypeptides** from a unique series of amino acids. The decoding of mRNA to make polypeptides is called **translation**. In the translation process, ribosomes and a particular mRNA form a complex, and the first tRNA (carrying a specific amino acid) binds to the start codon of the mRNA (initiation stage) (Figure 2.4). Ribosomes are complexes of proteins and RNA essential for translation (see Figure A.2 in the Appendix). **Codons** are various combinations of three nucleotides that encode a specific amino acid. All the known codons and their corresponding amino acids are organized in a table that comprises the **genetic code** (see Figure A.3 in the Appendix). Notice that some codons are not translated to an amino acid but signal the termination of translation (stop codons). A tRNA transfers an amino acid to the next codon in the mRNA sequence (elongation phase). Specific tRNAs contain anticodons for each amino acid. The ribosome continually moves along the mRNA template to the next codon in the sequence thereby forming a growing amino acid chain (translocation phase). The ribosome releases the amino acid chain when it encounters a stop codon (termination phase). The transition from genetic information to final product can be summarized in Figure 2.5.

nucleotides → DNA → genes → RNA → amino acids → polypeptides → proteins

(transcription)   (translation)

Figure 2.5. Flow chart illustrating the connection between nucleotides and amino acids in the cell

Amino acids are short chains of carbon with an amino group ($-NH_2$) and a carboxyl group ($-COOH$). Some amino acids have a functional (R) group that adds physical properties, such as charge or solubility in water. It is generally accepted that there are 20 common amino acids found in nature. During translation, ribosomes in the cell link amino acids in a linear chain, using the mRNA as a unique template, to make polypeptides. The amino acid sequence makes up the primary structure of a protein which is most often composed of a single polypeptide (Figure 2.6). The unique order of the four nucleotides (ACTG) in a gene results in a specific mRNA sequence that is translated to a unique sequence of amino acids in the polypeptide/protein. The polypeptide chain folds and twists to form a unique combination of α(alpha)-helixes and β(beta)-pleated sheets. This folding and twisting makes up the secondary structure of the protein. The secondary structure is characterized by hydrogen and ionic bonds and disulfide bridges (between closely spaced copies of the amino acid cysteine). The sequence and arrangement of α-helixes and β-sheets cause the protein to fold into a large-scale three-dimensional configuration known as the tertiary structure. Finally, multiple polypeptides, either duplicates of the same polypeptide or different polypeptides, can form a complex that makes up the quaternary structure of a protein.

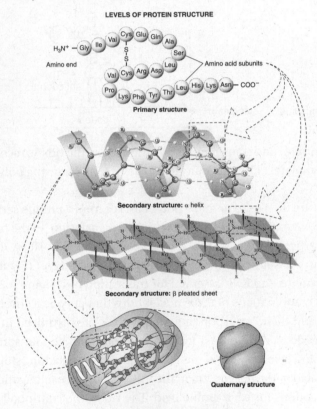

Figure 2.6. Protein structure

Enzymes are a special type of protein that convert one compound (substrate) into another (product) or hydrolyze a more complex compound to a simpler one through a chemical reaction. For example, the enzyme lactate dehydrogenase converts pyruvic acid to lactic acid in some fermentation reactions. Alternatively, collagenase breaks peptide bonds in collagen to yield smaller fragments. In general, enzymes work by binding to the substrate at a specific "active" site that mimics the shape of the substrate. This mechanism has been compared to the specific fit of a key in a lock. By forming the enzyme and substrate complex, the activation energy of the reaction is significantly lowered, thus increasing the rate of the catalyzed reaction. Some special enzymes that catalyze reactions in metabolic pathways are called **allosteric**. These enzymes contain a site for the binding of the substrate and a second site for the binding of an "effector" molecule. Effector molecules are often end products of a metabolic pathway. When the effector molecule binds to the enzyme, the conformation of the active site is altered thereby preventing the substrate from binding to the enzyme. This process is known as **feedback inhibition** and provides a way for cells to turn off metabolic pathways. Allosteric enzymes are essential for carrying out this type of control because the end product (effector) of a metabolic pathway is structurally distinct from the intermediate in the pathway that is the substrate for the enzyme.

A nonclassical type of enzyme has been termed **ribozyme**. A ribozyme is a RNA species that can catalyze specific types of chemical reactions such as processing of tRNA. Discovery of this type of enzymatic reaction has implications for the activity of viroids (*see Chapter 4*) and origin of life theories (*see Chapter 5*).

Phosphorylation of enzymes also plays a key role in many cell processes such as regulation and cell cycle. **Kinases** are specialized enzymes that add a phosphate group to other proteins or enzymes. In a generic example, enzyme 1 is phosphorylated by a kinase (Figure 2.7). The addition of the phosphate activates the enzyme which then converts substrate A to substrate B. In other reactions, regulatory proteins are phosphorylated by kinases. Phosphorylation changes the structural conformation of regulatory proteins to make them active or inactive.

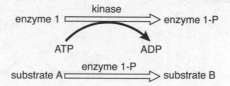

Figure 2.7. Example of how protein phosphorylation regulates an enzyme reaction

Coenzymes work with enzymes to increase reaction rates. They can carry various chemical groups. Coenzymes are recycled so that they can participate in repeated enzymatic reactions. An example of a common coenzyme is **nicotinamide adenine dinucleotide** (NAD^+), which carries electrons (e^-) in **oxidation-reduction reactions**. Oxidation-reduction or redox reactions are chemical reactions in which electrons are transferred between two molecules. The molecules lose or gain an electron. In coupled oxidation-reduction reactions, one molecule loses an electron and the other molecule gains an electron (Figure 2.8). This type of reaction is found in a number of biological pathways or processes (*see Chapter 3*).

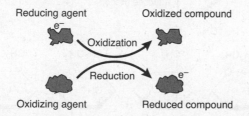

Figure 2.8. Oxidation-reduction (redox) reaction

Sugars or carbohydrates are molecules containing primarily carbon, hydrogen, and oxygen, with the latter two elements in a 2:1 ratio. The simplest sugar structure is a **monosaccharide** (Figure 2.9). Common examples include glucose, galactose, and fructose. Other common sugars, such as sucrose (table sugar), lactose (milk sugar), and maltose, are **disaccharides** composed of two identical or different monosaccharides. Some monosaccharides are charged because they contain an amino group (N-acetylglucosamine) or are sugar alcohols or alditols (xylitol). Monosaccharides can form longer (linear or highly branched) chains generally referred to as **polysaccharides**. Polysaccharides form structural polymers in some cells. A common complex form of sugar is the highly branched polysaccharide glycogen. Glycogen can be stored in the human body as a source of energy (*see Chapter 8*). Some proteins are termed glycoproteins because of the addition of carbohydrate to the basic amino acid structure.

Fatty acids are carboxylic acids that contain a long saturated (no double bonds in the carbon chain) or unsaturated (at least one double bond) aliphatic (C–H) chain (Figure 2.10). Examples of saturated fatty acids include palmitic and stearic acids. Linoleic acid is an example of a polyunsaturated fatty acid. Fatty acids are key components of **lipids**. There are various types of lipids, including **glycolipids**, **phospholipids**, sphingolipids, and sterols. Phospholipids, important components of biological membranes, contain glycerol modified with long chain fatty acids and phosphate. These types of lipids are **amphiphilic**, that is, they contain a **hydrophobic** (water-insoluble) end and a **hydrophilic** (water-soluble or polar) end.

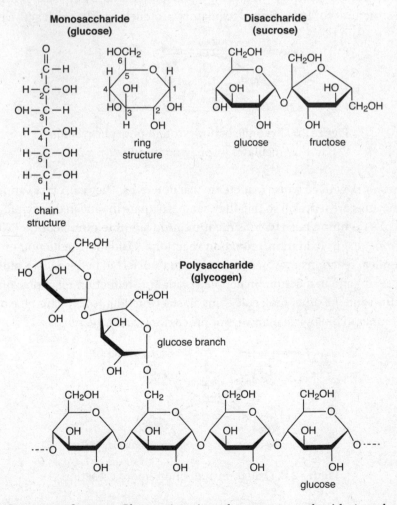

Figure 2.9. Structure of sugars. Glucose is a six carbon monosaccharide (see the numbers). Glycogen is an example of a polysaccharide that is composed of a very long chain of glucoses. Glucose chains branch from the main chain about every 8–12 glucoses.

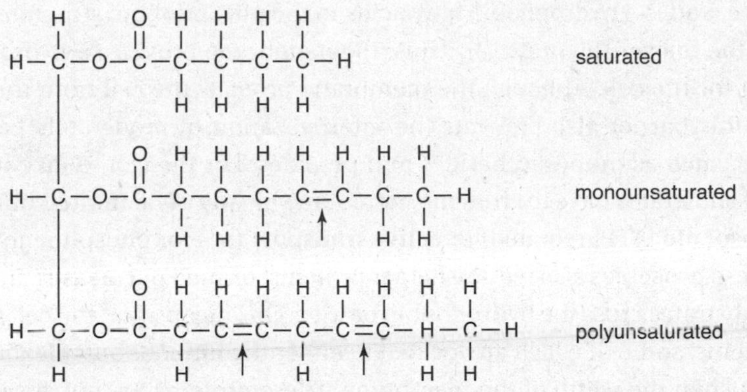

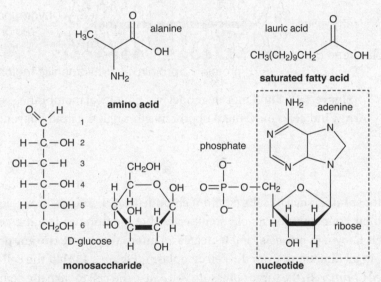

Figure 2.10. Example of a lipid containing saturated, monounsaturated, and polyunsaturated fatty acids. Arrows indicate the positions of double bonds that are characteristic of unsaturated compounds.

A comparison of the structures of simple organic compounds (amino acid, fatty acid, simple sugar, and nucleotide) are shown in Figure 2.11.

Figure 2.11. Comparison of the structures of a typical amino acid, saturated fatty acid, monosaccharide, and nucleotide. A nucleotide lacks the phosphate group (box).

BIOLOGICAL MEMBRANES

Membranes are essential components of all cells. This primary membrane surrounds the cell forming a protective barrier that holds together the material that makes up the cell. Some types of cells contain intracellular membrane-containing organelles that carry out very specific functions required for cell maintenance and energy production (*see Chapter 3*). Phospholipids make up the majority of the structure and composition of the cell membrane. Based on their properties, lipids naturally organize into a bilayer that forms a physical and hydrophobic barrier against the entry of compounds from the environment into the cell. The hydrophilic polar head groups of the lipids are arranged at the inner and outer surfaces of the membrane, and the hydrophobic fatty acids in the phospholipid structure extend toward the inside of the bilayer (Figure 2.12). Thus, the membrane provides a hydrophobic permeability barrier for the cell. Although the membrane protects the cell from the influx of toxic compounds, this barrier also prevents the internalization of moderately large water-soluble substrates, such as monosaccharides and peptides. For the cell to take up nutrients for growth, some substrates have to cross the membrane by way of **facilitated diffusion** (no adenosine triphosphate [ATP] required) or **active transport** (ATP or phosphoenolpyruvate [PEP] required). These processes also require helper proteins, termed **permeases**, in the membrane to help the substrates cross the hydrophobic barrier. This means that the cell membrane also contains proteins, some of which are located in either the inner or outer leaflet of the bilayer or others that span the width of the membrane. These proteins are not covalently linked to the lipids, which means they float free in the bilayer. This type of membrane organization, known as the fluid mosaic model, allows proteins to come together to form complexes in the membrane to carry out specific processes such as substrate transport.

Phospholipid Membrane

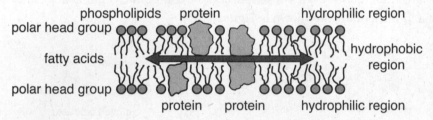

Figure 2.12. Fluid mosaic model of a biological membrane. Arrow indicates movement of proteins through the lipid bilayer.

Osmosis

It is natural for **solutes**, such as salts (sodium chloride [NaCl], magnesium chloride [$MgCl_2$]), to equalize their concentration across semipermeable membranes like the cell membrane. This process is known as **osmosis,** and it creates an internal pressure (**turgor pressure**) pushing outward, in all directions, from the cell cytoplasm (Figure 2.13A). If the cell does not have a cell wall (*see Chapter 3*), the turgor pressure will cause the cell to take the shape of a sphere. If the concentration of the solute is much higher in the cytoplasm of a cell than outside of the cell, water (**solvent**) will rush out of the cell through the membrane causing the cell to shrink or plasmolyze. Alternatively, if the concentration of the solute is much higher outside of the cell than in the cytoplasm, water will rush into the cell through the membrane. This rapid influx of water will cause the cell to swell and eventually burst or lyse due to the increased pressure (Figure 2.13B). This is why certain types of eukaryotic cells, that do not have a cell wall, have to live in an **isotonic** environment in which the solute concentration (and osmotic or turgor pressure) is equal on both the outside and the inside of the membrane. Cells that have a cell wall, such as bacteria (prokaryotic cells) and plant cells, can survive in hypertonic (high salt) and hypotonic (low salt) environments.

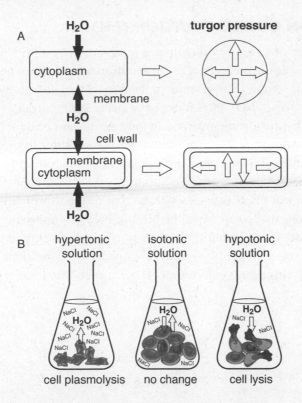

Figure 2.13. Effects of the flow of water (solvent) across a semipermeable biological membrane. (A) Effects of turgor pressure on a cell that lacks or has a cell wall. (B) Consequences of water flow in and out of a cell in various salt (solute) environments.

THERMODYNAMICS

Thermodynamics is actually a branch of physics that is concerned with the relationship of heat and temperature to the production of energy or the capacity to do work. However, thermodynamic concepts have important implications for the efficient functioning of living cells. The biochemists Hans Krebs and Hans Kornberg are credited with making the first observations on the thermodynamics of biochemical reactions in the 1957 treatise "Energy Transformations in Living Matter." The name of the first author may be familiar as the discoverer of key reactions in the Krebs cycle (*see Chapter 3*). Biological thermodynamics is the study of the conversion of energy that occurs in cells and structures and focuses on the principles of chemical thermodynamics in biological or biochemical reactions. Examples include essential energy-controlled pathways or processes involved in adenosine triphosphate (ATP) hydrolysis, protein stability, DNA binding, membrane diffusion, and enzyme kinetics. The amount of energy that potentially contributes to work during a chemical reaction is quantified by the change in Gibbs free energy. Concepts most important for understanding biological thermodynamics are the first and second laws of thermodynamics, Gibbs free energy, and reaction kinetics (rates of chemical processes). The First Law of Thermodynamics states that energy can be changed from one form to another but cannot be created or destroyed. This is known as the conservation of energy. The Second Law of Thermodynamics states that no natural process can occur unless it is accompanied by an increase in the **entropy** or degree of disorder of the universe.

HYDROGEN ION CONCENTRATION (pH)

The acidity or basicity of an aqueous solution is represented by a pH ("power of Hydrogen") value. pH is expressed as the measure of the **hydronium ion** (H_3O^+) concentration according to a standardized scale (values 1–14). Water molecules dissociate into hydroxide and hydronium ions: $2H_2O \leftrightarrows OH^- + H_3O^+$. Pure water has a pH of 7.0 (neutrality) because it contains an equal number of hydroxide and hydronium ions. Acidic and basic solutions have pH values less than and greater than 7.0, respectively. pH is important in biology. Many bacteria and other unicellular organisms cannot grow at pH values significantly above or below 7.0. Various cellular compartments, organs, and fluids need to maintain acid-base homeostasis or balance. Physiological pH is considered to be that of blood which is 7.35. Acidosis and alkalosis are conditions that occur when the pH falls below or above neutrality, respectively. Significant changes in pH can be harmful. For example, high acidic and basic pHs can denature proteins and decrease the activity of enzymes. And, acidic conditions in plaque can facilitate tooth decay. Buffering agents can control pH because they reversibly bind hydrogen ions.

The Cell

3

In Chapter 2, background information and concepts important for an understanding of the cell were concisely outlined. The cell is the fundamental unit of life. In this chapter, we will survey the structure, composition, and major properties of the two general types of cells found in organisms.

PROKARYOTIC CELL—BACTERIA

The prototypical **prokaryotic** (also spelled procaryotic) cell is the bacterium. **Bacteria** are single-celled organisms and represent the most abundant life forms comprising one-third or more of the Earth's biomass. There are at least ten times as many bacteria as cells in the human body. This conglomerate of bacteria is known as the human **microbiome**. Approximately twenty million bacteria reside in the human oral cavity. The average size of a bacterium is approximately 2 micrometers in length and 0.5–1 micrometers in diameter. However, nano-bacteria, 67 times smaller than a typical bacterium, represent some of the smallest living cells.

Composition and Structure

Bacteria come in many diverse shapes, including cocci, rods, and spirilla. Shapes other than coccoid or round are possible because bacteria contain a rigid cell wall that can overcome the osmotic forces inside the cell. The cell wall also allows bacteria to survive in **hypertonic** (high concentration of solute = high osmotic pressure) and **hypotonic** (low concentration of solute = low osmotic pressure) environments where mammalian cells cannot. This property contributes to the vast diversity of bacteria and colonization of a myriad of environmental niches. Like all cells, bacteria contain a lipid membrane that is located internal to the cell wall and protects the cytoplasm and nucleus. In general, the bacterium is devoid of intra-membranous structures or compartments (Figure 3.1). A major defining property of prokaryotes is that they lack a nuclear membrane. **Ribosomes**, which are necessary for protein synthesis, and the chromosome are free in the cytoplasm. Bacteria have 70S ribosomes (50S and 30S subunits; see Figure A.2 in the Appendix) and a single chromosome composed of a superhelix of double-strand DNA. Based on structural differences, almost all bacteria can be divided into two groups—Gram-positive and Gram-negative.

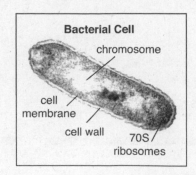

Figure 3.1. Enhanced thin section electron micrograph of a typical bacterial cell. Note that the chromosome is not enclosed in a membrane.

Physiology and Metabolism

Under ideal conditions, bacteria grow and divide relatively rapidly. The starting point for bacterial metabolism is typically **glycolysis** in which a carbohydrate (sugar) substrate is oxidized, through a series of chemical reactions, to produce usable forms of energy compounds such as adenosine triphosphate (ATP). The idealized goal is to completely oxidize the 6-carbon sugar glucose to carbon dioxide, a 1-carbon molecule. As discussed in Chapter 2, a sugar substrate has to be transported across the hydrophobic cytoplasmic membrane of the cell. Bacteria have a number of active transport systems to accomplish this. Once inside, the more complex sugars, such as disaccharides and trisaccharides, are hydrolyzed to monosaccharides. All of the monosaccharides are converted to glucose-6-phosphate, which is the required starting substrate for glycolysis. In the first series of reactions, the glucose-6-phosphate is oxidized to pyruvic acid, a three-carbon compound. Bacteria either require oxygen for growth (**aerobes**) or are killed in the presence of oxygen (**anaerobes**). Anaerobic bacteria can only grow in the absence of oxygen and further metabolize the pyruvic acid to acids, alcohols, and CO_2 in a process known as **fermentation** (Figure 3.2). In contrast, aerobic bacteria can use a respiratory type of metabolism to convert the pyruvic acid to carboxylic acid intermediates in the tricarboxylic acid (TCA) cycle. Reduced nicotinamide adenine dinucleotide (NADH) is then used by the electron transport chain in the cytoplasmic membrane to make ATP. In practice, the oxidation of pyruvic acid is not usually complete in either fermentation reactions or in the TCA cycle. Also, respiration is a more efficient process than fermentation yielding a maximum of 36–38, rather than 2 moles of ATP, per mole of glucose. Not all bacteria are capable of metabolizing carbohydrates. Some bacteria use peptides and amino acids as their primary source of carbon, further exemplifying the significant diversity of the prokaryotic kingdom.

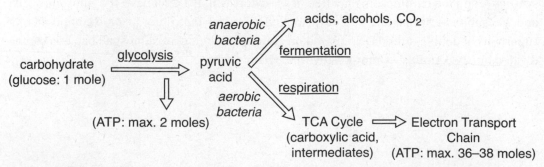

Figure 3.2. Flow chart illustrating the glycolytic path in anaerobic and aerobic bacteria

Reproduction

For the most part, bacteria multiply by binary fission. Prokaryotic cells are **haploid** (one set of chromosomes). The bacterial chromosome is replicated by the action of a series of enzymes that untwist and unwind the supercoiled double helix. The separated strands are used as templates for making two copies of the chromosome. The chromosome contains a specific site, known as the origin of replication, where DNA synthesis begins (initiation phase). Unwinding of the helix creates a replication fork, and each unwound strand serves as a template for the simultaneous synthesis of the new strands. Synthesis of the two new strands occurs bidirectionally. **DNA polymerase** directs the synthesis of each of the new strands by the ordered 5′ to 3′ addition of nucleotides complementary to those on the template sequence (elongation phase). A number of additional enzymes form a complex, known as the **replisome**, which carries out specific functions during the elongation phase (Figure 3.3). The chromosome of bacteria is circular, so DNA synthesis ends when the two replication forks meet (termination phase). It is essential that DNA replication is perfect to ensure that errors or mutations in gene sequences do not occur. Therefore, there are proofreading and error checking mechanisms to achieve this. Each new copy of the chromosome is segregated in the cell by the formation of a septum or a simple pinching off of the cell membrane and cell wall. Therefore, the bacterial population grows exponentially as one cell divides into two and two into four and so on.

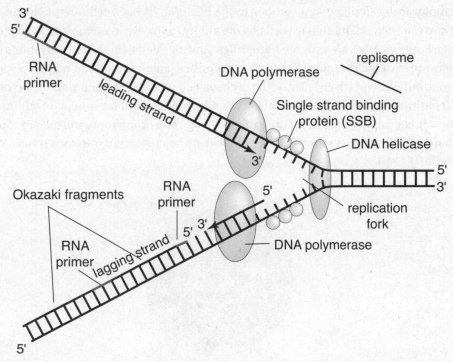

Figure 3.3. Enzymes and other components of the DNA replication machinery

Genetics

Bacteria carry several different types of extrachromosomal genetic elements that orchestrate the movement of genes within bacterial populations. The first type of genetic element is known as a **plasmid**. Plasmids are smaller versions of the chromosome. They consist of covalently closed circles of double-strand DNA that can be taken up by competent bacteria in the population. A specialized class of plasmid directs bacterial conjugation, or mating, in a sexual type of reproduction. The second type of extrachromosomal genetic element is the **transposon**. Transposons are linear sequences of double-strand DNA that have the ability to jump or transpose from one region of the DNA to another. Transposons can be passed to other cells either as insertions into larger pieces of DNA or in a conjugative mechanism. The third type of element is a type of virus, known as a **bacteriophage**, which can only infect a bacterial cell. The general composition and structure of bacteriophages is somewhat similar to that of typical animal viruses and will be reviewed in Chapter 4. All three genetic elements participate in the transfer of genes among bacterial populations outside of the normal process of cell division. The implications of this promiscuous transfer of genetic information is the more rapid and widespread dissemination of antibiotic resistance and toxins across bacterial species lines. Furthermore, the mechanisms by which plasmids, transposons, and bacteriophages operate has been exploited in the laboratory for the development of gene cloning and other molecular biology and recombinant DNA techniques.

PROKARYOTIC CELL—ARCHAEA

A second large group of single-celled organisms has been named the **archaea** (Figure 3.4). The archaea, which are a prokaryotic type of cell, were not considered as a group separate from the bacteria until relatively recently (1970s) due to similarities in appearance or phenotype. Although physically similar in appearance to the bacteria, archaea cells are phylogenetically distinct (*see Chapter 5*). The archaea cell has the ability to survive in exceptionally harsh environments. Some archaea are extreme **halophiles** (able to tolerate high concentrations of salt) and others are extreme **thermophiles** or **psychrophiles** (able to survive at relatively high and low temperatures, respectively). Thus, the archaea cell type has some unique catabolic and anabolic pathways and cell components, like enzymes, which have unusual stabilities and properties. It is probably safe to assume that if living cells or microorganisms are found on other planets in our solar system, they will most likely be more similar to the archaea than to the bacteria.

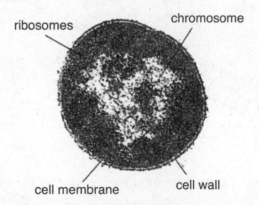

Figure 3.4. Thin section electron micrograph of a typical archaea cell. Note that the cell wall is similar in appearance to that in the bacterial cell and that the chromosome is not enclosed in a membrane.

EUKARYOTIC CELL

The **eukaryotes** (also spelled eucaryote) comprise a relatively large and diverse group of organisms with a cell type that is phenotypically and genetically distinct from that of the bacteria and archaea. The most obvious visual differences are a nuclear membrane and a highly compartmentalized internal organization marked by the presence of various membrane-containing organelles (Figure 3.5). Eukaryotic cells are highly complex and display significant diversity between and within organisms. For example, animal cells are different from plant cells, and human skin cells are different from human blood cells. Therefore, only the major features of the eukaryotic cell will be emphasized in this overview.

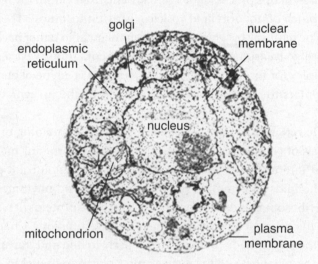

Figure 3.5. Thin section electron micrograph of a eukaryotic cell. Note the obvious membrane bound internal structures relative to the appearance of bacteria (Figure 3.1) and archaea (Figure 3.3). This intracellular compartmentalization suggests the segregation of cell processes.

Composition and Structure

Like prokaryotic cells, eukaryotic cells also contain ribosomes. However, eukaryotic-type **ribosomes** are 80S (60S and 40S subunits; see Figure A.2 in the Appendix). The difference in ribosome composition between prokaryotic and eukaryotic cells has important implications for the use and effectiveness of some antibiotics. Ribosomes are located free in the cytoplasm and can also be associated with the inner surface of the cell membrane.

The **nucleus** contains the genetic information of the cell and is protected by a membrane. Unlike prokaryotic cells, which have a circular chromosome, eukaryotic chromosomes are linear sequences of DNA. Eukaryotic cells can be haploid, **diploid** (two sets of chromosomes), or **multiploid** (more than one set of chromosomes) and can contain several to many chromosomes depending on the particular organism. For example, fruit flies have 8 chromosomes and humans have 23 pairs of chromosomes (46 total).

Mitochondria are membrane-enclosed structures found in all eukaryotic cells. Their primary function is to supply the cell with energy in the form of ATP. The Krebs cycle (TCA cycle in bacteria) and electron transport chain in the inner membrane of the mitochondrion produce the ATP required by the cell. The size, shape, and structure, as well as the protein and genetic compositions of the mitochondrion, are very similar to those of the bacteria and archaea. Overwhelming evidence suggests that mitochondria have evolved from a once free-living prokaryotic cell. This concept is known as the **endosymbiotic theory** and is discussed further in Chapter 5.

The **Golgi complex** is a membrane-bound organelle with internal layers of folded membranes that house enzymes required for the processing of cell proteins in preparation for delivery to their final locations. Proteins are modified within the Golgi apparatus by the addition of carbohydrates and phosphate and are sorted and packaged for secretion from the cell. The Golgi complex works in close association with the endoplasmic reticulum and cell membrane. A common way for molecules to enter the eukaryotic cell is by a process known as **endocytosis**. In this process molecules are enclosed within invaginations of the cell membrane, which pinch off to form lipid vesicles (early **endosomes**). The endosomes travel through the endocytic pathway by which they deliver their cargo either back to the surface for removal from the cell, to **lysosomes** (hydrolytic enzyme-containing vesicles) for degradation, or to the Golgi complex for further processing. **Pinocytosis** is a type of endocytosis in which extracellular fluid enters the nucleus in vesicles formed by the invagination of the nuclear membrane.

The **endoplasmic reticulum** (ER) is another membrane-containing organelle that functions in the synthesis of complex molecules and transport of proteins made in the cell. The organelle is divided into a smooth ER and a rough ER. The smooth ER participates in the synthesis of phospholipids and steroids and metabolism of carbohydrates. The rough ER is associated with the ribosomes and helps process newly made proteins. It works with the Golgi complex to deliver the processed proteins to their final destinations. Chaperone proteins in the ER ensure that the newly made proteins are properly folded and transported to the Golgi complex. The ER, in association with the nuclear and Golgi membranes, make up an intracellular membrane network.

Peroxisomes are membrane-enclosed organelles, found in almost all eukaryotic cells, that carry out a variety of metabolic reactions, including the breakdown of substrates such as fatty acids, amino acids, and uric acid. A myriad of enzymes are found in peroxisomes which supports their role in **catabolic** activities. Sequestering these types of reactions in the peroxisome may protect cytosolic components of the cell from the activity of highly oxidative enzymes.

Many eukaryotic cells lack a cell wall external to the cell or plasma membrane, therefore, their shape is maintained by a true **cytoskeleton**. The cytoskeleton is a network of filaments, composed of the proteins **actin** and **tubulin**, in the cytoplasm (Figure 3.6).

Plant cells and algae contain a membrane-containing structure known as a **chloroplast** (Figure 3.7). Like the mitochondrion, the main function of the chloroplast is to provide energy for the cell. However, energy production in the chloroplast is achieved, when sunlight is available, by the interaction of a **photosynthesis** pathway (light reactions), Calvin cycle (dark reactions), and the electron transport chain. Chloroplasts contain photosynthetic pigments, such as the chlorophylls, that help convert sunlight into chemical energy. Chloroplasts, like mitochondria, are thought to have evolved as explained by the endosymbiotic theory (*see Chapter 5*). Plant cells and algae also contain mitochondria which carry out ATP synthesis when light of the proper wavelength is not available. Photosynthetic bacteria, such as the **cyanobacteria**, were once thought to be eukaryotic cells. However, genetic analysis has been used to classify them as prokaryotes (*see Chapter 5*). The cyanobacteria do not contain chloroplasts.

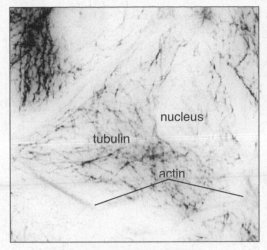

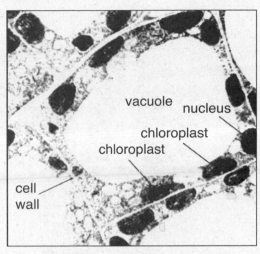

Figure 3.6. Eukaryotic cell stained to detect actin and tubulin filaments in the cytoskeleton

Figure 3.7. A thin section electron micrograph of a plant cell

Physiology and Metabolism

Most eukaryotic cells are **heterotrophs**, which means they require an external source of organic carbon (carbohydrates, peptides/amino acids) for growth. As in prokaryotic cells, glycolysis is the primary metabolic pathway leading to energy production with the flow of the overall glycolytic scheme very similar to that shown in Figure 3.2. More specifically, complex carbohydrates and disaccharides, such as sucrose and lactose, are enzymatically broken down into monosaccharides which are converted to glucose-6-phosphate to enter the phosphorylation stage of the Embden-Meyerhof-Parnas (EMP) pathway. In the EMP, pathway 2 moles of ATP are used to convert the sugar to fructose-1,6-diphosphate (Figure 3.8). In a splitting reaction, each 6-carbon intermediate is hydrolyzed to form two moles of 3-carbon intermediates. These 3-carbon molecules are ultimately oxidized to pyruvic acid in the oxidation-reduction stage of the pathway. In this stage, 2 moles of the coenzyme NAD^+ are reduced, and 4 moles of ATP are made. The fate of the pyruvic acid is determined by the environment of the cells. Under anaerobic conditions, the pyruvic acid is further reduced to small carbon number acids, acetaldehydes, alcohol, and/or carbon dioxide. Alcoholic fermentation by yeast is used as an example in Figure 3.8. Note that the NAD^+ that is reduced in the oxidation-reduction stage is recycled in the **fermentation** reactions. If conditions are aerobic, the pyruvic acid is converted to acetyl CoA, which enters the **citric acid/Krebs cycle/TCA cycle**.

In the citric acid cycle, 4-, 5-, and 6-carbon intermediates are made along with the reduction of NAD^+ and **flavin adenine dinucleotide** (FAD^+). **Anaerobic glycolysis**, the conversion of glucose to pyruvic acid, can occur under conditions in which the amount of oxygen is limited. This process is usually observed in muscle cells when they shift metabolism from aerobic respiration to anaerobic glycolysis. The shift occurs because the body cannot quickly replenish the oxygen that has been converted to carbon dioxide. Therefore, anaerobic glycolysis is only efficient for producing energy (ATP) for very short times due to the buildup of lactic acid. Some microorganisms use anaerobic glycolysis during fermentation.

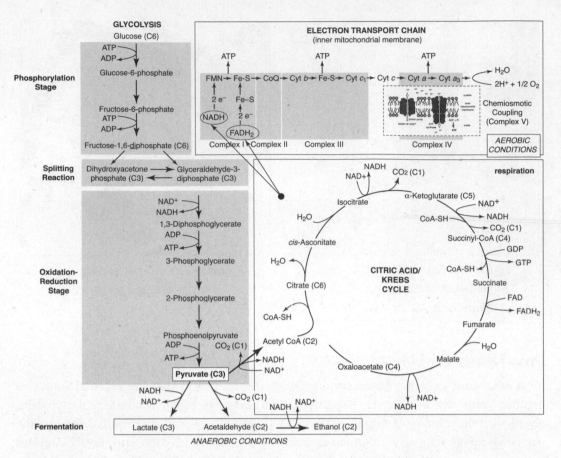

GLYCOLYSIS

ELECTRON TRANSPORT CHAIN
(inner mitochondrial membrane)

CITRIC ACID/ KREBS CYCLE

Figure 3.8. Glycolytic pathway in the eukaryotic cell functioning under anaerobic and aerobic conditions

High energy phosphate molecules are typically not made in the citric acid cycle except for a guanosine triphosphate (GTP). The majority of the ATP is made during the reactions of the **electron transport chain**. Electrons from the reduced NAD^+ and FAD^+ made in the citric acid cycle are transferred, via a series of carriers, such as flavin mononucleotide (FMN), iron-sulfur proteins (Fe-S), coenzyme Q, and cytochromes, to the terminal electron acceptor oxygen. During the coupled oxidation-reduction reactions, protons are released across the membrane. This sets up a proton gradient that drives the influx of protons back through a channel that is coupled to an ATP synthase. Energy obtained from the movement of the protons back across the membrane catalyzes the synthesis of ATP from ADP and inorganic phosphate. **Inorganic** compounds generally lack carbon and are from nonliving material. This process is known as the **chemiosmotic theory**. A theoretical maximum of 38 moles of ATP can be obtained from the metabolism of 1 mole of sugar (glucose).

In addition to the role of glycolysis in the conversion of carbohydrate to ATP and the recycling of NAD^+, intermediates in the EMP pathway and citric acid cycle are used by the cell to make amino acids (Figure 3.9). Not all cells are capable of synthesizing all twenty common amino acids. For example, humans have to obtain nine amino acids by dietary intake.

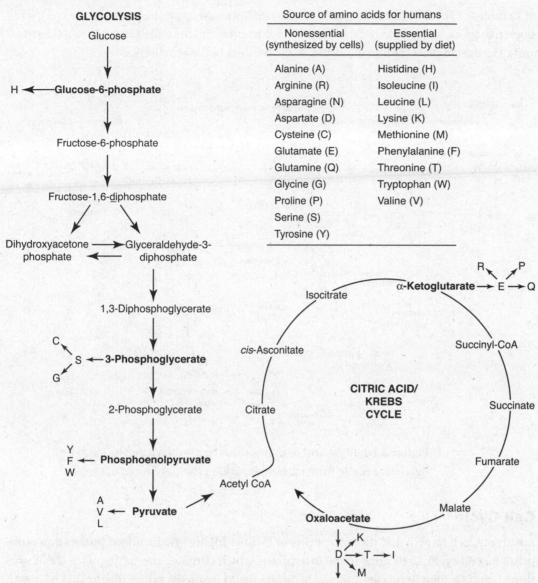

GLYCOLYSIS

Glucose

H ← **Glucose-6-phosphate**

Fructose-6-phosphate

Fructose-1,6-diphosphate

Dihydroxyacetone phosphate → Glyceraldehyde-3-diphosphate

1,3-Diphosphoglycerate

C
S ← **3-Phosphoglycerate**
G

2-Phosphoglycerate

Y
F ← **Phosphoenolpyruvate**
W

A
V ← **Pyruvate** → Acetyl CoA
L

Source of amino acids for humans	
Nonessential (synthesized by cells)	Essential (supplied by diet)
Alanine (A)	Histidine (H)
Arginine (R)	Isoleucine (I)
Asparagine (N)	Leucine (L)
Aspartate (D)	Lysine (K)
Cysteine (C)	Methionine (M)
Glutamate (E)	Phenylalanine (F)
Glutamine (Q)	Threonine (T)
Glycine (G)	Tryptophan (W)
Proline (P)	Valine (V)
Serine (S)	
Tyrosine (Y)	

CITRIC ACID/ KREBS CYCLE

R ↖ ↗ P
α-**Ketoglutarate** → E → Q

Isocitrate

cis-Asconitate

Succinyl-CoA

Citrate

Succinate

Fumarate

Malate

Acetyl CoA

Oxaloacetate

K
D → T → I
M

Figure 3.9. Glycolytic pathway showing how some intermediates in the EMP pathway and citric acid cycle are used for amino acid biosynthesis. Detailed enzymatic reactions in amino acid synthesis are not shown. The table illustrates which amino acids cannot be synthesized by humans.

Photosynthesis is carried out by **autotrophs**, that is, organisms that can use atmospheric carbon dioxide as the sole source of carbon for growth. All other organisms that use an organic source of carbon are known as **heterotrophs**. Energy from the absorption of sunlight is used to produce electrons that drive the synthesis of ATP via chemiosmotic coupling and the reduction of NADP$^+$ (Figure 3.10). The photosynthesis machinery is located in the chloroplast and in the thylakoid membrane in the cyanobacteria. The components of the electron transport chain and ATP synthesis complex in the chloroplast inner (thylakoid) membrane differ somewhat from those in the mitochondrial inner membrane. NADPH and ATP made in the electron transport chain is used with atmospheric CO_2 in the **Calvin cycle** to make glucose through a series of enzymatic steps. It takes 6 moles of CO_2, 18 moles of ATP, and the oxidation of 12 moles of NADPH to make 1 mole of glucose. Note that in photosynthesis, the cell makes sugar using CO_2 as the substrate. In glycolysis or respiration, the cell uses sugar as a substrate, and CO_2, the smallest carbon molecule, is a byproduct of the reactions.

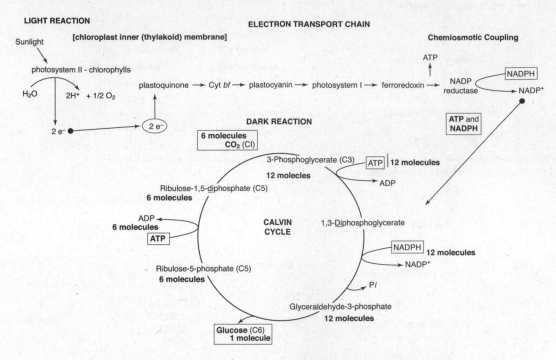

Figure 3.10. Light and dark reactions in photosynthesis. Sugars are made from carbon dioxide in the Calvin cycle.

Cell Cycle

Eukaryotic cell growth and division occurs in distinct highly synchronized phases that comprise the **cell cycle**. Cells grow in the **interphase**, which contains the G_1 (gap 1), S (DNA synthesis), and G_2 (gap 2) phases and divide during the M (**mitosis**) phase (Figure 3.11). Growth and DNA replication occur in a highly ordered fashion during **interphase** to get ready for cell division. The G_1 period represents the time between mitosis and initiation of DNA replication. Initiation of replication is controlled by the G_1/S checkpoint (restriction checkpoint). Cells that fail this checkpoint do not replicate their DNA. Cells that pass this checkpoint proceed to the S phase where the DNA is replicated. The mechanism of DNA replication is similar to that in the prokaryotic cell (see Figure 3.3). During the second gap period, G_2, the cells continue to grow and make proteins required for mitosis in the M phase. The length of time for each cell phase is dependent on cell type. Cell phases are identified, using a flow cytometer, by quantifying the amount of nuclear DNA labeled with a fluorescent dye. Cells having a DNA content of $2n$ are in the G_1 phase (see the inset in Figure 3.11). Cells having a DNA content of $4n$ are at the G_2/M interphase. Cells having a DNA content between $2n$ and $4n$ are in the S phase.

Progression of the cell cycle phase transitions are controlled by the interactions of two families of proteins called cyclins and cyclin-dependent kinases. Examples of these protein families are Cyclin B and Cdc2 (Cdk1), respectively. The primary action of protein kinases was reviewed in Chapter 2. If DNA in the cell is damaged by exposure to light in the ultraviolet wavelength (10–410 nanometers) or by some other chemical mechanism, the cell cycle is arrested to prevent the start of mitosis before DNA replication has been completed. Therefore, there are **cell cycle checkpoints** in the G_1 and G_2 phases to make certain that damaged chromosomes are not replicated and passed on in cell division. The checkpoints are controlled by the synthesis of specific proteins such as p53.

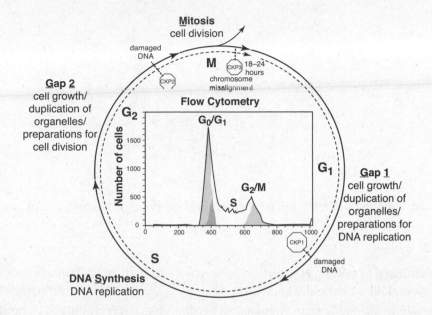

Figure 3.11. The eukaryotic cell cycle. The outer ring shows the four phases with the three checkpoints (CKP). The inner graph shows how flow cytometry can separate cells based on their DNA content (2*n* or 4*n*). On average, the cell cycle is completed in 18–24 hours.

Mitosis (M Phase)

During mitosis, or nuclear division, the chromosomes condense, the nuclear envelope in some organisms breaks down, the cytoskeleton reorganizes to form the **mitotic spindle,** and the chromosomes move to opposite poles of the nucleus. The mitotic spindle contains **centrioles,** which are cylindrical structures made up of the protein tubulin. These structural reorganization events are required for the cell to enter cell division or **cytokinesis**. There are four general stages in mitosis—**prophase**, **metaphase**, **anaphase**, and **telophase** (Figure 3.12). During prophase, the chromosomes condense and are represented by two sister **chromatids** (*see Chapter 7, Genetics*). The mitotic spindle begins to form by the movement of the **centrosomes** to opposite sides of the nucleus. The condensed sister chromatids are held together at the **centromere**. The nuclear envelope breaks down in the higher eukaryotes. In metaphase, the two centrosomes begin to pull the chromosomes via the centromeres to the opposite ends of the cell. This process stretches the chromosomes along a central plane in the cell. In anaphase, the sister chromatids are separated to become daughter chromosomes that are then pulled to the opposite ends of the cell. Finally, in telophase, the daughter chromosomes are attached to the ends of the cell. A new nuclear membrane is formed around each set of separated daughter chromosomes, and they lose their condensed form to return to **chromatin** (*see Chapter 7, Genetics*). Cell division is completed by the formation of a septum that separates the two nuclei into two **diploid** daughter cells.

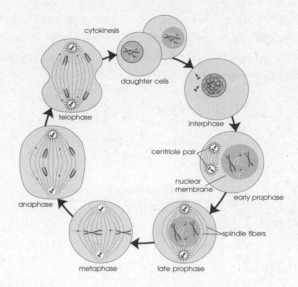

Figure 3.12. The stages of mitosis. The stages repeat every reproductive cycle or generation.

Meiosis

Meiosis, compared to mitosis, is a sexual type of reproduction in which **haploid** daughter cells arise from a **diploid** parent cell (Figure 3.13). The process is divided into two parts—Meiosis I and Meiosis II. In Meiosis I, each chromosome becomes two sister chromatids following DNA replication. Homologous chromosomes are paired and then segregated into two cells. In Meiosis II, the sister chromatids in each cell are separated to form four haploid daughter cells. These cells represent **gametes** (examples include sperm and egg cells). The two gametes join in fertilization to form a diploid **zygote** that now contains the original number of sets of chromosomes.

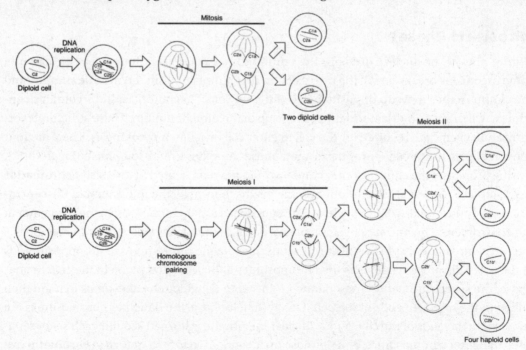

Figure 3.13. Comparison of the events in mitosis (top panel) and meiosis (bottom panel). Meiosis is divided into two phases. Chromosome sets are labeled C1 and C2, replicated chromosomes C1a (C2a) and C1b (C2b) and homologous paired chromosomes C1a′ (C2a′) and C1b′ (C2b′).

Viruses

4

Viruses have been around for millions of years. They do not have a typical prokaryotic or eukaryotic cell structure. They are comprised mostly of either DNA or RNA encased in a protein coat called a **nucleocapsid** and, in some cases, an additional lipid envelope. Viruses are among the smallest "life-forms," having an average diameter of 20–300 nanometers. Therefore, they can be viewed only with the aid of an electron microscope. They are not capable of carrying out metabolism or reproduction because they lack the enzymes, pathways, and structures required for these processes. Viruses must infect cells and use the host cell's transcription and translation processes in order to make new virus particles. Viruses have been found in almost every known type of cell. Those that infect prokaryotic cells are known as **bacteriophages**, and those that infect eukaryotic cells are grouped as animal, plant, or insect viruses.

BACTERIOPHAGES-PROKARYOTIC VIRUSES

Bacteriophages are classified according to the presence of single- or double-stranded DNA or single-stranded RNA and the type of protein coat structure. The DNA or RNA that makes up the viral genome is protected by a geometrically shaped nucleocapsid that is attached to tail fibers by a tail region that may or may not have a contractile sheath (Figure 4.1). Bacteriophages have a limited host range due to the presence of specific receptors on the bacterial or archaea cell surface that recognize and bind the tail fibers. After adsorption to the bacterial cell surface, the nuclear material is injected through the tail, and the bacteriophage genome is combined with the bacterial chromosome. Bacteriophages can be either virulent or temperate. The virulent type of bacteriophage particles are rapidly made in the host cell and the cell is destroyed. The genome of temperate bacteriophages is carried by the bacterium until a signal instructs the cells to make virus particles. The host cell is then destroyed to release the mature bacteriophages.

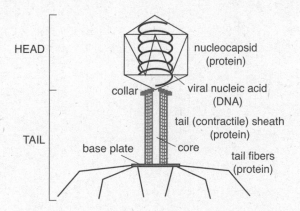

Figure 4.1. Structure of a typical bacteriophage

EUKARYOTIC VIRUSES

Like bacteriophages, animal and plant viruses are also grouped based on the nature of their genetic material. DNA viruses can contain either single- or double-stranded DNA. Examples of DNA viruses are the herpes viruses, including the virus that causes chicken pox and the virus that causes smallpox. Common examples of RNA viruses are those that cause polio and influenza in humans and the tobacco mosaic virus that infects plants. The close association of some plants and insects allows for the exchange of some viruses. Compared to bacteriophages, viruses that infect eukaryotic cells have complicated infection pathways and replication cycles.

VIROIDS

Smaller viruslike forms were discovered in plants in 1971. These **viroids** are composed of a very short piece (less than 500 nucleotides) of circular single-stranded RNA. The viroid RNA is used as a template by the infected host cell for replication. Some viroids act as ribozymes (*see Chapter 5*).

PRIONS

In 1982, Stanley Prusiner, a researcher at the University of California at San Francisco, isolated a small sialoglycoprotein that infects mammalian tissues and cells. This protein was named the Prion Protein (PrP) or simply, prion. Prions are transmissible, primarily through ingestion or inhalation, and cause several animal and human diseases when the normal protein folds in an abnormal fashion.

Relationships Among Organisms

5

The two general types of cells, prokaryotic and eukaryotic, reviewed in Chapter 3 form the foundation for establishing relationships among all living organisms. The concepts of evolution, phylogenetics, claudistics, systematics, and taxonomy are now highly interwoven due to rapid developments in molecular biology.

EVOLUTION—The process by which populations of organisms become altered over relatively long periods of time. Organisms may divide into separate groups or branches, combine to form hybrid organisms, or cease to exist due to extinction.

PHYLOGENETICS—The study of evolutionary relationships among organisms by comparing gene sequencing data and morphological data matrices.

CLADISTICS—The classification of organisms based on phylogenetic relationships of groups of organisms rather than on shared physical features as used in Linnaean classification (*see Taxonomy below*).

SYSTEMATICS—The study of the classification of organisms in order to reconstruct their evolutionary history and relationships.

TAXONOMY—The description, classification, identification, and naming of organisms. Organisms are grouped into units known as a taxon (plural form taxa) and are named using the binomial system (genus and species) of classification developed by Carolus Linnaeus (1707–1778), a Swedish botanist. The classification system that he developed is referred to as Linnaean taxonomy.

Relationships among organisms in phylogenetics and systematics are depicted as evolutionary "trees" or cladograms. Key features of evolutionary trees are branches, which indicate changes that occur among organisms or groups of organisms over time, and branch length, which indicates the amount of change or genetic distance from an immediate ancestor.

ORIGINS OF LIFE

Until the mid-1800s, a popular theory, known as **spontaneous generation**, supported the concept that life which did not come from the germination of seeds, eggs, or parents, arose from inanimate matter. Theodore Schwann (1810–1882) proposed the "cell theory of life" and, along with Louis Pasteur (1822–1895), helped disprove the theory of spontaneous generation. Current theory suggests that life began on the planet Earth in three stages: formation of biological monomers, formation of biological polymers, and evolution of cells from molecules. Monomers of life are basic small molecules such as amino acids. Other important monomers are the phospholipids that form lipid bilayers, which are the basic components of biological membranes, and nucleotides that can form RNA-based molecules such as ribozymes. These stages also required the presence of basic inorganic chemicals, such as methane (CH_4), ammonia (NH_3), water (H_2O), hydrogen sulfide (H_2S), carbon dioxide (CO_2) or carbon monoxide (CO), and phosphate ($PO_4{}^{3-}$). Organic molecules may have been created by (i) the action of ultraviolet light or electrical discharges on inorganic chemicals, (ii) from carbonaceous meteorites, or (iii) enhanced by impact shocks.

The formation of biological polymers could have occurred by numerous mechanisms. For example, the RNA world hypothesis, which proposes that early life was based on RNA rather than DNA, is a popular theory because RNA can be a carrier of genetic information as well as catalyze chemical reactions (ribozyme). In addition, laboratory experiments have shown that small peptides can be spontaneously formed from amino acids. Membranes, spontaneously formed from lipid bilayers, could have trapped and concentrated organic chemicals creating more complex biochemical "factories."

DEVELOPMENT OF CELLS

Formation of the cell is probably the most important stage in the origin of life. It is not clear exactly how the cell developed or evolved, but it is accepted that an early RNA world would have been important for the process. Current thinking promotes a model in which prokaryotic and eukaryotic cells evolved independently from a common ancestral cell (Figure 5.1). The older linear prokaryotic-eukaryotic model, in which eukaryotic cells evolved from prokaryotic cells, is now considered to be obsolete.

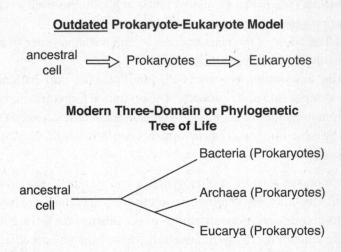

Figure 5.1. The three-domain model and rooted phylogenetic tree of life based on 16S ribosomal RNA gene sequence comparisons.

In 1977, Carl Woese (University of Illinois at Urbana-Champaign) began a phylogenetic study in which he compared 16S ribosomal RNA gene sequences among organisms. This led to the construction of the most up-to-date version of the phylogenetic tree of life (see Figure 5.1). The tree is composed of three branches that represent **three domains: bacteria**, **archaea**, and **eucarya**. Members of the bacteria and archaea domains have a prokaryotic cell composition and structure, and those in the eucarya domain have a eukaryotic cell configuration. It is interesting that this phylogenetic approach established that the archaea did not evolve separately from a common ancient ancestor nor do they appear to be a branch of the bacteria domain. Rather, the data indicates that the archaea are a branch of the eucarya. However, in 2010 an organism named Lokiarchaeota, discovered in deep ocean sediment, was subsequently determined to be a good candidate for a common ancestor of the archaea and eucarya. Viruses and viroids do not have a branch on the phylogenetic tree of life because they do not have the genetic and physical properties of "true" cells.

Endosymbiotic Theory

In 1966, Lynn Margulis (Boston University) published a paper "The Origin of Mitosing Eukaryotic Cells" in which she put forth the **endosymbiotic theory**. The basis of this theory is the interdependence and cooperative existence of multiple prokaryotic organisms evolving over millions of years in eukaryotic cells. This led to the process by which ancient cells acquired specific organelles such as mitochondria and chloroplasts. Therefore, the theory supports the idea that some prokaryotic cells were internalized by other cells and established a symbiotic relationship. Over time, the internalized prokaryotic cells lost their ability to independently replicate and became an integral part of the newly evolved eukaryotic type cell.

Cell Size

In general, neither prokaryotic nor eukaryotic cells have evolved to a "gigantic" size. If it is assumed that a typical cell is basically a sphere, then the volume (V) and surface area (SA) of a cell can be calculated using the formulas: $V = \frac{4}{3}\pi r^3$ and $SA = 4\pi r^2$. The greater the volume of a cell, the larger the number of enzymatic reactions that are required to take place in the cytoplasm to sustain the cell. The larger the surface area of a cell, the greater the amount of raw materials that can enter the cell over a certain period of time. However, as the volume of the cell increases, the ratio of surface area to volume decreases dramatically. At some point in the growth of the cell, the surface area to volume ratio becomes so small that the surface area of the cell cannot support the level of intake of raw materials needed to support the internal reactions. Therefore, a cell that reaches a relatively large size cannot survive due to a relatively low surface area to volume ratio. In addition to the importance of cell size, cell complexity is also related to the amount of genomic material (DNA) that it contains (Figure 5.2). On average, bacteria, which are relatively small (large surface to volume ratio), can grow faster than animal cells. And, animal cells are structurally, compositionally, and physiologically more complex than bacteria.

PHYLOGENESIS AND CLASSIFICATION OF ORGANISMS

The **three domains** have been described in Figure 5.1. Since the time of Linnaeus in the mid-1700s, when living organisms were divided into plant and animal kingdoms, classification of organisms has undergone many changes. Currently, there are **eight major taxonomic ranks**: domain, kingdom, phylum, class, order, family, genus, and species (Figure 5.3). A five-kingdom classification scheme (monera, protista, plantae, fungi, and animalia) proposed by Robert Whittaker in 1969 was popular until the Carl Woese 16S rRNA gene sequencing studies. Dr. Woese divided the monera into the bacteria and archaea. In the most recent scheme proposed by Thomas Cavalier-Smith, all organisms are divided into **six kingdoms**: bacteria, protozoa, chromista, plantae, fungi, and animalia (Figure 5.3). All of the kingdoms, except bacteria (and in some schemes the archaea), are part of the eucarya domain.

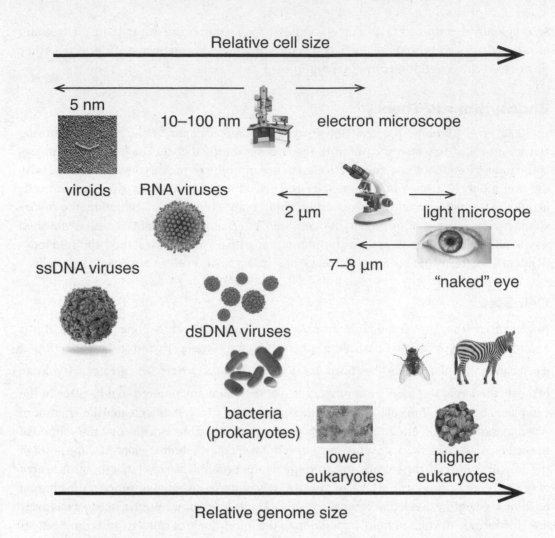

Relative cell size

5 nm

10–100 nm

electron microscope

viroids

RNA viruses

2 μm

light microsope

ssDNA viruses

7–8 μm

"naked" eye

dsDNA viruses

bacteria
(prokaryotes)

lower
eukaryotes

higher
eukaryotes

Relative genome size

Figure 5.2. Relationship of cell and genome size to organism complexity. Cell size is viewed with an electron microscope, light microscope, and the "naked" eye.

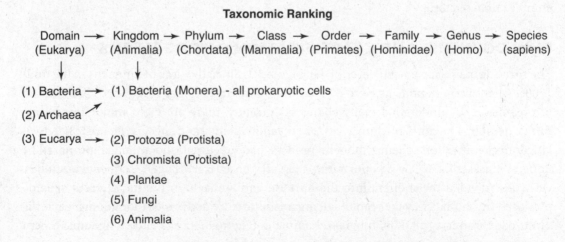

Taxonomic Ranking

Domain → Kingdom → Phylum → Class → Order → Family → Genus → Species
(Eukarya) (Animalia) (Chordata) (Mammalia) (Primates) (Hominidae) (Homo) (sapiens)

(1) Bacteria → (1) Bacteria (Monera) - all prokaryotic cells

(2) Archaea

(3) Eucarya → (2) Protozoa (Protista)

(3) Chromista (Protista)

(4) Plantae

(5) Fungi

(6) Animalia

Figure 5.3. The eight major taxonomic groups in hierarchical order. The taxonomic ranking of man, or *Homo sapiens,* is used as an example. The three domains and six kingdoms are also listed.

Bacteria

The **bacteria kingdom** (formerly **monera**) usually includes all prokaryotic cells—bacteria, archaea, and the cyanobacteria. All members of this kingdom have a single-celled prokaryotic composition and structure. It is believed that bacteria were first observed by Antony van Leeuwenhoek (1632–1732) using specially ground lenses. Members of the bacteria domain have many different shapes and sizes, live in a variety of environments, carry out many different types of metabolic reactions, and can be associated with health and disease. Bacteria are grossly divided into three types, Gram-positive, Gram-negative, and Acid-fast, based on structural and compositional differences in their cell wall and carbohydrate polymers on the cell surface. Unique characteristics of bacteria include (i) the absence of a nuclear membrane, (ii) a simple phospholipid membrane, (iii) 70S ribosomes, (iv) a peptidoglycan cell wall, and (v) a single circular chromosome. These and other properties of prokaryotic cells were reviewed in Chapter 3.

In some taxonomic schemes, the archaea are considered to be either a subkingdom within the kingdom bacteria or a separate kingdom in the three domain scheme. They have many of the prokaryotic features of the bacteria and a less diverse range of size and shape. There are differences in the composition of their cell wall and membrane compared to those of the bacteria, and the archaea can metabolize a wide variety of inorganic and organic compounds as sources of energy. Related to this property is their ability to survive in environments that are considered to be relatively inhospitable for other prokaryotes and eukaryotes. The archaea have some metabolic and replication genes that are more similar to those present in eukaryotes, which may explain their position as a branch of the eucarya on the phylogenetic tree (see Figure 5.1).

The cyanobacteria are also known as **cyanophyta** and blue-green algae. The older blue-green algae terminology comes from the observation that these cells produce the pigment phycocyanin. They have many of the features of bacteria, such as no nuclear membrane and a peptidoglycan cell wall. However, they contain a thylakoid membrane in which the photosynthetic reactions take place with gaseous oxygen as the end product (*see Chapter 3*). This property is thought to have had a major impact during the conversion of an oxidizing atmosphere on early Earth. This change most likely had a profound effect on evolution due to the increase in populations of aerobic organisms. Cyanobacteria are excellent candidates for the initial structures that led to the evolution of chloroplasts in eukaryotic cells as proposed in the endosymbiotic theory. The cyanobacteria have a broad range of habitats and can be **endosymbionts** (organisms that live in other cells; *see Chapter 8*) in some members of the protozoa and plantae.

Protozoa (Protista)

There is significant debate and confusion over the proper terminology for the classification of mostly unicellular organisms that have a eukaryotic cell type. The Whittaker and Woese taxonomic schemes reviewed on page 39 use the term **protista**, whereas the more recent Cavalier-Smith scheme uses protozoa. This kingdom is exceptionally diverse. Included in this kingdom are organisms that (i) use internal cytoplasmic flow for motility (amoebas), (ii) use cilia for motility (ciliates), (iii) move through the action of a single posterior flagellum (flagellates), and (iv) have two, four, or more flagella and a ventral feeding groove. Flagella are long structures composed of self-assembling protein subunits that function in motility. **Protozoa** can replicate by binary fission, multiple fission, a sexual or asexual process, or by a combination of these mechanisms.

Chromista (Protista)

In earlier schemes, the **protozoa** and **chromista** kingdoms were included in a single kingdom termed Protista. In current classification, the chromista kingdom contains all algae that have chloroplasts with chlorophylls a and c. This group includes unicellular and multicellular algae (unicellular green algae), cells that contain two heterogeneous flagella, and algae that contain an anterior groove and plastids. Plastids are chloroplast-like organelles that contain photosynthesis pigments. Green algae are eukaryotic organisms that reproduce by a process known as **alteration of generations**. In this process, the organism switches between a haploid multicellular **gametophyte** stage and a diploid multicellular **sporophyte** stage (Figure 5.4). The **zygote**, produced when a haploid egg cell is fertilized by a haploid sperm, develops into a sporophyte that has two sets of chromosomes, one from each parent. The sporophyte contains a cuticle, or outer layer, that provides protection from desiccation and derives nutrients from the gametophyte. Meiosis in the sporophyte produces spores. Mitotic cell division of the spores leads to formation of gametophytes. Gameophytes produce both haploid male and female gametes during mitosis. Identical cells can fuse in a sexual process in which haploid algal cells combine to form diploid zygotes. When this process occurs in filamentous algae, it is known as conjugation because bridges are formed between the joining cells. Alternatively, a large nonmotile cell can be fertilized by a smaller motile cell.

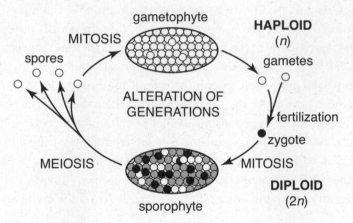

Figure 5.4. Alteration of generations between a diploid sporophyte and haploid gametophyte in the life cycle of algae

Plantae

The plantae kingdom is a very large group of multicellular organisms including the flowering plants, multicellular green algae, mosses, conifers and other gymnosperms, ferns, club mosses, hornworts, and liverworts. The current list of land plant phyla is shown in Table 5.1.

Table 5.1. Land Plant Phyla or Divisions

Phylum	Common Name	Properties
Anthocerotophyta	Hornworts	Horn-shaped sporophytes, no vascular system
Bryophyta	Mosses	Persistent unbranched sporophytes, no vascular system
Marchantiophyta Hepatophyta	Liverworts	Ephemeral unbranched sporophytes, no vascular system
Lycopodiophyta Lycophyta	Club mosses & spikemosses	Microphyll leaves, vascular system
Pteridophyta	Ferns & horsetails	Prothallus gametophytes, vascular system
Pinophyta Coniferophyta	Conifers	Cones containing seeds and wood composed of tracheids
Cycadophyta	Cycads	Seeds, crown of compound leaves
Ginkgophyta	Ginkgo, Maidenhair	Seeds not protected by fruit (single living species)
Gnetophyta	Gnetophytes	Seeds and woody vascular system with vessels
Flowering plant Anthophyta	Flowering plants, angiosperms	Flowers and fruit, vascular system with vessels

A subkingdom of the plantae kingdom is composed of the green plants or **embryophytes**, which make up the majority of the vegetation on Earth (Figure 5.5). The green plants have cell walls composed of **cellulose** (a polysaccharide composed of glucose), carry out photosynthesis using chloroplasts with chlorophylls a and b, and store food as **starch** (a complex carbohydrate composed of the glucose polymers **amylose** and **amylopectin**). Some plants exhibit **heliotropism**, the ability to turn toward the sun as it moves across the sky. This subkingdom contains the vascular plants (flowering plants, ferns, and conifers) and the bryophytes (mosses and liverworts). The embryophytes or land plants have specialized reproductive organs that are protected by nonreproductive tissues. Bryophytes are relatively small members of the embryophyte subkingdom, contain nonvascular tissue, and primarily inhabit moist or humid environments. They have small differentiated stems and atypical leaves but lack roots. Like the green algae, the embryophytes reproduce using an alteration of generations process.

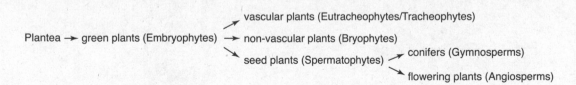

Figure 5.5. Flow chart showing the general organization of the plantae kingdom

Vascular plants, or **eutracheophytes/tracheophytes**, are characterized by the development of a complex tissue system comprised of leaves, roots, and stems. The vascular system, known as xylem, transports water and nutrients upward from the roots. Phloem is the vascular system that carries sugars and other metabolic products downward from the leaves. Vascular plants have strong cell walls, and the more advanced species have a protective cuticle. These properties have allowed the vascular plants to diversify and spread into many different terrestrial environments. The sporophyte is usually large, branched, and nutritionally independent from the gametophyte. The gametophyte has less importance in the life cycle as evidenced by its reduction in size compared to that in the bryophytes.

Plants that produce seeds are known as **spermatophytes**. Seeds represent an encapsulated reproduction unit that is resistant to desiccation. The sporophyte contains one of two spore-forming organs or **sporangia**. The **megasporangium** is enclosed by an integument or a protective layer that constitutes the seed coat. In this structure, a single megaspore develops into a small gametophyte that produces one or more egg cells within the seed coat. The megasporangium and its coat are known as an ovule prior to fertilization and as a seed following fertilization. In contrast, microspores are made in the microsporangium. Each small gametophyte, made in the microspore wall, becomes a grain of pollen that can be easily dispersed in the environment by air currents and insects. The fertilization process begins when a pollen grain encounters and enters an ovule. Sperm cells, produced by the gametophyte within the pollen grain, then fertilize an egg cell. The advantage of this mechanism is enhanced survival and reproduction in very dry environments.

Seed plants are divided into **gymnosperms** (conifers) and **angiosperms** (flowering plants). Enclosure of the ovules or seeds in ovaries in angiosperms distinguishes this group of plants from the gymnosperms. Other unique features of angiosperms are the usual presence of petals and flowers. The flower is the reproductive organ of angiosperms. In a double fertilization process, pollen which is produced in the stamen, sticks to the stigma of the pistil (Figure 5.6). A long pollen tube is formed, and a haploid generative cell moves down the tube. The generative cell divides by mitosis to form two haploid sperm cells. The growing pollen tube reaches the ovary and ovule where it deposits the sperm cells. One sperm cell fertilizes the egg cell resulting in a diploid zygote. The other sperm cell fuses with two cell nuclei forming a triploid cell. An embryo develops from the zygote, and the triploid cell forms the endosperm which provides nutrients. The ovule becomes a seed, and the ovary forms the fruit of the plant.

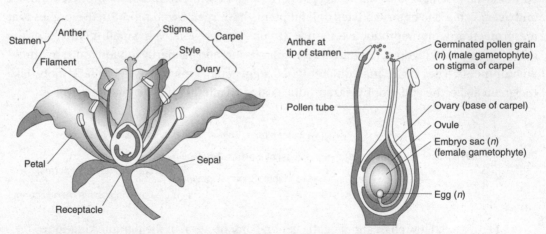

Figure 5.6. Reproductive organ of the flowering plant and the fertilization process

Fungi

The **fungi** kingdom includes yeasts, molds, and mushrooms, all of which have cell walls composed of glucan and chitin, a long-chain polymer of N-acetylglucosamine (Figure 5.7).

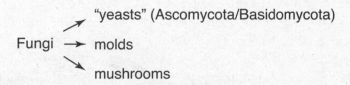

Figure 5.7. Flow chart showing the organization of the fungi kingdom

The term "**yeast**" does not represent a taxonomic or phylogenetic grouping. The two main phylogenetic groups are ascomycota and basidiomycota. Yeasts are typically unicellular and average 3–4 micrometers in size, but they can form **pseudohyphae** made up of linear arrangements of budding cells. Budding yeasts are members of the order saccharomycetales. Asexual reproduction by budding is the most common method of replication. The process begins when the cell forms a bleb or small bud (Figure 5.8). The cell nucleus divides, and one copy migrates to the budding portion of the cell. Once the bud reaches its final size, it separates to form a new, slightly smaller, cell. Alternatively, some yeasts can reproduce by conjugation (sexual reproduction). In some cases, under conditions of stress, haploid cells in the population die, and diploid cells form spores that then undergo conjugation to form new diploid cells.

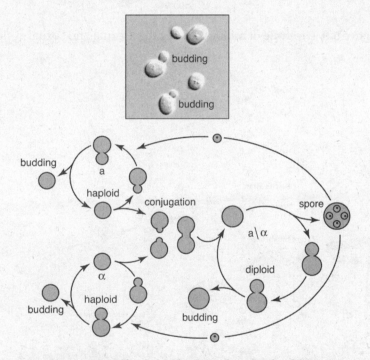

Figure 5.8. Life cycle of yeasts showing budding,
conjugation, and sporulation pathways

Molds typically grow as very narrow, long threadlike structures known as hyphae. The hyphae elongate from their tips and new hyphae form by branching. The combination of apical growth and branching leads to the formation of an interconnected network of filaments termed mycelium. Cross walls, or septa, form in some hyphae creating compartments. Reproduction occurs asexually by mycelial fragmentation or sporulation and sexually by meiosis (Figure 5.9). Some fungi form rhizomorphs—linear, parallel assemblies of hyphae that can function like the roots of vascular plants. Dimorphic fungi can reproduce based on environmental conditions by switching between a yeast phase and a hyphal phase.

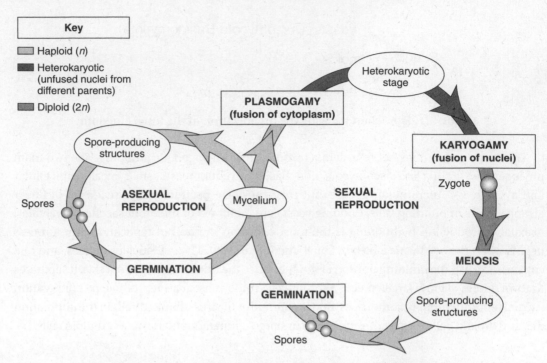

Figure 5.9. Life cycle of molds showing the asexual and sexual cycles

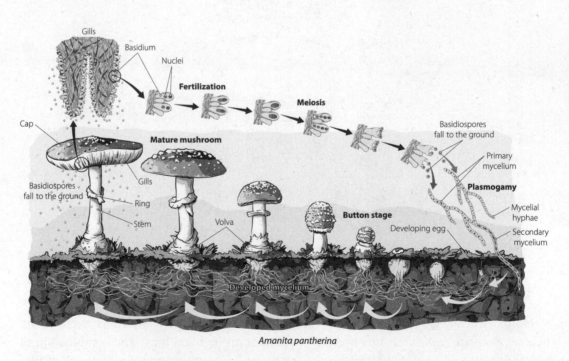

Figure 5.10. Life cycle of the mushroom

Mushrooms represent the spore-containing fruiting body of a fungus that resides above the surface of the soil or a food source. Typical parts of the mushroom include a cap, gills, and a stem (Figure 5.10). Spores are produced in the gills. A nodule, known as a **primordium**, develops within the mycelium and grows into a mass of interwoven hyphae to initiate formation of the mushroom. As this mass of hyphae expands, it surrounds the developing fruit body. Some mushroom species either lack a stem or have a supporting base. The stem, when present, supports the cap. There is extensive variation in the way the gills attach to the stem in different mushroom species.

Animalia

The sixth kingdom, **animalia**, is made up of eukaryotic multicellular organisms that have an early developmental stage or a later metamorphosis stage. An outdated, but occasionally seen, term for the animalia is **metazoa**. This extremely large group includes, but is not limited to, organisms ranging from sponges, jellyfish, shellfish, nontetrapod craniates ("fish"), insects, arachnids, amphibians, birds, and mammals. Except for sponges, these organisms have bodies composed of various tissues. An internal digestive chamber, with one or two openings, is also present. In place of cell walls, the cells of the animalia are surrounded by a collagen and elastic glycoprotein matrix that can be calcified (shells or bone) in some organisms. A current list of 35 animal phyla is listed in Table 5.2.

Most members of the animalia are motile and must ingest other organisms or the products of organisms to grow and survive. Many members of this kingdom propagate by sexual reproduction by which specialized reproductive cells in each parent undergo meiosis to produce nonmotile **ova** and motile **spermatozoa** that fuse to form zygotes. Zygotes, which contain DNA from both parents, are the earliest stage in the formation of **embryos**. The zygote forms a **blastula** or hollow sphere that usually invaginates to form a **gastrula** having two, and in most cases three, germ layers (**ectoderm**, **mesoderm**, and **endoderm**) and a digestive chamber. The germ layers differentiate to form tissues and organs. Certain members of the animalia kingdom can also reproduce by asexual means, such as **parthenogenesis**, which is the development of an embryo from an unfertilized egg.

The animalia can be divided into the **invertebrates** and **vertebrates** (Tables 5.3A–C). Invertebrates fail to develop a vertebral column from the **noto–chord** and include organisms such as worms, insects, snails, crabs, lobsters, clams, octopuses, starfish, and sea urchins. The lower invertebrates do not have defined organs. The higher invertebrates have a true central body cavity, or **coelom**, that encloses the digestive tract. Vertebrates have a vertebral column, characterized by a segmented series of parts (vertebrae) separated by joints, and a defined brain. The vertebral column replaces the notochord found in the invertebrates. Basal vertebrates, those lowest on the phylogenetic tree of life, use gills to breathe. During vertebrate development, the **pharyngeal pouches** that form in the neck region become **gills** in fish.

Table 5.2. Animal Phyla

Phylum	Common Name	Properties
Acanthocephala	Thorny-headed worms	Reversible, spiny proboscis that bears many rows of hooked spines
Acoelomorpha	Acoels	No mouth or alimentary canal (alimentary canal = digestive tract in digestive system)
Annelida	Segmented worms	Multiple circular segment
Arthropoda	Arthropods	Segmented bodies and jointed limbs, with chitin exoskeleton
Brachiopoda	Lamp shells	Lophophore and pedicle
Bryozoa	Moss animals, sea mats	Lophophore, no pedicle, ciliated tentacles, anus outside ring of cilia
Chaetognatha	Arrow worms	Chitinous spines on either side of head, fins
Chordata	Chordates	Hollow dorsal nerve cord, notochord, pharyngeal slits, endostyle, post-anal tail
Cnidaria	—	Nematocysts (stinging cells)
Ctenophora	Comb jellies	Eight "comb rows" of fused cilia
Cycliophora	Symbion	Circular mouth surrounded by small cilia, sac-like bodies
Echinodermata	Echinoderms	Fivefold radial symmetry in living forms, mesodermal calcified spines
Entoprocta	Goblet worm	Anus inside ring of cilia
Gastrotricha	—	Two terminal adhesive tubes
Gnathostomulida	Jaw worms	
Hemichordata	Acorn worms, pterobranchs	Stomochord in collar, pharyngeal slits
Kinorhyncha	Mud dragons	Eleven segments, each with a dorsal plate
Loricifera	Brush heads	Umbrella-like scales at each end
Micrognathozoa	—	Accordion-like extensible thorax
Mollusca	Mollusks / molluscs	Muscular foot and mantle round shell
Nematoda	Round worms	Round cross section, keratin cuticle
Nematomorpha	Horsehair worms	
Nemertea	Ribbon worms	
Onychophora	Velvet worms	Legs tipped by chitinous claws
Orthonectida		Single layer of ciliated cells surrounding a mass of sex cells
Phoronida	Horseshoe worms	U-shaped gut
Placozoa		Differentiated top and bottom surfaces, two ciliated cell layers, amoeboid fiber cells in between
Platyhelminthes	Flatworms	
Porifera	Sponges	Perforated interior wall
Priapulida	Penis worm	
Rhombozoa	—	Single anteroposterior axial cell surrounded by ciliated cells
Rotifera	Rotifers	Anterior crown of cilia
Sipuncula	Peanut worms	Mouth surrounded by invertible tentacles
Tardigrada	Water bears	Four-segmented body and head
Xenoturbellida	Strange worms	Ciliated deuterostome

Table 5.3A. Subdivision of the Kingdom Animalia

		Lower Invertebrates			
Phylum	Porifera	Ctenophora/ Cnidara	Nematoda	Platyhelminthes	Acanthocephala
Common members	Sponges	Sea anemones, corals, jellyfish	Roundworms	Flatworms	Spiny-headed worms
Distinguishing features	Cells are differentiated but usually not organized into distinct tissues	Radially symmetric; digestive chambers with a single opening; have distinct tissues that are not organized into organs; only ectoderm and endoderm	Microscopic; found in most aquatic environments; many are important parasites	Lack a body cavity	Inside-out probiscus with spines; complex life cycles requiring two hosts; parasitic

Table 5.3B. Subdivision of the Kingdom Animalia

		Higher Invertebrates		
Phylum	Mollusca	Annelida	Arthropoda	Echinodermata
Common members	Snails, slugs, clams, squids, cuttlefish, octopus	Earthworms, leeches	Insects, spiders, crabs	Starfish, sea urchins, brittle stars, sea cucumbers, feather stars
Distinguishing features	Mantle with pronounced breathing/ excretion cavity; radula; neurologically advanced	Segmented	Body divided into repeating segments; paired appendages; hardened exoskeleton	Radially symmetric; found exclusively in marine environments

Table 5.3C. Subdivision of the Kingdom Animalia

	Vertebrates						
Subphylum	Vertebrata						
Class	Agnatha	Chondrichthyes	Osteichthyes	Amphibia	Reptilia	Aves	Mammalia
Common name	Jawless fishes	Cartilaginous fishes	Bony fishes	Amphibians	Reptiles	Birds	Mammals
Common members	Lampreys, hagfishes	Sharks, rays, skates	Ray-finned and bone-finned fishes	Salamanders, frogs, toads	Turtles, snakes, lizards, crocodilians	Many species	Many species
Distinguishing features	Round mouths that lack jaws but have retractable horny teeth	Jawed; paired fins and nares; scales; heart with chambers in series; skeleton made of cartilage	Skeleton made of bone	Ectothermic; skin is secondary respiratory surface; aquatic larval stage	Four limbs or descended from four-limbed ancestors; oviparous	Feathered; winged; two-legged; warm blooded; egg-laying	Endothermic; hair; three middle ear bones; mammary glands; neocortex; four-chambered heart; teeth replaced once or never; most give birth to live young

Evolution 6

In the beginning of Chapter 5, evolution was defined in relation to phylogenetics and the use of modern molecular methods to assemble organisms into a hierarchal scheme showing relationships. A more detailed definition of evolution includes the concepts of heredity and variation. That is, the process of evolution is the change in inherited characteristics that occurs in populations of organisms as these populations proceed through subsequent generations.

HEREDITY

Traits, or characteristics, of an organism are passed from one generation to the next in a highly predictable fashion due to the assortment and segregation of genes. This concept of **inheritance** was first observed by the Augustinian friar, **Gregor Mendel** (1822–1884), who used the crossbreeding of pea plants to develop "**laws of inheritance**" and the concepts of "recessive" and "dominant" traits (which we now know are controlled by genes). This idea that very small specific parts of the parents of an organism are responsible for heredity replaced the popular **pangenesis** theory of Darwin, who felt that the entire organism was involved in the transfer of characteristics from parent to offspring. Acceptance of Mendel's laws of inheritance was aided by the ideas of **August Weismann** (1834–1914), who proposed that traits are passed only through germ cells (sperm and egg) and not through somatic (body) cells.

Deoxyribonucleic acid (DNA) is the molecule that carries the genetic information of an organism and, therefore, is the vehicle by which inheritable traits are passed from parents to offspring. The genetic information is organized into functional units known as genes (*see Chapter 2*). A copy of the DNA template is made in a cell prior to cell division to ensure that the parent and daughter cells each contain a full complement of the DNA. The DNA is arranged in the cell nucleus as condensed strands or chromosomes on which the genes are aligned in a linear array. The exact position of a gene on the chromosome is a **locus**. **Alleles** represent variations in the DNA sequence of different copies of the same gene or genetic locus. Genes carry the inherited traits of an organism, and the genome (complete set of genes) makes up the organism's **genotype**. The collection of traits that comprise the appearance and behavior of an organism, and are therefore visible, make up the **phenotype**. Some phenotypic traits are not inherited because they are the result of interactions between the genotype and environment.

Traits that are not the result of changes in gene sequences can be inherited during mitosis or meiosis and are referred to as **epigenetic inheritance systems**. These changes can occur in some cases due to differences in patterns of DNA methylation or can be due to the alteration of gene expression by gene silencing directed by RNA interference (RNAi). In this process, small RNA molecules known as microRNA (micRNA) and small interfering RNA (siRNA) increase or decrease the expression of genes by binding to the messenger RNA (mRNA).

VARIATION—POPULATION GENETICS

Genotype and the effects of environment influence the phenotype of an organism. **Phenotypic variation** in a population is due to differences among the genotypes of the organisms that comprise that population. Four predominant processes in evolution (natural selection, mutation, genetic drift, and gene flow) impact the distribution of alleles (gene variants) and alteration of their frequencies in populations.

The number of copies of a particular gene variant or allele divided by the number of copies of all alleles at a specific locus in a population represents the allele or gene frequency. Allele frequencies are used to measure the amount of genetic diversity or variation in an individual or population. Natural selection, mutation, genetic drift, and gene flow will result in evolution only if there is significant genetic variation in a population. However, allele frequencies will remain constant in a population from one generation to the next in the absence of these evolutionary modulators. This is known as genetic equilibrium. The **Hardy-Weinberg principle** mathematically explains the connection between genetic equilibrium and evolution in a population and is represented by the equation: $p^2 + 2pq + q^2 = 1$. In this equation, p represents the frequency or percentage of all the dominant alleles (A) in a population. This variable counts all of the **homozygous dominant** individuals (AA) and half of the **heterozygous** individuals (Aa). q represents the frequency or percentage of the recessive alleles, and, therefore, it counts all of the **homozygous recessive** individuals (aa) and half of the heterozygous individuals (Aa). p^2 stands for all homozygous dominant individuals, q^2 stands for all homozygous recessive individuals, and $2pq$ is all heterozygous individuals in a population. Everything is set equal to 1 because all individuals in a population equal 100% of that population. This equation can accurately determine whether or not evolution has occurred between generations and in which direction the population is heading. Typically, variation among members of a species is relatively low because the genomes are identical in all individuals of that species. However, small genotypic differences can appear as obvious differences in phenotype.

Natural Selection

Natural selection is a process by which those members of a species in a population that have traits that allow them to more favorably adapt to a specific environment survive and reproduce (Figure 6.1). Thus, the "advantageous" genes are passed to members of the next generation. Natural selection will only cause evolution if there is enough genetic variation in a population. **Charles Darwin** (1809–1882) based his theory of evolution on the process of natural selection. His study of species and populations included three key observations that supported his theory: (i) more offspring are produced than can possibly survive, (ii) traits vary among individuals leading to different rates of survival and reproduction, and (iii) trait differences are heritable. Members of a population who die are replaced by the progeny of parents who are better adapted to survive and reproduce. Therefore, this selection process maintains traits that are most beneficial for their functions and leads to adaptation.

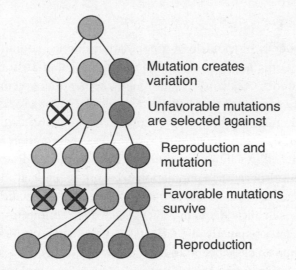

Figure 6.1. In this example, natural selection of a mutation creates a population with darker pigmentation.

Mutation

Mutations are changes in the genetic information (DNA) of a genome. Typically, mutations result in the addition, deletion, or substitution of one or more nucleotides in a gene sequence. These changes may have no effect (null mutation) or may change expression of the gene or function of the gene product. Therefore, in some instances mutations can produce new alleles that alter the phenotype of the organism. Mutation can be a nonadaptive cause of evolution. However, some traits are complex requiring the interaction of multiple gene products.

Mutations can occur spontaneously through errors in DNA replication or can be induced by some chemical agents or light of specific wavelengths, such as in the ultraviolet range. Gene function can be disrupted by the insertion of new genetic information through the action of extrachromosomal elements called transposons (*see Chapter 3*). Barbara McClintock (1902–1992) made the initial observation that the insertion of these mobile pieces of DNA were the cause of pigment variation in maize (the various patterns of colored kernels in ornamental corn). Multiple genes can become duplicated or exchanged by a process known as **genetic recombination**, which results in the production of a new combination of alleles through the pairing of homologous chromosomes and exchange of genetic information. In some cases, extra copies of genes are produced leading to the evolution of new genes. In sexual reproduction, homologous recombination produces offspring having new combinations of alleles that increases genetic variation and may increase the rate of evolution (Figure 6.2).

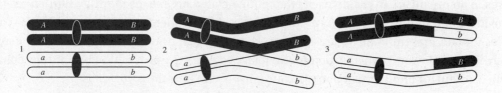

Figure 6.2. A cross-over event in genetic recombination

Genetic Drift

A change in the frequency of an allele in a population due to random sampling is known as **genetic drift**. Each organism in a population has alleles that are a random sampling of those alleles of the parents. Chance also determines whether or not members of a population survive and reproduce to pass on those alleles. As reviewed on page 52, the Hardy-Weinberg principle states that in relatively large populations, allele frequencies remain constant from generation to generation unless the equilibrium is upset by mutation or selection. Genetic variation may be reduced in a limited population because alleles disappear due to genetic drift. Over time, genetic drift causes a population to become genetically uniform because random sampling can cause the loss of alleles but cannot replace a specific allele. Also, random reductions or increases in allele frequency affect allele distributions for the next generation. An allele is fixed or lost in a population when it attains a frequency of 100% or 0%, respectively. Genetic drift ends when an allele becomes fixed. Allele frequency cannot change until a new allele enters the population due to mutation or gene flow. Like mutations, genetic drift can be a cause of nonadaptive evolution.

Gene Flow

The movement of alleles or genes from one species or population to another has been termed **gene flow**, or migration, and can have a pronounced affect on allele frequencies. Migration, either the movement of animals among populations or the transport of plant seeds, is the most common cause of gene flow. Natural formations such as mountains and oceans, as well as manmade obstacles, can impede or slow down the rate of gene flow. The consequences of gene flow are the creation of hybrid organisms and **horizontal gene transfer**. Horizontal gene transfer is the passage of genetic material from one organism to another and is most frequently observed in, but not limited to, bacteria. Conjugative plasmids and transposons and viruses significantly increase the frequency of horizontal gene transfer.

OUTCOMES OF EVOLUTION

In the scientific view, as apposed to a religious view, the results of the four processes that drive evolution are not attained by a predetermined organizational scheme or plan. The results of evolution are adaptation, speciation, or extinction.

Adaptation

Organisms can become "better suited" to their environment by adapting. **Adaptation** is an evolutionary process and is capable of causing either the acquisition of a new trait or the loss of an ancestral trait. The process occurs by the relatively slow modification of existing structures in an organism. In examples of adaptation, related organisms may have structures that provide different functions but have similar internal components. In other cases, some structures remain present in an organism but become vestigial or nonfunctional over the course of evolution. However, when structures that have adapted to one function become, by coincidence, useful for another function, they are known as **exaptations**.

Speciation

Processes that drive evolution can lead to the formation of new species. **Speciation** is defined as a process by which a "species" separates into two or more new or descendant species. However, the definition of what constitutes a species is somewhat dependent upon the type of organism. The definition of a species can take into account interbreeding, ecology, and phylogenetics. For example, using a definition based on interbreeding, the biological species concept states that "species are groups of actually or potentially interbreeding natural populations, which are reproductively isolated from other such groups." When populations within the same species become separated by a geographical event (loss of a land bridge, glacial movement, island formation) such that they can no longer exchange genetic material, they undergo **allopatric speciation**. This reproductive isolation means that the primary and newly isolated populations are affected by different selective pressures, acquire different mutations, and are independently subjected to genetic drift leading to the development of a new species. **Parapatric speciation** occurs when immediately adjacent organisms, whose ranges do not overlap, develop into closely related but distinct species.

Extinction

The disappearance of an entire species is known as **extinction**. Extinction is not a rare process because a great majority of the plant and animal species that have lived on our planet are now extinct. Many extinctions have been driven by competition between species for limited materials required for survival. If one species out competes another, the species that is most fit survives, and the other is forced to extinction.

MODERN EVOLUTIONARY SYNTHESIS

Arguably, the most current view of evolution, having its beginnings in the 1920s–1930s, is known as modern evolutionary synthesis. The name for this new concept of evolution was taken from the book, *Evolution: The Modern Synthesis* published in 1942 by Julian Huxley. This concept unified findings based on the ideas of heredity, natural selection, and mutation to define evolution. Modern evolutionary synthesis updates Darwin's "Theory of Evolution through Natural Selection" (published in *On the Origin of Species* in 1859) by recognizing that (i) other mechanisms, such as genetic drift, can be just as important as natural selection, (ii) characteristics are passed from parents to offspring on genes, (iii) variation between members of a species is due to the presence of multiple alleles of a gene, and (iv) speciation is most likely the result of the gradual accumulation of mutations in genes.

Vertebrate Organisms

7

As shown in Table 5.3C, vertebrates are members of the subphylum **vertebrata** in the second subdivision of the kingdom animalia. Members of this subphylum characteristically have segmented backbones or spinal columns. All vertebrates have a chordate construction composed of a vertebral column or notochord (relatively stiff rod extending the length of the animal), a spinal cord (hollow tube containing tissue of the nervous system), and a gastrointestinal tract. The anterior end of the gastrointestinal tract contains the mouth, and the anterior end contains the anus. The vertebrae and spinal cord typically extend beyond the length of the gastrointestinal tract forming a tail. In most, but not all, vertebrates the vertebrae have replaced the notochord found in all chordates. Evolution of the vertebrata is summarized in Figure 7.1.

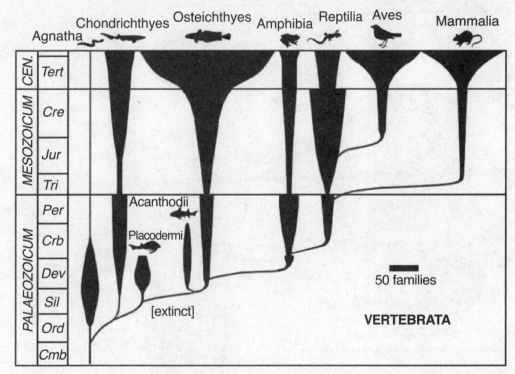

Figure 7.1. Spindle diagram showing the evolution of the common vertebrate classes (Table 5.3C). Eras of the Phanerozoic eon (from newest to oldest): Cenozoic (CEN.), Mesozoic, Paleozoic. Geological periods (from newest to oldest): Tertiary (Tert), Cretaceous (Cre), Jurassic (Jur), Triassic (Tri), Permian (Per), Carboniferous (Crb), Devonian (Dev), Silurian (Sil), Ordovian (Ord), Cambian (Cmb). Use of the Period name Tertiary is common, but more modern schemes divide the Cenozoic era into the Paleocene, Eocene, Oligocene, Miocene, Pliocene, Pleistocene, and Holocene. The extant Vertebrata classes are defined in Table 5.3C.

EMBRYOLOGY AND DEVELOPMENT

In sexual reproduction or meiosis (*see Chapter 3*), a diploid zygote is formed when two gametes join due to the **fertilization** of an egg cell by a sperm. The developing multicellular diploid zygote is known as an **embryo** from the instance of fertilization to germination. This process of the development of the embryo is referred to as **embryogenesis** (Figure 7.2). In human development, an embryo develops between 1–8 weeks after fertilization. Development of the zygote in animals goes through three ordered stages. In the first stage, the cells in the zygote divide multiple times to form a ball of cells (**morula**) with a fluid-filled cavity (**blastocoele**). The embryo is now a **blastula** (**blastocyst** in mammals). During this blastocyst stage, the human embryo is traveling down the Fallopian tube. The embryo is encased in a zona pellucida or glycoprotein shell. The zona pellucida lyses to release the blastocyst for attachment to the uterus (zona hatching) by approximately the fifth day postfertilization. Trophectoderm cells in the blastocyst adhere to endometrial cells in the uterus (implantation). The placenta and embryonic membranes are formed from the trophectoderm. Implantation occurs around 8–10 days after ovulation or release of the egg from the ovary.

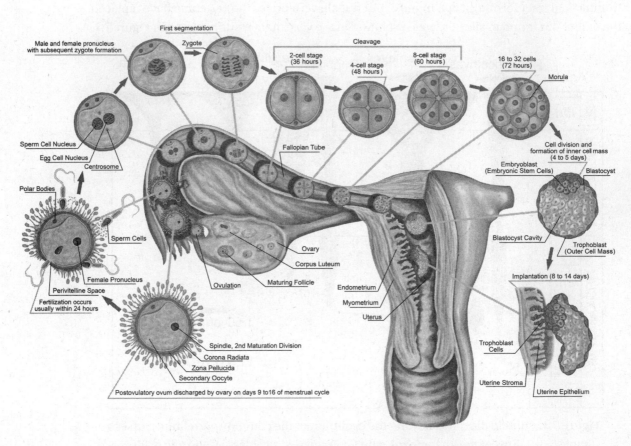

Figure 7.2. Summary of the general steps in embryogenesis

The blastula develops into a **gastrula** to allow the formation of the **germ layers** (**ecto-derm**, **mesoderm**, and **endoderm**) of the embryo. Gastrulation patterns differ greatly among members of the vertebrata. However, all exhibit five basic types of cell movements: invagination, involution, ingression, delamination, and epiboly (thinning and spreading of cells). In addition, the **primitive node or knot** (**Hensen's node** in birds and **Spemann's organizer** in amphibians) is a primary cell organizing structure of gastrulation in this subphylum. Another hallmark of gastrulation is the formation of a digestive tube or **archenteron**. Following gastrulation, individual organs develop in each of the germ layers through **organogenesis**. The epidermis, pigment cells, neural crest, and other nervous system tissues and specifically tooth enamel and dentin are formed from the ectoderm. According to some sources, the neural crest is considered to be a fourth germ layer. Muscle, cartilage, dermis, notochord, blood, blood vessels, and bone develop from the mesoderm. The **conus arteriosus** and **sinus venosus** are two key precursor compartments formed early in the development of the chordate heart. However, these structures do not persist in mammals. The endoderm develops into epithelium that comprises the digestive and respiratory systems as well as the liver, pancreas, and thyroid. The archenteron develops into a digestive tract. The development of tissues can potentially be affected by other tissues. This phenomenon is known as **embryonic induction**. For example, the lens of the eye develops from epidermis that comes into contact with tissue that forms the eye cup that grows toward the skin from the brain. This induction is now known to be due to the regulation of gene expression. Therefore, embryonic induction is an outdated term.

In the 9th week after fertilization, the human embryo is now called a **fetus**, but there is no defined stage or group of characteristics to distinguish between the two. Development between weeks 8 and 9 postfertilization is a continuous process. During weeks 9–16, the fetus exhibits breathing-like activity to stimulate lung development. Tooth development (**odontogenesis**) begins from cells derived from the ectoderm of the first pharyngeal arch. Extremities, muscles, heart, and brain, as well as other organs, begin to develop. During weeks 26–28, the lungs and bones fully develop, and thalamic brain connections for sensory input are formed. The fetus is full-term or able to sustain life outside the uterus between weeks 35 and 38.

GENETICS (CLASSICAL MENDELIAN)

Information that dictates the make-up and properties of all organisms, including the vertebrates, is contained in sequences of DNA known as genes (*see Chapter 2*). Genes are responsible for passing the traits or characteristics of an organism from one generation to the next. Vertebrate or eukaryotic chromosomes are coiled pieces of double-stranded DNA that contain a series of defined regions that encode structural and regulatory proteins (genes), as well as other regulatory and noncoding sequences. The DNA is packaged, by proteins (histones), into a condensed structure in the cell nucleus known as **chromatin**. Condensing the structure of chromosomes is required to fit these very long structures in the nucleus and plays an important role in cell division during mitosis or meiosis (*see Chapter 3*). In 1902, the "chromosome theory of inheritance" proposed by Theodor Boveri (1862–1915), Walter Sutton (1877–1916), and Edmund Beecher Wilson (1856–1939) extended the discoveries of Gregor Mendel. To transfer traits or genes among generations, chromosomes are replicated and divided. Therefore, chromosomes can exist in either an unduplicated or duplicated state. In the unduplicated state the chromosome is a single linear strand of DNA. In the duplicated state there are two identical copies of the chromosome known as chromatids. The chromatids are connected by a centromere that is located at either the middle or near the ends of the complex to create a structure with four arms or two arms, respectively.

Autosomes and Sex Chromosomes

The number of chromosomes varies significantly among the eucarya. The characteristic pattern of chromosomes in an organism is called the **karyotype**. An illustration of all the human chromosomes during metaphase (see Figure 3.12), arranged by length and location of the centromere is known as the karyotype (Figure 7.3). Humans have two copies of 22 autosomes and single copies of 2 sex chromosomes (X and Y) for a total of 46. Remarkably, the correct number of human diploid chromosomes was not confirmed until 1954! Examination of an individual's karyotype by staining can reveal regions of chromosomal deletions, insertions, duplications, inversions, and translocations. A karyotype can also be helpful for diagnosing some genetic disorders. Missing or extra chromosomes (**aneuploidy**) are readily detected in a normal karyotype. Genetic diseases that result from a specific mutation in a gene on a specific chromosome (for example, Down syndrome marked by mutation C on chromosome 21) cannot be observed in a karyotype. **Sex chromosomes** carry the genetic information that dictates the sex of offspring. Human males are heterologous because they have X and Y chromosomes, and human females are homologous having two X chromosomes. **Autosomes** carry the genetic information for all other traits. All chromosomes behave in the same way during meiosis (see Figure 3.13). Offspring that receive the X chromosome from the father and either X chromosome from the mother will be female. Offspring that receive the Y chromosome from the father and either X chromosome from the mother will be male.

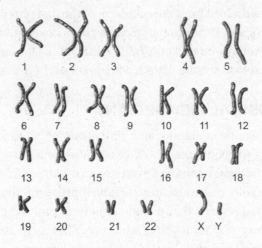

Figure 7.3. Karyotype of a human male

Alleles

Vertebrates contain two sets of chromosomes (autosomes in humans), so they are diploid. Diploid organisms contain one copy of each gene on each chromosome. **Alleles** are alternate forms of the same gene. Therefore, diploid organisms contain one allele on each chromosome. If a pair of chromosomes contains the same allele, the organism is **homozygous** for that specific gene. If within a pair of chromosomes each chromosome contains a different allele, the organism is **heterozygous** for that gene. For example, the genotype for black hair is BB (homozygous) or Bb (heterozygous). Using test genetic crosses of plants, Gregor Mendel found that alleles can be dominant or recessive. A **dominant allele** will be expressed over a

recessive allele in a heterozygous offspring. By convention, dominant alleles are designated by capital letters and recessive alleles by lowercase letters. In our example, the allele for black hair (B) is dominant, and the allele for brown hair (b) is recessive. Therefore, an offspring must acquire a recessive allele from each parent to have brown hair (bb). Several genetic crosses between parents with black or brown hair would yield the following probable offspring as depicted in **Punnett squares** (Figure 7.4).

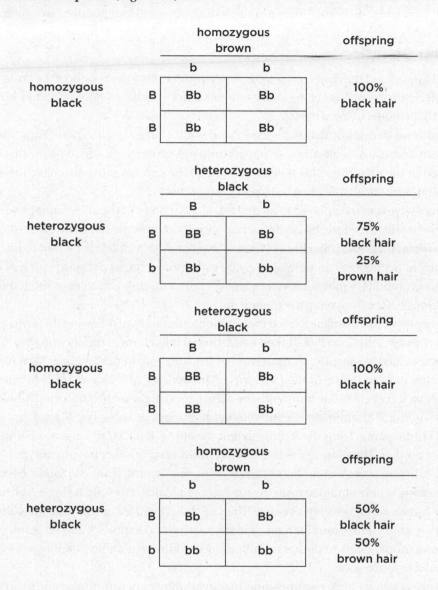

Figure 7.4. Examples of theoretical genetic crosses performed in Punnett squares

The examples shown above represent simple allelic patterns. Most genetic loci contain multiple alleles or are said to be **polymorphic**. The frequencies of these multiple alleles vary among populations. A significant degree of allelic variation cannot be observed because of alleles that fail to produce obvious phenotypic differences. The number of alleles or polymorphism that exists or the proportion of heterozygotes in the population is used to determine allelic variation. The frequency of alleles in a diploid population can be used to predict the frequencies of the genotypes according to the Hardy-Weinberg principle (*see Chapter 6*).

Mendel formulated three principles of inheritance. In the **fundamental theory of heredity**, inheritance is dictated by the passage of discrete units of inheritance (which we now know as alleles) from parents to offspring. The principle of segregation stated that during reproduction, the inherited factors (alleles) that determine traits are separated into reproductive cells by a process called meiosis (*see Chapter 3, Eukaryotic Cell*) and randomly reunite during fertilization. In the **principle of independent assortment**, Medel predicted that inherited factors (alleles) located on different chromosomes will be inherited independently of each other.

Human Genetics

Mendel formulated the concepts of inheritance by observing the results of the cross-breeding of plants. Human genetics is the study of inheritance specific to human beings but is based on Mendel's model of inheritance.

Autosomal dominant traits are associated with a single gene on an autosome and are dominant because a single allele, inherited from either parent, is adequate for this trait to be observed in the offspring. This means that one of the parents must also have the same trait unless it is introduced due to an unlikely new mutation.

If a recessive trait is displayed in an individual, two copies of the allele must be present. The trait or gene will, therefore, be located on a nonsex chromosome. This characteristic is known as **autosomal recessive inheritance**. It takes two copies of an allele for a trait to be displayed; therefore, many people can unknowingly be carriers of certain conditions such as a disease. From an evolutionary perspective, a recessive trait or disease can remain hidden for several generations before displaying the phenotype.

The expression of an allele related to the chromosomal sex of offspring is known as sex linkage. Sex linkage inheritance (**X-linked and Y-linked inheritance**) differs from the inheritance of traits specified by autosomal chromosomes because both males and females have the same probability of inheritance in the latter case. The number of X-linked traits is much greater than Y-linked traits because humans have more genes on the X chromosome. X-linked genes, present on the X chromosome, can be either dominant or recessive. Male offspring obtain their X chromosome from the female parent, resulting in all X-linked genes being inherited from the mother. Therefore, recessive X-linked traits usually affect the phenotype of male offspring. X-linked traits cannot be obtained by male offspring from the father because the Y chromosome is only obtained from the male parent. Males only have a single X chromosome, so they cannot be carriers for recessive X-linked traits. Females are carriers for X-linked traits when they are heterozygous for a particular genotype and express X-linked genes when they are homozygous. X-linked dominant inheritance exhibits the same phenotype as a homozygote and a heterozygote.

A process known as **X chromosome inactivation** occurs during the embryonic stage in females (XX) to prevent the duplication of normal proteins produced from the expression of X chromosome genes. X-inactivation will eliminate the expression of all but one X chromosome in disorders that are characterized by the presence of three X chromosomes. Males that have disorders in which there is an extra X chromosome also exhibit X chromosome inactivation.

Y-linked traits are only inherited by male offspring from the male parent because Y chromosomes are present only in males. Maleness, controlled by the "testis determining factor" gene located on the Y chromosome, is an example of a Y-linked inherited trait.

The passage of genetic traits over generations in a family is represented by a standard **genogram**. Males and females are depicted by squares and circles, respectively, and the offspring of mating pairs are shown by connecting lines (Figure 7.5). Genograms are useful for predicting the inheritance of a specific trait and to follow the transmission of genetic diseases. Autosomal dominant and autosomal recessive traits and X-linked or Y-linked inheritance can be tracked by the analysis of a genogram. The outcome of matings between closely related individuals (inbreeding) can be observed as is commonly found among early generations of royal families. Pedigrees can also be used by genetic counselors to predict the health of offspring. Another way to display detailed genetic information about members of a family is in a **pedigree chart** (Figure 7.5).

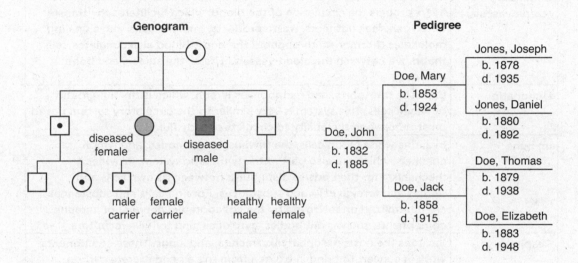

Figure 7.5. Examples of a genogram and pedigree chart

ORGAN SYSTEMS

The vertebrate body is organized into a number of organ, circulating, and signaling systems that have distinct structures and carry out specific functions related to maintaining the life of the organism. These systems are summarized in Table 7.1.

Integumentary System

The **integumentary system** is the largest "organ" in the human body and is made up of the skin and various appendages that include hair and nails. Animal appendages that are part of this system are scales, feathers, and hooves. The skin acts as a protective barrier against invading microorganisms, dehydration, and ultraviolet light. It also helps eliminate waste (perspiration), regulates temperature (perspiration and homeostasis), and houses receptors for detecting temperature, pressure, pain, and sensation. The skin can also store water, fat, and glucose, as well as make vitamin D when exposed to ultraviolet light.

Table 7.1. Summary of Human Vertebrate Systems

System	Description
Integumentary	Skin (covering of the body), hair, nails and other functionally important structures, such as the sweat glands and sebaceous glands. The skin provides containment, structure, and protection for the other organs. It also serves as a major sensory interface with the environment.
Musculoskeletal (skeletal and muscular)	Human skeleton, including bones, ligaments, tendons, cartilage, and attached muscles. The skeleton is the basic structure of the body and allows for movement. Bone marrow contained in the larger bones of the body functions in the production of blood cells. Calcium and phosphate are also stored in bones. In some sources, this system is divided into the skeletal and muscular systems.
Circulatory (cardiovascular)	Heart and blood vessels, including arteries, veins, and capillaries. The heart propels the circulation of the blood, which facilitates the transfer of oxygen, fuel, nutrients, waste products, immune cells, and signaling molecules (hormones) throughout the body. Blood also circulates cells that move between the blood vessels, tissue, the spleen, and bone marrow.
Lymphatic	Extracts, transports, and metabolizes lymph, which is the fluid found between cells. This system is very similar to the circulatory system based on structure and the ability to circulate a body fluid.
Immune	Includes white blood cells, the thymus, lymph nodes, and lymph channels, which are also part of the lymphatic system. Provides a mechanism for the body to distinguish between its own cells and tissues and foreign cells and substances. Foreign cells and substances are neutralized or destroyed by the collaborative network of immune components, such as antibodies, cytokines, and toll-like receptors.
Respiratory	Includes the nose, nasopharynx, trachea, and lungs. These components work in concert to bring in oxygen from the air and excrete carbon dioxide and water back into the environment.
Digestive	Includes the mouth, tongue, teeth, salivary glands, esophagus, stomach, gastrointestinal tract, small and large intestines, rectum, liver, pancreas, and gallbladder. Food is converted into small, nutritional, non-toxic molecules for circulation to all tissues of the body. Unusable components of the food are secreted as waste.
Urinary	Includes the kidneys, ureters, bladder, and urethra. Water is removed from the blood to produce urine, which carries a variety of waste molecules and excess ions, and water out of the body.
Nervous	Includes the central nervous system (brain and spinal cord) and the peripheral nervous system. The brain is the organ of thought, emotion, memory, and sensory processing. It also functions in communication and controls various systems and activities. The senses include vision, hearing, taste, and smell. The eyes, ears, tongue, and nose help collect information about the environment.
Endocrine	Includes the primary endocrine glands—the pituitary, thyroid, adrenals, pancreas, parathyroids, and gonads. All organs and tissues produce specific endocrine hormones that serve as signals among body systems. Exocrine glands (sweat, salivary, mammary) secrete products through ducts.
Reproductive	Includes the internal and external sex organs and the gonads. Gametes in each sex are produced, a mechanism for their combination is maintained, and a nurturing environment is provided for the first 9 months of development of the embryo/infant.

There are three major layers of tissue in the human skin: **epidermis**, **dermis**, and **hypodermis** (Figure 7.6). The epidermis is in contact with the environment and, therefore, carries out the major functions of the skin. There are five layers (stratum corneum, stratum lucidium, stratum granulosum, stratum spinosum, and stratum basale) composed primarily of **epithelial cells** or **keratinocytes** (cells that contain a fibrous, water-shedding protein known as keratin) that form a keratinized stratified squamous epithelium. In addition to keratinocytes, the epidermis also contains **melanocytes** (a type of pigment-producing cell), **Merkel cells** (sensory cells), and **Langerhans' cells** (antigen-presenting immune cells). Dead keratinocytes are constantly sloughed off of the epidermis layer, except for the nonkeratinized lining of the inside of the mouth. Nails are formed by the strengthening of epidermal tissue with additional keratin.

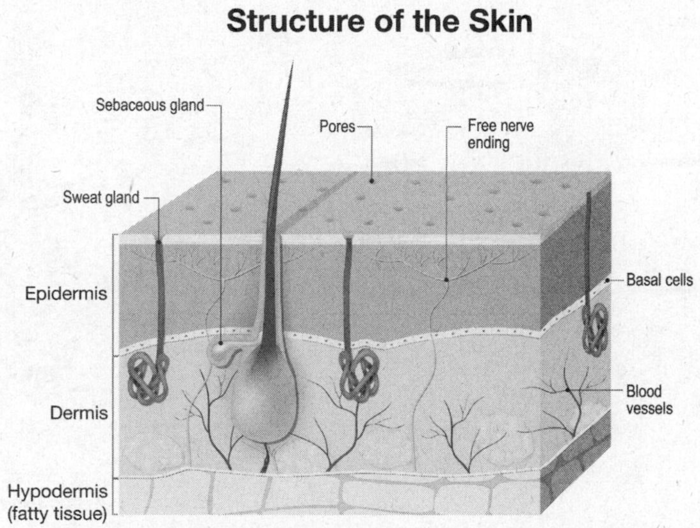

Structure of the Skin

Figure 7.6. Layers of the skin

The dermis layer underlies the epidermis and is composed of dense irregular connective tissue and areolar connective tissue. The latter type of tissue contains collagen and elastin, a stretchable protein. The outermost region of the dermis is known as the papillary layer and consists of the areolar connective tissue. The reticular layer, which is underneath the papillary layer, contains the dense irregular connective tissue. The function of these layers is to make the skin flexible and prevent wrinkling. Blood vessels and nerves that serve the skin end in the dermal layer. In addition, the dermis is an anchor point for hair (follicles), feathers, and glands (**sebaceous** and **sweat**) depending on the type of vertebrate animal. Additional pigment-containing cells known as chromatophores also reside in the dermis layer. The hypodermis is the deepest and thickest layer of the skin. It is attached to the collagen and elastin fibers of the dermis and is composed primarily of fat storage cells called adipocytes.

Musculoskeletal System

The human **musculoskeletal system** (sometimes referred to as the locomotor system or activity system) provides form, support, protection, stability, and movement. This system is comprised of the bones of the skeleton, muscles, joints, and the connective tissues **cartilage** (flexible), **tendons** (tough and fibrous), and **ligaments** (fibrous) that support and bind tissues and organs together. Calcium, phosphorus, and components of the hematopoietic system (blood-forming cells) are stored in the skeleton. The musculoskeletal system is often divided into two subsystems: skeletal and muscular.

An average adult skeleton contains approximately 206 bones. This number has some flexibility based on the methods used to count bones that may have fused together since birth (over 300 bones). The skeleton is divided into two parts called the **axial skeleton** (bones that form the head, rib cage, sternum, and vertebral column) and the **appendicular skeleton** (bones that form the appendages) (Figure 7.7A). Bones are classified as **long**, **short**, **flat**, **irregular**, and **sesamoid** (Figure 7.7B). The human skeleton contains both bones that are fused and others that are independent. Bones in the skeleton are supported by ligaments, tendons, muscles, and cartilage.

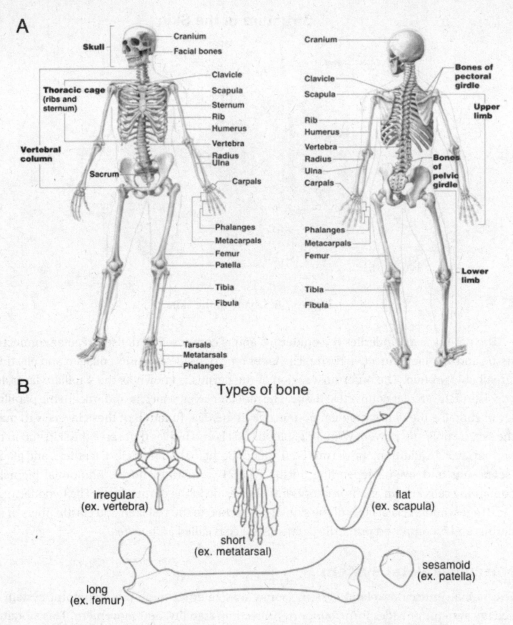

Figure 7.7. (A) Skeletal system. Front and rear views. (B) Types of bone.

Tissues and organs are attached to the skeleton which forms a framework and protects these structures. Bones contain a membranous coating, the **periosteum**, a hard external layer containing compact or cortical bone, and a softer internal material known as cancellous bone (Figure 7.8). Long bones contain yellow and red bone marrow. Yellow marrow is made up of fatty connective tissue that serves as an energy source during times of starvation. Blood cells (leukocytes, erythrocytes) and platelets are produced in the red marrow (also see section on *Circulatory System*, on page 70). These cells migrate to the circulatory system from the bone marrow. The storage of calcium and phosphorus in bones regulates the balance of minerals in the blood.

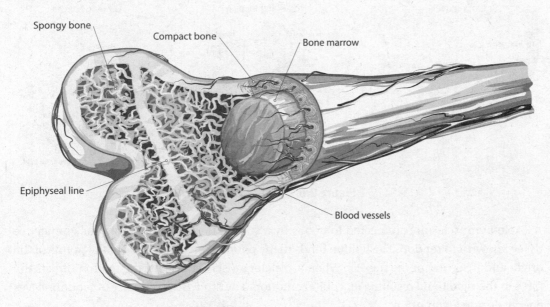

Spongy bone

Compact bone

Bone marrow

Epiphyseal line

Blood vessels

Figure 7.8. Structure of long bones

Muscles are divided into three types: smooth, skeletal, and cardiac (Figure 7.9). The movement of substances through hollow organs (**peristalsis**) is controlled by smooth muscles. These muscles contract and relax to form a wave motion that propels the substance in a forward motion along the tract. Smooth muscles have one nucleus per cell and are controlled involuntarily. Skeletal muscles have multiple nuclei and are attached, in an opposing arrangement, to bones at joints. Communication between nerves and these muscles induce electrical currents that cause voluntary contraction. Only skeletal muscles function in body movement, and only these and smooth muscles are considered to be part of the musculoskeletal system. Cardiac muscles have a single nucleus per cell and are confined to the heart where they function to circulate blood. Cardiac muscles are under involuntary control and, along with skeletal muscles, have a striated structure or appearance. Skeletal muscles are made up of tubular-shaped muscle cells that contain myofibrils. Myofibrils are composed of repeating units called **sarcomeres**. Myosin and actin are fibrous proteins present in the sarcomeres. Contraction is described by the **sliding filament theory**, which explains how a thin actin filament slides over a thick myosin filament to create a tension that causes Z disks (bands bound to actin in the sarcomere) to be pulled toward each other (Figure 7.10). To initiate a skeletal muscle contraction, a motor neuron from the somatic nervous system sends a message to the muscles. The motor neuron is depolarized (change in the electrical state) causing neurotransmitters (chemicals that transmit signals across a synapse) to be released from the nerve terminal. The neurotransmitters travel across the space (neuromuscular junction) between the nerve channel and the muscle and bind to receptors on the surface of the muscle fiber. This signal causes a change in the electrical membrane potential of a muscle cell leading to a change in the permeability of the membrane. This allows calcium (Ca^{2+}) to enter the cells and activate actin. Activated actin binds myosin, which causes the Z bands to be pulled together (**contraction**). This process also releases ADP and inorganic phosphate. ATP that is formed [ADP + Pi → ATP] binds to myosin causing it to release the actin allowing the Z bands to move apart (**relaxation**).

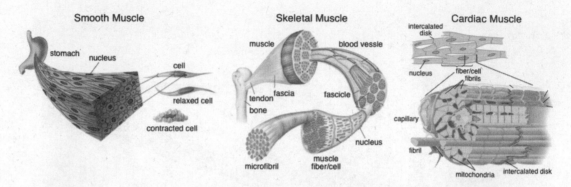

Figure 7.9. Types of muscle

Skeletal muscles are connected to bones by a strong, flexible band of fibrous connective tissue known as a tendon. The tendon binds to the periosteum of the bone at the points of the origin and insertion of the muscle. When a skeletal muscle contracts, the tendon directs the force to the rigid bone resulting in a pulling motion. The stretching property of tendons saves energy during locomotion.

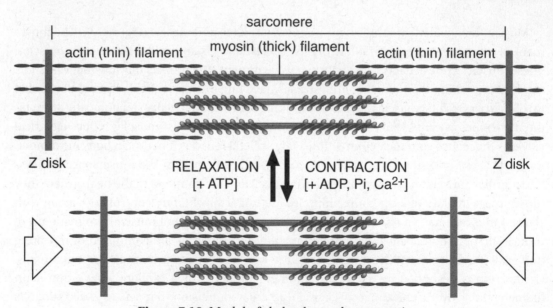

Figure 7.10. Model of skeletal muscle contraction

Joints connect bones and function to permit bones to move against each other. A synovial joint, or **diarthrosis**, is the most common type of joint and permits extensive mobility between two or more articular heads (Figure 7.11A). **Amphiarthrosis** joints allow a slight continuous movement. False joints, or **synarthroses**, permit a small amount or no movement. **Synovial** joints are not joined but have a solution (synovial fluid) between the bones to lubricate the movement. The synovial fluid is contained in a bursa, or sac, composed of white fibrous tissue. Bursae provide a cushion between the bones, tendons, and muscles. Joints are formed when skeletal bones are connected by ligaments, which are bands of dense white fibrous elastic tissue (Figure 7.11B). In general, ligaments prevent joints from dislocating under reasonable forces.

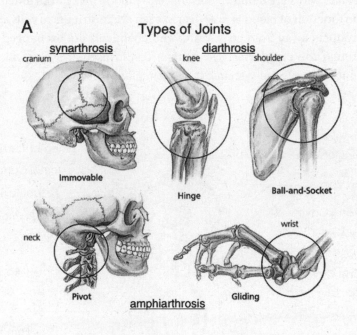

A   Types of Joints

synarthrosis   diarthrosis

cranium   knee   shoulder

Immovable   Hinge   Ball-and-Socket

neck   wrist

Pivot   Gliding

amphiarthrosis

B   Anatomy of a Hinge Joint

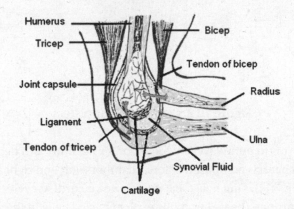

Humerus

Tricep

Joint capsule

Ligament

Tendon of tricep

Cartilage

Bicep

Tendon of bicep

Radius

Ulna

Synovial Fluid

Figure 7.11. Human joints. (A) Types of joints. (B) Structure of a hinge joint (elbow).

Circulatory System

The **circulatory**, **or cardiovascular system**, functions to move blood and blood cells around the body and to transport oxygen, carbon dioxide, hormones, and nutrients to and from tissues and cells. In some cases, the circulatory system is viewed as being composed of two independent systems: cardiovascular for the dissemination of blood and lymphatic for the circulation of lymph.

The human cardiovascular system is composed of blood, the heart, and blood vessels (Figure 7.12). **Blood** is composed of plasma (dissolved proteins, glucose, electrolytes, hormones, clotting factors), red (**erythrocytes**) and white (**leukocytes**) blood cells, and platelets (**thrombocytes**) (Figure 7.13). These components are circulated by the heart through blood vessels. **Arteries** and **veins** are blood vessels that carry blood away from and toward the heart, respectively. The function of blood is to deliver oxygen and nutrients to cells and to carry metabolic waste products away from cells. Water and chemicals are exchanged between blood and tissues through the **capillaries**. The human cardiovascular system includes coronary (heart), pulmonary (lungs), and systemic (body) circulation.

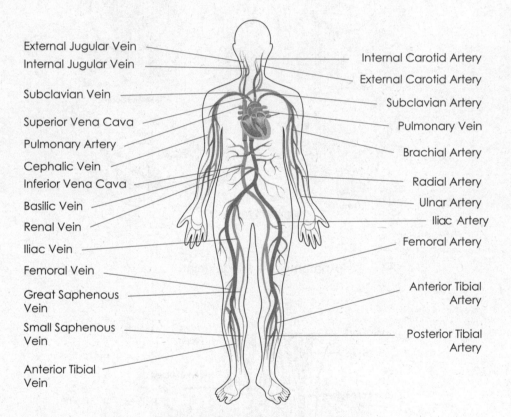

Figure 7.12. Cardiovascular system

The role of the heart is to pump oxygenated blood to the body and deoxygenated blood to the lungs. The human heart is composed of four chambers: left and right atriums and left and right ventricles (Figure 7.14). One heartbeat constitutes a **cardiac cycle**, and its frequency is determined as the heart rate (beats per minute). Specialized cells in the atrioventricular and sinoatrial nodes produce electrical pulses that coordinate the cardiac cycle. Each beat of the heart has five stages. In stage 1 (early diastole), the semilunar valves (pulmonary and aortic) close and the atrioventricular valves (mitral and tricuspid) open. In stage 2 (atrial systole), the atriums contract to force blood from the atriums to the ventricles. In stage 3 (isovolumic contraction), the ventricles contract and the atrioventricular and semilunar valves close. In stage 4 (ventricular ejection), the semilunar valves open and the blood leaves the ventricles. In stage 5 (isovolumic relaxation time), the semilunar valves close.

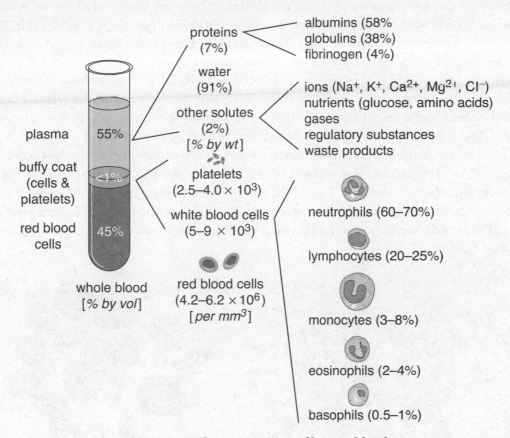

Figure 7.13. The composition of human blood

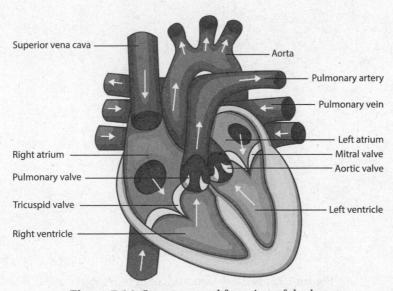

Figure 7.14. Structure and function of the heart

Deoxygenated blood enters the right atrium and passes into the right ventricle for delivery through the pulmonary artery to the lungs for oxygenation and removal of carbon dioxide (**pulmonary circulation**). The oxygenated blood from the lungs re-enters the heart through the left atrium. From there, the blood is passed to the left ventricle and is pumped to various organs through the aorta (**systemic circulation**). The valves that separate the chambers prevent back-flow. In **coronary circulation**, a supply of oxygen-rich blood is delivered to the myocardium (cardiac or heart muscle) via the coronary arteries. The blood is then returned to the heart through the coronary veins. In humans and other vertebrates, the blood never leaves the cardiovascular network; this is referred to as a "closed" system. However, oxygen and nutrients diffuse across the blood vessels and capillaries entering the **interstitial fluid** (fluid that surrounds cells) to feed cells. Carbon dioxide and waste from cells enters the interstitial fluid and is carried in the blood plasma back to the lungs for expulsion.

Most oxygen in the body is transported by the iron-containing metalloprotein **hemoglobin** (Figure 7.15). Hemoglobin is composed of four subunits. Each subunit carries a Fe^{2+} ion-containing cofactor known as heme. The high oxygen-binding capacity of hemoglobin significantly increases total blood oxygen levels. Hemoglobin is the most abundant protein in red blood cells (erythrocytes) and is also involved in the transport of other gases, such as carbon dioxide.

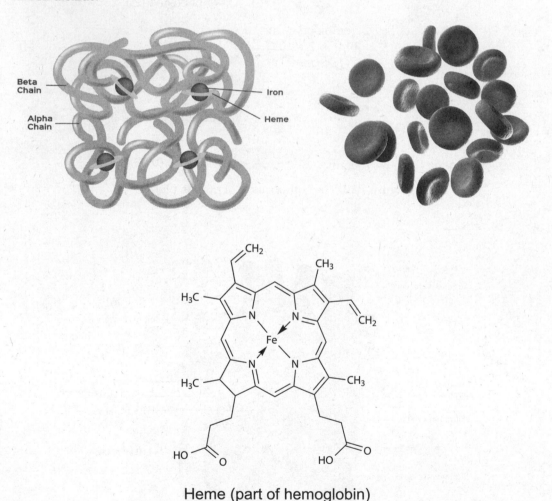

Heme (part of hemoglobin)

Figure 7.15. Tertiary structure of hemoglobin

Red blood cells contain inherited (*see Chapter 6*) antigens, such as proteins, carbohydrates, or glycolipids (see section on *Immune System*, page 76), on their surface. These antigens have been used to type or group individuals primarily for the purpose of donating blood for transfusions. The four main blood groups are A, B, AB, and O (Table 7.2). Note that individuals who have blood types AB and O are universal blood recipients and universal blood donors, respectively. The cardiovascular system is a "closed" system. If the endothelial lining of a blood vessel is damaged, the blood rapidly coagulates or **clots** (**thrombus**; changes form from a liquid to a gel). Clotting factors (platelets and proteins) are found in all mammals and provide a safety feature to limit the extent of blood loss when a blood vessel is damaged.

Table 7.2. Blood Groups

Blood Type	Average Percentage in Population	Antigen(s) on Red Blood Cell	Serum Antibodies	Can Receive Blood from Donor	Can Donate Blood to Recipient
A	40	A	Anti-B	A and O	A and AB
B	10	B	Anti-A	B and O	B and AB
AB	4	A and B	none	A, B, AB, and O	AB
O	46	none	Anti-A and anti-B	O	A, B, AB, and O

Lymphatic System

The **lymphatic system** is made up of a network of vessels that carry **lymph** directly toward the heart (Figure 7.16). Lymph is created when interstitial fluid is filtered through lymph capillaries. The lymph is then transported through vessels to the **lymph nodes** and is delivered to the right or the left subclavian vein. Lymph moves through vessels by the coordinated actions of intraluminal valves, to ensure a unidirectional flow, and lymphatic muscle cells. At the end of the journey, the lymph is mixed back with blood. Therefore, lymph represents filtered blood plasma returned from the interstitial fluid. Unlike the cardiovascular system, the lymphatic system is an "open" system responsible for maintaining balance of body fluids and providing an alternative route for excess interstitial fluid and blood plasma components to be returned to the blood.

Lymph also contains **lymphocytes** and other white blood cells (**leukocytes**) of the immune system (see section on *Immune System*, page 76), as well as waste products, cell debris, and bacterial components. Lymphocytes play an important role in cell-mediated, humoral, innate, and adaptive immunity. Lymphocytes are produced by organs composed of lymphoid tissue, such as the spleen and thymus (immune system) and the tonsils (digestive system). They are concentrated in the lymph nodes, which are organized collections of lymphoid tissue located at various intervals (chest, neck, pelvis, armpits, groin, and abdominal areas) along the lymphatic system (Figure 7.16).

To summarize, interrelated functions of the lymphatic system include (i) the removal of interstitial fluid from tissues, (ii) the absorption and transport of fatty acids and fats from the digestive system, (iii) the transport of white blood cells to and from the lymph nodes into the bones, and (iv) the transport of antigen-presenting cells (dendritic cells) to the lymph nodes to stimulate an immune response.

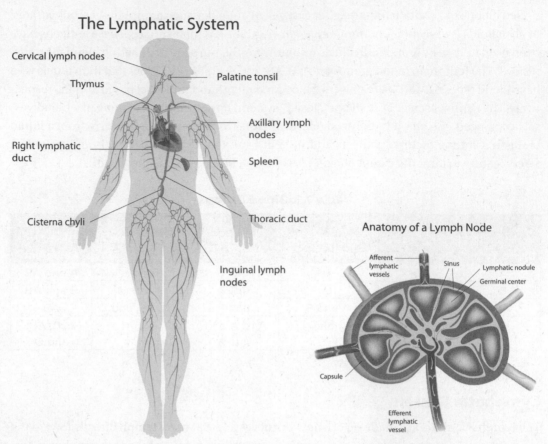

The Lymphatic System

Cervical lymph nodes

Thymus

Palatine tonsil

Axillary lymph nodes

Right lymphatic duct

Spleen

Cisterna chyli

Thoracic duct

Inguinal lymph nodes

Anatomy of a Lymph Node

Afferent lymphatic vessels

Sinus

Lymphatic nodule

Germinal center

Capsule

Efferent lymphatic vessel

Figure 7.16. Lymphatic system and structure of a lymph node

Respiratory System

The **respiratory system** includes those structures and organs required for the transport of oxygen from the external atmosphere to tissues and cells (Figure 7.17). Another important function of this system is to transport carbon dioxide from the cells and tissues of the body to the outside. Respiration in mammals occurs in the lungs, which are located on both sides of the heart near the backbone. The main function of the lungs is to transport oxygen to and remove carbon dioxide from the bloodstream. The lungs are made up of small, thin-walled **alveoli** (air sacs) that provide the necessary extensive surface area required for the exchange of gases.

In mammals, breathing is achieved by contraction and expansion of the **diaphragm** (sheet of skeletal muscle), which is located at the base of the thorax or rib cage. When the diaphragm contracts, the bottom of the chest cavity is pulled downward drawing air into the nasal (and oral) cavity, trachea, and lungs by increasing volume and decreasing pressure. This process is known as **inhalation**. For **expiration**, the diaphragm relaxes. Air entering the trachea of humans passes into two bronchi to enter the bronchioles in the lungs and reach the alveolar sacs. Alveoli in the sacs are engulfed by blood vessels (Figure 7.18A) to allow **gas exchange** by diffusion (Figure 7.18B). This process also occurs in the gills in fish and some invertebrates. Deoxygenated blood from the heart reaches the lungs via the pulmonary artery. Oxygen diffuses into the blood through the blood vessels that are associated with the alveolar sacs. There it is exchanged for carbon dioxide by binding to hemoglobin that is carried by the red blood cells (erythrocytes). The newly oxygenated blood enters the heart through the pulmonary veins and is delivered to tissues and cells through the circulatory system (Figure 7.18C).

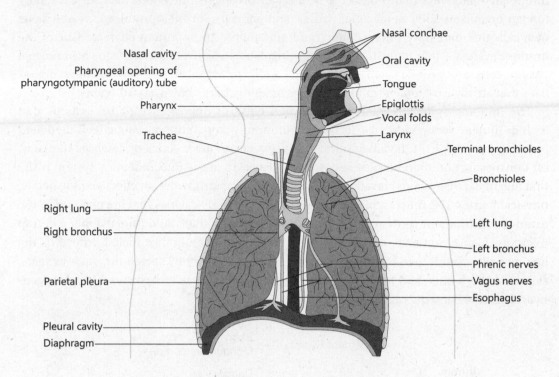

Figure 7.17. Components of the respiratory system

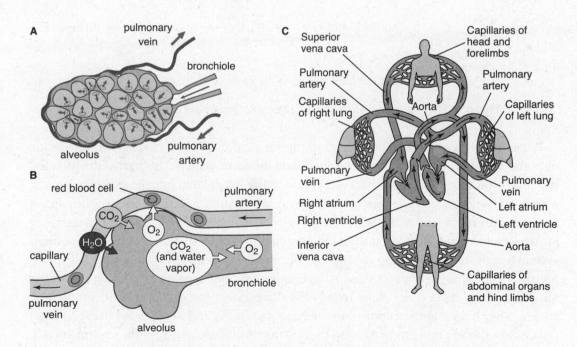

Figure 7.18. Mechanism of gas exchange in the lungs and the transport of oxygen through the circulatory system

Immune System

The **immune system** is made up of a complex assortment of cells, biological substances, and interrelated pathways that protect the host organism against infectious diseases caused by foreign organisms such as bacteria, viruses, and parasites (or their products), as well as its own cells that may have undergone harmful mutations. An important characteristic of the immune system is that it must be able to distinguish between a host organism's own normal tissues, cells, and proteins (**self**) and those of a foreign organism (**nonself**). Foreign organisms that are invasive and harmful to humans or animals are known as **pathogens**.

The immune system is made up of several types of opposing response systems that include innate versus adaptive (acquired) immunity and humoral versus cell-mediated immunity (Figure 7.19). Invading microorganisms encounter a series of defenses that start off nonspecific and then become very specific. The skin of the integumentary system is the first line of defense against invaders and, unless damaged, provides an effective nonspecific physical barrier. The mucous membranes that line the body cavities that are exposed to the external environment contain an epithelium and secrete a thick fluid (**mucus**) that can trap microorganisms. Some examples of protective mucous membranes include those of the lips, nostrils, eyelids, genital area, and anus. A number of bodily secretions, such as tears, saliva, mother's milk, and mucus, contain an enzyme known as **lysozyme**, which attacks or hydrolyzes the bacterial cell wall (*see Chapter 3*).

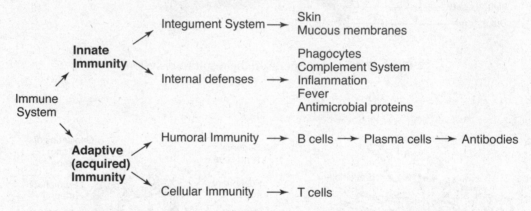

Figure 7.19. Flow chart showing the organization of the immune system

When a pathogen successfully breaches the physical barriers, a rapid and non-specific response to the invasion is initiated by the **innate immune system**. This part of the immune system is evolutionarily ancient because it is found in multicellular organisms, fungi, insects, plants, and animals. The vertebrate innate immune system organizes the recruitment of immune cells to the site of the infection. Cells, such as macrophages, release cell signaling proteins called **cytokines** that mediate the immune process. In addition, the **complement system** is activated. This system is a complex biochemical cascade of proteins that help identify and clear pathogens by recruiting inflammatory cells and tagging or marking pathogens for clearance by other cells. White blood cells (leukocytes) are part of the innate immune system. They help identify, capture, and remove pathogens and debris from damaged host cells. Some specific types of leukocytes include **macrophages**, **neutrophils**, and **mast cells**. Therefore, cells of the innate immune system nonspecifically recognize pathogens. The purpose of this system is to rapidly respond to an infection, but it does not provide long term or protective immunity to the host organism.

The **adaptive immune system**, unique to vertebrates, is available if pathogens successfully defeat the innate immune response. In contrast to the innate immune system, the adaptive or **acquired immune system** is very specific for each pathogen. The adaptive immune system is activated by the innate immune response and is designed not only to enhance recognition of invading pathogens, but also to retain the ability to recognize the same pathogens after the infection has been cleared. This concept is known as **immunological memory** and is the underlying principle of **vaccination**. This memory allows the organism to deliver a more rapid and effective response if repeatedly infected with the same pathogen. Like innate immunity, adaptive immunity relies on the ability of the immune system to recognize pathogens as non-self. A major type of non-self molecule is known as an **antigen** (antibody generator). More specifically, antigens can be proteins and carbohydrate polymers that make up pathogens. These antigens bind to specific immune receptors on cells to initiate an immune response. The adaptive immune response is carried out by B and T lymphocytes.

T lymphocytes (T cells) are made in the bone marrow but mature in the thymus or tonsils. T cells are divided into multiple types. The major types are helper, suppressor or regulatory, memory, and cytotoxic. T cells are important in the type of adaptive immunity known as **cell-mediated immunity** which involves the activation of specific types of cells and the release of various cytokines in response to an antigen. Therefore, unlike B cells, T cells do not make antibodies.

The adaptive immune system is turned on in vertebrates when a pathogen, encountering the innate immune system, accumulates to produce a threshold level of antigen and induces signals that activate **dendritic cells** (Figure 7.20). The dendritic cells engulf the pathogen, degrade the pathogen to smaller molecules (antigens), and migrate to T cell-enriched lymph nodes. The antigens are then displayed on the surface of the dendritic cells by binding to **major histocompatibility complexes** (MHC or human leukocyte antigen). Dendritic cells and B cells are professional antigen-presenting cells. The exposed and immobilized antigens are then recognized by some types of T cells. When T helper cells are activated in this manner, they rapidly divide and secrete cytokines to facilitate different types of immune responses (T cell activation). Activated cytotoxic T cells destroy virus-infected and tumor cells. Memory T cells remain after an infection has been cleared and are activated when re-exposed to the specific antigen.

B lymphocytes (B cells) are made in the bone marrow, and their job is to make **antibodies** that recognize specific antigens. They also function as antigen-presenting cells and develop to form memory B cells after the native B cells have been activated by binding to antigen in the blood or lymph. B cells are important in the type of adaptive immunity known as **humoral immunity**. Humoral immunity is directed by macromolecules present in bodily fluids (humours) and involves the production of antibodies or **immunoglobulins**. Therefore, the primary function of B cells is to make antibodies that recognize soluble antigens. B cells are activated by either a T cell-independent or -dependent mechanism (Figure 7.20). In T cell-independent activation, an antigen-presenting B cell delivers a processed antigen to a T helper cell resulting in the release of cytokines which activates the B cell (B cell activation). The mature B cell then proliferates and terminally differentiates into antibody-producing **plasma cells**.

Antibodies, or immunoglobulins, are glycoproteins secreted in large quantities by the plasma cells that were derived from antigen-activated B cells. Antibodies are part of the acquired immune system and play a role in humoral immunity. They are found in the blood, tissue fluids, and various bodily secretions, such as saliva. The basic structure of antibodies consists of two heavy chains and two light chains (polypeptides) arranged in a Y-shaped configuration

(Figure 7.21A). Every antibody has two identical light and heavy chains. The heavy chains are each composed of constant and variable regions. The constant region is the same in all antibodies having the same isotype. The variable region is identical in those antibodies produced by a single B cell. However, each B cell produces antibodies that have distinct variable regions. The variable regions on different antibodies bind to specific parts (**epitopes**) of an antigen (Figure 7.21B). This binding specificity is the basis for the ability of antibodies to recognize different antigens and for the production of **monoclonal antibodies**. The variable region controls the specificity of the antigen-binding site at the end of the heavy and light chain region (Fab fragment). The ends of the two heavy chains form the Fc fragment that controls the appropriate immune response for each antigen by binding to a specific class of Fc receptor on various types of cells. These cells include B lymphocytes, macrophages, neutrophils, and mast cells. The Fc fragment also interacts with other immune molecules and components of the complement system. The complement system, or cascade, is a signaling pathway made up of small blood proteins that helps clear pathogens as part of the innate immune system. Activation of this cascade by the binding of antigen-antibody complexes to complement proteins can result in enhanced **phagocytosis** (**opsonization**) and lysis of invading bacteria.

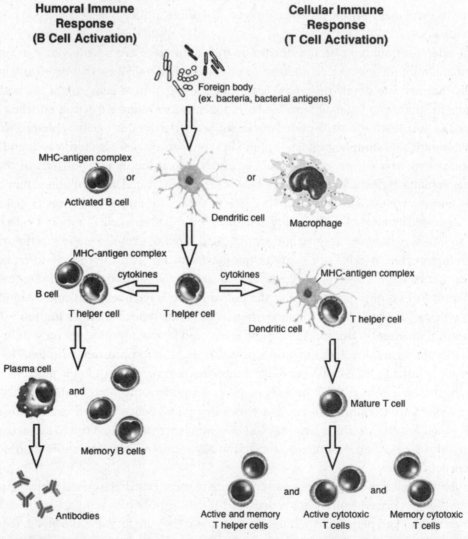

Figure 7.20. Comparison of the humoral immune response (B cell activation) and cellular immune response (T cell activation). MHC, major histocompatibility complex.

There are various **isotypes** or classes of antibodies based on the form of the heavy chains in the structure. Mammals produce five isotypes called IgA, IgD, IgE, IgG, and IgM (Ig stands for immunoglobulin and A–M represent the different heavy chains) (Figure 7.21C). The isotypes have different properties, recognize different types of antigens, and work in different regions of the body.

Therefore, antibodies are part of the humoral branch of the acquired immune system and help identify and neutralize pathogens and their products. Each antibody recognizes a specific antigen as well as distinct parts (epitopes) of the same antigen. Antibodies bind to antigens, forming a heavy complex that precipitates (protein antigens) or agglutinates (whole bacteria or viruses). These heavy complexes are engulfed by macrophages and other phagocytic cells to clear the nonself substances from the body. These complexes also stimulate protective responses by immune cells and pathways such as the complement cascade. The ability of antibodies to bind antigens also helps neutralize the activity of toxic secreted and surface-bound molecules produced by pathogens.

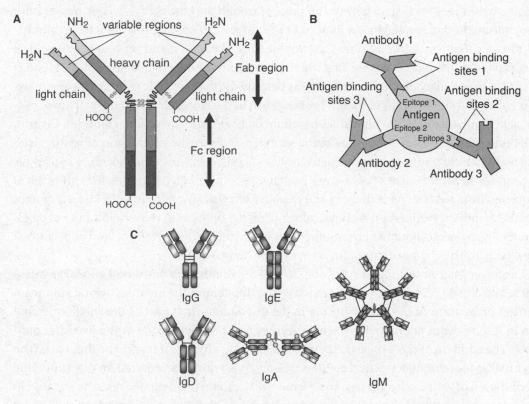

Figure 7.21. Structure and activities of antibodies. (A) General structure of an immunoglobulin. (B) Recognition and binding of antibodies to epitopes on an antigen. (C) Antibody isotypes.

Digestive System

The function of the **digestive system**, or alimentary canal, is to convert food into smaller components that can be easily absorbed to feed cells in the body. The first steps in the processing of food into nutrients takes place in the mouth (Figure 7.22). Much of the mouth is lined with an oral mucosa that produces a mucus, known as mucin, which serves as a lubricant. The palate separates the oral and nasal cavities. The tongue, composed mostly of muscle, is primarily a sensory organ but is also important for speech. Three pairs of relatively large **salivary glands** (**parotid**, **submandibular**, and **sublingual**) secrete components of **saliva** that help digestion by softening and breaking down food, maintaining the health of the tissues and structures of the oral cavity, and providing lubrication. Human saliva is made up of mostly water and smaller amounts of mucus, enzymes, glycoproteins, electrolytes, and secretory IgA. Enzymes in saliva, such as lysozyme and amylase, have antibacterial properties and help convert the starch or complex carbohydrates in food to smaller units. Specialized teeth, such as incisors and molars, have various roles in the process of mastication or the chewing of food to create smaller pieces. **Teeth** are relatively hard structures composed of enamel and dentin and are tightly anchored in bone in the mouth (Figure 7.22 inset). Mastication, along with the actions of mucus and saliva, prepare food for swallowing by creating a soft **bolus**.

The upper gastrointestinal tract is delineated by the **esophagus**, **stomach**, and **duodenum** (Figure 7.22). The **pharynx** connects the mouth to the esophagus. It is divided into the naso-pharynx, oropharynx, and laryngopharynx. Only the latter two structures are considered to belong to the digestive system because air passes through the nasopharynx. Food passes from the pharynx to the esophagus on its way to the stomach. Esophageal sphincters (cylindri-cal muscles that constrict an orifice) control the flow of the food and prevent backflow. The epiglottis prevents food from entering the trachea. From the esophagus, the bolus of food is passed to the stomach by a process known as **peristalsis** (the rhythmic contraction and relax-ation of muscles). The bolus of food is broken down in the stomach due to the activity of gas-tric acid (a mixture of hydrochloric acid, sodium chloride, and potassium chloride). Gastrin, a peptide hormone made by G cells in the stomach, induces the production of gastric acid. The hydrochloric acid in gastric acid activates the digestive enzyme pepsinogen by hydrolysis to produce **pepsin**. Pepsin digests large proteins to form smaller peptides. The stomach is protected from the actions of the acid and digestive enzymes by secretion of a layer of mucus. Peristalsis enhances digestion by physically mixing the bolus with these acids and enzymes. Ultimately, a viscous liquid known as **chyme** is produced in the pylorus or lowest portion of the stomach. The chyme at this point is very acidic (low pH).

The lower gastrointestinal tract is composed of the **duodenum** and **small** and **large intes-tines**. The chyme passes from the stomach to the duodenum through the pyloric sphincter. Further breakdown of the chyme occurs in the duodenum (first part of the small intestine) where it mixes with additional digestive enzymes and products made in the liver and pan-creas. The addition of these digestive components makes chyme more alkaline (high pH). The **liver** makes proteins, biochemical compounds, and bile which are required for digestion. **Bile** is composed of water, salts, mucus, and pigments. The main pigment, bilirubin, is released in the spleen as a result of the breakdown of blood cells in that organ. Bile made in the liver is carried to the **gallbladder** via the bile ducts. It is stored in the gallbladder and released into the duodenum when chyme enters that part of the small intestine. Bile functions as a surfactant that facilitates the emulsification of fats in the chyme. The emulsified fats are further digested into fatty acids and a monoglyceride for absorption through the intestinal wall. The liver is a secondary digestive gland that, among the number of functions noted above, also helps to breakdown carbohydrates. The pancreas is also an accessory digestive gland that produces enzymes that help breakdown chyme in the duodenum.

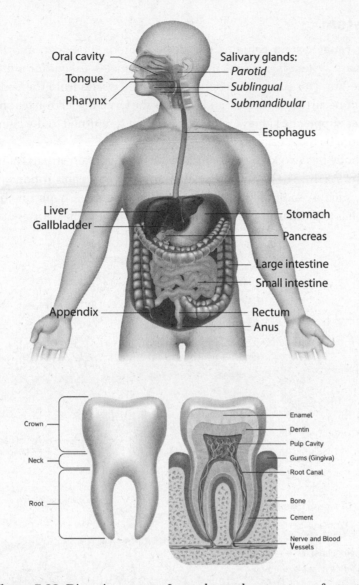

Crown

Neck

Root

Enamel

Dentin

Pulp Cavity

Gums (Gingiva)

Root Canal

Bone

Cement

Nerve and Blood
Vessels

Figure 7.22. Digestive system. Inset shows the structure of a tooth.

The **jejunum**, or second part of the small intestine, is the primary site of digestion. Mucus lubricates the walls of the intestine. When the chyme is completely digested, the nutrient components are absorbed by the intestinal wall and are passed into the bloodstream through surrounding blood vessels. The bloodstream carries the nutrients to cells and tissues. The **ileum**, or last part of the small intestine, absorbs bile salts and products that are not absorbed in the jejunum.

The division between the small and large intestine is identified by the **caecum**, a pouch that receives the chyme from the ileum. In the **colon** of the large intestine, the unabsorbed portion of the chyme, called feces, is metabolized by local bacteria (gut flora). Water and minerals are also reabsorbed back into the bloodstream. Undigested fecal waste is passed to the **rectum** by peristalsis and is defecated through the anal canal and anus.

Urinary System

The **urinary or renal system** contains the kidneys, ureters, bladder, and urethra (Figure 7.23A). The urinary system is identical in males and females, except for a difference in the length of the urethra. This system functions to eliminate wastes from the body; regulate the body's blood volume, pressure and pH; and controls the levels of electrolytes and metabolites. The renal arteries supply the kidneys with blood, which is returned to the circulatory system following filtration, by the renal vein.

The human body has two **kidneys** (right and left) that contain structural units known as **nephrons** (Figure 7.23B). The nephrons function to carry out reabsorption and secretion of various solutes, such as sodium ions, glucose, and glutamate. A nephron contains a **renal corpuscle**, which is the initial filtering part and the **renal tubule** that carries out reabsorption and secretion.

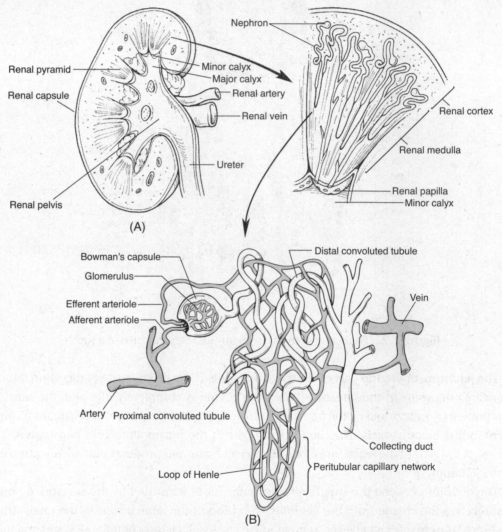

Figure 7.23. Urinary system and kidney function. (A) Overall view of the urinary system. (B) Structure and function of nephrons.

The renal corpuscle contains the glomerulus, a tuft of capillaries, and the **Bowman's capsule**, which surrounds the glomerulus. Fluids from the blood that enters the glomerulus are filtered through the Bowman's capsule. The filtrate enters the renal tubule and is passed to the distal convoluted tubule and the collecting duct system. The **Loop of Henle**, which is a U-shaped tube containing descending and ascending branches, is a major part of the renal tubule. The Loop of Henle is connected to the Bowman's capsule by the **proximal tubule** and is surrounded by the **vasa recta renis**, which is a series of capillaries. The primary function of this loop is to concentrate the salt in the surrounding tissue. This results in the formation of a concentration gradient in the central part of the kidney leading to production of a highly concentrated renal filtrate. During this process, solutes from the blood are filtered out by the renal corpuscle that is located in the renal cortex. The filtrate passes through the papillary ducts where water is reabsorbed and the concentrated urine, containing urea, is stored in the **bladder** waiting for secretion through the **urethra**. The distal convoluted tubule also secretes ammonium and hydrogen ions to regulate pH.

Nervous System

The nervous system coordinates voluntary and involuntary actions by transmitting signals between various parts of the body. The nervous system is divided into the **central nervous system** (CNS), which is composed of the spinal cord and brain, and the **peripheral nervous system** (PNS), which contains the nerves that link the CNS to all other parts of the body (Figure 7.24).

The CNS contains two major parts: the **spinal cord** and the **brain**. The spinal cord is a relatively long tubular bundle of nervous tissue and supporting cells that starts at the **medulla oblongata** in the brain stem and extends to the lumbar region of the vertebral column. The main function of the spinal cord is to transmit neural signals between the brain and other parts of the body. The spinal cord also contains neural circuits that can independently control reflexes and **central pattern generators** (biological neural networks that produce rhythmic patterned outputs without sensory feedback). Therefore, the spinal cord acts as a pathway for motor information away from the brain, as a pathway for sensory information that flows toward the brain, and as a control center for coordinating specific reflexes. The brain is an organ that controls sensory processing, memory, thought, emotion, and communication. The largest part of the brain is the cerebral cortex which is composed of neural tissue. The **cerebral cortex** is made up of four "lobes": frontal, parietal, temporal, and occipital. Specific functions, such as vision, motor control, and language, are associated with a particular lobe. The medulla oblongata sits at the base of the brain stem and contains the cardiac, respiratory, vomiting, and vasomotor centers. Therefore, this organ is involved with the autonomic (involuntary) functions of breathing, heart rate, and blood pressure.

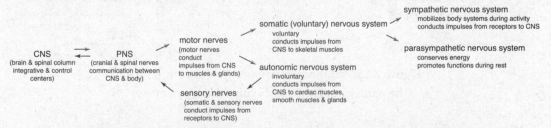

Figure 7.24. Flow chart showing the organization and communication of the subsystems of the nervous system in vertebrate animals. CNS, central nervous system; PNS, peripheral nervous system.

The PNS is further divided into the **motor neurons** that control voluntary movements, the **autonomic nervous system** that controls involuntary movements (heart rate, digestion, respiratory rate, pupillary response, urination, sexual arousal), and the **enteric nervous system** that controls the gastrointestinal system. The autonomic nervous system is divided into the sympathetic and parasympathetic systems (Figure 7.25). The **sympathetic nervous system** originates in the spinal cord and functions to maintain physiology related to stress stimuli. This system is important for the "fight-or-flight" response when danger is detected. The **parasympathetic nervous system** originates in the spinal cord and medulla and controls "resting" activities of the body, such as salivation, lacrimation, urination, and digestion.

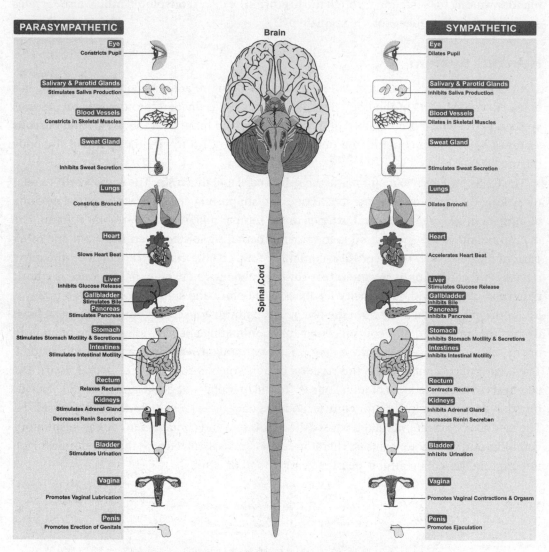

Figure 7.25. Autonomic nervous system comparing
the parasympathetic and sympathetic systems

Neurons (nerve cells) are the central functional component of the nervous system (Figure 7.26). This specialized type of cell sends electrochemical signals along **axons**, which are thin fibers of protoplasm often found in bundles. The electrochemical signals regulate the release of **neurotransmitters** (chemicals) at **synapses**, or junctions, between cells. Signals are sent from a presynaptic to a postsynaptic cell. The presynaptic cell contains small spherical synaptic vesicles that contain the neurotransmitter. When this cell is electrically stimulated, the contents of the synaptic vesicles are released. The neurotransmitter is now free to bind to receptors on postsynaptic cells. The binding excites, inhibits, or modulates the postsynaptic cells based on the type of neurotransmitter receptor. **Sensory neurons** convert physical stimuli (light, sound, touch, taste) into neural signals. Motor neurons adapt neural signals to activate muscles or glands.

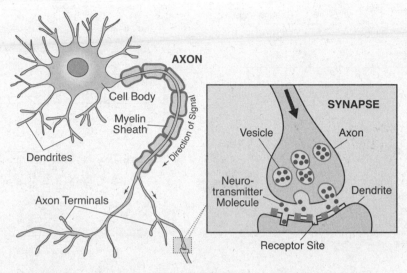

Figure 7.26. Structure of a neuron and the signaling pathway

   Glial cells, or neuroglia, are nonneuronal structural and metabolic support cells found in the nervous system. These cells function to support and hold neurons in place, supply nutrients and oxygen to neurons, electrically insulate neurons, destroy pathogens, and remove dead neurons. To electrically insulate cells of the CNS and PNS, glial and Schwann cells, respectively, wrap axons with layers of **myelin** (a fatty mixture of lipids, cholesterol, and proteins). Myelin increases electrical resistance and the speed of travel of electrical impulses along the axon fibers and decreases capacitance (ability to store an electrical charge).

   An electrochemical signal travels along an axon as a wave known as an **action potential** (Figure 7.27A). Action potentials are created by a type of voltage-gated ion channel present in the cell membrane (Figure 7.27B). The channels are closed when the membrane potential is close to the **resting potential** (–70 mV) of the cell. The channels begin to open when the membrane potential increases to a defined threshold value. There is an influx of sodium ions when the channels open resulting in a change in the electrochemical gradient. This leads to a greater increase in the membrane potential causing additional channels to open further increasing the electric current across the membrane. The process continues until all available ion channels are open and maximum membrane potential is reached at +40 mV. The polarity of the membrane is quickly reversed due to the rapid influx of the sodium ions which inactivates the ion channels. Closure of the ion channels causes the sodium ions to be actively transported out of the membrane. An efflux of potassium ions then occurs due to the activation of potassium channels. This efflux of potassium ions returns the electrochemical gradient to the resting state (Figure 7.27C).

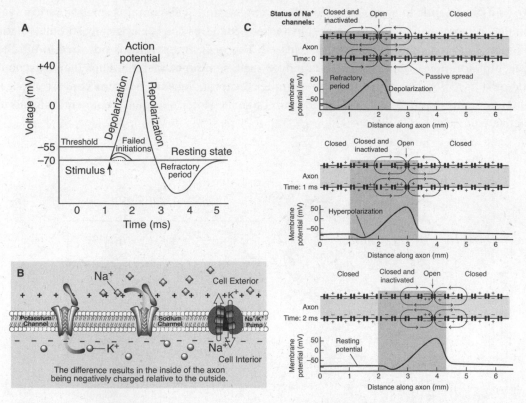

Figure 7.27. How an action potential works in a nerve cell. (A) Plot of voltage versus time showing the action potential of an electrochemical signal traveling along an axon. (B) Voltage-gated ion channels present in the cell membrane. (C) The fate of ion channels in the membrane in response to an action potential.

The ability of neurons to send signals to other cells also suggests that neurons can exchange signals with other neurons. These "neural networks" provide a significant capacity for many different functions and types of processing of information. The function of the nervous system was traditionally viewed as an association between a stimulus and a response. That is, neural processing starts with a stimulus that activates sensory neurons that produce signals that multiply through a network of connections in the spinal cord and brain. This chain of events leads to the activation of motor neurons and muscle contraction representative of an obvious response. However, by the 1940s it was found that the nervous system is capable of carrying out a number of mechanisms for producing patterns of activity without needing an external response. That is, without an external stimulus, neurons can produce regular sequences of action potentials. That means there is the greater possibility of producing detailed temporal patterns when these natively active neurons are connected in complex networks. Therefore, a more modern view is that the nervous system functions, in part, as stimulus-response chains but also as intrinsically generated activity patterns. Furthermore, these two types of mechanisms work together to provide the entire range of behavior.

A **reflex arc** is the simplest example of a neural circuit based on a stimulus-response chain. A sensory input is passed through a sequence of neurons connected in series and ends with a motor output. For example, when one touches a hot pan, sensory receptors in the skin are activated by the dangerous elevation in temperature. The electrical field across the membranes of the exposed cells changes in response to the heat stimulus. If the change in electrical potential reaches the given threshold, an action potential is initiated and transmitted along the axon of the receptor cell reaching the spinal cord. The axon in the spinal cord makes excitatory synaptic contacts with other cells. Some of these cells send axonal output to the same region of the spinal cord and others to the brain. The spinal cord neurons send the axonal output to motor neurons controlling the arm muscles. If the excitation level is strong enough, some of the motor neurons generate action potentials along their axons and make excitatory synaptic contacts with muscle cells. This cascade of activity induces contraction of the muscle cells causing the arm to pull away. This example is a simplification of a reflex arc. Even though there are relatively short neural paths from sensory to motor neurons, other neurons in close proximity can be part of the neural circuit and can modulate the response. In addition, axonal output from the brain to the spinal cord can affect the reflex.

The nervous system is also capable of carrying out **intrinsic pattern generation** or control of body activities that do not require an external stimulus. Instead, control is carried out by internally generated rhythms of activity. Various types of neurons can, in isolation, generate rhythmic sequences of action potentials or rhythmic alternations between high-rate bursting and quiescence. A common example of intrinsic pattern generation is the environmental oscillation of activity based on a 24-hour period known as circadian rhythm.

Endocrine System

The group of glands that secrete hormones for distribution throughout the body by the blood and lymph circulatory subsystems comprise the **endocrine system**. **Hormones** are chemical signaling molecules which can be steroids, eicosanoids (high carbon number fatty acids), proteins, or peptides. Hormones are made in the endocrine glands, or in special types of cells, and work as communication molecules between tissues and organs. Hormones regulate the physiology and behavior of many organs and systems, such as those involved in respiration, digestion, metabolism, sensory perception, growth and development, movement, and reproduction. Hormones work by binding to specific receptors on the surface of target cells. The binding activates signaling pathways.

The most important glands in this system include the pituitary, thyroid, parathyroid, hypothalamus, adrenal, and pineal glands, as well as the pancreas, testes, and ovaries (Figure 7.28). In vertebrates, the hypothalamus is the central signaling control center. Hormones released by several major endocrine glands are summarized in Table 7.3. Endocrine glands characteristically are vascular (contain blood vessels), store hormones in granules, and do not use ducts to transport hormones. Glands, such as the salivary, sweat, prostate and those in the gastrointestinal tract, are part of the **exocrine system**. Exocrine glands are less vascular than those of the endocrine system and contain ducts or a lumen (hollow area in a tube). Some organs of the body, such as the pancreas, kidneys, liver, gonads, and bone, have secondary endocrinelike functions. The **pancreas** is considered to be both an endocrine and exocrine gland. As an endocrine gland, the pancreas contains hormone-producing cells in the **islets of Langerhans**. **Insulin**, an example of an endocrine hormone, is secreted when blood sugar levels are high. As an example of an exocrine gland, the pancreas produces **glucagon** when the blood sugar level is low. Insulin aids the absorption of glucose from the blood to be used by muscles and tissues. Glucagon tells the liver to convert stored glycogen into glucose for transport through the bloodstream to balance sugar levels.

Several different signaling mechanisms exist in the endocrine system. In **autocrine signaling**, a hormone or other chemical molecule secreted by a cell binds to autocrine receptors on the same hormone-producing cell. This process results in cellular changes. In

paracrine signaling, the hormone-releasing cell induces changes in adjacent cells that alters their behavior. In contrast, hormones typically have to travel extensively through the body via the circulatory system to exhibit their effects. In **juxtacrine signaling**, communication is mediated by oligosaccharide, protein, or lipid components of a cell's membrane and requires physical contact between the interacting cells. The effects of the communication can be intercellular (between different cells) or intracellular (within the same cell). Hormone levels are controlled in the body by positive and negative feedback.

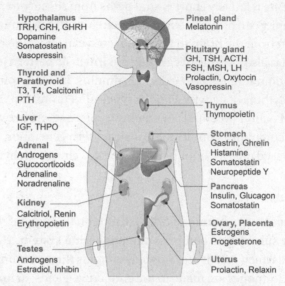

Figure 7.28. Endocrine system. PTH, parathyroid hormone; prolactin (luteotropin); GH, growth hormone; ACTH, adrenocorticotropic hormone; ADH, antidiuretic hormone (vasopressin); LH, luteinizing hormone; FSH, follicle-stimulating hormone.

Table 7.3. Some Examples of Hormones Secreted by Major Endocrine Glands

Gland	Hormone	Effect of Hormone
Hypothalamus	Corticotropin-releasing	Stimulates release of adrenocorticotropic hormone from the anterior pituitary
	Dopamine	Inhibits prolactin released from the anterior pituitary
	Gonadotropin-releasing	Stimulates release of follicle-stimulating hormone from the anterior pituitary; stimulates release of luteinizing hormone from the anterior pituitary
	Growth hormone-releasing	Stimulates release of growth hormone from the anterior pituitary
	Somatostatin	Inhibits release of growth hormone from the anterior pituitary; inhibits release of thyroid-stimulating hormone from the anterior pituitary
	Thyrotropin-releasing	Stimulates release of thyroid-stimulating hormone from the anterior pituitary
	Vasopressin	Promotes water reabsorption and blood volume by increasing water permeability in the distal convoluted tubule and collecting ducts of nephrons

Table 7.3. Some Examples of Hormones Secreted by Major Endocrine Glands (cont'd.)

Gland	Hormone	Effect of Hormone
Pituitary	Corticotropin (adrenocorticotropic hormone)	Stimulates synthesis and release of corticosteroid and androgen from adrenocortical cells
	Beta-endorphin	Inhibits the perception of pain
	Follical-stimulating hormone	Stimulates maturation of ovarian follicles in the ovary; Stimulates maturation of seminiferous tubules, spermatogenesis and production of androgen-binding protein from Sertoli cells in the testes
	Somatotropin (growth hormone)	Stimulates growth and reproduction of cells; Stimulates release of insulinlike growth factor 1 from the liver
	Lutenizing hormone	Stimulates ovulation and formation of corpus luteum (in females); Stimulates synthesis of testosterone by Leydig cells (in males)
	Melanocyte-stimulating	Stimulates synthesis and release of melanin from skin, hair, and melanocytes
	Oxytocin	Uterine contraction during birthing; lactation when nursing
	Prolactin	Stimulates synthesis and release of milk from mammary glands; mediates sexual gratification
	Thyrotropin (thyroid-stimulating)	Stimulates synthesis and release of thyroxine and triiodothyronine from the thyroid gland; stimulates adsorption of iodine by the thyroid gland
	Casopressin	Promotes water reabsorption and blood volume by increasing water permeability in the distal convoluted tubule and collecting ducts of nephrons
Thyroid	Calcitonin	Stimulates bone synthesis and controls calcium (Ca^{2+}) release from bone
	Thyroxine	Stimulates oxygen and energy consumption and protein synthesis
	Triiodothyronine	Stimulates oxygen and energy consumption and protein synthesis
Pineal	Melatonin	Antioxidant; monitors circadian rhythm and core body temperature

Reproductive System

The **reproductive system** of humans is composed of a group of sex organs unique to males and females that function in the process of sexual reproduction. The uniqueness of the male and female reproductive systems permits genetic material from two different individuals to be combined with an assurance that offspring exhibit genetic fitness (the ability to survive, reproduce, and expand the gene pool of the next generation).

The reproductive system of the female is composed of a group of organs centered around the pelvic region and residing mostly inside the body (Figure 7.29). A hormone secreted by the pituitary gland, on an average 28-day cycle, stimulates **ova** (female gametes or eggs) to develop and grow in one of the ovaries. A single ovum is released and travels through one of the **fallopian tubes** into the uterus. Other hormones made in the ovaries prepare the uterus wall for eventual attachment of the ovum. If the ovum is not fertilized, the **endometrium** or lining of the uterus and the ovum are shed during **menstruation**. This 28-day menstruation cycle results in the discharge, through the vagina, of blood and mucosal tissue. The menstrual cycle is linked to the production of ova and functions in the maintenance of the uterus. The cycle is present only in female primates and is active in human females from the first occurrence (**menarche**) until **menopause**. The ovarian part of the menstrual cycle is divided into a follicular phase, ovulation, and luteal phase. Menstruation and the proliferative and secretory phases all occur in the uterine part of the cycle.

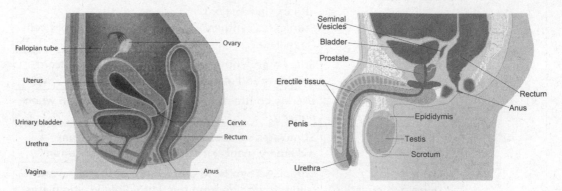

Figure 7.29. Male and female reproductive systems

The entire menstruation cycle is regulated by the endocrine system (Figure 7.30A). During the follicular stage, menstrual bleeding is controlled by the release of increasing amounts of the hormone **estrogen**. Following the secretion of the menses or blood, the lining of the uterus becomes thicker, and a combination of hormones, including the **follicle-stimulating hormone (FSH)**, cause the primordial follicles in the ovary to develop into primary oocytes. This is the first step in **oogenesis** or creation of an ovum (egg cell) in the ovary. The **primary oocyte** (female gametocyte or germ cell) divides by meiosis to form an ootid (mature oocyte) (Figure 7.30B). However, meiosis is stopped at the prophase I (meiosis I) step. Once a female menstruates for the first time, around puberty, a few primary oocytes continue to develop every menstrual cycle. Pairing of homologous chromosomes (synapsis) occurs as meiosis continues and tetrads are formed. The primary oocyte develops into the secondary oocyte and the first **polar body**. The haploid secondary oocyte then proceeds to meiosis II. The process is stopped at the metaphase II stage until fertilization occurs. An ootid and a second polar body are formed at the end of meiosis II. During oocyte development, the primordial ovarian follicle is developing into a pre-ovulatory follicle. At the end of meiosis II, both polar bodies disintegrate and the ootid becomes a mature ovum. The purpose of the formation of the polar bodies is to eliminate the extra haploid set of chromosomes that were formed during meiosis.

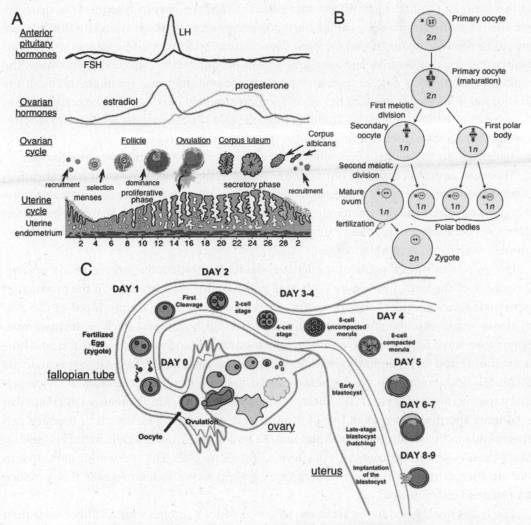

Figure 7.30. Hormones and female reproduction.
(A) Menstruation cycle. (B) Oogenesis. (C) Ovulation.

One, or sometimes two, follicles mature or become dominant during the follicular stage. At the start of ovulation, around the mid-point of the menstrual cycle, the **luteinizing hormone (LH)** produced by the pituitary gland induces the mature follicle to release an ovum into the oviduct (Figure 7.30A and C). The rapid increase in the level of LH is thought to be controlled by the stimulation of the hypothalamus, by estrogen, to secrete the **gonadotropin-releasing hormone (GnRH)**. **Estradiol**, a human sex hormone, is also thought to be involved in the regulation of LH production. There is no pattern to ovulation. The release of a mature ovum from either the left or right ovary is a random event. In a rare occurrence, both ovaries may release a mature egg resulting in fraternal twins, provided that both eggs are fertilized. The egg enters the fallopian tube following its release from the ovary. The egg will fall apart or dissolve if unfertilized. Embryogenesis occurs when the egg is fertilized by a **spermatozoon** (motile sperm cell) (*see Chapter 7, Embryology and Development*). The fertilized egg travels from the fallopian tube to the uterus where it implants in the endometrium as a blastocyst. In the last phase of the ovarian cycle (luteal phase), FSH and LH induce the remaining structure of the dominant follicle to transform into what is called the **corpus luteum**. This structure produces significant quantities of the hormone **progesterone**, which stimulates the adrenal glands to produce estrogen and prepares the endometrium for possible implantation of an embryo. In the proliferative and secretory phases of the uterine cycle, estrogen causes the endometrium to grow and progesterone prepares the endometrium for implantation of the blastocyst. If implantation does not occur in approximately two weeks, hormones made in the corpus luteum suppress the production of FSH and LH causing the structure to disintegrate. This process reduces the amount of progesterone and estrogen leading to another cycle of menstruation. Therefore, fertilization of the egg prevents atrophy of the corpus luteum.

The most common forms of birth control suppress ovulation. Hormonal contraceptives disrupt the menstrual cycle. Progestogen, a steroid hormone that activates the progesterone receptor, can decrease the frequency of release of GnRH by the hypothalamus. This action decreases the release of FSH and LH by the anterior pituitary, which inhibits follicular development thereby preventing ovulation.

In contrast to those organs of the female, the male reproductive organs reside primarily outside of the body (see Figure 7.29). One group of organs is involved in the production (**spermatogenesis**) and storage of sperm. **Spermatozoa** (sperm) are produced in the pair of **testes** (male gonads) along with androgens (steroid hormones) such as **testosterone**. Spermatogenesis and hormone production by the testes is controlled by gonadotropic hormones produced in the pituitary gland. Male primordial germ cells develop into spermatozoa by mitosis and meiosis. Spermatogonia or initial sperm cells undergo mitosis to create primary spermatocytes (Figure 7.31). Each spermatocyte divides during meiosis I to create two secondary spermatocytes. Each one of these cells divides during meiosis II to produce two **spermatids** in the **seminiferous tubules** located in the testes. **Sertoli cells** in the epithelium of the tubules provide nutrients for the developing sperm cells. The spermatids develop into mature spermatozoa. Therefore, each primary spermatocyte yields two cells that produce four haploid spermatozoa.

The testes are housed in the **scrotum**, which provides a temperature slightly cooler than that of the internal temperature of the body. Higher temperatures may damage the sperm. Immature spermatozoa in the testes enter the **epididymis** in the scrotum where they mature and are stored. In preparation for ejaculation, the sperm are transported by peristalsis through the **vas deferens** to the ejaculatory ducts. The sperm mix with fluids from the seminal vesicles and prostate gland to form **seminal fluid**, or semen. The role of the seminal and prostate secretions are to enhance survival of the sperm.

To fertilize an ovum, the ejaculated seminal fluid, containing mature motile sperm, undergoes changes in the female reproductive tract to prepare it for travel along the tract and fusion with the egg. Enzymes carried by the sperm help degrade the outer coat of the egg and allow the sperm to bind to the plasma membrane of the egg. Additional enzymes harden the surface of the egg to ensure that it will be fertilized by only a single sperm. The sperm loses its tail and mitochondria, and its nucleus fuses with the ovum. The male and female chromosomes form a mitotic spindle and undergo mitosis. The fertilized egg, or zygote, proceeds through the stages of development (*see Chapter 7, Embryology and Development*) until the blastocyst implants in the wall of the uterus for further progression into an embryo.

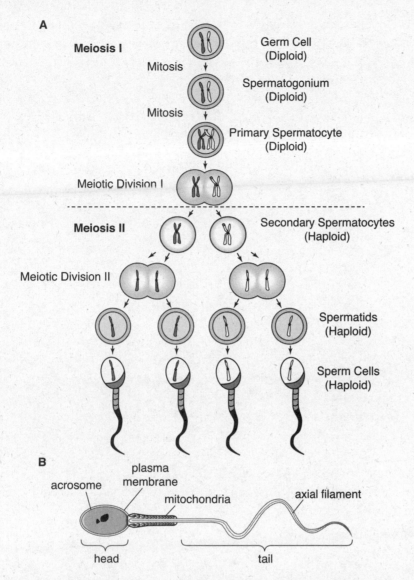

A

Meiosis I

Mitosis

Mitosis

Germ Cell (Diploid)

Spermatogonium (Diploid)

Primary Spermatocyte (Diploid)

Meiotic Division I

- -

Meiosis II

Secondary Spermatocytes (Haploid)

Meiotic Division II

Spermatids (Haploid)

Sperm Cells (Haploid)

B

acrosome

plasma membrane

mitochondria

axial filament

head

tail

Figure 7.31. Spermatogenesis. (A) Production of sperm. (B) Structure of sperm.

Ecology and Behavior 8

The interdisciplinary study of the interactions among organisms and between organisms and their environments is known as **ecology**. The term "ecology" was devised by the German scientist Ernst Haeckel (1834–1919) in 1866. Prior to that time, the science of ecology was viewed as natural history and was focused on observational approaches. Since the time of Haeckel, the study of ecology grew to utilize more experimental approaches. Modern approaches have shown how evolutionary biology and ethology (study of animal behavior) are tightly associated with ecological concepts. Ecology and evolution, especially the topics of natural selection, inheritance, adaptation, and populations (*see Chapter 6*), are closely integrated. Morphological, genetic, and behavioral traits can be used to construct evolutionary trees for studying species development, or **organic evolution**. The study of ecology is organized in a hierarchal scheme (Figure 8.1). The scheme, as depicted in Figure 8.1, flows from the most basic to the most complex unit of ecological organization.

genes $\longrightarrow$ cells $\longrightarrow$ tissues $\longrightarrow$ organs $\longrightarrow$ organisms $\longrightarrow$ species $\longrightarrow$

populations $\longrightarrow$ communities $\longrightarrow$ ecosystems $\longrightarrow$ biomes $\longrightarrow$ biosphere

Figure 8.1. Flow chart of ecological organization. The flow is in the direction from the smallest component of ecosystems to the largest.

ORGANIZATION OF THE BIOSPHERE

The **biosphere** includes all of the biomes present on Earth. Fluctuations in climate, nutrient levels, and energy on the planet are controlled by ecological relationships. For example, the changing composition of the earth's atmosphere over time has been controlled by the respiration and photosynthesis of evolving organisms. In the 1970s, James Lovelock, a chemist, and Lynn Margulis, a microbiologist (*also see Chapter 6*), co-developed a hypothesis (Gaia) proposing that conditions for maintaining life on planet Earth are self-regulating through the interactions of organisms and their environment. This hypothesis attempted to explain how the biosphere and evolution of organisms make life sustainable on the planet by tightly controlling important environmental properties such as the stability of atmospheric oxygen levels, the salinity of the oceans, and the global temperature. That is, organisms influence the nonliving part of their environment, and that the environment affects the sum total of all living things on the planet. Therefore, the hypothesis assumes that Earth is a self-regulating system, or "living being," in which living organisms and nonliving environmental factors comprise a single evolving system called Gaia. There is significant debate concerning the validity of this hypothesis. Current opinion points out the lack of empirical evidence to support the hypothesis but considers it a good framework for developing new ideas about Earth and for applying holistic approaches to the study of our planet.

Biomes are relatively large regions, or zones, of the planet or globe defined by the plant and animal groups that are highly adapted to the physical environment of the distribution area. The distribution area is identified by characteristics such as geographical location, climate, and the dominant vegetation. There are terrestrial (forests, grasslands, desert, tundra), freshwater (ponds, lakes, rivers, streams, wetlands), marine (oceans, estuaries, coral reefs), and anthropogenic (manmade) biomes. **Microbiomes**, an ecological community of microorganisms, are a relatively new type of biome having been discovered and characterized using molecular genetics and DNA sequencing techniques. The human microbiome is one example representing a summation of microorganisms that live on and in the skin, in the oral cavity, and in the gastrointestinal tract.

Ecosystems are systems, or habitats within biomes, composed of living organisms (**biotic** component) that interact with the nonliving components (**abiotic** component). Examples of abiotic components include energy, nitrogen, water, soil minerals, temperature, humidity, and pH. A **habitat** is any component of the environment that is directly or indirectly involved in the use of a location by the organism. An ecosystem can be any size, but typically encompasses a limited area within the biome. There is some redundancy in the naming of biomes and ecosystems. Ecosystems have been classified as **terrestrial** (forest, littoral zone, riparian zone, subsurface lithoautotrophic microbial ecosystem, urban, grassland, tundra, desert) and **aquatic** (marine, freshwater [lake, river, wetland]). Ecosystems produce organic matter from inorganic carbon sources primarily through photosynthesis (*see Chapter 3*). Plants convert energy from light and use this energy to produce organic carbon compounds (carbohydrates or sugars) and oxygen from carbon dioxide and water. The **carbon cycle** (Figure 8.2) is dependent upon the energy produced from light and affects the temperature, and, therefore, the climate of the planet based on the amount of thermal radiation that is produced, absorbed by atmospheric gasses, and transferred back to the lower atmosphere (**greenhouse effect**). The natural greenhouse effect of the planet makes it possible to sustain life. However, a significant increase in the amount of thermal radiation produced on the planet increases the greenhouse effect leading to global warming. **Desertification**, in which a relatively dry land region becomes devoid of water, vegetation and wildlife, is a significant problem due to global warming.

The Carbon Cycle

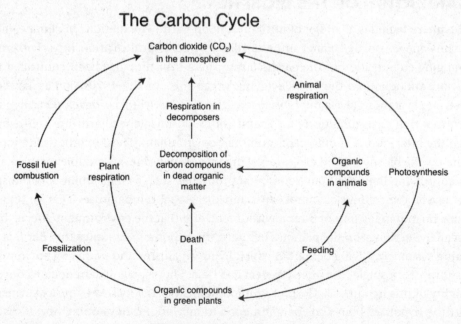

Figure 8.2. The carbon cycle

The most abundant component of the present atmosphere of the earth is nitrogen gas (N_2). Nitrogen is essential for the synthesis of amino acids (proteins), nucleic acids (RNA and DNA), and chlorophyll (in plants). The N_2 form of nitrogen cannot be used by plants. It must be converted, or fixed, into other reactive forms, such as ammonia (NH_4^+) or nitrate (NO_3^+). Microorganisms have various important jobs in these reactions. Therefore, like the carbon cycle, the **nitrogen cycle** (Figure 8.3) plays an essential role in ecosystems.

The Nitrogen Cycle

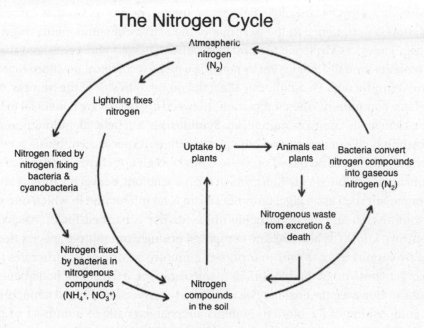

Figure 8.3. The nitrogen cycle

The best example of an ecological network is illustrated by a **food web** (formerly known as a food cycle). Food webs contain autotrophs that produce complex organic carbon compounds from the single carbon compound CO_2, and heterotrophs that cannot fix carbon from CO_2 but must use organic carbon for growth (Figure 8.4A). Autotrophs (defined in Chapter 3) are the primary **energy producers** using either chemical reactions or photosynthesis. The heterotrophs, represented by the **herbivores** (plant eaters), **carnivores** (meat eaters), **omnivores** (plant and meat eaters), and **detritivores** (decomposers that break down dead or decaying organisms), are consumers rather than energy producers. The heterotrophs cycle the flow of energy and nutrients from the self-feeding autotrophs. The linear sequence of links in a food web is known as a **food chain**. A food chain typically begins with a producer species (plant) and ends with a top-level predator. The organisms in a food chain comprise trophic levels that form a pyramid (Figure 8.4B). **Keystone species** are linked to a very large number of other species in a food web. Thus, they play a very important role in the structure of an ecological community, such that their loss can lead to the extinction of other species.

Communities are associations of populations made up of two or more different species occupying the same space (geographical area) and time. Change in the composition of those species that make up a community, over time, is known as **ecological succession**. Succession is driven by the impact of established species on their own environments. Orderly and predictable changes in an existing community can usually occur after the initial colonization of a habitat or after an **environmental disruption**. Species in a community can exhibit various types of interactions including **competition**, **predation**, **parasitism**, **mutualism**, and

commensalism. Species can compete over a limited amount of resources. Neither species benefits from this interaction. Although competition can help limit population size and the number of different species in a community, there is little evidence to support its role in the evolution of large groups. A predator species can hunt a prey species. Some species kill their prey before feeding, but others, known as parasites, feed on living prey. This type of interaction benefits one species and harms the other. A highly specialized form of parasitism occurs between a host organism and an invading pathogen. A **pathogen**, as discussed in Chapter 7 in the *Immune System*, is typically a bacterium, fungus, or protozoan that causes disease. The association is detrimental to the host due to the activity of components or products of the pathogen, known as **virulence factors**, that cause damage to host cells and tissues. The pathogen benefits from the interaction by creating a **niche** (ecological position) that favors its survival and reproduction. Predation can affect the population size of the number of species that coexist in a community. When interactions between organisms are beneficial to both species, the relationship is known as mutualism. **Symbiosis** is a beneficial, intimate, and permanent association between at least two biologically different species. Symbiosis is considered to be a persistent mutualism based on these characteristics. A classic example of a symbiotic relationship is exhibited by lichens, which are associations between a fungus and photosynthetic organism such as an alga. Commensalism is an interaction in which one organism benefits (commensal) and the other neither benefits nor is harmed (host). Associations of microorganisms, known as **biofilms**, are composed of single or multiple species that stick to each other by various mechanisms to form a community on tissues or structures in a host. The microorganisms within the biofilm, in many instances, derive metabolic benefits from the association. However, the host may be unaffected or adversely affected depending on the microbial composition of the biofilm. Biofilms are characteristic of a number of microbial infections or colonizations of the human body. **Dental plaque** is one of the most well-known examples.

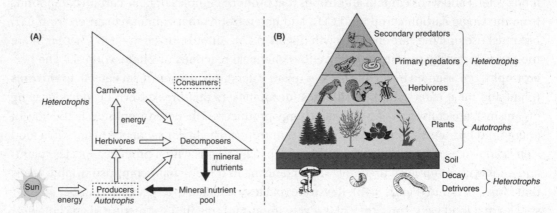

Figure 8.4. Movement of food through ecosystems. (A) food cycle. (B) food web.

A **population** is composed of individuals of the same species that interact in the same habitat and niche or conditions under which a species can establish a stable population size. A population will increase in numbers of individuals or lose individuals exponentially as long as the environment remains constant for all the individuals in the population. This **Malthusian**

growth model is the primary law of population ecology. In a closed population, in which **immigration** and **emigration** does not occur, the rate of population change is calculated by

$$\frac{dN}{dT} = bN - dN = (b-d)N = rN$$

In this equation, N is the total number of individuals in the population, b and d are the per capita rates of birth and death, respectively, and r is the per capita rate of population change. A model known as the **logistic equation** was developed from the Malthus model:

$$\frac{dN}{dT} = aN\left(1 - \frac{N}{K}\right)$$

In this model, N is the number of individuals measured as biomass density, a is the maximum per capita rate of change, and K is the carrying capacity (the maximum population size of the species that the environment can sustain indefinitely) of the population. The formula states that the rate of change in population size $\left(\frac{dN}{dT}\right)$ is equal to growth (aN) that is limited by carrying capacity $\left(1 = \frac{N}{K}\right)$.

ETHOLOGY (ANIMAL BEHAVIOR)

Ethology is the objective study of movement that can be observed behavior in animals, usually in natural rather than laboratory environments. All animals are capable of exhibiting **behaviors**. Behaviors can be documented as traits and can, therefore, be inherited like physical attributes. A central unifying theme in behavioral ecology is **adaptation**. Adaptive traits that provide functional utilities that increase reproductive fitness can evolve according to natural selection. For example, prey species can use behavioral adaptations to avoid, flee from, or defend against predators.

Animal communication is thought to be influenced by instinctive behavioral responses that occur due to the action of "sign" or "releasing" stimuli. These instinctive responses are known as **fixed action patterns (FAP)**, **behavioral patterns**, or **behavioral acts**. FAPs are important because they are the most simple kind of behavior in which a specific stimulus results in a "hard-wired" response that, once initiated, is not influenced by the environment. FAPs are examples of instinctive or innate behavior. An animal's physical nondirectional response to a stimulus is known as **kinesis**. A directional response or movement toward or away from a stimulus is **taxis**. A simple turning response, such as growth, is a **tropism**. Instinct is inherited, cannot be altered, and is not subject to reason. Behavior is instinctive if it is not driven by prior experience or learned. Releasing stimuli that trigger an instinctive behavior can act as communication signals among members of the same species. These signals are known as releasers. In some instances, releasers trigger amplified or exaggerated behavior and are termed supernormal stimuli. Humans respond to supernormal stimuli for nurturing, social, and sexual instincts.

LEARNING

The probability of survival and reproduction of a species would be significantly reduced if behavior consisted only of FAPs. This type of behavior would be too inefficient and inflexible. Therefore, **learning** and the ability to change behavioral responses based on experience, rather than on FAPs, is very important. A simple form of learning found in many animal species is **habituation**. In habituation, an animal learns not to respond to stimuli that have become irrelevant or unimportant. This reduces the expenditure of energy by the animal. When a new response becomes associated with a specific stimulus, the process is known as **associative learning**. A well-known example of associative learning comes from experiments on the "conditioned reflex" or **conditioned response** in dogs performed by the Russian physiologist Ivan Pavlov (1849–1936). Some animal species can identify or recognize members of their own species. This type of learning behavior, most commonly observed in birds, is known as **imprinting**. Imprinting occurs at a specific stage in the life of an animal and can be very important for assuring reproductive success. There are several forms of **observational learning**, including **imitation**, **stimulus enhancement**, and **social transmission**. In imitation, one animal exactly mimics the behavior of another. In stimulus enhancement, one animal becomes interested in an object by observing other animals that are interacting with that object. This can lead to "object manipulation" that can stimulate new behaviors related to the object based on learning by trial-and-error. In social transmission, reciprocally beneficial behaviors develop among related animals or kin. These behaviors stem from kin and group selection. **Kin selection** is an altruistic behavior that ensures the reproductive success of an animal's relatives over that of the individual. The altruistic individual endures a fitness loss, and the receiving individual experiences a fitness gain in this behavior. This sacrifice of one individual to benefit the other is common among insects, such as ants, bees, and wasps, because colonies of these species contain male drones that are genetically identical. This type of behavior is more properly referred to as **group selection** because the social structure is such that interactions occur more frequently between groups of individuals rather than between individuals and groups. In this case, natural selection is imposed on the group instead of on the individual. **Teaching** is also a very special type of learning. An individual manipulates its behavior (teacher) to increase the probability that another individual (pupil) will learn the behavior. Teaching behavior, once thought to be exhibited only by a few select species, has been observed in a wider number of animals and insects.

Appendix

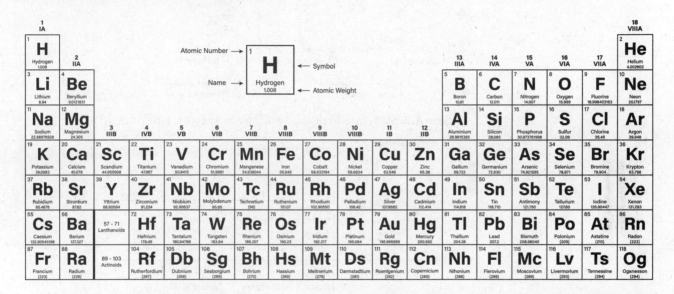

Figure A.1. Periodic table of the elements

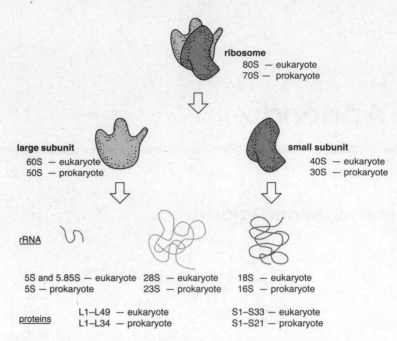

ribosome
80S — eukaryote
70S — prokaryote

large subunit
60S — eukaryote
50S — prokaryote

small subunit
40S — eukaryote
30S — prokaryote

rRNA

5S and 5.85S — eukaryote   28S — eukaryote   18S — eukaryote
5S — prokaryote   23S — prokaryote   16S — prokaryote

proteins   L1–L49 — eukaryote   S1–S33 — eukaryote
            L1–L34 — prokaryote   S1–S21 — prokaryote

Figure A.2. Structure of prokaryotic and eukaryotic ribosomes

The Genetic Code*

Second Letter

First Letter	U	C	A	G	Third Letter
U	Phenylalanine	Serine	Tyrosine	Cysteine	U
	Phenylalanine	Serine	Tyrosine	Cysteine	C
	Leucine	Serine	STOP	STOP	A
	Leucine	Serine	STOP	Tryptophan	G
C	Leucine	Proline	Histidine	Arginine	U
	Leucine	Proline	Histidine	Arginine	C
	Leucine	Proline	Glutamine	Arginine	A
	Leucine	Proline	Glutamine	Arginine	G
A	Isoleucine	Threonine	Asparagine	Serine	U
	Isoleucine	Threonine	Asparagine	Serine	C
	Isoleucine	Threonine	Lysine	Arginine	A
	Methionine (Start)	Threonine	Lysine	Arginine	G
G	Valine	Alanine	Aspartate	Glycine	U
	Valine	Alanine	Aspartate	Glycine	C
	Valine	Alanine	Glutamate	Glycine	A
	Valine	Alanine	Glutamate	Glycine	G

* The amino acids encoded by mRNA triplets (codons). Although the code depicted above is used by most organisms, subcellular organelles and some ciliate protists show minor variations. The code is also said to be degenerate because more than one triplet may code for a single amino acid.

Codon-Anticodon Pairing

5′ end of anticodon	3′ end of codon
G	U or C
C	G only
A	U only
U	A or G
I	U, C, or A

Figure A.3. Codon usage table. The table includes both the three letter and one letter designations for the amino acids. During the translation of most genes, ATG also represents the start codon.

PART TWO

General Chemistry

General Format on How to Approach a Problem

1. Determine what information is given.
2. Ask "What is the question asking for?"
3. Check the units given in the question and what unit is required in the answer.
4. Some problems are just unit conversions and do not need an equation. Balanced chemical equations are necessary when converting from one substance to another.
5. Evaluate the answer to make sure it seems reasonable.

General Advice on Avoiding Common Mistakes

1. Pay particular attention to units.
2. Set up and **write down** the unit conversions to make sure units cancel out as necessary. Do not try to do this in your head.
3. Practice!

Atoms

9

STATES OF MATTER

Matter occurs in three common states: solid, liquid, and gas. Solids have a fixed macroscopic shape and a packed, organized microscopic structure. The rigid molecular structure of solids restricts molecular motions to vibrations, which are low energy. Liquids have a fixed volume and adopt the shape of their container. Molecules in the liquid state are free to move around. They have both vibrational and rotational energies. Liquid molecules are still closely packed, but they are disorganized. Gases are the most energetic of the common states of matter. These molecules are far apart, disorganized, and form both to the shape and volume of the container.

CLASSIFICATIONS OF MATTER

Matter is anything that occupies space and has mass. Matter can be organized into four different classifications: pure element, pure compound, homogeneous mixture, and heterogeneous mixture. A pure element cannot be broken down any further through physical or chemical means. Pure compounds cannot be separated by physical means, but chemically they can be separated into their respective elements. Mixtures can be physically separated into pure compounds or elements depending on the composition of the mixture. Homogeneous mixtures contain elements and/or compounds that, in solution, have a continuous distribution. An example of a homogeneous mixture is coffee with sugar and milk. Heterogeneous mixtures contain an assortment of elements and/or compounds that are nonuniform throughout, such as dirt with rocks.

STRUCTURE OF THE ATOM

An atom is the smallest basic particle of an element. It is comprised mostly of space and has electrons that orbit around a positively charged nucleus. Protons are positively charged subatomic particles found inside the nucleus. Each proton has a mass of 1.67262×10^{-27} kg. Neutrons are subatomic particles with a neutral charge found inside the nucleus. Each neutron has a mass of 1.67493×10^{-27} kg. Electrons are negatively charged subatomic particles that orbit the nucleus. Each electron has a mass of 0.00091×10^{-27} kg. Notice that the mass of an electron is much smaller than the mass of a proton or neutron.

The **atomic mass** is the mass of a single atom of a specific element. Since the mass of an electron is so small in comparison to the mass of a proton and neutron, the atomic mass is based on the number of protons and neutrons. The **periodic table** is arranged by atomic number (number of protons) and shows the average atomic mass of an element (average of all isotopes, weighted by their respective abundance). **Isotopes** of an element have the same number of protons but a different number of neutrons, thus resulting in a different mass. For example, the most abundant form of carbon (carbon-12) has 6 protons and 6 neutrons and an atomic mass of 12. However, the radioactive isotope carbon-14 has 6 protons and 8 neutrons. If the number of protons changes, then the atom is no longer carbon. Isotopes are typically written in the following notation:

$$_Z^A X$$

Where A represents the atomic mass (protons + neutrons), Z is the atomic number (protons), and X represents the elemental symbol. Using this notation, carbon-14 can be written as $_6^{14}C$, where 14 is the mass, 6 is the number of protons, and C represents carbon. Reactions involving radioactivity usually follow this notation.

TYPES OF RADIOACTIVITY AND BALANCING NUCLEAR REACTIONS

Radioactivity is the emission of particles from the nucleus due to unstable particles disintegrating into more stable ones. There are several different types of radioactive reactions. The most common are alpha decay, beta decay, and gamma emissions.

Alpha decay occurs when an alpha particle is emitted. Of the three types of radioactive reactions, alpha decay has the lowest penetrating power. **Alpha particles** are comprised of two protons and two neutrons, which is similar to the helium (He) atom. For this reason, there are two ways to represent alpha particles: α and $_2^4 He$. An example of an element undergoing alpha decay is shown below using both ways to represent the alpha particle:

$$_{92}^{236}U \rightarrow _{90}^{232}Th + \alpha$$

or

$$_{92}^{236}U \rightarrow _{90}^{232}Th + _2^4 He$$

Notice that the mass (236) and the number of protons (92) on the reactant side is the same as the total mass (232 + 4) and total number of protons (90 + 2) on the product side. This is because the law of conservation of mass requires that matter cannot be neither created nor destroyed.

A beta particle (β or $_{-1}^0 e$) is emitted when a neutron inside the nucleus breaks down into a proton and an electron:

$$_0^1 n \rightarrow _1^1 p + _{-1}^0 e$$

Where $_0^1 n$ is a neutron, $_1^1 p$ is a proton, and $_{-1}^0 e$ is an emitted electron (beta particle). The beta particle has a charge of -1 and is about 100 times more powerful than an alpha particle. An example of a beta decay is shown in the following equation:

$$_6^{14}C \rightarrow _7^{14}N + _{-1}^0 e$$

Gamma emission is different from alpha and beta decay because it releases only a high-energy photon that is about 1,000 times more penetrating than an alpha particle. Gamma rays do not have either mass or charge $\left(_0^0 \gamma\right)$. An example of a gamma emission is shown in the following equation:

$$_{56}^{137}Ba \rightarrow _{56}^{137}Ba + _0^0 \gamma$$

Gamma emissions commonly occur with other decays:

$$_{56}^{137}Ba \rightarrow _{54}^{133}Xe + _2^4 He + _0^0 \gamma$$

All of the examples shown on page 110 are considered to be **nuclear fission** reactions, a process by which a single particle splits apart into several smaller particles. The reverse process can also happen when two or more particles combine to form a single, bigger particle. This is called **nuclear fusion**.

APPLICATIONS OF RADIOCHEMISTRY TO MEDICINE

Radiation is typically considered dangerous, but it is also a powerful tool used in medicine. For example, radioactive isotopes, such as $^{131}_{53}I$, can be used to image parts of the body such as the thyroid. Radiation is also used to sterilize surgical devices and food because it is extremely effective at killing infectious bacteria. These are just a few examples of how radioactivity is used in the medical field.

Scientific Measurement and the Mole Concept

10

SI UNITS AND CONVERSIONS

The International System of Units, which is also known as the Système International (SI), has seven basic units as shown in Table 10.1.

Table 10.1. Standard SI Base Units

Common Physical Quantity	Unit and Unit Abbreviation	Common Non-SI Units
Mass	Kilogram (kg)	Gram (g)
Length	Meter (m)	
Time	Second (s)	
Temperature	Kelvin (K)	
Amount of substance	Mole (mol)	
Electric current	Ampere (A)	
Luminous intensity	Candela (cd)	
Volume*	Cubic meter (m³)	Liter (L)

*Not an SI unit but a metric unit that is commonly used in chemistry

Depending on the quantity of a physical measurement, using either scientific notation or prefixes can be beneficial. For example, 0.0000000091 g of carbon is easier to represent in scientific notation as 9.1×10^{-9} g or with the corresponding prefix, 9.1 nanograms, abbreviated 9.1 ng. Table 10.2 shows common prefixes that are used in chemistry.

Table 10.2. Common Prefixes

Prefix	Prefix Symbol	Exponential Notation	Conventional Notation
Mega-	M	1×10^{6}	1,000,000
Kilo-	k	1×10^{3}	1,000
—	—	1×10^{0}	1
Centi-	c	1×10^{-2}	0.01
Milli-	m	1×10^{-3}	0.001
Micro-	μ	1×10^{-6}	0.000001
Nano-	n	1×10^{-9}	0.000000001

SCIENTIFIC NOTATION

Having a working understanding of exponents is essential to understanding scientific notation:

    a. $10^1 = 10$
    b. $1 \times 10^1 = 1 \times 10 = 10$
    c. $2 \times 10^1 = 20$
    d. $1 \times 10^2 = 1 \times 10 \times 10 = 100$

If the exponent is positive, move the decimal to the right:

    a. $1 \times 10^2 = 100$
    b. $2.5 \times 10^2 = 250$

Negative exponents can be represented as the reciprocal:

    a. $10^{-1} = \dfrac{1}{10^1} = 0.1$
    b. $1 \times 10^{-1} = 0.1$
    c. $2 \times 10^{-1} = 0.2$

If the exponent is negative, move the decimal to the left:

    a. $2 \times 10^{-3} = 0.002$
    b. $3.24 \times 10^{-3} = 0.00324$

SIGNIFICANT DIGITS/FIGURES AND UNCERTAINTY

Accuracy is how close experimental measurements are to the true value. **Precision** is when repeated experimental measurements are close to one another. Every instrument or device comes with limitations to its measurements; these all have some degree of uncertainty. Measurements are reported with digits that have certainty, except for the last digit, which is estimated. The measured digits, including the estimated digit, are called **significant digits** or **significant figures**. To determine if a digit in a number is significant or not, use the following general rules to guide you.

    RULE 1. All nonzero digits are significant.
    RULE 2. Any zeros to the left of the first nonzero number are insignificant.
    RULE 3. Any zeros *between* nonzero digits are significant.
    RULE 4. Any zeros to the right of the first nonzero number are significant IF there is a decimal point in the number.

EXAMPLES OF SIGNIFICANT FIGURES

100 has 1 significant figure since there is no decimal point. (See rules #1 and #4.)

100. has 3 significant figures since there is a decimal point. This indicates the measuring instrument was able to measure to the ones position accurately. (See rules #1 and #4.)

0.02050 has 4 significant figures. All nonzero digits, 2 and 5, are significant. (See rule #1.) The first two zeros are not significant because they are to the left of the first nonzero digit. (See rule #2.) The zero between 2 and 5 is significant because it is between nonzero digits. (See rule #3.) The last zero is significant because it is to the right of a nonzero number and *there is a decimal point*. (See rule #4.)

To determine the number of significant digits in an answer to an equation, one of two sets of rules must be used. The rules used depend on the type of mathematical function performed in the equation. With multiplication and division, the final answer must have the same number of significant figures as the number multiplied or divided that has the least significant digits. With addition and subtraction, the final answer depends on the least precise number added or subtracted.

➡ **Example** _____

Calculate the answer to the following equation: $20.05 \times 124 \div 0.00010$. Make sure the answer has the correct number of significant digits.

$$20.05 \times 124 \div 0.010 = 248{,}620 = 250{,}000 \text{ or } 2.5 \times 10^5$$

Solution

There are 4 significant digits in 20.05. There are 3 significant digits in 1.24. There are 2 significant digits in 0.010. So, the answer must have 2 significant digits.

➡ **Example** _____

Calculate the answer to the following equation: $20.05 + 1.24 - 0.0010$. Make sure the answer has the correct number of significant figures.

$$20.05 + 1.24 - 0.0010 = 21.289 = 21.29$$

Solution

The first and second numbers, 20.05 and 1.24, each measure out to the hundredths place, whereas 0.0010 measures out to the ten thousandths place. Both the first and second number are the least precise. Therefore the answer can go out only to the hundredths place.

INTRODUCTION TO UNIT CONVERSION

The ability to perform unit conversions is an essential skill in math, engineering, chemistry, and physics. Mastery of this topic will prevent most common and simple mistakes and will eliminate incorrect answers on the exams designed specifically to test this skill. Manipulating units is very similar to manipulating numbers. Units can be multiplied, divided, added, subtracted, and canceled out.

➡ **Example** _____

$$2.4 \text{ cm} \times 2.4 \text{ cm} = (2.4 \text{ cm})^2 = 5.76 \text{ cm}^2 = 5.7 \text{ cm}^2$$
$$2.4 \text{ cm} \div 2.4 \text{ cm} = 1 \text{ (both the numbers and units cancel out)}$$
$$2.4 \text{ cm}^2 \div 2 \text{ cm} = 1.2 \text{ cm} \ (2.4 \div 2 = 1.2 \text{ and cm}^2 \div \text{cm} = \text{cm})$$

Sometimes the definitions of units have to be manipulated to cancel out correctly. For example, there are 1,000 mL in 1 L. However, $1{,}000 \text{ mL}^2 \neq 1 \text{ L}^2$. The conversion factor that must be used in this case is $\left(\dfrac{1{,}000 \text{ mL}}{1 \text{ L}}\right)^2 = \dfrac{1{,}000^2 \text{ mL}^2}{1^2 \text{ L}^2} = \dfrac{1{,}000{,}000 \text{ mL}^2}{1 \text{ L}^2}$.

Density can be used to convert between volume and mass (density = mass/volume):

$$5.78 \text{ g Al} \cdot \frac{1 \text{ mL Al}}{2.70 \text{ g Al}} = 2.14 \text{ mL Al}$$

MASS AND WEIGHT

Mass and weight are different.
Mass is constant.
Weight = Mass × Gravitational Force

Another common unit conversion is the *mole*. For example, if you baked a dozen muffins, you baked 12 muffins. However, if you baked a mole of muffins, you baked 6.022×10^{23} muffins. In chemistry, the mole is typically used to count atoms, molecules, ions, and electrons.

➡ **Example** _____

How many atoms of F are in 12.3 mol F?

Solution

$$12.3 \text{ mol F} \times \frac{6.022 \times 10^{23} \text{ atoms F}}{1 \text{ mol F}} = 7.41 \times 10^{24} \text{ atoms F}$$

Quantum Mechanical Model of the Atom

11

ELECTROMAGNETIC RADIATION AND INTERACTIONS WITH MATTER

Electromagnetic radiation has both wavelike and particlelike properties. Its wavelike properties include wavelength (λ) and frequency (v). Wavelength is the distance between crests of a wave in meters (m). Frequency is the number of crests that pass through a single point in a second. The units for frequency are 1/s or s^{-1}, which is also known as Hz (hertz). The equation that relates the wavelength and frequency is $v = \dfrac{c}{\lambda}$, where c = speed of light (3.00×10^8 m/s). The electromagnetic spectrum shows all wavelengths in electromagnetic radiation. Electromagnetic radiation is made up of photons. The *energy of a photon* depends on the frequency of that photon:

$$E = hv = \frac{hc}{\lambda}$$

In this equation, E is the energy of a photon, h is Planck's constant (6.626×10^{-34} J · s), v is frequency, c is speed of light (3.00×10^8 m/s), and λ is wavelength (in m).

ATOMIC SPECTRA AND THE BOHR MODEL

Atoms can absorb energy, which causes an electron in the atom to jump to an excited state. When the electron goes back to the ground state, it re-emits the energy as light. In the visible region, this can be observed with the emission of certain colors. One way to understand this phenomenon is using the Bohr model. The Bohr model shows electrons orbiting around the nucleus at specific distances, where each orbit contains a fixed energy (quantized). This can be thought of like the rungs of a ladder—there are steps where your feet can land, but they cannot land between the rungs. Electrons orbit around the nucleus at defined energies, like rungs. The electrons need to absorb exactly the right amount of energy to be excited to another energy level. The following is the equation used to calculate the amount of energy an electron needs to be excited to or the amount of energy released when an electron transfers from one energy level to another:

$$\Delta E = -2.18 \times 10^{-18} \text{ J} \left(\frac{1}{n_f^2} - \frac{1}{n_i^2} \right)$$

In this equation, n_f is the final energy level and n_i is the initial energy level of the electron. Since each element has a different number of protons and energy levels, the distance that electrons orbit around a nucleus is unique to the particular element. This allows scientists to use unique emission spectra to identify specific elements.

The de Broglie wavelength equation shows the relationship between the kinetic energy of an electron with the electron's wavelength:

$$\lambda = \frac{h}{mv}$$

In this equation, h is Planck's constant (6.626×10^{-34} J · s), m is the mass of an electron in kg, and v is the velocity of the electron. As the speed of an electron increases, its wavelength decreases.

ATOMIC ORBITALS: ENERGIES AND SHAPES

Atomic orbitals are the 3D probability of finding an electron at a specific location. Nodes in an orbital are points where the probability of finding an electron at that location is zero.

Quantum numbers are used to identify each electron as a specific and unique electron. To do this, the energy level, the orbital, and the spin of an electron have to be known. The principle quantum number n is used to represent the energy level, where $n = 1$ for energy level one, $n = 2$ for energy level two, and so on. The shape of an orbital is represented by the angular momentum quantum number, l. For every energy level, there is a new type of orbital gained. For example, in energy level 1 ($n = 1$), there is only an s-orbital ($l = 0$). In the second energy level ($n = 2$), there are both s-orbitals and p-orbitals ($l = 0$ and $l = 1$, respectively). The relationship between n and l are $l = 0, 1, 2, \ldots, n - 1$. The quantum numbers, n and l, are different for each set of orbitals listed below:

$5s$	$5p$	$5d$	$5f$	$5g$
$4s$	$4p$	$4d$	$4f$	
$3s$	$3p$	$3d$		
$2s$	$2p$			
$1s$				

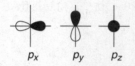

Within the p-subshell are three different types of p-orbitals: p_x, p_y, and p_z. The difference among these is where the p-orbital lies: on the x-, y-, or z-axis, respectively. The magnetic quantum number, m_l, is used to differentiate among the various orientations of orbitals. For example, to represent the three different orientations for the p-subshell, m_l can be –1, 0, or 1. For the d-subshell, there are five different orientations of d-orbitals. The different orientations are represented by m_l = –2, –1, 0, 1, or 2. Last but not least is the spin of the electron, where m_s is the electron spin quantum number. The spin of an electron can be either $+\frac{1}{2}$ or $-\frac{1}{2}$. **The Pauli exclusion principle** states that two electrons cannot occupy the same orbital with the same spin and instead must have opposite spins in order to pair. This is represented in Figure 11.1, where each half arrow depicts an electron with either a $+\frac{1}{2}$ or $-\frac{1}{2}$ spin. Figure 11.1 also shows Hund's rule, which states that electrons will half-fill any orbitals that have the same energy before completely filling an orbital.

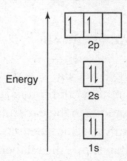

Figure 11.1. Orbital energy diagram that depicts Hund's rule and the Pauli exclusion principle. Each label represents a subshell, each box represents an orbital, and each arrow represents an electron.

Periodic Properties of Elements Arise from the Structure of the Atom

12

OVERVIEW OF THE PERIODIC TABLE

The structure of an atom determines its properties. The periodic table is organized by atomic number (number of protons). However, the physical and chemical behavior of an element is based on the arrangement of electrons.

ELECTRON CONFIGURATION OF ATOMS

Electron configuration describes the electrons in an atom with their placement in specific orbitals. For example, hydrogen has one electron in the lowest energy orbital ($1s$). In $1s$, the coefficient (1) represents the energy level and the letter (s) represents the type of orbital. To represent that this atom has one electron, the superscript is added ($1s^1$), as shown in Figure 12.1.

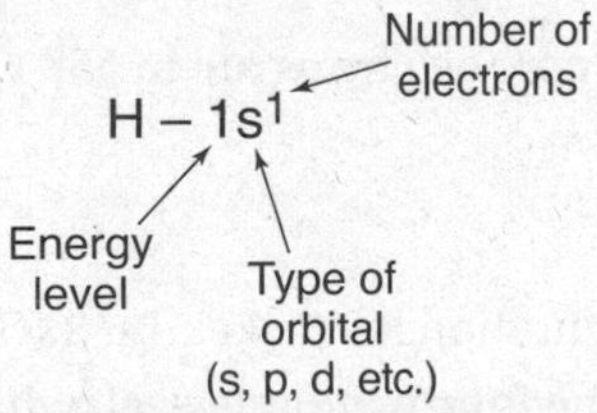

Figure 12.1. The electron configuration of hydrogen

Each orbital can hold up to 2 electrons. Depending on the subshell, the number of different orientations for each type of orbital can vary. For example, the p-subshell has 3 orbitals: p_x, p_y, and p_z. Therefore, the p-subshell can hold up to 6 electrons. When writing electron configurations, the order the orbitals are filled must be considered. Fortunately, the periodic table can be used as a guide, as shown in Figure 12.2.

Note in Figure 12.2 that the $3d$ orbitals are not filled until after the $4s$ orbitals have been filled. Recall that for each energy level, a new orbital is introduced. This means that energy level 3 has d-orbitals. The energy difference between $4s$ and $3d$ orbitals is small, allowing electrons to transition easily between the two. In general, subshells are the most stable when they are completely filled, then half-filled is second best.

Noble gas configuration is a shorthand notation for writing electron configuration. For example, boron has 5 electrons. Its electron configuration is $1s^2 2s^2 2p^1$. Helium (He), which is a noble gas, has 2 electrons. Its electron configuration is $1s^2$. The electron configuration for He can be written as part of boron's electron configuration: $1s^2 2s^2 2p^1 = [He]2s^2 2p^1$. This is especially useful with larger elements, like manganese (Mn). The shorthand electron configuration for Mn is $[Ar]4s^2 3d^5$ where $[Ar] = 1s^2 2s^2 2p^6 3s^2 3p^6$.

$1s^1$																	$1s^1$
$2s^1$	$2s^2$												$2p^1$	$2p^2$	$2p^3$	$2p^4$	$2p^5$	$2p^6$
$3s^1$	$3s^2$												$3p^1$					
$4s^1$	$4s^2$	$3d^1$	$3d^2$	$3d^3$	$3d^4$	$3d^5$	$3d^6$	$3d^7$	$3d^8$	$3d^9$	$3d^{10}$	$4p^1$					
$5s^1$	$5s^2$	$4d^1$										$5p^1$					
$6s^1$	$6s^2$	$5d^1$										$6p^1$					
$7s^1$	$7s^2$	$6d^1$										$7p^1$					

Figure 12.2. Guide to orbital filling

VALENCE ELECTRONS AND THE FORMATION OF IONS

Valence electrons are found in the outermost energy level. For example, carbon has a total of 6 electrons. However, 2 electrons are in the first energy level and 4 electrons are in the second energy level. This can also be seen in carbon's electron configuration: $1s^2 2s^2 2p^2$. There are four electrons in the outermost energy level ($n = 2$), which means there are 4 valence electrons. The other 2 electrons are considered core electrons.

➡ Example _____

How many valence electrons and core electrons are in Ni?

Solution

First, write out the electron configuration for nickel: $1s^2 2s^2 2p^6 3s^2 3p^6 4s^2 3d^8$ or $[\text{Ar}]4s^2 3d^8$. There are 2 valence electrons in the fourth energy level, which is the outermost energy level. The remaining electrons ($28 - 2 = 26$) are 26 core electrons. When nickel becomes a cation, it first loses its valence electrons. For example, when Ni becomes Ni^+, the new electron configuration is $[\text{Ar}]4s^1 3d^8$. Notice that the electron was lost from the $4s$ (outermost) orbital before the $3d$ orbital.

In the example above, Ni has 8 of the allowed 10 electrons in the d-orbital. All orbitals are filled in the lowest energy state. For Ni, this will lead to 3 paired electrons (6 total electrons) and 2 unpaired electrons in order to fill all of the d-orbitals. When an atom or an ion has unpaired electrons, it is paramagnetic. Atoms or ions that have all of their electrons paired are diamagnetic, which generally occurs only for atoms or ions that have completely filled subshells (s, p, d, etc.).

ELECTRON CONFIGURATIONS DETERMINE ATOMIC PROPERTIES

Chemical properties are generally based on the number of electrons an atom has in its valence orbital. The noble gases have completely filled valence orbitals and are very stable, which is why the noble gases are typically unreactive. All group 1 elements (alkali metals) only have 1 valence electron. (The electron configurations of all alkali metals end in s^1 but with varying energy levels.) These metals can be easily stripped of their outer electron (s^1) to make a +1 cation. This occurs because once the lone electron in the s^1 orbital is lost, the alkali metal has the same electron configuration as a noble gas, which is energetically stable. For example, the electron configuration for Na is $1s^22s^22p^63s^1 = $ [Ne]$3s^1$. Once Na loses one electron to become Na$^+$, the electron configuration becomes $1s^22s^22p^6$ or [Ne]. Alkali metals are much more stable after losing an electron, which makes them the most reactive group on the periodic table. Group 2 elements (alkaline earth metals) have an electron configuration that ends with s^2. They typically lose 2 electrons to attain the energetically favored noble gas electron configuration, which is why alkaline earth metals usually form +2 cations. Group 17 elements (halogens) end with p^5 and are only 1 electron away from having a completely filled p-orbital. For this reason, halogens usually form –1 ions. Transition metals usually make a variety of cations (+1, +2, +3, etc). This occurs because the valence electrons of transition metals are in the s- and d-subshells, which are similar in energy. For example, Ni is [Ar]$4s^23d^8$. Even though the 4th energy level is higher than the 3rd energy level, having either a completely filled or a half-filled orbital is more stable. It is easier to achieve this by filling the one s-orbital first before filling all five d-orbitals. Transition metals typically lose electrons from the s-orbital first since these electrons are in the outmost shell, which is why +1 and +2 charges are very common.

SPECIFIC TRENDS IN THE PERIODIC TABLE

The periodic table is arranged by atomic number. Since atomic properties are based on the number of protons and electrons, trends are found within the periodic table. One periodic trend is the atomic radius of a neutral atom, which increases with more electron shells (going down a column) and decreases going from left to right. Therefore, the smallest neutral atom is He. The atomic radius decreases in the same row due to a higher attraction between protons and electrons (effective nuclear charge). Effective nuclear charge (Z) can be calculated using this formula: $Z = $ number of protons – core electrons. Going from left to right within a row, the number of protons increases but the number of core electrons stays the same. When the atom becomes charged (and therefore becomes an ion), the ionic radius changes. In general, cations are smaller than the neutral atomic radii, whereas anions are larger due to electron repulsion.

Another periodic trend is electron affinity, which is the energy change when an atom gains another electron. In general, electron affinity increases going up a column and from left to right within a row, where the atom with the highest electron affinity is F. Electronegativity measures the ability of an atom to pull electrons toward it in a bond. The most electronegative atom is also F, which makes sense since electronegativity and electron affinity are closely related. Ionization energy is the energy required to remove an electron. The first ionization energy is the energy needed to remove the first electron, second ionization energy is the energy needed to remove the second electron, etc. In general, the first ionization energy increases going up a column and going from left to right within a row. This trend predicts that He has the highest first ionization energy. Recall that subshells (s, p, d, etc.) are the most stable when these are completely filled and second most stable when these are half-filled. The ionization energies reflect this. All of these trends are summarized in Figure 12.3.

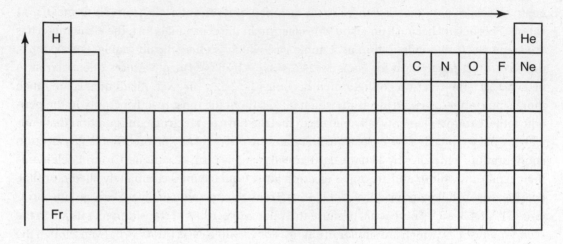

Figure 12.3. Periodic trends. The arrows show (1) an increase in electronegativity, (2) an increase in electron affinity, (3) a decrease in neutral atomic size, and (4) an increase in first ionization energy.

➡ Example

What element on the 2nd row of the periodic table has the following ionization energies?

$$1st = 900 \text{ kJ/mol}, 2nd = 1{,}757 \text{ kJ/mol}, 3rd = 14{,}849 \text{ kJ/mol}$$

Solution

Look for the biggest jump between ionization energies. The biggest jump is from the 2nd ionization energy to the 3rd. Atoms/ions with the same electron configuration as a noble gas are the most stable. After losing two electrons, this element's electron configuration now resembles that of a noble gas. This would place the element in the 2nd column of the 2nd row (given). As such, the element must be Be.

Molecules and Compounds

13

INTRAMOLECULAR BONDS

Intramolecular bonds occur within a compound. There are three different types of intramolecular bonds: ionic, covalent, and metallic. An **ionic bond** forms between a metal and a nonmetal when the electronegativity difference is great enough that one atom *transfers* one or more electrons to another. This results in the formation of a cation and an anion. The cation is a positively charged ion (gives up one or more electrons). The anion is a negatively charged ion (gains one or more electrons). Unlike ionic bonds, a **covalent bond** forms between a nonmetal and nonmetal when the electrons are *shared* between the atoms. **Metallic bonding** occurs between two or more metal atoms. The best way to visualize this is to think of positively charged metals held together by a "sea" of delocalized electrons, as shown in Figure 13.1.

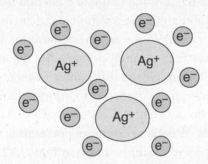

Figure 13.1. Metallic bonding. Positively charged metals are held together by a "sea" of delocalized electrons.

CHEMICAL FORMULAS AND MOLECULAR MODELING

Chemical formulas are representations of the elements and ratios of atoms that form a compound. An **empirical formula** shows the lowest whole-number ratio of atoms within a compound and may or may not be the actual formula. In contrast, the **molecular formula** is the actual ratio of atoms in a compound. For example, $C_6H_{12}O_6$ is the molecular formula for the sugar glucose. However, the smallest whole-number ratio for glucose is CH_2O (the empirical formula). Sometimes the empirical formula and the molecular formula are the same. Chemical formulas, however, do not give information about how the atoms are attached. Instead, structural formulas are used to show which atoms are bound to other atoms. For example, the chemical formula of H_2O doesn't show how the hydrogens and oxygen atoms are connected, but the structural formula for water does. See Figure 13.2.

Figure 13.2. Structural formula of water

The structure shows that the hydrogen atoms are NOT bonded to one another. Instead, they are each bonded to the oxygen atom. The lines between atoms are covalent bonds, where each single line represents 2 electrons. Molecular modeling shows how the atoms are bonded to each other in relation to space (3D representation of a molecule). The section "Lewis Dot Structures" goes into detail on how to draw three-dimensional molecules.

CHEMICAL NOMENCLATURE

Different compounds have different naming conventions.

Naming Ionic Compounds

A compound is named based on the type of intramolecular bonding present. For ionic compounds, which have a cation and an anion, the convention is to name the cation first, followed by the anion. The cation name stays the same as the element name. For example, Li is the symbol for lithium. When Li is found in an ionic compound, the cation name for Li^+ is still lithium. Exceptions to this rule are transition metals, which need an additional step. Transition metals are in the *d*-block of the periodic table and usually form multiple charges (*see Chapter 12*). Therefore, the charge of a transition metal ion must be included in the name by using Roman numerals. For example, the cation ion name for Ni^{2+} is nickel (II). When naming the anion, it starts the same as the neutral element, but the ending is dropped and "-ide" is added. For example, F is fluorine. When it becomes negatively charged as F^-, the name becomes fluoride. Oxygen (O) becomes oxide (O^{2-}). One exception to this naming convention is polyatomic anions, which do not change. Carbonate (CO_3^{2-}) is a polyatomic ion. In ionic compounds, its name stays as carbonate. Common polyatomic ions are listed in Table 13.1. An overview of naming cations and anions is shown in Table 13.2.

Table 13.1. Common Polyatomic Ions

Polyatomic Ion Name	Polyatomic Ion Formula
Ammonium	NH_4^+
Bicarbonate (hydrogen carbonate)	HCO_3^-
Carbonate	CO_3^{2-}
Chlorate	ClO_3^-
Chlorite	ClO_2^-
Hydrogen phosphate	HPO_4^{2-}
Hydroxide	OH^-
Hypochlorite	ClO^-
Nitrate	NO_3^-
Nitrite	NO_2^-
Perchlorate	ClO_4^-
Phosphate	PO_4^{3-}
Sulfate	SO_4^{2-}
Sulfite	SO_3^{2-}

Table 13.2. Overview of Naming Cations and Anions in Ionic Compounds

Element	Element Name	Ion	Ion Name
Cations			
Li	Lithium	Li^+	Lithium
Na	Sodium	Na^+	Sodium
Be	Beryllium	Be^{2+}	Beryllium
Mg	Magnesium	Mg^{2+}	Magnesium
Ni	Nickel	$*Ni^{2+}$	Nickel (II)
Ni	Nickel	$*Ni^{3+}$	Nickel (III)
Fe	Iron	$*Fe^{2+}$	Iron (II)
Fe	Iron	$*Fe^{3+}$	Iron (III)
Cu	Copper	$*Cu^+$	Copper (I)
Cu	Copper	$*Cu^{2+}$	Copper (II)
Anions			
O	Oxygen	O^{2-}	Oxide
N	Nitrogen	N^{3-}	Nitride
F	Fluorine	F^-	Fluoride
Cl	Chlorine	Cl^-	Chloride

*Ni, Fe, and Cu have multiple different ions. The ions listed in this table are just some examples.

➡ Example

Name the following ionic compound: NaCl.

Solution

The cation, Na, is the first element listed and is followed by the anion. The cation name stays the same as the element's name (Na and $Na^+ \rightarrow$ sodium). Cl is the anion. When naming anions in ionic compounds, take the elemental name (chlorine), drop the ending (-ine), and add -ide (chloride). Put the cation and anion name together: sodium chloride.

➡ Example

Name the following ionic compound: $CrBr_3$.

Solution

Cr is a transition metal that forms multiple different ions, which means it requires Roman numerals to specify the charge. To determine the charge on Cr, recall that ionic compounds must have charge neutrality. The charge of Br can be determined from the periodic table. Br makes a 1– charge. There are 3 Br– and only 1 Cr, which means Cr must have a 3+ charge to make the overall compound neutral. The name for $CrBr_3$ is chromium (III) bromide.

➡ Example

Name the following ionic compound: NH_4OH.

Solution

This is an ionic compound formed by two polyatomic ions. When naming a compound, polyatomic ion names do not change. Therefore, the name for this compound is ammonium hydroxide.

➡ Example

Name the following ionic compound: $CaSO_3$.

Solution

The name for $CaSO_3$ is calcium sulf*ite*, NOT sulf*ide*. Remember that sulfide is the anion name for sulfur (S). In this compound, it has the polyatomic ion sulfite (SO_3^{2-}). Like all polyatomic ions, it does not change its name in an ionic compound.

To write the molecular formula of ionic compounds from names, the charge of each ion will need to be known. Molecular formulas are typically neutral overall. This means the ratio of cations to anions is based on the charge on each ion.

➡ Example

What is the molecular formula for barium chlorite?

Solution

Barium is the cation and forms a 2+ charge (Ba^{2+}). Chlorite is a polyatomic ion that has a 1– charge (ClO^-). To balance the overall charge, 2 chlorites are needed. To show that there are 2 chlorites, use parentheses and a subscript of 2: $(ClO)_2$. The molecular formula for barium chlorite is $Ba(ClO)_2$.

➡ Example

What is the molecular formula for calcium sulfate?

Solution

The first word is the cation, and the second is the anion. Calcium makes a 2+ charge, whereas sulfate makes a 2– charge. Since the charges are already balanced (2+ and 2– added together equal zero), only one of each are needed (Ca^{2+} and SO_4^{2-}). The molecular formula is $CaSO_4$.

➡ Example

What is the molecular formula for tin (IV) chlorite?

Solution

Roman numerals are used for metals that form multiple charges. So the IV represents the charge on tin. Chlorite is a polyatomic ion (ClO_2^-), and 4 of these are needed to balance with the 4+ charge on tin. The molecular formula is $Sn(ClO_2)_4$.

Naming Hydrates

Some ionic compounds will form with a specific ratio of water attached. This is called a hydrate. For these cases, the number of water molecules plus "hydrate" is added at the end of the name. For example, $BaCl_2 \cdot 6H_2O$ is called barium chloride hexahydrate. Barium chloride is an ionic compound and therefore uses the ionic naming system. The prefix "hexa-" is used to represent the number 6 in $6H_2O$. Hydrate is the name for water. A list of numbers and their prefixes are listed in Table 13.3.

Table 13.3. Prefixes Used for Numbers

Number	Prefix
$\frac{1}{2}$	hemi-
1	mono-
2	di-
3	tri-
4	tetra-
5	penta-
6	hexa-
7	hepta-
8	octa-
9	nona-
10	deca-

Naming Covalent (Molecular) Compounds

Since covalent compounds are comprised of nonmetals bound to nonmetals, charges do not form and cannot be used to help predict the ratio of atoms when bound together. Therefore, the ratio of atoms has to be included in the name (as shown in Table 13.3). For example, NO_3 (*not* NO_3^-, which is a polyatomic ion called nitrate) is nitrogen trioxide. Notice that the ending for the last element is still changed—from oxygen to oxide—just like in ionic compounds. However, to indicate how many nitrogen and oxygen atoms are found in the compound, the prefix "tri-" is added to oxide to represent the 3 oxygens. (Using the prefix "mono-" is optional for the first element.)

➡ Example _____

Name the following covalent compound: CO.

Solution

CO is carbon monoxide. Using the "mono-" prefix for the first element is optional but is required for the second element.

Example _____

Name the following covalent compound: P_4S_{10}.

Solution

P_4S_{10} is tetraphosphorus decasulfide. "Tetra-" is 4, and "deca-" is 10. The word "phosphorus" is left alone just like the cations in ionic compounds. The last element is changed from "sulfur" to "sulfide," just like the anions in ionic compounds.

Example _____

What is the molecular formula for dinitrogen pentoxide?

Solution

N_2O_5

COMPOSITION OF COMPOUNDS BY MASS PERCENT

Mass percent is used to determine how much of a compound's mass originates from a certain element. The formula below is used to calculate mass percent:

$$\text{mass percent of element } X = \frac{\text{mass of element } X \text{ in 1 mole of compound}}{\text{molecular mass of 1 mole of compound}} \times 100$$

Example _____

What is the mass percent of H in $C_6H_{12}O_6$?

Solution

First, determine the mass coming from just H. The molar mass of H = 1.01 g/mol. There are 12 mol of H in $C_6H_{12}O_6$. Therefore, calculate the total mass of H in $C_6H_{12}O_6$:

$$12 \text{ mol H} \cdot \frac{1.01 \text{ g H}}{1 \text{ mol H}} = 12.1 \text{ g H}$$

Second, determine the total mass of $C_6H_{12}O_6$:

$$\left(6 \text{ mol C} \cdot \frac{12.01 \text{ g C}}{1 \text{ mol C}}\right) + \left(12 \text{ mol H} \cdot \frac{1.01 \text{ g H}}{1 \text{ mol H}}\right) + \left(6 \text{ mol O} \cdot \frac{16.00 \text{ g O}}{1 \text{ mol O}}\right)$$

$$= (72.06 \text{ g}) + (12.1 \text{ g}) + (96.00 \text{ g}) = 180.2 \text{ g } C_6H_{12}O_6$$

Third, plug into the mass percent equation and solve:

$$\text{mass percent of element H} = \frac{12.1 \text{ g}}{180.2 \text{ g}} \times 100 = 6.71\%$$

It is important to check what type of formula the question is asking for: an empirical formula or a molecular formula. Remember that an empirical formula has the lowest whole-number ratio of elements possible and that a molecular formula is the actual formula for a compound. Recall that sometimes the empirical formula is the same as the molecular formula. If the mass percent composition is given, assume that there is a 100 g sample. This makes the percentages given equal to the mass of each compound.

➥ **Example** _____

A compound with only C and H has a carbon mass percent of 74.97%. What is the empirical formula?

Solution

If carbon has a mass percent of 74.97%, the remaining mass percent is due to hydrogen (100.00% – 74.97% = 25.03% hydrogen). Assume there is a 100.00 g sample. That means there are 74.97 g of C and 25.03 g of H. The empirical formula shows the *mole* ratios of each element, which means that each of these masses needs to be converted to moles:

$$74.97 \text{ g C} \cdot \frac{1 \text{ mol C}}{12.01 \text{ g C}} = 6.242298 \text{ mol C}$$

$$25.03 \text{ g C} \cdot \frac{1 \text{ mol H}}{1.01 \text{ g H}} = 24.78217 \text{ mol H}$$

Next, a ratio of each element to each other is needed. There are only whole-number ratios in chemical formulas. This means the moles of each element have to be divided by the smaller number. In this example, the number of moles of carbon is smaller and will be used to calculate the mole ratios:

$$\frac{6.242298}{6.242298} = 1.000 \text{ mol C}$$

$$\frac{24.78217}{6.242298} = 3.97 \text{ mol H}$$

3.97 moles of H is close enough to 4 that it can be rounded up to 4, which means the empirical formula is CH_4.

As a general rule, if the mole ratio is within 0.1 of a whole number, it can be either rounded up or down to the nearest whole number. Otherwise, a multiplication factor is needed to reach a whole-number ratio for all elements. For example, let's say instead of 3.97 moles of H, it was 3.799 moles of H. This cannot be rounded up to 4. Instead, 3.799 must be multiplied by a factor until it is within 0.1 of a whole number:

$$3.799 \times 2 = 7.598$$
$$3.799 \times 3 = 11.397$$
$$3.799 \times 4 = 15.196$$
$$3.799 \times 5 = 18.995 = 19.00$$

To keep the ratios the same, carbon also has to be multiplied by 5. Therefore, the empirical formula for this compound is C_5H_{19}.

If the question is asking for the molecular formula, then more information is needed. For example, if CH_4 is determined to be the empirical formula, the question might also state that the compound has a molecular mass of 48.15 g/mol. To determine the molecular formula, do the following.

1. First, divide the molar mass of the molecular formula by the molar mass of the empirical formula:

$$\frac{48.15\,\frac{g}{mol}\,C_xH_y}{16.05\,\frac{g}{mol}\,CH_4} = 3.00$$

2. Multiply the ratio throughout the empirical formula:

$$C_{1\times3}H_{4\times3} = C_3H_{12}$$

Always double-check the answer by calculating the molar mass of the molecular formula.

Lewis Dot Structures

14

HOW TO DRAW MOLECULES AND IONS

A Lewis dot structure is a simplistic way of representing how atoms bond together. It starts with the number of valence electrons each atom contains. A single dot is used to represent one valence electron.

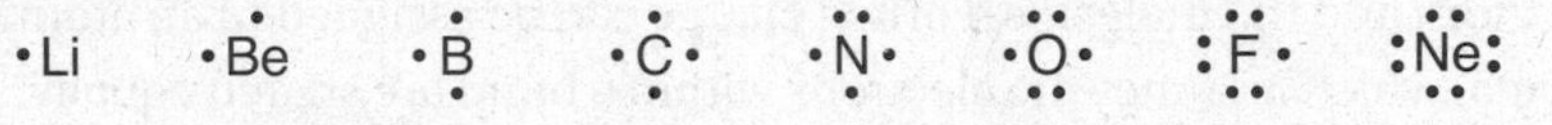

$$\cdot Li \qquad \cdot Be \qquad \cdot \overset{\cdot}{B} \qquad \cdot \overset{\cdot}{C} \cdot \qquad \cdot \overset{\cdot}{\underset{\cdot}{N}} \cdot \qquad \cdot \overset{\cdot \cdot}{\underset{\cdot \cdot}{O}} \cdot \qquad : \overset{\cdot \cdot}{\underset{\cdot \cdot}{F}} \cdot \qquad : \overset{\cdot \cdot}{\underset{\cdot \cdot}{Ne}} :$$

Figure 14.1. Lewis dot structures of several atoms

Lines are used to show when 2 electrons are being shared between atoms, as in covalent bonds. Figure 14.2 shows the Lewis dot structures of two covalent molecules.

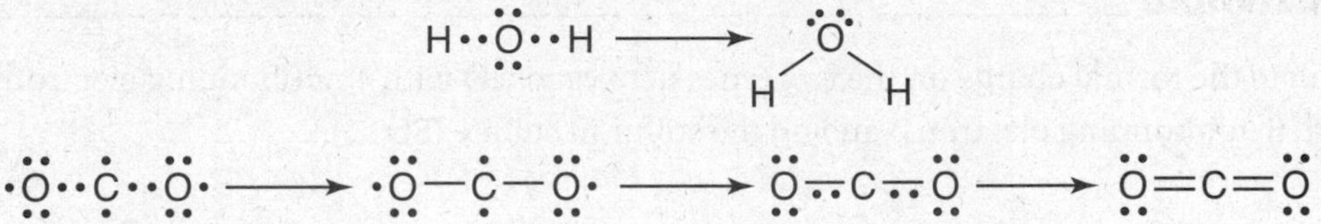

$$H \cdot \cdot \overset{\cdot \cdot}{\underset{\cdot \cdot}{O}} \cdot \cdot H \longrightarrow \overset{\overset{\cdot \cdot}{O}}{\underset{H \qquad H}{}}$$

$$\cdot \overset{\cdot \cdot}{\underset{\cdot \cdot}{O}} \cdot \cdot \overset{\cdot}{C} \cdot \cdot \overset{\cdot \cdot}{\underset{\cdot \cdot}{O}} \cdot \longrightarrow \cdot \overset{\cdot \cdot}{\underset{\cdot \cdot}{O}} - \overset{\cdot}{C} - \overset{\cdot \cdot}{\underset{\cdot \cdot}{O}} \cdot \longrightarrow \overset{\cdot \cdot}{\underset{\cdot \cdot}{O}} \cdots C \cdots \overset{\cdot \cdot}{\underset{\cdot \cdot}{O}} \longrightarrow \overset{\cdot \cdot}{\underset{\cdot \cdot}{O}} = C = \overset{\cdot \cdot}{\underset{\cdot \cdot}{O}}$$

Figure 14.2. The Lewis dot structures of water (H_2O) and carbon dioxide (CO_2)

Once the number of electrons has been determined, follow the octet rule, which states that atoms are more stable when they have or share a total of 8 electrons. This rule originates from the stability of an atom when it has a full energy level ($2s^2 2p^6 \rightarrow 8$ outer electrons). There are a few exceptions to this rule.

1. Hydrogen (H) wants only a total of 2 electrons. This means it can form only 1 bond because the $1s$ orbital can hold only 2 electrons.
2. Boron (B) prefers to form only 3 bonds, resulting in 6 electrons instead of 8.
3. Beryllium (Be) prefers to form only 2 bonds, resulting in 4 electrons.
4. Atoms that can expand the octet rule (having more than 8 electrons) are any atoms at or above the third energy level. These atoms have d-orbitals into which the electrons can be placed.

For example, sulfur is on the third energy level and therefore has the d-orbitals to expand the octet rule. Figure 14.3 is a Lewis dot structure for the sulfate ion, SO_4^{2-}, starting with neutral SO_4.

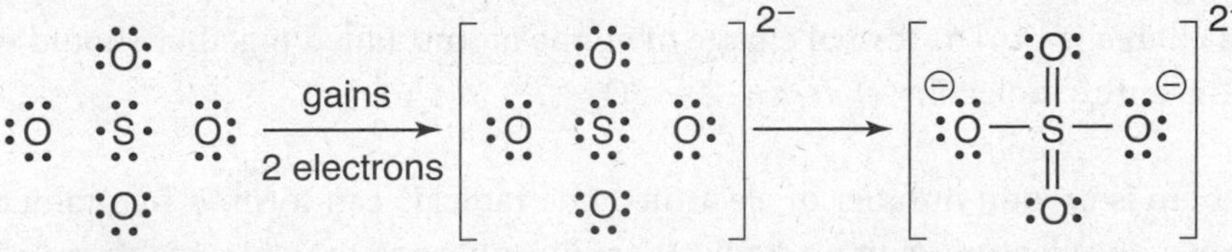

Figure 14.3. The Lewis dot structure for the sulfate ion, SO_4^{2-}

There can be multiple ways to represent how atoms are bonded. If the connectivity between atoms does not change but the electrons do change, *resonance structures* are formed (see Figure 14.4). If a molecule has resonance, the actual structure is an average of all resonance structures.

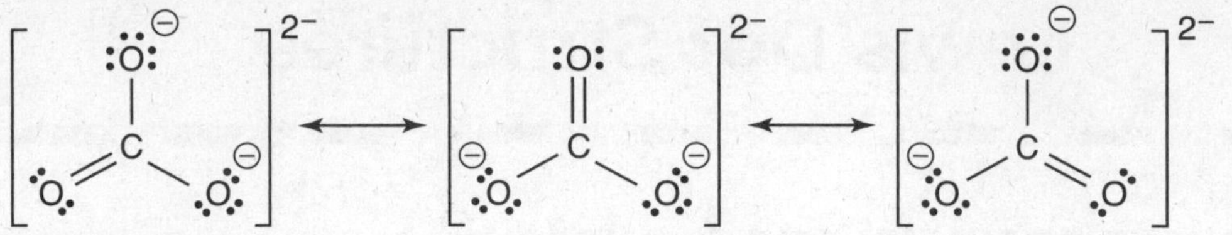

Figure 14.4. The resonance structures of the carbonate ion (CO_3^{2-})

Previously, sulfate was drawn with an expanded octet. When is it known if an atom is more stable with an expanded octet? If an atom has a formal charge of zero, then that is more stable for both the atom and the molecule. Formal charge can be assigned to an atom using the following formula, which assumes the electrons within a bond are shared equally:

$$\text{Formal charge on atom} =$$
$$\text{\# of valence electrons for atom} - (\text{\# of nonbonding electrons} + \text{\# of bonds})$$

➡ **Example** _____

Calculate the formal charge on the two types of oxygens (O with 4 nonbonding electrons and O with 6 nonbonding electrons) and on the sulfur in sulfate (SO_4^{2-}).

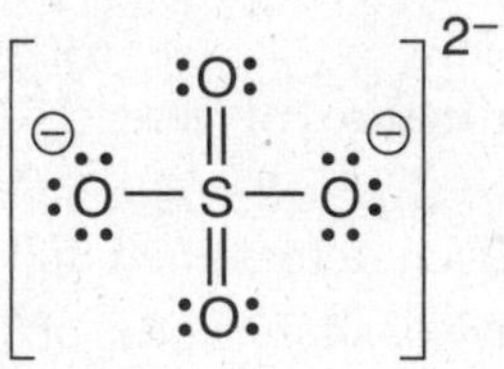

Solution

Formal charge (FC) on sulfur:

$$FC_S = 6 - (0 + 6) = 0$$

Formal charge (FC) on oxygen with 4 nonbonding electrons:

$$FC_O = 6 - (4 + 2) = 0$$

Formal charge (FC) on oxygen with 6 nonbonding electrons:

$$FC_O = 6 - (6 + 1) = -1$$

The two oxygens that have 6 nonbonding electrons are shown with a negative charge because the formal charge is –1. The formal charge of all the atoms added together should equal the charge of the entire molecule ($-1 + -1 = -2 \rightarrow SO_4^{2-}$).

When there is an odd number of electrons, free radicals can form. A free radical occurs when not all of the electrons pair up. Radicals are unstable and therefore highly reactive. NO_3, which has no charge, is an example of a free radical. The arrow in the following figure is pointing at the unpaired electron.

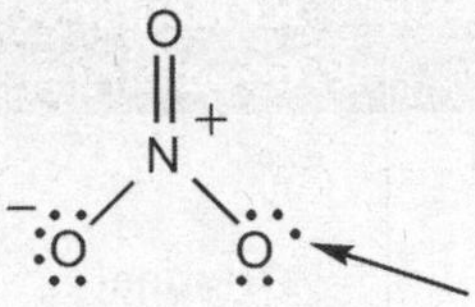

VSEPR THEORY

Valence shell electron-pair repulsion (VSEPR) theory predicts the 3D geometry around a single atom based on electron repulsion. It can be used to determine electron and molecular geometry. Electrons repel each other, which causes bonds and lone pairs to spread as far apart from one another as possible. This means the electron geometry of compounds can be predicted depending on the number of electron regions. Bonds, whether they are single, double, or triple, count as one electron region. Lone pairs count as one electron region. The molecular geometry of a compound includes only the geometry of the atoms. Table 14.1 summarizes the electron and molecular geometries for compounds with up to 6 electron regions.

Table 14.1. VSEPR Geometry

Electron Regions	Electron Geometry	Lone Pairs	Molecular Geometry	Examples
2	Linear 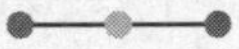	0 or 1	Linear	$H-C\equiv N$ $H-C\equiv C-H$
3	Trigonal planar 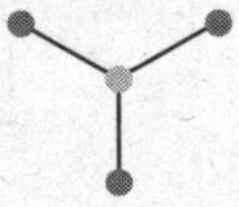	0	Trigonal planar	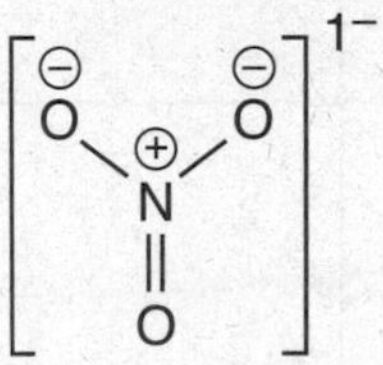
		1	Bent	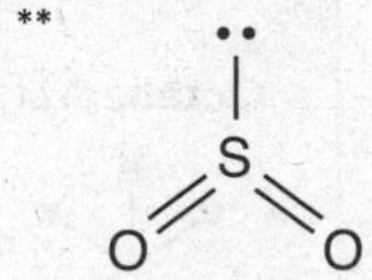
4	Tetrahedral* 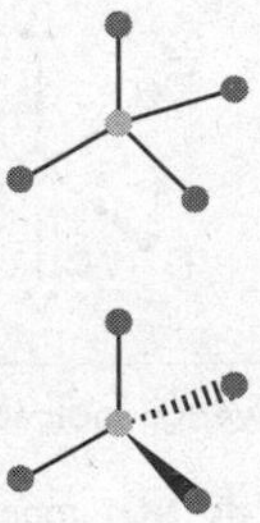	0	Tetrahedral	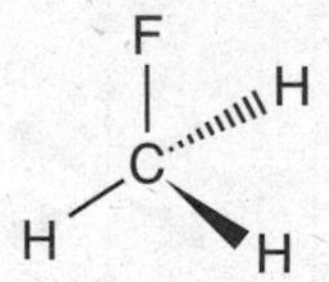
		1	Trigonal pyramidal	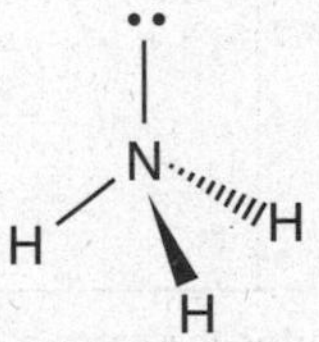
		2	Bent	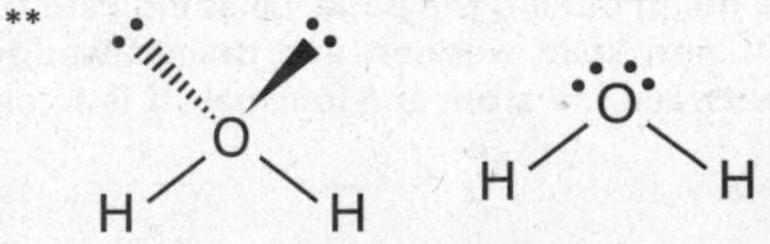

Table 14.1. VSEPR Geometry (continued)

Electron Regions	Electron Geometry	Lone Pairs	Molecular Geometry	Examples
5	Trigonal bipyramidal*	0	Trigonal bipyramidal	Cl, $Cl-P-Cl$, Cl, Cl
		1	Seesaw	$Cl-S-Cl$, Cl, Cl
		2	T-shape	$F-Cl-F$, F
		3	Linear	$F-Xe-F$
6	Octahedral*	0	Octahedral	F, F, F, S, F, F, F
		1	Square pyramidal	F, F, Br, F, F, F
		2	Square planar	F, F, Xe, F, F

*A solid wedge indicates a 3D bond that is coming out of the page. The dashed wedge indicates a 3D bond that is going behind the page. Lines indicate the bond is on the page.
**Lines, solid wedges, and dashed wedges connecting an atom to a lone pair do NOT mean there is a bond between the atom and lone pair. It is solely there to help visualize the 3D formation better.

DETERMINING POLARITY FROM A LEWIS STRUCTURE

Polar covalent bonds are formed when two atoms share electrons unequally. When one atom is more electronegative than the other, the more electronegative atom has a slightly negative charge (δ^-), leaving the other atom to have a slightly positive charge (δ^+). This occurs because the more electronegative atom pulls the shared electron closer to itself. This forms polarity within the bond, much like a magnet has a north pole and a south pole. For example, oxygen is more electronegative than carbon. So when carbon is bound to oxygen, a polar bond forms: $^{\delta+}C—O^{\delta-}$. In general, if the two atoms bound together are not the same, the covalent bond is polar, except for C—H bonds. Carbon and hydrogen have similar electronegativities and result in a nonpolar covalent bond.

If there are polar bonds in a molecule, the whole molecule is not necessarily polar. A molecule can have polar bonds and be nonpolar if each polar bond is canceled out by another. For example, each As—F bond in AsF_5 is polar. As shown in Figure 14.5, the As is completely surrounded with F. So each As—F polar bond cancels out another As—F polar bond, making the whole molecule nonpolar.

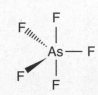

Figure 14.5. The nonpolar molecule AsF_5, which contains 5 polar covalent bonds

When the polar bonds do not cancel out each other, the molecule itself is polar. Lone pairs do not cancel out with polar bonds. For example, if two As—F bonds were replaced with lone pairs as in AsF_3, there would be a slightly negative charge density around the lone pairs, making the molecule polar. This is shown in Figure 14.6.

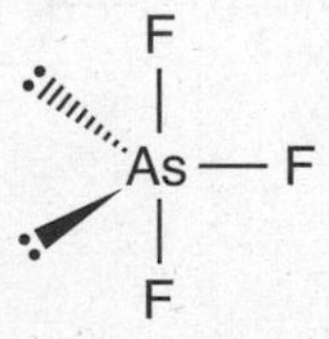

Figure 14.6. The polar molecule AsF_3, which contains 3 polar covalent bonds and 2 lone pairs of electrons

If the molecule contains only nonpolar bonds, as in Figure 14.7, the molecule itself is nonpolar.

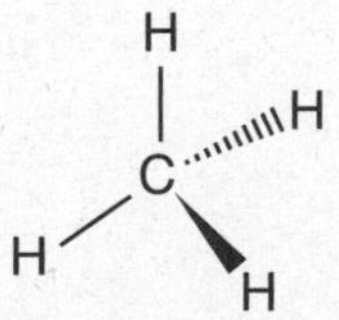

Figure 14.7. The nonpolar molecule CH_4, which contains 4 nonpolar covalent bonds

Valence Bond and Molecular Orbital Theory

15

VALENCE BOND THEORY

Valence bond theory states that covalent bonds form when two electrons pair from overlapping atomic orbitals. In order for the electrons to pair, they must have opposite spins (the Pauli exclusion principle). The strength of the bond is related to the amount of orbital overlap; more overlap between atomic orbitals leads to stronger bonds.

Hybrid orbitals form when two or more atomic orbitals mix. The initial orbital type determines which hybridization is used. For example, there are three different *p*-orbitals in the *p*-subshell (p_x, p_y, and p_z). If an *s*-orbital hybridizes with *one* of the three *p*-orbitals, it's called *sp* hybridization, as shown in Figure 15.1. If the *s*-orbital mixes with *two* of the three *p*-orbitals, it's called sp^2 hybridization, and so forth. There are also *d-*, *f-*, and *g*-orbitals available for hybridization.

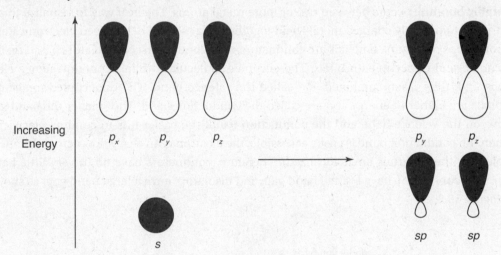

Figure 15.1. *sp* hybridization leaves two available *p*-orbitals. Notice that there are four orbitals before hybridization and that there are still four orbitals after hybridization.

A **sigma bond** (σ) is formed when two atomic orbitals directly overlap in such a way that the bond can freely rotate. A **pi bond** (π) is formed when two *p*-orbitals "bend" to form a bond that cannot rotate. Single bonds have one sigma bond. Double bonds have one sigma and one pi bond. Triple bonds have one sigma and two pi bonds. Figure 15.2 shows both sigma and pi bonds.

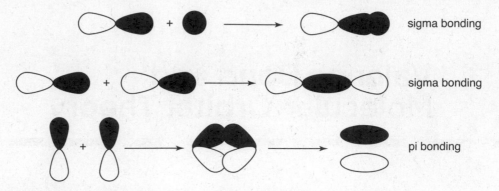

Figure 15.2. Various types of atomic overlap and their respective bonding

ELECTRON DELOCALIZATION

In valence bond theory, the two bonding electrons are assumed to be localized between the two atomic nuclei. However, **molecular orbital theory** states that the electrons are delocalized across the entire molecule in an electron cloud. Even though molecular orbital theory is a more accurate representation of molecular bonding, it is harder to visualize than the valence bond theory. Therefore, both are still used.

METALLIC BONDING AND SEMICONDUCTORS

Metallic bonding occurs between two or more metal atoms. The best way to visualize this is to think of positively charged metals held together by a "sea" of delocalized electrons. Band theory helps determine if metals are conductors, semiconductors, or insulators based on the occupied and unoccupied orbitals. The occupied molecular orbitals contain valence electrons and, thus when combined, are called the valence band. The unoccupied molecular orbitals are higher in energy and are called the conduction band. The smaller the band gap between the valence band and the conduction band, the easier it is to conduct electricity. When the conduction band is easily accessible, the electrons can easily flow across the entire molecule (the electrons are delocalized). Therefore, conductors have no or very little band gap, semiconductors have a small band gap, and insulators have a large band gap, as shown in Figure 15.3.

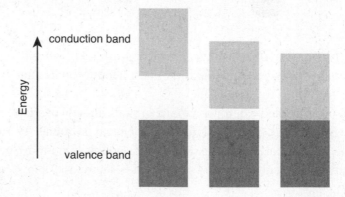

Figure 15.3. There are three general types of metals: insulators (left), semiconductors (middle), and conductors (right). These different properties arise from the band gap between the valence band and the conduction band.

Introduction to Chemical Reactions

16

Atoms and molecules are too small for the naked eye to see. When a chemical reaction occurs, though, there are visible signs that a reaction took place. For example, the formation of a gas when baking soda reacts with vinegar is a visible clue that a reaction occurred. Other signs that indicate a chemical reaction occurred are color changes, formation of a solid (precipitation), emission of light, and emission or absorption of heat. Part of understanding chemical reactions is writing and balancing equations.

WRITING AND BALANCING REACTIONS

A chemical equation is a mathematical representation of a chemical reaction that expresses the *identities* and *quantities* of the substances involved in the reaction. Atomic symbols are used to represent the atoms or molecules reacting and being produced. The phases are represented by using the following abbreviations: (s) for solid, (l) for liquid, (g) for gas, and (aq) for aqueous.

➡ **Example** _____

Write a balanced chemical equation for an aqueous solution containing potassium bromide and lead(II) nitrate that react to form solid lead(II) bromide and aqueous potassium nitrate.

Solution

(STEP 1) Use symbols to represent each cation, anion, and polyatomic ion found in the reaction:

Name of Cation, Anion, or Polyatomic Ion	Symbol and Charge of Cation, Anion, or Polyatomic Ion
Potassium	K^+
Bromide	Br^-
Lead(II)	Pb^{2+}
Nitrate	NO_3^-

(STEP 2) Balance the charges within each compound using the smallest ratios possible.

Potassium bromide is formed from K^+ and Br^-. One of each ion is needed to form a neutral compound: KBr.

Lead(II) nitrate is formed from Pb^{2+} and NO_3^-. One Pb^{2+} and two NO_3^- are needed to form a neutral compound: $Pb(NO_3)_2$.

Lead(II) bromide is formed from Pb^{2+} and Br^-. One Pb^{2+} and two Br^- are needed to form a neutral compound: $PbBr_2$.

Potassium nitrate is formed from K^+ and NO_3^-. One of each is needed to form a neutral compound: KNO_3. Note that parentheses are not needed if only one polyatomic ion is present.

STEP 3 Write the reactants on the left and the products on the right with their respective phases:

$$KBr(aq) + Pb(NO_3)_2(aq) \rightarrow PbBr_2(s) + KNO_3(aq)$$

STEP 4 Use coefficients to balance the number of atoms. There is one Br on the left side and two Br on the right side. To balance this, put a coefficient of 2 in front of KBr. Do NOT put KBr_2 because that is not a neutral compound:

$$2KBr(aq) + Pb(NO_3)_2(aq) \rightarrow PbBr_2(s) + KNO_3(aq)$$

Now there are two K on the reactant side and only one K on the product side. So place a 2 in front of KNO_3:

$$2KBr(aq) + Pb(NO_3)_2(aq) \rightarrow PbBr_2(s) + 2KNO_3(aq)$$

STEP 5 Check and double-check that all cations, anions, and polyatomic ions are balanced on both sides of the equation:

Reactant Side	$\rightarrow$	Product Side
2K	$\rightarrow$	2K
2Br	$\rightarrow$	2Br
1Pb	$\rightarrow$	1Pb
$2NO_3$	$\rightarrow$	$2NO_3$

The charges are balanced within each compound, the number of ions is balanced on each side of the chemical reaction, and the phases are included. This is a balanced chemical equation for the chemical reaction.

TYPES OF REACTIONS

There are four main classes of chemical reactions—synthesis (combination), decomposition, single displacement, and double displacement. In synthesis reactions, atoms or molecules combine to form a more complex compound. A decomposition reaction is the reverse. Single displacement reactions have one element displacing another. In double displacement reactions, both elements (either a single element or a group of elements) are exchanged. The general format and an example of each type of reaction is summarized in Table 16.1.

Table 16.1. Four Types of Chemical Reactions

Type of Reaction	General Format	Example
Synthesis (combination)	$A + B \rightarrow AB$	$CaO(s) + CO_2(g) \rightarrow CaCO_3(s)$
Decomposition	$AB \rightarrow A + B$	$2KClO_3(s) \rightarrow 2KCl(s) + O_2(g)$
Single Displacement	$A + BC \rightarrow AC + B$	$Zn(s) + CuCl_2(aq) \rightarrow ZnCl_2(aq) + Cu(s)$
Double Displacement	$AB + CD \rightarrow AD + CB$	$CaCl_2(aq) + Li_2SO_4(aq) \rightarrow CaSO_4(s) + 2LiCl(aq)$

REACTION STOICHIOMETRY

In chemical reactions, specific ratios of compounds are required to react and produce a product. An analogy can be drawn with cooking and following a recipe. For example, in order to make 3 pancakes, you need 1 cup of flour and 2 eggs:

$$1 \text{ cup flour} + 2 \text{ eggs} \rightarrow 3 \text{ pancakes}$$

To make 6 pancakes, double the amount of flour (2 cups flour) and eggs (4 eggs). Chemical reactions are similar in that specific ratios of reactants are required to form the end product(s). In the balanced chemical equation below, the reactant to product ratios are 1 mole HCl to 1 mole NaOH to 1 mole NaCl to 1 mole H_2O:

$$HCl(aq) + NaOH(aq) \rightarrow NaCl(aq) + H_2O(l)$$

In other words, for every 1 mole of HCl, 1 mole of NaOH is needed to react to form 1 mole of NaCl and 1 mole of H_2O. If, instead, there are 2 moles of HCl, then 2 moles of NaOH are needed to react completely with all of the HCl. By using the factor-label method, this can easily be seen:

$$2 \text{ mol HCl} \cdot \frac{1 \text{ mol NaOH}}{1 \text{ mol HCl}} = 2 \text{ mol NaOH}$$

The ratio of 1 mole of NaOH per 1 mole HCl is taken from the balanced chemical equation. In the example above, mol HCl is divided by mol HCl and therefore cancels out, leaving only mol NaOH as the remaining unit. The factor-label method is very useful when the mole to mole ratios are not 1:1. For example, look at the following balanced combustion reaction:

$$2C_2H_6(g) + 7O_2(g) \rightarrow 4CO_2(g) + 6H_2O(l)$$

In this reaction, every 2 moles of C_2H_6 produces 6 moles of H_2O. If 0.158 moles of C_2H_6 completely react, how many moles of H_2O will be produced? To determine this amount, use the factor-label method and the balanced chemical equation:

$$0.158 \text{ mol } C_2H_6 \cdot \frac{6 \text{ mol } H_2O}{2 \text{ mol } C_2H_6} = 0.474 \text{ mol } H_2O$$

There will be 0.474 moles H_2O produced if all 0.158 moles of C_2H_6 react.

LIMITING REACTANTS, THEORETICAL YIELD, AND PERCENT YIELD

Let's go back to the pancake example to define liming reactants. If there are 5 cups of flour and 6 eggs, how many pancakes can be made?

$$1 \text{ cup flour} + 2 \text{ eggs} \rightarrow 3 \text{ pancakes}$$

To figure out how many pancakes can be made, determine which ingredient will run out first, flour or eggs:

$$5 \text{ cups flour} \cdot \frac{3 \text{ pancakes}}{1 \text{ cup flour}} = 15 \text{ pancakes}$$

$$6 \text{ eggs} \cdot \frac{3 \text{ pancakes}}{2 \text{ eggs}} = 9 \text{ pancakes}$$

We learn that 6 eggs can be used to make 9 pancakes and that 5 cups of flour can be used to make 15 pancakes. So unless we get more eggs, we can make only 9 pancakes. Therefore, eggs are the *limiting reactant*, which makes the least amount of product. If all 6 eggs are used (none were broken in the process), then ideally 9 pancakes can be made. This is the *theoretical yield*, which is the amount of product made based on the limiting reactant. Even though 9 pancakes can be made with the ingredients available, let's say that 1 pancake is burned in the process. This means only 8 edible pancakes are actually made. To calculate the percent yield, take the actual amount produced divided by the theoretical amount and multiply by 100:

$$\frac{8 \text{ pancakes}}{9 \text{ pancakes}} \cdot 100 = 88.9\% \text{ yield}$$

Now apply this method to chemical equations.

➡ **Example** _____

What is the limiting reactant if 1.63 moles of Cr and 1.35 moles of O_2 react together? What is the percent yield if 104.6 g of Cr_2O_3 are produced? The balanced chemical equation is:

$$4Cr(s) + 3O_2(g) \rightarrow 2Cr_2O_3(s)$$

Solution

First, determine the amount of product that can be made with 1.63 moles of Cr:

$$1.63 \text{ mol Cr} \cdot \frac{2 \text{ mol Cr}_2O_3}{4 \text{ mol Cr}} \cdot \frac{151.99 \text{ g Cr}_2O_3}{1 \text{ mol Cr}_2O_3} = 123.9 \text{ g Cr}_2O_3$$

Then use a similar calculation to determine the amount of product that can be made with 1.35 moles of O_2:

$$1.35 \text{ mol O}_2 \cdot \frac{2 \text{ mol Cr}_2O_3}{3 \text{ mol O}_2} \cdot \frac{151.99 \text{ g Cr}_2O_3}{1 \text{ mol Cr}_2O_3} = 136.8 \text{ g Cr}_2O_3$$

In this scenario, Cr is the limiting reagent, which means the theoretical yield is 123.9 g Cr_2O_3. To calculate the percent yield, divide the actual amount produced (104.6 g Cr_2O_3) by the theoretical yield (123.9 g Cr_2O_3) and multiply by 100:

$$\frac{104.6 \text{ g Cr}_2O_3}{123.9 \text{ g Cr}_2O_3} \cdot 100 = 84.4\% \text{ yield}$$

The Gas Phase of Matter

17

██

PRESSURE

Pressure is defined as the number of collisions among gas molecules and surrounding surfaces. Another way to explain pressure is the force of gas molecules that results from collisions over a certain area. The greater the force in a smaller area, the higher the pressure:

$$\text{Pressure} = \frac{\text{Force}}{\text{Area}}$$

Table 17.1 lists common units for measuring pressure.

Table 17.1 Common Units of Pressure

1 atmosphere (atm)* = 760 torr
1 atm = 760 mmHg
1 atm = 14.7 pounds per square inch (psi)
1 torr = 1 mmHg
1 pascal = 1 newton per square meter (N/m²)

*Atmospheric pressure is based on the average pressure at sea level.

SIMPLE GAS LAWS

The **simple gas laws** relate two of the four common measurable properties of gases: pressure (P), volume (V), temperature (T), and/or moles (n).

When temperature and number of moles are constant, **Boyle's law** shows the inverse relationship between pressure and volume. As pressure increases, volume decreases. As volume increases, pressure decreases. When comparing the same substance under changing pressure and volume conditions, Boyle's law states:

$$P_1 V_1 = P_2 V_2$$

In the formula, P_1 and V_1 are the pressure and volume, respectively, for one condition, and P_2 and V_2 are the pressure and volume, respectively, for the second condition.

When pressure and number of moles are constant, **Charles's law** shows the direct relationship between temperature and volume. As temperature increases, so does the volume. As temperature decreases, so does the volume. When comparing the same substance under changing volume and temperature conditions, Charles's law states:

$$\frac{V_1}{T_1} = \frac{V_2}{T_2}$$

In the formula, V_1 and T_1 are the volume and temperature (in kelvins), respectively, for one condition, and V_2 and T_2 are the volume and temperature (in kelvins), respectively, for the second condition.

➡ Example

A balloon expands from 1.80 L to 2.10 L when initially at 23.5°C. What is the final temperature of the gas in °C?

Solution

Recognize that only volume and temperature are changing. Charles's law shows the relationship for two sets of conditions where only volume and temperature (in kelvin) are changing:

$$\frac{V_1}{T_1} = \frac{V_2}{T_2}$$

You are given $V_1 = 1.80$ L, $T_1 = 23.5°C + 273.15 = 296.65K$, and $V_2 = 2.10$ L. Plug these into the equation and solve for T_2:

$$\frac{1.80 \text{ L}}{296.65K} = \frac{2.10 \text{ L}}{T_2}$$

$$T_2 = \frac{(2.10 \text{ L})(296.65K)}{1.80 \text{ L}} = 346.\underline{09}K$$

Now convert back to °C:

$$346.\underline{09}K - 273.15 = 72.\underline{94}°C = 73°C$$

When temperature and pressure are held constant, **Avogadro's law** states that the volume and number of moles for a substance are directly proportional. As one doubles, so does the other. For example, when inflating a balloon, the volume doubles as the amount of gas molecules inside doubles. The relationship between temperature and the number of moles can be expressed as:

$$\frac{V_1}{n_1} = \frac{V_2}{n_2}$$

In the equation, V_1 and n_1 are the volume and number of moles, respectively, for one condition, and V_2 and n_2 are the volume and number of moles, respectively, for the second condition.

The **combined gas law** combines Boyle's and Charles's laws. If the number of moles of a substance is constant, the pressure, volume, and temperature (in kelvin) are related:

$$\frac{P_1 V_1}{T_1} = \frac{P_2 V_2}{T_2}$$

In this equation, the subscript 1 designates one condition and the subscript 2 designates the second condition.

DERIVATION AND USE OF THE IDEAL GAS LAW

When all three gas laws are combined, it forms the *ideal gas law* equation:

$$PV = nRT$$

In the ideal gas law, R is a universal constant where $R = 0.0821 \dfrac{\text{L} \cdot \text{atm}}{\text{K} \cdot \text{mol}}$. This equation assumes that gases behave ideally, which means the gas molecules are far enough apart that there are no interactions among them. At standard temperature (273K) and pressure (1 atm) for 1 mole of gas, the volume of 1 mole of gas can be calculated from the ideal gas law equation:

$$V_{\text{gas}} = \frac{(1 \text{ mol gas})\left(0.0821 \dfrac{\text{L} \cdot \text{atm}}{\text{K} \cdot \text{mol}}\right)(273\text{K})}{1 \text{ atm}} = 22.4 \text{ L}$$

This conversion factor (22.4 L gas per 1 mole gas) can be used if the substance is a gas and if the conditions are at STP (standard temperature and pressure).

DALTON'S LAW OF PARTIAL PRESSURES

Dalton's law of partial pressures states that the sum of the partial pressures of each gas component in a mixture is the total gas pressure of the mixture:

$$P_{\text{total}} = P_a + P_b + P_c + \ldots$$

In this formula, P_a, P_b, P_c, etc. are the partial pressures of individual gases (and only gases). To calculate the partial pressures of, for example, gas A:

$$P_a = \frac{\text{pressure of gas molecule } A}{\text{total pressure of all gas molecules in the reaction}}$$

Make sure the pressures of gases (both on top and bottom of the fraction) are in the same units.

KINETIC-MOLECULAR THEORY OF GASES

The kinetic-molecular theory is used to simplify the understanding of gas molecules. This theory states the following.

1. Gas molecules do not interact; they only collide.
2. There is a lot of empty space between gas molecules; the space a gas molecule occupies is negligible in comparison to the container.
3. The average kinetic energy (motion) of the gas molecules depends on only temperature (in kelvin).

Using these assumptions, this theory makes several predictions about basic gas molecule behavior.

1. Gases are compressible.
2. Gases fill the shape and volume of the container.
3. Gases have low densities.

Condensed Phases of Matter

18

TYPES OF INTERMOLECULAR FORCES

Intermolecular forces are an important part of chemistry that influence how molecules interact. These forces affect boiling points, melting points, and viscosity. Intermolecular forces are the attractions among *two or more* molecules. Do not confuse *inter*molecular forces with *intra*molecular bonds, which are bonds within *one* molecule (i.e., ionic or covalent). Instead, intermolecular forces look at how electron density around molecules affects the physical and chemical properties of those molecules. London dispersion force (a type of van der Waals force) is an attractive force found among all molecules and atoms, both nonpolar and polar. Recall that electrons are delocalized across a molecule or atom. This means that in any one instant, there might be a side of the molecule or atom that has a slightly higher electron density than the other. This causes the molecule or atom to have in an instance where it has a dipole moment. The larger the surface area of a molecule, the stronger the London dispersion force.

There are multiple types of intermolecular forces. However, the basics can be understood if the naming of the intermolecular forces are explained. Induced dipoles describe nonpolar molecules that are somehow being "forced" into a dipole moment from another molecule. Permanent dipoles occur within a polar molecule, where there are slightly positive and slightly negative charges (dipole) that stay on atoms within the molecule. If there is a mixture of polar and nonpolar molecules, then there will be dipole-induced dipole interactions among the polar molecules (dipole) and nonpolar molecules (induced dipole).

Dipole-dipole forces occur among two or more polar molecules. When a polar molecule comes near another polar molecule, the slightly negative charge on one molecule is attracted to the slightly positive charge on the other. Hydrogen bonding, as shown in Figure 18.1, is a special case of dipole-dipole interactions where there is a slightly positive charge on a hydrogen interacting with a slightly negative charge on a nitrogen, oxygen, or fluorine (NOF). Hydrogen bonding occurs between a H and only a N, O, or F.

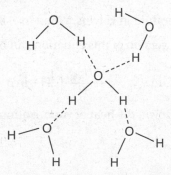

Figure 18.1. Hydrogen bonding among water molecules. Hydrogen bonding (dotted lines) is an intermolecular force that can occur among atoms that have a H attached to a N, O, or F, only. The solid O–H bonds are **covalent** bonds.

Ions can also participate in intermolecular forces. If an ion is interacting with a polar molecule, this is an ion-dipole interaction. For example, when a salt is dissolved in water, the salt splits into ions and interacts with the polar water molecules instead. If the ion is interacting with a nonpolar molecule, this is an ion-induced dipole interaction.

PROPERTIES OF CONDENSED PHASES

Condensed phases (that is, the liquid and solid phases) have macroscopic physical properties that are influenced by intermolecular interactions. Examples of these properties include surface tension, melting point, boiling point, vapor pressure, and viscosity.

Surface tension is the amount of energy required to increase the surface area by a certain amount. When surface tension is present, molecules inside and not at the surface are more stable due to the neighboring molecules with which the interior molecules have to interact. Therefore, the substance tries to decrease the surface's area as much as possible. This creates surface tension. In general, the stronger the intermolecular attraction, the higher the surface tension.

When enough energy is added to a solid, the molecules break free and start to move around in a liquid state. This is called the *melting point*. The heat of fusion, ΔH_{fusion}, is the amount of energy needed to melt 1 mole of a specific substance. Another similar property is *boiling point*, which occurs when the external atmospheric pressure is equal to the vapor pressure. At this point, the molecules in the liquid phase are able to escape into the gaseous phase. More specifically, the *normal boiling point* is the boiling point of a liquid at 1 atm. This means at a minimum, the vapor pressure has to be 1 atm. The heat of vaporization, ΔH_{vap}, is the amount of energy needed to vaporize 1 mole of a specific substance.

Another property of condensed phases is vapor pressure. *Vapor pressure* is the amount of pressure exerted on a solution due to the escaping gaseous molecules. If the boiling point of a solution is low, it is easier for the liquid molecules to escape into the gaseous phase. The result is a high vapor pressure. The opposite is also true; a high boiling point means a low vapor pressure. This occurs because as the intermolecular force increases, the number of molecules escaping into the gas phase decreases, resulting in a lower vapor pressure. The Clausius-Claperyron equation relates the effects of temperature changes on vapor pressure:

$$\ln \frac{P_2}{P_1} = \frac{-\Delta H_{vap}}{R}\left(\frac{1}{T_2} - \frac{1}{T_1}\right)$$

In this equation, P is pressure, R is the gas constant $8.314 \frac{J}{mol \cdot K}$, ΔH_{vap} is enthalpy (heat) of vaporization, and T is temperature in kelvins. When $\ln P$ is plotted on the y-axis and $\frac{1}{T}$ is plotted on the x-axis, the linear version of this equation can be determined:

$$\ln P_{vap} = \frac{-\Delta H_{vap}}{R}\left(\frac{1}{T}\right) + \ln \beta$$

If the slope of the equation is known, the heat of vaporization can be calculated.

Calculate the heat of vaporization based on the given data.

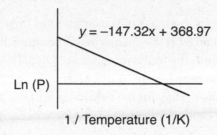

$$y = -147.32x + 368.97$$

Ln (P)

1 / Temperature (1/K)

Solution

When the axes are ln P and 1/temperature (in kelvin), the slope of the line equals $\dfrac{-\Delta H_{vap}}{R}$.

In this equation, R is 8.314 $\dfrac{J}{mol \cdot K}$. Plug in the values and solve for ΔH_{vap}:

$$-147.32 = \frac{-\Delta H_{vap}}{8.314 \text{ J/mol}}$$

$$-\Delta H_{vap} = -147.32(8.314 \text{ J/mol})$$

$$\Delta H_{vap} = 1,224 \text{ J} = 1.224 \text{ kJ}$$

Condensed phases also have viscosity, which measures the resistance to flow. Viscosity increases with stronger intermolecular forces and with bulkiness.

PHASE DIAGRAMS

Phase diagrams show the relationship between pressure and temperature with the phases of a substance. The solid lines are phase boundaries where the two touching phases are in equilibrium. For example, if the solid line is separating a solid and a liquid, the temperatures and pressures along that line will be various melting points for that substance. There is one place on the diagram where all three phases touch and the lines intersect. This is called the *triple point* and is where a substance can exist as a solid, liquid, and gas at that particular temperature and pressure. There is also a *critical point*, which occurs at the end of a phase boundary. More specifically, the critical point usually occurs at the end of a liquid-gas phase boundary, where the liquid and gas densities are the same. This causes both to coexist as a supercritical fluid instead of a liquid and a gas in equilibrium. The temperature and pressure at the critical point are the critical temperature (T_c) and critical pressure (P_c).

HEATING AND COOLING CURVES

Heating and cooling curves are designed to help visualize the addition or removal of heat from a specific compound or solution. Figure 18.2 shows water starting as a solid, melting into a liquid, and lastly evaporating into a gas. The type of equation used to calculate the amount of energy needed to heat or cool a substance varies based on if there was a temperature change and whether or not the substance undergoes a phase change. Going from left to right in Figure 18.2, water in the solid form starts at –5°C and warms up to 0°C. Since no phase change occurs during this portion of the graph, the following equation is used to find the amount of heat used:

$$q = mC_s\Delta T$$

In this equation, q is heat, m is the mass of the compound in grams, C_s is the specific heat capacity for the compound, and ΔT is the change in temperature. Remember that ΔT is always the final temperature (T_f) minus the initial temperature (T_i). The specific heat capacity is the amount of energy required to heat 1 gram of the substance by 1°C. The specific heat capacity is a constant that varies depending on the substance and the phase of the substance. For Figure 18.2, the specific heat capacity of ice is needed for the change in heat from –5°C to 0°C.

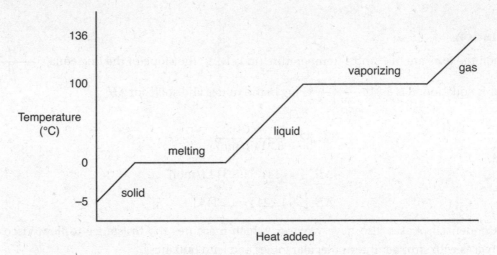

Figure 18.2. Heating curve for water heated from –5°C to 136°C. Water starts off as ice at –5°C. The water is then heated to 0°C, where it begins to melt. The water is further heated until the liquid vaporizes into gas at 100°C. Then the gas reaches a final temperature of 136°C.

Once the solid has been heated to 0°C, it begins to melt. During the phase change from solid to liquid, a separate equation must be used to calculate the amount of heat used during this process:

$$q = n\Delta H_{\text{fusion}}$$

In this equation, n is the number of moles of substance and ΔH_{fusion} is the heat of fusion (melting) for 1 mole of substance. ΔH_{fusion} can also be used for freezing, but the sign will have to be changed. The same amount of heat is released during freezing as is absorbed during melting. If the phase change is from a liquid to a gas, then the necessary equation is very similar:

$$q = n\Delta H_{\text{vap}}$$

In this equation, n is the number of moles of substance and ΔH_{vap} is the heat of vaporization for 1 mole of substance. Again, ΔH_{vap} is positive for vaporization and is negative for condensation.

The process repeats at different points throughout the heating curve. Any time there is a temperature change, the specific heat equation should be used ($q = mC_s\Delta T$). Don't forget to use the correct specific heat constant! Any time there is a phase change, use the correct ΔH equation.

➦ Example _____

How much heat is required to heat 2.47 g of ice from –9°C to 83°C? Use Figure 18.2 as a visual if needed.

Solution

STEP 1 Calculate the amount of heat needed to heat ice from –9°C to 0°C. The specific heat of ice is 2.06 J/mol · °C:

$$q = mC_s\Delta T$$

$$q = (2.47\ g)\left(\frac{2.06\ J}{mol \cdot °C}\right)(0°C - (-9°C))$$

$$q = 45.8\ J$$

STEP 2 Calculate the amount of heat needed to melt ice. The $\Delta H_{fusion} = 6.02$ kJ/mol:

$$q = n\Delta H_{fusion}$$

$$2.47\ g\ H_2O \cdot \frac{1\ mol\ H_2O}{18.0\ g\ H_2O} = 0.137\ mol\ H_2O$$

$$q = (0.137\ mol)\left(\frac{6.02\ kJ}{mol}\right) = 0.825\ kJ = 825\ J$$

STEP 3 Calculate the amount of heat needed to heat liquid water from 0°C to 83°C. The specific heat of liquid water is 4.18 J/mol · °C:

$$q = mC_s\Delta T$$

$$q = (2.47\ g)\left(\frac{4.18\ J}{mol \cdot °C}\right)(83°C - 0°C)$$

$$q = 857\ J$$

STEP 4 Add the results from all the steps to calculate the total amount of heat required to heat ice from –9°C to 83°C:

$$\text{step 1 + step 2 + step 3 = total energy needed}$$

$$45.8\ J + 825\ J + 857\ J = 1,727.8\ J = 1.728\ kJ$$

Therefore, 1.728 kJ of heat is needed to heat ice from –9°C to 83°C.

CRYSTAL STRUCTURES

Compounds can crystallize in a small, repeating pattern. The smallest repeatable portion of a crystalline lattice is called the *unit cell*. There are three main types of unit cells that can form depending on the compound: simple cubic, body centered, and face centered.

A simple cubic unit cell packs in a way where there is an atom at each corner of the cube and only 1/8 of each atom is inside the cube. This means a lattice that has a simple cubic unit cell has one full atom per unit cell. (There are 8 corners in a cube and 1 atom is at each corner: $1/8 \times 8$ atoms = 1 atom.) A body-centered cubic unit cell is like a simple cubic unit but has another atom in the center of the cube. Therefore, the body-centered cubic unit cell contains 2 atoms: $1/8 \times 8$ corners = 1 atom + 1 atom in the very center. A face-centered cubic unit cell is like a simple cubic unit but has another 1/2 atom at each face (side) of the cube. This means a face-centered cubic unit cell contains 4 atoms: 1/8 atom × 8 corners = 1 atom and 1/2 atom × 6 sides = 3 atoms, giving a total of 4 atoms. The packing efficiency increases when the number of atoms packed inside each unit cell increases. Table 18.1 gives more details about the three different types of unit cells.

Table 18.1. Unit Cells

Unit Cell Type	Number of Atoms in Unit Cell	Edge Length of Cell in Terms of Atomic Radius (*r*)	Pictorial Representation
Simple Cubic	1 atom There are 8 atoms located at each corner with 1/8 of each atom INSIDE the unit cell.	$l = 2r$	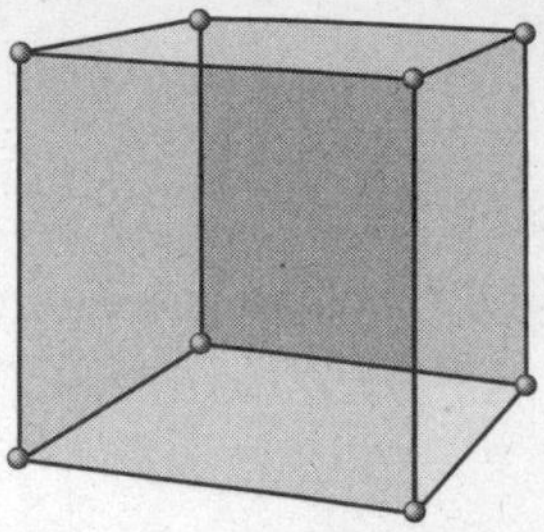
Body Centered	2 atoms There are 8 atoms located at each corner with 1/8 of each atom INSIDE the unit cell + 1 atom in the middle.	$l = \dfrac{4r}{\sqrt{3}}$	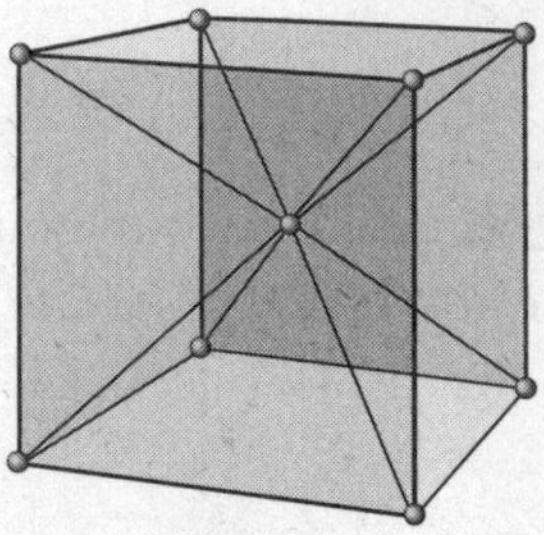
Face Centered	4 atoms There are 8 atoms located at each corner with 1/8 of each atom INSIDE the unit cell + 6 atoms located at each side with 1/2 of each atom INSIDE the unit cell.	$l = 2r\sqrt{2}$	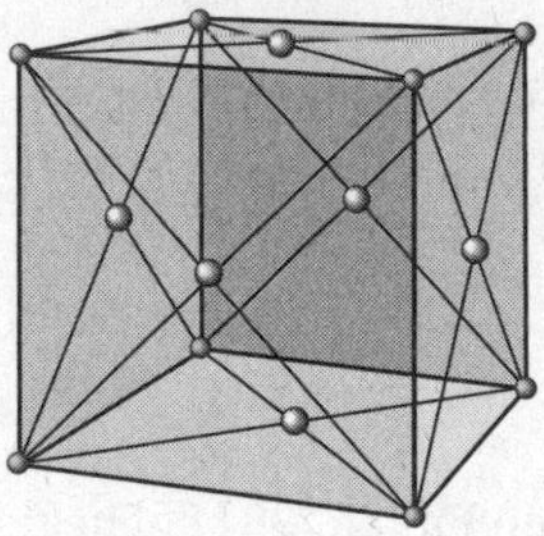

Solution Chemistry 19

CONCENTRATIONS AND UNITS

A solution is a homogenous mixture where the **solvent** is the compound in excess and the **solute** is the compound in lesser amount. More specifically, aqueous solutions are solutions with water as the solvent. There are various ways to measure the amount of solute and solvent (or concentration) in a solution: molarity, molality, mass percent, volume percent, mole fraction, and parts per million (ppm) are just a few. The following gives the definitions and formulas for the various ways to calculate the concentration of a solution.

$$M \text{ (molarity)} = \frac{\text{moles of solute}}{\text{liters of solution}}$$

When calculating molarity, the liters of solution include the volume of both the solute and the solvent.

$$m \text{ (molality)} = \frac{\text{moles of solute}}{\text{kg of solvent}}$$

In contrast to molarity (M), molality (m) includes only the solvent in the denominator. This means the mass of the solute has to be subtracted from the mass of the solution to get the mass of the solvent alone (mass of solvent = mass of solution – mass of solute).

$$\text{Mass percent} = \frac{\text{mass of solute}}{\text{mass of solution}} \cdot 100$$

When calculating the mass percent, the units for mass of solute and mass of solution do not matter as long as they are in the *same* units.

$$\text{Volume percent} = \frac{\text{volume of solute}}{\text{volume of solution}} \cdot 100$$

Again, the units for volume of solute and volume of solution do not matter as long as they are in the *same* units.

$$\text{mole fraction of solute } (X_{\text{solute}}) = \frac{\text{moles of solute}}{\text{moles of solute} + \text{moles of solvent}} \cdot 100$$

$$\text{PPM (parts per million)} = \frac{\text{mass of solute}}{\text{mass of solution}} \times 10^6$$

Parts per million is sometimes a hard concept to grasp. One way to approach ppm is to compare it to percent. Percent means how much is there in a cent, where cent means 100. Using ppm is similar. Instead of comparing the amount to 100, you are seeing how much there is in

1 million (10^6). To convert a number into percent, the number is multiplied by 100. To change a number into ppm, it is multiplied by 10^6.

Certain terms can be used to describe the general concentration of a solute in a solution. If a solution is **saturated**, the maximum amount of solute that can be dissolved without causing precipitation has been reached. This means if any more solute is added, the solute will start precipitating out. Once solute is precipitating out of solution, the solution is **supersaturated**. An **unsaturated** solution is when there is solute dissolved in solution but more solute can easily be added without precipitation.

Sometimes a solution has too much solute and needs to be diluted. When a solution is diluted, the number of moles of solute stays the same. The following formula relates the volume and concentration of the undiluted solution to that of the diluted solution.

$$C_1 V_1 = C_2 V_2$$

In the formula, C_1 and C_2 are the concentrations of the original and diluted solution, respectively, and V_1 and V_2 are the FINAL volumes that correspond to the original and diluted solution, respectively.

➡ Example

What is the final concentration of a 1.7 M solution after a 1:15 dilution?

Solution

First, it's necessary to understand what a 1:15 dilution means. This means 1 part of the original solution was diluted to 15 parts. The word "parts" can be any volumetric unit (mL, L, uL, etc.) as long as they are the same. For example, 1 mL of 1.7 M solution could have been diluted to 15 mL. Alternatively, 1 L of 1.7 M solution could have been diluted to 15 L. It doesn't matter which volumetric unit is used as long as they are the same. Now let's use mL and plug the numbers into the dilution equation:

$$C_1 V_1 = C_2 V_2$$

$$(1.7\ M)(1\ \text{mL}) = (C_2)(15\ \text{mL})$$

$$C_2 = \frac{(1.7\ M)(1\ \text{mL})}{15\ \text{mL}} = 0.11\ \text{M}$$

Solubility and Precipitation (K_{sp})

K_{sp} is the equilibrium solubility for the maximum amount of a solute that can dissolve in a solvent at a certain temperature—the higher the K_{sp} number, the more soluble the compound (*see Chapter 21 for more information on equilibrium*). Some compounds ionize very easily in water, such as NaCl. Other compounds may be only slightly soluble, such as CaF_2. To write a K_{sp} expression, include only the products since the reactant is a solid and solids are not included in equilibrium reactions. Note that the square brackets indicate the concentration of a particular ion.

$$CaF_2(s) \rightleftharpoons Ca^{2+}(aq) + 2F^-(aq)$$

$$K_{sp} = [Ca^{2+}][F^-]^2$$

The solubility of a solid can be expressed in terms of **molar solubility** (S), which is the molar concentration of solute dissolved in solution before the solute starts precipitating. Using the same equilibrium equation from page 154, the K_{sp} equation in terms of molar solubility can be expressed as shown here:

$$K_{sp} = [S][2S]^2$$

Since there are 2 F^- for every 1 Cu^{2+}, the molar solubility of F^- is $2s$ and Ca^{2+} is $1s$.

Sometimes solubility deals with how soluble a gas is in solution, such as carbon dioxide in soda. The solubility of that gas can be calculated using Henry's law.

$$S_{gas} = k_H P_{gas}$$

In this equation, S_{gas} is the solubility of a gas, k_H is Henry's law constant, and P_{gas} is the partial pressure of a gas (*see Chapter 17*).

Factors that affect the solubility of either a compound into solution or a gas into solution are concentration of solute (including common ion effect), temperature, and pressure (Henry's law). If the concentration of the solute particles is lower than the molar solubility, more solute can still dissolve in solution. If another salt is added to a solution that has the same ion, the solubility of the original solute decreases. For example, adding NaF to a solution that already contains CaF_2 decreases the solubility of CaF_2. This is due to Le Châtelier's principle (*see Chapter 21*), where an increase in concentration of a product ion (F^-) shifts the equilibrium toward the reactants (CaF_2). Temperature also affects the solubility of a solute—as temperature increases, the amount of solid that can dissolve also increases. When it comes to the solubility of gases, an increase in pressure forces more gas to stay dissolved in solution.

When solutions are **miscible**, two solutions make a homogenous mixture. For example, vinegar is miscible in water but oil is not. This is due to intermolecular forces. When different molecules have similar intermolecular forces (and therefore polarity), they are miscible, such as vinegar and water. However, if one is polar and the other is not, such as water and oil, the solutions will stay as two separate layers (immiscible). A general saying that describes if a solution is miscible in another solution or not is "like dissolves like." As long as the two solutions are similar with respect to types of intermolecular forces, the solutions will most likely be miscible.

COLLIGATIVE PROPERTIES OF SOLUTIONS

Colligative properties, such as vapor pressure, depend on only the number of particles and not the identity of those particles. To determine how many particles or ions are in a solution, you first have to identify if the compound is an electrolyte or a nonelectrolyte.

Electrolytes are substances that dissociate into ions when placed into water. **Strong electrolytes** dissociate **completely** in water (i.e., salts, strong acids, and strong bases). When compounds partially dissociate into ions when placed into water but do not dissociate completely, they are **weak electrolytes** (i.e., weak acids and weak bases). **Nonelectrolytes** do not break up into ions at all when placed into water. These particles can still dissolve in water, but they do not form ions in the process. For example, sugar dissolves in water. However, it is breaking down into individual sugar molecules instead of staying grouped together in a sugar cube. Nonelectrolytes are usually comprised of only covalent bonds.

The following properties are affected by the number of particles dissolved in solution: vapor pressure lowering, boiling point elevation, freezing point depression, and osmotic pressure. Recall that vapor pressure is the pressure of the gaseous form of a compound on the liquid form in a closed container. According to **Raoult's law**, the vapor pressure of a solvent is lowered as shown in the following formula.

$$P_{\text{solvent}} = X_{\text{solvent}} P°_{\text{solvent}}$$

In the equation, P_{solvent} is the vapor pressure of solvent in the solution, X_{solvent} is the mole fraction of solvent in the solution, and $P°_{\text{solvent}}$ is the vapor pressure of pure solvent. If there are at least two substances present, the mole fraction is less than 1 and causes the vapor pressure to decrease. Therefore, vapor pressure is lowed when the number of particles dissolved in a solvent increases. This can be further supported by the fact that boiling points of solvents increase, and therefore vapor pressure decreases, when the number of particles dissolved in a solvent increases. The following formula shows how to calculate the increase in boiling point (ΔT_b).

$$\Delta T_b = iK_b m$$

In this equation, ΔT_b is the temperature of the solute/solvent mixture minus the temperature of pure solvent, i is the van 't Hoff factor, K_b is the boiling point elevation constant, and m is the molality of the solute. The van 't Hoff factor can be calculated using the following equation.

$$i = \frac{\text{moles of particles dissociated}}{\text{moles of formula units dissolved}}$$

In general, $i = 1$ for substances that dissolve in water but do not dissociate into ions, i.e., sugar. In addition, i generally equals moles of particles dissociated. For example, $MgCl_2$ has $i = 3$ because $MgCl_2$ dissociates into 1 Mg^{2+} ion and 2 Cl^- ions.

During cold temperatures, it is common to put salt on the roads to help keep water from freezing. This is due to freezing point depression. When the number of particles dissolved or dissociated in water increases, the freezing point decreases. In other words, salt on icy roads makes the ice melt by decreasing the freezing point. To calculate how much the freezing point is lowered, use the following equation.

$$\Delta T_f = iK_f m$$

In this equation, ΔT_f is the temperature of the pure solvent minus the temperature of the solute/solvent mixture, i is the van 't Hoff factor, K_f is the freezing point depression constant, and m is the molality of the solute.

Osmosis is the flow of water from lower-concentrated solutions to higher-concentrated solutions that are separated by a semipermeable membrane. The semipermeable membrane must allow the water to pass through while preventing the solute from passing through. The following equation calculates the pressure associated with the water flow.

$$\Pi = iMRT$$

In this equation, Π is the osmotic pressure or the pressure difference between the two solutions, i is the van 't Hoff factor, M is the molarity of the solute, R is the ideal gas constant 0.0821 atm · L/mol · K, and T is the temperature in kelvins.

In general, the concentration, whether molarity (M) or molality (m), and the number of particles the compounds dissociate into (i) affect the colligative properties—vapor pressure lowering, boiling point elevation, freezing point depression, and osmotic pressure.

Kinetics of Chemical Reactions

20

DEFINITION OF RATES

A **rate** is how fast a reaction occurs with respect to time. A rate has to be measured experimentally. Usually to calculate an **average rate**, specific concentrations at certain time intervals are given, which can be determined from a graph or given from a table.

$$\text{rate} = \frac{\Delta \text{ concentration}}{\Delta \text{ time}}$$

This formula can also be written using the symbol [ ] for concentration in molarity of compound A.

$$\text{rate} = \frac{\Delta[A]}{\Delta \text{ time}}$$

The average rates of reactants and products can all be related by using the following balanced chemical equation.

$$aA + bB \rightarrow cC + dD$$

In this equation, the rate of reactants and products can be found as follows.

$$\text{rate} = -\frac{1}{a}\frac{\Delta[A]}{\Delta t} = -\frac{1}{b}\frac{\Delta[B]}{\Delta t} = \frac{1}{c}\frac{\Delta[C]}{\Delta t} = \frac{1}{d}\frac{\Delta[D]}{\Delta t}$$

The rate is always positive, but reactants decrease over time. Therefore, reactants require a negative sign in front of them to keep the rate positive.

HOW PARTICULATES AFFECT REACTION RATES

In order for a reaction to occur, the reactant particles must do the following:

1. Collide
2. Collide in the correct orientation to break and/or form bonds
3. Collide with enough energy to overcome the activation barrier

There are experimental factors that can be changed to help increase the rate of a reaction. One factor is increasing the concentration of reactants, which increases the chance for reactant molecules to collide. Increasing the temperature also increases the probability for reactant molecules to collide but also helps increase the energy of the molecules to overcome the activation barrier. Lastly, a catalyst can be added to the reaction, where the catalyst effectively lowers the activation barrier making it easier for the reaction to proceed (and thus increasing the rate of reaction).

THE RATE LAW AND REACTANT CONCENTRATION

Rate laws relate the rate of the reaction to the concentration of reactants only (not products). This is because it is assumed that the reaction goes only in the forward direction where reactants go to products and the reverse reaction is negligible.

$$\text{reaction 1: A} \rightarrow \text{B}$$

$$\text{reaction 2: } a\text{A} + b\text{B} \rightarrow c\text{C} + d\text{D}$$

The rate law for reaction 1 is rate = $k[\text{A}]^n$ where k is the rate constant and n is the reactant order. The rate law for reaction 2 is rate = $k[\text{A}]^m[\text{B}]^n$ where m and n are the reactant order for each reactant. Notice that the concentrations of products are not included in the rate law for either reaction. This is because the rate of these reactions depend only on how the reactants collide and react to form products.

REACTION TYPES AND INTEGRATED RATE LAWS

A *zero-order reaction* means that the concentration of the reactant does not affect the rate of the reaction.

$$\text{rate} = k[\text{A}]^0 = k$$

Anything to the 0th power = 1, which means the concentration of [A] has no affect on the rate of the reaction.

For a *first-order reaction*, the concentration of the reactant is directly proportional to the rate of the reaction.

$$\text{rate} = k[\text{A}]^1 = k[\text{A}]$$

If the concentration of A doubles, so does the reaction rate. If the concentration of [A] halves, so does the reaction rate.

For a *second-order reaction*, the rate of the reaction is proportional to the square of the concentration of the reactant.

$$\text{rate} = k[\text{A}]^2$$

In this case, if the concentration of [A] doubles, the reaction rate quadruples ($2^2 = 4$). If the concentration of [A] halves, the reaction rate decreases by $\frac{1}{4}$ because $\left(\frac{1}{2}\right)^2 = \frac{1}{4}$.

The reaction orders of the reactants must be determined experimentally. Typically, this is done by running a set of reaction conditions where one reactant is held constant while the other is varied to see how it affects the overall reaction rate. The overall reaction order is the sum of each reactant order ($m + n + \ldots$).

➡ **Example** _____

What is the overall reaction order for a reaction that has rate = $k[\text{A}]^3[\text{B}]^0[\text{C}]^{\frac{1}{2}}$? What happens to the rate if [A] triples?

Solution

The overall reaction order is the order of each reactant added together: $3 + 0 + 0.5 = 3.5$. (Yes, it is possible to have an overall reaction order of 3.5. The overall reaction order does not need to be a whole number.)

If the concentration of [A] triples and the reactant order is to the 3rd power:

$$[A]^3 = (3)^3 = 27$$

When the concentration of [A] triples, the rate will be 27 times faster than when the reaction had the original concentration of [A].

The rate law can also be expressed in the integrated forms, which show the relationship with rate, concentration, and time in a linear form ($y = mx + b$). For example, the following is the integrated rate law for the 0th order:

$$[A]_t = -kt + [A]_0$$

In this equation, $[A]_t$ is the concentration of A at time t, k is the rate constant, t is time, and $[A]_0$ is the initial concentration of [A]. By plotting $[A]_t$ on the y-axis and plotting t on the x-axis, there will be a linear line with a negative slope ($-k$). The reactant order, rate law, and integrated rate laws for 0th, 1st, and 2nd orders are listed in Table 20.1. The table also includes the half-lives for each reactant order. Half-lives are the amount of time to decrease the concentration of the reactant by half (1/2). For example, if the half-live for compound X is 10 days, then after 10 days, half of compound X will decompose. After another 10 days, another half will decompose.

Table 20.1. An Overview of Zero-, First-, and Second-Order Reactions

Reaction Order	Rate Law	Integrated Rate Law	Half-life
0	$\text{rate} = k[A]_0 = k$	$[A]_t = -kt + [A]_0$	$t_{\frac{1}{2}} = \dfrac{[A]_0}{2k}$
1	$\text{rate} = k[A]^1 = k[A]$	$\ln[A]_t = -kt + \ln[A]_0$ $\ln\dfrac{[A]_t}{[A]_0} = -kt$	$t_{\frac{1}{2}} = \dfrac{0.693}{k}$
2	$\text{rate} = k[A]^2$	$\dfrac{1}{[A]_t} = kt + \dfrac{1}{[A]_0}$	$t_{\frac{1}{2}} = \dfrac{1}{[A]_0 k}$

ARRHENIUS LAW

The rate law shows how the rate is affected by concentration, but it is not obvious how rates are affected by temperature. Experimentally, it can be shown that the rate constant k changes at various temperatures. An equation used to show how temperature affects the rate is the Arrhenius equation.

$$k = Ae^{-E_a/RT}$$

In the Arrhenius equation, k is the rate constant, A is the frequency factor (constant), e is the base for natural logarithms, E_a is the activation energy (or the minimum energy required for a reaction to occur), R is the gas constant $8.314 \ \dfrac{J}{mol \cdot K}$, and T is the absolute temperature in kelvins. The linear version of this equation can also be written.

$$\ln k = \frac{-E_a}{R}\left(\frac{1}{T}\right) + \ln A$$

A plot of $\ln k$ on the y-axis versus $\dfrac{1}{T}$ on the x-axis gives a slope equal to $\dfrac{-E_a}{R}$ and a y-intercept of $\ln A$. If the concentration of A is not known, the rate of the reaction can be measured at two different temperatures to calculate E_a.

$$\ln \frac{k_2}{k_1} = \frac{-E_a}{R}\left(\frac{1}{T_2} - \frac{1}{T_1}\right) = \frac{E_a}{R}\left(\frac{1}{T_1} - \frac{1}{T_2}\right)$$

The activation barrier is a crucial step that has to be overcome in order for reactions to go to completion. As the reactants are transitioning to products, they form a high-energy transition state, as shown in Figure 20.1. The energy difference between the reactants and the transition state is the minimum energy required for the reaction to occur. This energy difference is called the **activation energy**. The transition state is always higher in energy than either the reactants or the products.

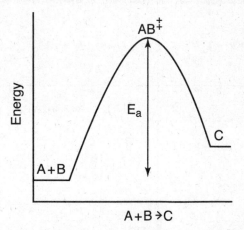

Figure 20.1. Reaction diagram. The minimal amount of energy required to transition from reactants (A + B) to products (C) is the activation energy (E_a). $AB^{\ddagger}$ is the high energy transition state between reactants and products.

REACTION MECHANISMS

A balanced chemical reaction may show only the overall reaction that occurs and does not necessarily show what individual steps occur in the process. Instead, the reaction mechanism must be given. For example, the overall reaction may be:

$$3A + B \rightarrow D$$

but the reaction mechanism may be:

$$\text{step 1: } 2A + B \rightarrow C$$

$$\text{step 2: } A + C \rightarrow D$$

In this case, C is an intermediate that is formed during the reaction and then consumed to complete the reaction. The individual steps in a reaction are also called the elementary steps. To check that the elementary steps represent the correct overall equation, first add all the reactants together. Then add all the products together. Cancel anything that's found on both sides, and see if it is the same as the overall reaction.

$$\text{step 1: } 2A + B \rightarrow C$$

$$\text{step 2: } A + C \rightarrow D$$

$$\text{sum of products: } 2A + B + A + C \rightarrow C + D$$

In this equation, $2A + A$ can be simplified to $3A$ and the C on the reactant side cancels out with the C on the product side. This gives an overall reaction of $3A + B \rightarrow D$. The rate of the overall reaction depends on the rate-determining step, which is the slowest elementary step. This is the same concept as you are traveling only as fast as the car in front of you. If something is slow, then it determines the rate of the overall reaction. Go back to the elementary steps and determine the rate-limiting step.

$$\text{step 1(slow): } 2A + B \rightarrow C$$

$$\text{step 2 (fast): } A + C \rightarrow D$$

Step 1 is the rate-limiting step, which means the rate of the overall reaction depends on step 1. If the elementary steps are given, the rate law can be determined directly from the rate-limiting reaction. The rate law for the above reaction can be written as:

$$\text{rate} = k[A]^2[B]$$

Chemical Equilibriums 21

EQUILIBRIUM AND THE EQUILIBRIUM CONSTANT

Previously, the rates of reactions were discussed based on the assumption that the reverse reaction was negligible. In chemical equilibriums, however, this is not the case. In fact, a reaction reaches equilibrium when the rate of the forward reaction is equal to the rate of the reverse reaction. This does not mean the concentrations of products equal the concentrations of reactants. Instead, only the formation and breakdown of reactants is equal to the formation and breakdown of products once a certain concentration of each has been achieved.

A different arrow is used to show that the reaction can proceed in both the forward and reverse direction, which is shown in the following example.

$$N_2O_2(g) \rightleftharpoons 2NO(g)$$

By looking at the equation in the forward direction, the rate is expressed as:

$$rate_{fwd} = k_{fwd}[N_2O_2]$$

By looking at the equation in the reverse direction, NO is now the reactant and the rate is expressed as:

$$rate_{rev} = k_{rev}[NO]^2$$

The equilibrium constant (K or K_{eq}) represents both the forward and the reverse rates. The equilibrium divides the concentration of products by the concentration of reactants.

$$K = \frac{[products]}{[reactants]} = \frac{[NO]^2}{[N_2O_2]}$$

If K is large, the products are favored and there will be a higher concentration of products than reactants at equilibrium. If K is small, the reactants are favored. If K is equal to 1, both the reactants and products are favored equally.

Recall that rates are affected by temperature, which means that equilibrium constants (K) are temperature dependent as well. Unless otherwise stated, assume the K constant is measured at 25°C.

WRITING EQUILIBRIUM CONSTANTS

When writing the equilibrium constant, be careful about what the phases are for each compound.

$$A(s) + B(aq) \rightleftharpoons 2C(g) + D(l)$$

For solids and liquids, their concentrations do not change over the course of the reaction and are therefore not included. The correct equilibrium expression for the above reaction is shown in the following equation.

$$K = \frac{[C]^2}{[B]}$$

Gases are included in the equilibrium expression because their concentrations can change by changing the volume of the container. In contrast, the concentrations of solids and pure liquids do not change by changing the volume of the container. If the overall reaction contains gases and only the gases are included in the equilibrium expression, the equilibrium constant can be expressed in terms of K_p, where K_p is the equilibrium constant with respect to partial pressures. Look at the reaction below.

$$2NO(g) + O_2(g) \rightleftharpoons 2NO_2(g)$$

The K_p expression can be written as:

$$K_p = \frac{\left(P_{NO_2}\right)^2}{\left(P_{NO}\right)^2 \left(P_{NO_2}\right)}$$

where P_{NO_2} is the partial pressure of NO_2 gas, P_{NO} is the partial pressure of NO gas, and P_{O_2} is the partial pressure of O_2 gas. K_p is related to the equilibrium constant, K_c by:

$$K_p = K_c(RT)^{\Delta n}$$

In this equation, K_c is the equilibrium constant with respect to concentrations, R is the gas constant $0.0821 \frac{L \cdot atm}{mol \cdot K}$, T is temperature in kelvins, and Δn is the change in moles of gas molecules (total moles of gas on product side – total moles of gas on reactant side). The Δn for the reaction $2NO(g) + O_2(g) \rightleftharpoons 2NO_2(g)$ is $2 - (2 + 1) = -1$.

If a reaction is reversed, products now become reactants and the reactants become products. Table 21.1 shows how K can be manipulated if the equation is reversed, summed, subtracted, and either multiplied or divided by a number.

Table 21.1. Manipulating the Equilibrium Constant (K)

Equation	K Expression	Relationship to K_{ref}
Reference equation: $A \rightleftharpoons B$	$K = \dfrac{[B]}{[A]}$	K_{ref}
Reverse reference equation: $B \rightleftharpoons A$	$K = \dfrac{[A]}{[B]}$	$K = \dfrac{1}{K_{ref}}$
Sum of reactions equals reference equation: Reaction 1: $A \rightleftharpoons C$ Reaction 2: $C \rightleftharpoons B$ Overall reaction: $A \rightleftharpoons B$	K for Reaction 1: $K_1 = \dfrac{[C]}{[A]}$ K for Reaction 2: $K_2 = \dfrac{[B]}{[C]}$ K for overall reaction: $K_{overall} = \dfrac{[C]}{[A]} \times \dfrac{[B]}{[C]} = \dfrac{[B]}{[A]}$	$K_1 \times K_2 = K_{ref}$
Subtraction of reactions equals reference equation (Reaction 2 – Reaction 1): Reaction 1: $2A \rightleftharpoons B + C$ Reaction 2: $3A \rightleftharpoons 2B + C$ Overall reaction: $A \rightleftharpoons B$	K for Reaction 1: $K_1 = \dfrac{[C][B]}{[A]^2}$ K for Reaction 2: $K_2 = \dfrac{[B]^2[C]}{[A]^3}$ K for overall reaction: $K_{ref} = \dfrac{\frac{[B]^2[C]}{[A]^3}}{\frac{[C][B]}{[A]^2}} = \dfrac{[B]}{[A]}$	$K_2 \div K_1 = K_{ref}$
Reference equation multiplied by a factor: $3A \rightleftharpoons 3B$	$K = \dfrac{[B]^3}{[A]^3} = \left(\dfrac{[B]}{[A]}\right)^3$	$K = (K_{ref})^3$
Reference equation divided by a factor: $\dfrac{A}{2} \rightleftharpoons \dfrac{B}{2}$ or $\dfrac{1}{2}A \rightleftharpoons \dfrac{1}{2}B$	$K = \dfrac{[B]^{\frac{1}{2}}}{[A]^{\frac{1}{2}}} = \sqrt{\dfrac{[B]}{[A]}}$	$K = (K_{ref})^{1/2} = \sqrt{K_{ref}}$

FINDING K_{eq} FROM EXPERIMENTAL DATA

One way to determine the value of K_{eq} is to measure the concentrations of all the reactants and products at equilibrium and plug those values into the equilibrium expression. For example, imagine the equilibrium concentrations are 0.12 M, 0.34 M, and 1.2 M for A, B, and C, respectively, for the following reaction at 25°C.

$$A(aq) + B(aq) \rightleftharpoons 2C(aq)$$

The equilibrium constant is found using the following equation.

$$K_{eq} = \frac{[C]^2}{[A][B]} = \frac{(1.2)^2}{(0.12)(0.34)} = 35.29 = 35$$

FINDING EQUILIBRIUM CONCENTRATIONS FROM K_{eq}

If the initial concentrations and K_{eq} are known, these can be used to calculate the equilibrium concentrations. A common way to set up these problems is using an **ICE** table, where **I** stands for initial, **C** stands for change, and **E** stands for equilibrium. Let's say the initial concentration for the following reaction is 0.45 M for A and the K_c (equilibrium constant with respect to concentrations) is given.

	A(aq)	$\rightleftharpoons$	2B(aq)	$K_c = 5.7 \times 10^{-2}$ at 25°C
Initial concentrations	0.45 M		0 M	
Change in concentrations	$-x$		$+2x$	
Equilibrium concentrations	0.45 M $- x$		$+2x$	

The change in concentration is in stoichiometric amounts, which means the change is in relation to the number of moles. If 1 mole of A is used up, 2 moles of B will form. Since there isn't any product, in order to reach equilibrium the reactant (A) has to convert into the product (B). This means that as the concentration of A decreases, the concentration of B increases. If the change is unknown, then x can be used in the calculation.

Once the equilibrium concentrations are known, they can be plugged into the equilibrium expression.

$$K_c = \frac{[B]^2}{[A]} = \frac{(2x)^2}{(0.45 - x)} = 5.7 \times 10^{-2}$$

Rearrange the equation so it equals zero. Then use the quadratic equation to solve for x. To avoid confusion with the variable x, the multiplication sign in 5.7×10^{-2} is being changed to a multiplication dot.

$$\frac{(2x)^2}{(0.45 - x)} = 5.7 \cdot 10^{-2}$$

$$4x^2 + 5.7 \cdot 10^{-2}x - 2.\underline{565} \cdot 10^{-2} = 0$$

$$x = \frac{-b \pm \sqrt{b^2 - 4ac}}{2a} = \frac{-5.7 \cdot 10^{-2} \pm \sqrt{\left(5.7 \cdot 10^{-2}\right)^2 - 4(4)\left(-2.\underline{565} \cdot 10^{-2}\right)}}{2(4)}$$

$$x = 0.073 \text{ or } -0.088$$

Since there cannot be a negative concentration (B = 2*x*), then *x* has to be 0.073 *M*. Therefore, the equilibrium concentration for *A* is 0.45 − *x* = 0.45 − 0.073 = 0.377 *M* and for B is 2*x* = 2(0.073) = 0.146 *M*. The section *Acids and Bases* shows a shortcut for solving these equilibrium concentrations.

THE REACTION QUOTIENT, Q

The reaction quotient, *Q*, is used in place of *K* if it is unknown whether or not the reaction is at equilibrium. *Q* is set up the same way as *K*, with products over reactants. *Q* can then be compared to *K*:

1. If $Q < K$, then there is too much reactant, and the reaction needs to proceed in the forward direction to produce more products.
2. If $Q = K$, then the reaction is at equilibrium, and the forward rate is equal to the reverse rate.
3. If $Q > K$, then there is too much product, and the reaction needs to proceed in the reverse direction to produce more reactants.

➡ **Example** _____

The concentrations for A, B, and C are 1.3 M, 0.75 M, and 4.3 M, respectively. Will the reaction shift to the left, right, or no change if the $K_{eq} = 81.9$?

$$2A(aq) + B(aq) \rightarrow 3C\ (aq)$$

Solution

Because it is not known if the reaction is at equilibrium, *Q* is used instead of K_{eq}. *Q* is set up exactly the same way as K_{eq}: $Q = [C]^3/[A]^2[B] = [4.3]^3/[1.3]^2[0.75] = 62.7$.

$Q < K_{eq}$, which means the concentration of reactants are too high, and the reaction will shift toward the products (shifts to the right).

LE CHÂTELIER'S PRINCIPLE

Le Châtelier's principle states that when something is added or taken away to a reaction that is at equilibrium, it will shift in a direction (toward reactants or toward products) that will counteract the disturbance to go back to equilibrium. Factors that can change equilibrium are:

1. **CHANGING THE CONCENTRATION OF A REACTANT OR PRODUCT**

$$AB(aq) \rightleftharpoons 2C(aq)$$

If the concentration of AB was increased, then to counteract that addition, the equilibrium would shift towards the products. If a salt was added, i.e., AX, then this is the same as increasing the concentration of A^+, and the equilibrium would shift toward the products. This is called the **common ion effect**. The opposite can also happen when a metal chelating agent is added, and it will bind to a specific metal. As an example, let's say the metal chelating agent binds to A^+. By adding the chelating agent, it will decrease the concentration of A^+ (by binding to it), and in order to counteract this disturbance, the equilibrium will shift toward the reactants.

2. CHANGING THE VOLUME/PRESSURE

$$AB(g) \rightleftharpoons C(g) + D(g)$$

Changing the volume and/or pressure will only affect gas molecules. Looking at the equation above, there is one gas molecule on the reactant side (AB) and two gas molecules on the product side (C + D). If the pressure is decreased, the reaction will counteract that by shifting toward the side that has more gas molecules (more gas molecules = increase in pressure). If the volume is decreased, then the pressure will go up. To counteract that, the equilibrium will shift toward the reactants (the side with less gas molecules will decrease the pressure).

3. CHANGING THE TEMPERATURE

$$AB(aq) \rightleftharpoons 2C(aq) \qquad \Delta H_{rxn} = -145 \text{ kJ}$$

In order to determine which side will be affected if temperature is increased or decreased, it has to be known if the reaction is exothermic or endothermic. If a reaction is endothermic, then heat is absorbed and can be placed on the reactant side. If a reaction is exothermic, then heat is released and can be placed on the product side. For this example, the reaction releases heat ($-\Delta H$) and, therefore, places heat on the product side:

$$AB(aq) \rightleftharpoons 2C(aq) + heat \qquad \Delta H_{rxn} = -145 \text{ kJ}$$

Now, if the temperature is increased, it is the same as increasing the "concentration" of heat. To counteract that, the equilibrium will shift toward the reactants.

➥ Example

An endothermic reaction was placed in a hot bath. According to Le Châtelier, which direction will the reaction shift to go back to equilibrium?

Solution

First, write out a generalized reaction, where heat is placed on the reactant side (endothermic reactions require heat in order for the reaction to proceed): Heat + A $\rightleftharpoons$ B. Now, treat heat as a reactant. A hot bath will increase the "concentration" of heat. Therefore, the reaction will shift toward the product side.

Acids and Bases 22

Acid-base chemistry often involves water, which is a weakly ionizing compound. This means it can dissociate to its ions, but only to a very small extent. The reaction can be represented as: $H_2O(l) \rightleftharpoons H^+(aq) + OH^-(aq)$ or $2H_2O(l) \rightleftharpoons H_3O^+(aq) + OH^-(aq)$. In this case, the reverse direction (H_2O) is strongly favored. If water is the only source of either ion, then the $[H^+]$ and $[OH^-]$ are very small and are equal. A solution in which this condition is true is neutral; it is neither acidic nor basic. Other substances added to the water can change the ratio of these ions by increasing either the $[H^+]$ or the $[OH^-]$. A solution in which $[H^+] > [OH^-]$ is acidic, and if $[OH^-] > [H^+]$, the solution is basic.

THREE THEORIES OF ACID-BASE CHEMISTRY

What determines if a compound is an acid or a base? Several different theories define acids and bases using different criteria.

Arrhenius Acid-Base Theory

The simplest view of acid-base chemistry defines an acid as a chemical species that releases H^+ into water, and a base releases OH^-.

➡ Example _____

An Arrhenius acid dissolving in water: $HCl(aq) \rightarrow H^+(aq) + Cl^-(aq)$
An Arrhenius base dissolving in water: $NaOH(aq) \rightarrow Na^+(aq) + OH^-(aq)$

This theory does not explain why some compounds, such as NH_3, function as bases in water, causing OH^- concentration to increase.

Brönsted-Lowry Acid-Base Theory

This theory identifies acids as compounds that release H^+ into water (same as Arrhenius), but bases are defined differently. In Brönsted-Lowry theory, a base is any substance that increases the OH^- concentration, whether OH^- is part of the formula or not. A base can do this by accepting H^+ from other species, including water itself (i.e., base hydrolysis of water). According to B-L theory, an **acid** is an **H^+ donor** and a **base** is an **H^+ acceptor**.

Lewis Acid-Base Theory

This is the most general acid/base theory and focuses on lone pair electrons rather than a proton, H^+. Therefore, Lewis theory includes acid-base chemistry in aqueous as well as non-aqueous solutions, and even gas phase reactions. A **Lewis acid** is an electron pair acceptor; a **Lewis base** is an electron pair donor. A classic example of Lewis acid/base chemistry is:

$$BF_3 + :NH_3 \rightleftharpoons F_3B:NH_3$$

Lewis acid Lewis base acid-base adduct boron in BF_3 (a Lewis acid) accepts the lone pair electrons from lone pair donor NH_3 (a Lewis base) forming a coordinate covalent bond.

AQUEOUS ACID-BASE CHEMISTRY

The rest of this discussion focuses on aqueous (water-based) solutions and the proton transfer reactions that occur in them using Brönsted-Lowry theory. A proton (H^+ ion) is exchanged between interacting chemical species. A typical reaction is:

1. $HNO_2(aq) + NH_3(aq) \rightleftharpoons NH_4^+ (aq) + NO_2^- (aq)$

   donates H^+ accepts H^+ a new   a new H^+
                              H^+ donor   acceptor

   the acid   *the base*   *conjugate*   *conjugate*
                              acid   *base*

This reaction can also occur between two water molecules, in the "autoprotolysis of water":

2. $H_2O + H_2O \rightleftharpoons OH^- + H_3O^+$

   donates H^+ accepts   a new   a new
              H^+ H^+ donor H^+ acceptor

   the acid   *the*   *conjugate*   *conjugate*
                        base   *base*   *acid*

The autoprotolysis of water occurs to a very limited extent. Only about 1.00×10^{-7} mole/L of each ion are formed in pure water at 25°C. The equilibrium constant for the autoprotolysis of water is:

$$K_w = [H_3O^+][OH^-] = 1.00 \times 10^{-14} \text{ at } 25°C$$

In reactions (1) and (2) above, the new base results from loss of a single H^+ from the original acid. These pairs, H_2O/OH^- and H_2O/H_3O^+, are called **conjugates**, or a **conjugate acid/base pair**. They always differ by (1) one and only one H^+ and (2) one and only one charge unit. In each pair, the acid is listed first and the base second. Notice, every pair differs by one H^+ and one charge unit:

$$HNO_2/NO_2^- \qquad NH_4^+/NH_3 \qquad H_2O/OH^- \qquad H_3O^+/H_2O$$

It is important in buffer chemistry to be able to recognize such conjugate acid/base pairs.

THE pH AND pOH SCALES

In water, the concentrations of the chemical species $H^+(aq)$ and $OH^-(aq)$ can vary over many orders of magnitude, therefore a logarithmic scale is used to express the acidity or basicity of aqueous solutions. The "p" is a mathematical operator that means "–log" of the concentration it is operating on. The square brackets indicate concentration as mol/L. For example, $p[Na^+]$ means "$-\log_{10}[Na^+]$." Common "pX" equations are pH and pOH.

$$pH = -\log[H^+] \qquad pOH = -\log[OH^-]$$

Logarithms are exponents. Therefore, to find $[Na^+]$ or $[H^+]$ from pNa or pH, use the antilog operator.

$$[H^+] = 10^{-pH} \qquad [Na^+] = 10^{-pNa}$$

➡ Example

Find the pH of a solution that has $[H^+] = 3.0 \times 10^{-4}$ mol/L.

Strategy

$$pH = -\log[H^+] = -\log(3.0 \times 10^{-4}\, M) = 3.52$$

To go from pH back to $[H^+]$: $[H^+] = 10^{-pH} = 10^{-3.52} = 3.0 \times 10^{-4}\, M$

THE ION PRODUCT OF WATER In the autoprotolysis reaction for water (reaction (2) on page 170), the products are the two ions of water, $H^+(aq)$ and $OH^-(aq)$. Their concentrations are related to each other by the equilibrium constant equation, which can be solved for either concentration provided K_w is known. To find pOH and/or $[OH^-]$ when either H^+ or pH are known, use the K_w equation.

➡ Example

Find $[OH^-]$, when $[H^+] = 3.0 \times 10^{-4}\, M$.

$$K_w = [H^+][OH^-] \Rightarrow [OH^-] = \frac{K_w}{H^+} = \frac{1.00 \times 10^{-14}}{3.0 \times 10^{-4}\, M} = 3.33 \times 10^{-11}\, M$$

$$pOH = -\log[OH^-] = -\log(3.33 \times 10^{-11}\, M) = 10.48$$

RELATIVE STRENGTHS OF ACIDS AND BASES

Strong acids are strong electrolytes and dissociate ~100% in water to release H^+ in the same amount as their concentration in the solution. The following five acids are very strong in water:

$$HCl \quad HBr \quad HI \quad HNO_3 \quad HClO_4$$

The LOWER the pH, the MORE ACIDIC the solution and the greater the concentration of H^+.

At 25°C, the acid range is pH < 7.00.

The HIGHER the pH, the MORE ALKALINE (basic) the solution and the greater the concentration of OH^-.

At 25°C, the basic (alkaline) range is pH > 7.00.

The product of these two ion concentrations always equals the K_w **at the given temperature**.

$$K_w = 1.00 \times 10^{-14} \text{ at } 25°C$$

Also, the first H^+ is lost from H_2SO_4 as a strong acid. The second H^+ from the HSO_4^- anion is not strong and is only partially dissociated from the SO_4^{2-} anion.

The anions of the five strong acids are *technically* bases: Cl^-, Br^-, I^-, NO_3^-, ClO_4^-, but they are so weak they do not function as bases in water (cannot accept H^+). These anions (conjugate bases) are considered **pH neutral ions**; they do not affect the pH of the solution. A typical reaction of a strong acid in water is:

$$HNO_3(aq) + H_2O(l) \xrightarrow{\sim100\%} NO_3^-(aq) + H_3O^+(aq)$$

The products of the reaction are strongly favored as indicated by the single-headed arrow. The equilibrium constant for the strong acid dissociation, K_a, is very large. To find the pH for a strong acid: $pH = -\log(C_A)$, where C_A is the concentration of the acid.

➡ Example

Find the pH of a nitric acid solution when $[HNO_3] = 7.4 \times 10^{-4} \, M$.

Strategy

Recognize nitric acid as one of the six strong acids. Assume $\sim100\%$ dissociation to its ions in water. Therefore, $7.4 \times 10^{-4} \, M \, HNO_3$ produces $7.4 \times 10^{-4} \, M$ of H^+ (1:1 ratio)

$$pH = -\log[H^+] = -\log(7.4 \times 10^{-4}) = 3.13$$

Weak acids are weak electrolytes, meaning they do not dissociate 100% to their ions. There is a wide range of relatively stronger and weaker "weak acids," and their relative strength is expressed by the special equilibrium constant for acid dissociations, K_a. The larger the K_a, the more H^+ is released and the stronger that weak acid is. For example, a weak acid with $K_a = 1 \times 10^{-3}$ is stronger (releases more H^+) than one with $K_a = 1 \times 10^{-8}$. The generic weak acid dissociation in water is:

$$HA(aq) \rightleftharpoons H^+(aq) + A^-(aq) \qquad K_a = \frac{[H^+][A^-]}{[HA]}$$

where $HA(aq)$ is the acid and $A^-(aq)$ is its conjugate base.

VARIABLES THAT AFFECT THE STRENGTH OF ACIDS

1. The strength of the bond between H^+ and the rest of the molecule determines how readily the H^+ is lost and, therefore, how strong the acid is. In this sequence, the bond strength and acid strength are the inverse.

   Bond Strength increasing $\longrightarrow$

   HI   HBr   HCl   HF

   $\longleftarrow$ ——————————— Acid strength increasing

   In the hydrohalic acids above, the weakest bond occurs in HI, therefore, the H^+ is most readily lost. HI, HBr, and HCl are all strong acids. HF is a weak acid because the HF bond is the strongest.

2. The greater the number of electron withdrawing groups, such as oxygen, the stronger the acid. The electron withdrawing effect weakens the attraction of H^+ for the corresponding anion.

← —————————————— Number of electron withdrawing atoms increasing

$HClO_4$	$HClO_3$	$HClO_2$	$HClO$
perchloric acid	chloric acid	chlorous acid	hypochlorous acid

← —————————————— Acid strength increasing

3. Increased electronegativity of an anion increases acid strength:

← —————————————— Electronegativity of bonded atom increasing

HF H_2O H_3N H_4C

← —————————————— Acid strength increasing

To find the pH of a weak acid solution, use a K_a expression for the acid and fill in the equilibrium concentrations for the species in the square brackets: $K_a = \dfrac{[H^+][A^-]}{[HA]}$. If starting concentration is known, make a table showing the result of dissolving the weak acid in water.

➥ **Example** _____

The initial concentration of HClO is 0.015 M. What is the pH of this solution?

Strategy

Let "x" be the unknown amount of weak acid that dissociates to produce an H^+ ion.

$$HClO(aq) \quad \rightleftharpoons \quad H^+(aq) \quad + \quad ClO^-(aq)$$

	HClO(aq)	H⁺(aq)	ClO⁻(aq)
Initial concentration	0.015 M	0	0
Change in concentration	$-x$	$+x$	$+x$
Equilibrium concentration	$0.015 - x$	x	x

The equilibrium concentrations are used in the K_a expression to find the value of x.

$$K_a = \frac{[H^+][A^-]}{[HA]} \qquad 3.0 \times 10^{-8} = \frac{x^2}{0.015 - x}$$

Make a simplifying assumption: A very small value of K_a means very little product is formed. Therefore, the value of x will be correspondingly small, so small that the value of $0.015 - x \approx 0.015$ M. Check to see if the assumption is valid after calculating a value for x ($x \le 5\%$).

With the simplifying assumption, the math is:

$$x^2 = (0.015)(3.0 \times 10^{-8}) \Rightarrow x = \sqrt{(0.015)\left(3.0 \times 10^{-8}\right)} = 2.12 \times 10^{-5} \ M$$

Notice that when this assumption is applied, the shortcut equation is $[H^+] = \sqrt{C_A K_A}$.

$$x \leq 5\% \text{ of original number} \Rightarrow \frac{2.12 \times 10^{-5}}{0.015}(100) = 0.14\% \Rightarrow \text{assumption is good } ☺$$

"x" was defined as the amount of H^+ released by this weak acid:

$$pH = -\log(2.12 \times 10^{-5}) = 4.67$$

STRONG BASES

Strong bases are strong electrolytes and dissociate ~100% in water to release $OH^-(aq)$, in a stoichiometric amount corresponding to their chemical formula. Hydroxides of Group I alkali metals are strong bases, i.e. NaOH, KOH. Also, hydroxides of *heavier* atoms of Group II alkaline earth metals are strong bases, i.e., $Ca(OH)_2$, $Ba(OH)_2$. Other metal hydroxides are weak electrolytes and, therefore, weak bases.

Analogous to strong acids, to find the pH for a strong base solution, assume ~100% dissociation to the ions. Note the stoichiometry of the compound: NaOH *vs.* $Ba(OH)_2$. Take the negative log of the OH^- ion concentration. Let $C_{Ca(OH)_2}$ represent the analytical concentration of the strong base, $Ca(OH)_2$.

➥ Example _____

Find the pH of calcium hydroxide solution when $C_{Ca(OH)_2} = 8.1 \times 10^{-4}\ M$.

Recognize calcium hydroxide as a strong base. Assume ~ 100% dissociation to its ions in water. Since there is a 1:2 ratio, $8.1 \times 10^{-4}\ M\ Ca(OH)_2$ produces $2(8.1 \times 10^{-4})$ of $OH^-(aq)$.

$$pOH = -\log(1.6 \times 10^{-3}) = 2.79$$

Either find $[H^+]$ from $K_w = [H^+][OH^-]$ and take the negative log, or use the logarithmic form of K_w:

$$pH + pOH = 14$$

Therefore, $pH = 14 - pOH = 11.21$.

WEAK BASES

There are several kinds of weak bases:

- conjugate bases of all weak acids are weak bases, i.e., F^- is a weak base
- metal hydroxides other than the strong bases, i.e., $Cr(OH)_3$
- nitrogen-containing molecules (the lone pair on N must be available), i.e., :NH_3

To calculate the pH of a weak base solution, the approach is analogous to the weak acid. Write the balanced chemical equation for the base hydrolysis of water, and use an ICE table to determine equilibrium concentrations of the participants. Put these values into the equilibrium constant K_b.

➡ Example

What is the pH of a 0.546 M acetate ion solution. The $K_b = 5.71 \times 10^{-10}$.

Strategy

Recognize acetate ion as the conjugate weak base of acetic acid. Use the shortcut (assume x is really small) and the equation becomes $[OH^-] = \sqrt{C_B K_B}$.

$$x = \sqrt{(0.546)(5.71 \times 10^{-10})} = 1.77 \times 10^{-5} M$$

Check the assumption: x has to be less than 5% of 0.546.

$$\frac{1.77 \times 10^{-5}}{0.546} (100) = 0.0032\% \Rightarrow \text{assumption is good} ☺$$

"x" was defined as the amount of OH^- produced by this weak base:

$$pOH = -\log(1.77 \times 10^{-5}) = 4.75$$

There is one more step to find the pH. Either find $[H^+]$ from $K_w = [H^+][OH^-]$ and take the negative log, or use the logarithmic form of K_w: $14 = pH + pOH$. Therefore, $pH = 14 - pOH = 9.25$.

POLYPROTIC ACIDS AND POLYFUNCTIONAL BASES

Polyprotic acids have more than one acidic ("removable") proton. One example important in biological systems is carbonic acid, H_2CO_3. It has two acid dissociation steps:

$$H_2CO_3 \rightleftharpoons H^+ + HCO_3^- \qquad K_{a_1} = 4.3 \times 10^{-7}$$

$$HCO_3^- \rightleftharpoons H^+ + CO_3^{2-} \qquad K_{a_2} = 5.6 \times 10^{-11}$$

A comparison of the magnitude of the two K_a's shows that the first proton is a stronger acid than the second one. Note that HCO_3^- acts as both a conjugate weak base (in step one) and a conjugate weak acid (in step two). A species that is both a weak acid and a weak base is called amphiprotic.

The carbonate ion is a weak base and has two base hydrolysis reactions. It is a "polyfunctional base."

$$CO_3^{2-} + H_2O \rightleftharpoons HCO^- + OH^- \qquad K_{b_1} = \frac{K_w}{K_{a_2}} = \frac{1.00 \times 10^{-14}}{5.6 \times 10^{-11}} = 1.8 \times 10^{-4}$$

$$HCO_3^- + H_2O \rightleftharpoons H_2CO_3 + OH^- \qquad K_{b_2} = \frac{K_w}{K_{a_1}} = \frac{1.00 \times 10^{-14}}{4.3 \times 10^{-7}} = 2.3 \times 10^{-8}$$

Polyprotic acids and polyfunctional bases generate amphiprotic species in water. These include acids like H_3PO_4, H_2SO_4, bases like S^{2-}, and amino acids, which are important in biological systems.

AMPHIPROTIC SPECIES

Some acids have more than one acidic H^+ in the chemical formula. These acids generate a series of deprotonation species, some of which function as either acid or base in water depending on the other species present. An example is phosphoric acid that has three protons and makes four possible forms:

$$H_3PO_4 \xrightarrow{-H^+} H_2PO_4^- \xrightarrow{-H^+} HPO_4^{2-} \xrightarrow{-H^+} PO_4^{3-}$$

weak acid, only   *amphiprotic*   *amphiprotic*   *weak base, only*

The fully protonated form H_3PO_4 is only a weak acid, and the fully deprotonated form PO_4^{3-} can only function as a base. The two middle amphiprotic forms can both donate and accept H^+, making them both acid and base. They participate in two equilibrium processes in water and, therefore, their solution pH depends on both. In many cases, concentration is not a factor, and the pH is calculated from the K's:

$$[H^+]_{amphiprotic} = \sqrt{K_{a_1} \cdot K_{a_2}} \text{ or in logarithmic form: } pH_{amphiprotic} = (pK_{a_1} + pK_{a_2})/2$$

➡ Example

Calculate the pH of a solution that is 0.4775 M NaHCO$_3$. The pK_a's for the carbonic acid system are: $pK_{a_1} = 6.351$; $pK_{a_2} = 10.329$.

Strategy

Recognize that the salt sodium bicarbonate is a strong electrolyte and dissolves as its two ions, Na^+ and HCO_3^-. After dissolving, the amphiprotic bicarbonate ion undergoes its two acid/base equilibrium processes, able to both gain H^+ forming H_2CO_3 and lose H^+ forming CO_3^{2-}. The pH of the solution depends on the K_a's but not on the concentration.

$$pH_{bicarbonate\ ion} = (6.351 + 10.329)/2 = 8.340$$

REACTIONS OF ACIDS AND BASES: TITRATIONS

The production of the very weakly ionizing molecule H_2O from its ions H^+ and OH^- is a major driving force for the reactions of acids and bases with each other. Titration analysis can be used to determine an unknown acid or base concentration if the balanced chemical equation for the reaction is known, and the titrant concentration is also known.

The unknown is usually placed in a flask, and the titrant is added from a buret. A color indicator or other method is used to determine when **stoichiometric amounts** of the acid and base have been combined. That point is taken to be the reaction. When concentration is in moles/L and volume is in L, the product (volume) × (concentration) has the units of moles.

> The equivalence point is when stoichiometric amounts of acid and base have been combined.

➡ Example

25.00 mL of sulfuric acid solution is titrated to the 2nd equivalence point (both H^+ ions on each molecule are titrated) requiring 37.06 mL of 0.0975 M sodium hydroxide according to the equation:

$$H_2SO_4 + 2\ NaOH \rightarrow 2\ H_2O + 2\ Na^+ + SO_4^{2-}$$

What is the concentration of the sulfuric acid in the original solution?

Solution

Notice the stoichiometry. It requires two moles of NaOH for each mole of H_2SO_4.

1. Find moles NaOH required:

$$37.06 \text{ mL} \cdot \frac{1 \text{ L}}{1000 \text{ mL}} \cdot \frac{0.0975 \text{ mol NaOH}}{1 \text{ L}} = 3.61 \times 10^{-3} \text{ mol NaOH}$$

2. Find moles H_2SO_4 reacted:

$$3.61 \times 10^{-3} \text{ mol NaOH} \cdot \frac{1 \text{ mol } H_2SO_4}{2 \text{ mol NaOH}} = 1.81 \times 10^{-3} \text{ mol } H_2SO_4$$

3. Find the original concentration of the H_2SO_4:

$$\frac{1.81 \times 10^{-3} \text{ mol } H_2SO_4}{0.02500 \text{ L}} = 0.0723 \text{ } M$$

MIXTURES OF CONJUGATE ACID-BASE PAIRS: BUFFERS

A pH buffer is a solution that resists change in pH with the addition of an acid, a base, and/or a solvent (dilution). The most common type of pH buffer in water consists of a weak acid and its conjugate weak base. The buffer pH is found from a logarithmic form of the weak acid K_a expression—the **Henderson-Hasselbalch equation:**

$$pH_{buffer} = pK_a + \log\left(\frac{[\text{conjugate base}]}{[\text{conjugate acid}]}\right)$$

Because the volume term in both concentrations must be the same, either moles or mol/L may be used.

➡ **Example** _____

Find the pH of a buffer consisting of 0.345 M acetic acid (CH_3COOH) and 0.177 M sodium acetate ($CH_3COO^- Na^+$). The K_a for acetic acid is 1.75×10^{-5}.

Strategy

Recognize acetic acid and the acetate ion as a weak conjugate acid/base pair. Calculate the pK_a for the acid and use the Henderson-Hasselbalch relationship to find the pH.

$$pK_a = -\log K_a = -\log (1.75 \times 10^{-5}) = 4.757$$

$$pH_{buffer} = pK_a + \log\left(\frac{[\text{conjugate base}]}{[\text{conjugate acid}]}\right) = 4.757 + \log\left(\frac{0.177 \text{ } M}{0.345 \text{ } M}\right) = 4.467$$

Notice that the pH did not change very much, as expected in a buffer.

Thermochemistry and Thermodynamics 23

LAWS OF THERMODYNAMICS

There are three laws of thermodynamics that allow chemists to make some assumptions. The **first law of thermodynamics** is the law of conservation of energy, which states that energy is neither created nor destroyed. This means that energy must be transferred. The **second law of thermodynamics** states that the entropy of the universe is always increasing for spontaneous reactions ($\Delta S_{univ} = \Delta S_{surr} + \Delta S_{sys}$). The **third law of thermodynamics** states that the entropy of a perfect crystal is 0 at 0 K (absolute zero), which allows chemists to measure standard entropies.

Entropy (S) is a measurement of randomness and disorder of molecules, which is based on the number of energetically equivalent arrangements available to the molecule. An increase in entropy (or an increase in disorder) will occur when a substance goes from a solid to a liquid, a liquid to a gas, a solid to a gas, or when the reaction produces more gas molecules. An example of the latter is given below:

$$A(g) + B(l) \rightleftharpoons 2C(g)$$

The reaction started off with one molecule of gas, but produces two molecules of gas. This increases disorder, which means the change in entropy is positive ($\Delta S > 0$).

Standard molar entropies ($S°$) of specific substances can be used to calculate the standard entropy changes of a reaction ($\Delta S°_{rxn}$) by using the following equation:

$$\Delta S°_{rxn} = \sum n_p S°(\text{products}) - \sum n_r S° (\text{reactants})$$

where $\sum$ means the sum, n is the number of moles, and $S°$ is the standard molar entropy. The difference between entropy, S, and standard molar entropies, $S°$, is that S is measured under any condition where the standard has to be at 25°C and 1 atm. Throughout this section, whenever the nought symbol (°) is used, it indicates that the value was measured under standard conditions.

➥ Example

What is the standard molar entropy for the following reaction?

$$2H_2S(g) + 3O_2(g) \rightarrow 2H_2O(g) + 2SO_2(g) \qquad \Delta S°_{rxn} = ?$$

Compound	$\Delta S° \left(\dfrac{J}{mol \cdot K} \right)$
$H_2S(g)$	205.6
$O_2(g)$	205.0
$H_2O(g)$	188.7
$H_2O(l)$	70.0
$SO_2(g)$	248.2

Solution

First, identify the correct compound with the correct *phase*. $H_2O(l)$ is not used in this reaction, so the correct number to use for $H_2O(g)$ is 188.7 J/mol · K. Next, calculate the molar entropy for each compound including the stoichiometric amounts:

Reactants: $2 \text{ mol } H_2S \cdot \dfrac{205.6 \text{ J}}{1 \text{ mol} \cdot K} = 411.2 \text{ J}; \ 3 \text{ mol } O_2 \dfrac{205.0 \text{ J}}{1 \text{ mol} \cdot K} = 615.0 \text{ J}$

Products: $2 \text{ mol } H_2O \cdot \dfrac{188.7 \text{ J}}{1 \text{ mol} \cdot K} = 377.4 \text{ J}; \ 2 \text{ mol } SO_2 \dfrac{248.2 \text{ J}}{1 \text{ mol} \cdot K} = 496.4 \text{ J}$

Now, the sum of the reactants can be subtracted from the sum of the products:

$\Delta S°_{rxn} = \Sigma n_p S° \text{ (products)} - \Sigma n_r S° \text{ (reactants)} = (377.4 \text{ J} + 496.4 \text{ J}) - (411.2 \text{ J} + 615.0 \text{ J}) = -152.4 \text{ J}$

Therefore, the standard molar entropy of the above reaction is –152.4 J, which is not a favorable change in entropy.

ENERGY IN RELATION TO HEAT AND WORK

The first law of thermodynamics states that energy cannot be created or destroyed, which means energy is transferred from one form into another. The change in energy (ΔE) can be explained in terms of heat and work:

$$\Delta E = q + w$$

where q is heat and w is work. Work can also be expressed as:

$$w = -P\Delta V$$

where P is pressure (atm) and V is volume (L). Typically, energy is measured in joules (J) and not pressure and volume. To convert work into J, use the conversion factor $\dfrac{101.3 \text{ J}}{1 \text{ L} \cdot \text{atm}}$.

HEAT TRANSFER AND SPECIFIC HEAT

Heat (q) is the transfer of thermal energy, where temperature measures that transfer. Temperature is often used to measure the heat transfer from one compound to another:

$$q = mC_s\Delta T$$

where q is heat, m is mass (g), C_s is the specific heat capacity of a compound (J/g°C), and ΔT is final temperature (T_f) minus the initial temperature (T_i). Temperature is often used to measure the heat transfer from one compound to another:

$$q_{sys} = -q_{surr}$$

where q_{sys} is the heat of the system, and will always be the opposite sign as the heat of the surroundings (q_{surr}). Basically, this is stating that heat is transferred from one to the other, where one gains heat and the other loses the *same* amount of heat.

ΔE AND ΔH: CONSTANT VOLUME AND CONSTANT PRESSURE PROCESSES

When heat transfer is measured under specific conditions, it can give us some valuable information about compounds. Bomb calorimetry, for example, is used to measure the amount of energy released when a compound undergoes combustion. Since bomb calorimeters have a constant volume, the change in energy is only due to heat released from the reaction (recall $\Delta E = q + w$ and $w = -P\Delta V$). The heat equation for bomb calorimetry is:

$$q_{cal} = C_{cal}\Delta T$$

where q_{cal} is the heat absorbed in the bomb calorimeter and C_{cal} is the heat capacity of the bomb calorimeter. Since the bomb calorimeter is closed off (constant volume), the heat absorbed by the bomb calorimeter is the heat released during the combustion reaction:

$$q_{cal} = -q_{rxn}$$

Bomb calorimetry has constant volume, but when heat is released or absorbed at constant pressure, the heat evolved is enthalpy (ΔH). When enthalpy is positive, this is indicative of an endothermic reaction where heat is absorbed. Exothermic reactions, on the other hand, release energy and, therefore, have a negative ΔH. A typical lab experiment that measures if a reaction is exothermic or endothermic is coffee-cup calorimetry. A reaction is most likely monitored through the change in temperature of the water:

$$q_{rxn} = -q_{soln}$$

where q_{rxn} is the heat absorbed or released by the reaction, and q_{soln} is the same amount of heat that was transferred to or from the reaction. The heat of the reaction is related to the enthalpy of the reaction as such:

$$\frac{q_{rxn}}{\text{experimentally determined mol of ``}X\text{''}} = \frac{H_{rxn}}{\text{stoichiometric mol of ``}X\text{''}}$$

where experimentally determined mol of "X" was the amount of the compound used in the experiment that gave off that amount of heat (q_{rxn}), and stoichiometric mol of "X" is the amount of compound "X" in the balance chemical equation. For coffee-cup calorimetry to be valid, it has to be done at constant pressure (i.e., room pressure).

➡ Example _____

24.8 g of NaOH was dissolved in 100 mL of water. Through calculations, it was determined that the water absorbed 147 J of heat. What is the enthalpy of the reaction?

$$NaOH \rightarrow Na^+ + OH^- \qquad \Delta H_{rxn} = ?$$

Solution

Recall that the water will *absorb* the amount of heat that is *released* from the reaction ($q_{soln} = -q_{rxn}$), which means the reaction *released* 147 J ($q_{rxn} = -147$ J). The relationship between an experimentally determined heat and enthalpy of a reaction is:

$$\frac{q_{rxn}}{\text{experimentally determined mol of ``}X\text{''}} = \frac{\Delta H_{rxn}}{\text{stoichiometric mol of ``}X\text{''}}$$

Next, convert grams of NaOH to moles using the molecular weight:

$$24.8 \text{ g} \times 1 \text{ mol}/40.0 \text{ g} = 0.62 \text{ mol NaOH}$$

Plugging in the values gives:

$$\frac{-147 \text{ J}}{0.62 \text{ mol NaOH}} = \frac{\Delta H_{rxn}}{1 \text{ mol NaOH}} \Rightarrow \Delta H_{rxn} = \frac{-147 \text{ J}}{0.62 \text{ mol NaOH}} \times 1 \text{ mol NaOH} = -23\underline{7} \text{ J} = -240 \text{ J}$$

Therefore, ΔH_{rxn} for NaOH dissolving in water is -240 J.

BOND ENERGIES AND ENTHALPY OF REACTIONS

The bond energy is the amount of energy that is released or absorbed when a bond forms or breaks. The enthalpy of a reaction can also be calculated from bond energies:

$$\Delta H_{rxn} = \Sigma (\Delta H \text{ of bonds broken}) - \Sigma (\Delta H \text{ of bonds formed})$$

where Σ is the sum. ΔH_{rxn} will be positive (endothermic) when ΔH of bonds broken is greater than the energy released when bonds are formed, and vice versa for exothermic reactions ($-\Delta H$).

Standard heat of formation (H_f°) of specific substances can be used to calculate the standard enthalpy changes of a reaction (ΔH_{rxn}°) by using the following equation:

$$\Delta H_{rxn}^\circ = \Sigma n_p H_f^\circ \text{ (products)} - \Sigma n_r H_f^\circ \text{ (reactants)}$$

where Σ means the sum, and n is the number of moles. The standard heat of formation (H_f°) for a pure substance is zero. An example problem for this would be the same setup as the previous example problem for (ΔS_{rxn}°).

➡ **Example** _____

Is the following reaction exothermic or endothermic based on the given bond energies?

$$2H_2(g) + O_2(g) \rightarrow 2H_2O(g)$$

Bond Type	Bond Energies (kJ/mol)
H—H	432
O=O	495
H—O	467

The equation that will be used to determine if this reaction is exothermic or endothermic is:

$$\Delta H_{rxn} = \Sigma (\Delta H \text{ of bonds broken}) - \Sigma (\Delta H \text{ of bonds formed})$$

On the reactant side, there are H–H bonds and O=O bonds. More specifically, there are 2 H–H bonds and 1 O=O bond. The sum of these energies are

$$2 \text{ mol H}_2 \text{ (432 kJ/mol)} + 1 \text{ mol O}_2 \text{ (495 kJ/mol)} = 1{,}359 \text{ kJ}$$

On the product side, 2 H–O bonds are formed for EACH H_2O molecule. Therefore, in total, there are 4 H–O bonds formed: 4 mol (467 kJ/mol) = 1,868 kJ. Plug these values into the equation and solve:

$$\Delta H_{rxn} = (1{,}359 \text{ kJ}) - (1{,}868 \text{ kJ}) = -509 \text{ kJ}$$

Since the reaction released heat, this is an exothermic reaction.

HESS'S LAW

Hess's law states that if the sum of multiple reaction steps equals the overall reaction, then the sum of each individual ΔH_{rxn} will equal the overall ΔH_{rxn}. The table below generalizes this law.

Equation	ΔH Expression	Relationship to ΔH_{ref}
Reference equation: $A \rightarrow B$	ΔH_{ref}	ΔH_{ref}
Reverse reference equation: $B \rightarrow A$	ΔH_{rev}	$\Delta H_{rev} = -\Delta H_{ref}$
Sum of reactions equals reference equation: Reaction 1: $A \rightarrow C$ Reaction 2: $C \rightarrow B$ Overall reaction: $A \rightarrow B$	ΔH_1 ΔH_2	$\Delta H_1 + \Delta H_2 = \Delta H_{ref}$
Subtraction of reactions equals reference equation: Reaction 3: $3A \rightarrow 2B + C$ Reaction 4: $2A \rightarrow B + C$ Overall reaction: $A \rightarrow B$	ΔH_3 ΔH_4	$\Delta H_3 - \Delta H_4 = \Delta H_{ref}$
Multiplied by a factor: $3A \rightarrow 3B$	ΔH_5	$\Delta H_5 = 3 \times \Delta H_{ref}$
Divided by a factor: $\dfrac{A}{2} \rightarrow \dfrac{B}{2}$ Or $\dfrac{1}{2}A \rightarrow \dfrac{1}{2}B$	ΔH_6	$\Delta H_6 = \dfrac{1}{2} \times \Delta H_{ref}$

GIBBS FREE ENERGY AND K_{eq}

The Gibbs free energy (G_{rxn}) of a reaction can be measured from the change in enthalpy and the change in entropy at a specific temperature (K). The Gibbs free energy equation is:

$$G_{rxn} = \Delta H_{rxn} - T\Delta S_{rxn}$$

If ΔG is negative, then the reaction is spontaneous. If it is positive, energy is required and it is nonspontaneous. A **spontaneous** reaction is a reaction that, once started, will continue to go without outside help because it is moving toward a lower energy state. A **nonspontaneous** reaction is moving toward a higher energy state and will, therefore, require outside intervention to proceed. Depending on the conditions, a reaction can be spontaneous at one temperature and nonspontaneous at another. Different conditions are summarized in the table below.

Equation: $\Delta H_{rxn} - T\Delta S_{rxn} = \Delta G_{rxn}$			
ΔH_{rxn}	T	ΔS_{rxn}	ΔG_{rxn}
positive	large	positive	negative due to large $-T\Delta S$
positive	small	positive	positive due to $\Delta H > -T\Delta S$
positive	large	negative	Always positive due to
positive	small	negative	$(+\Delta H) - T(-\Delta S) = (+\Delta H) + T(\Delta S)$
negative	large	positive	Always negative due to
negative	small	positive	$(-\Delta H) - T(+\Delta S) = (-\Delta H) - T(\Delta S)$
negative	large	negative	positive due to large $-T(-\Delta S) = T(\Delta S)$
negative	small	negative	negative due to $(-\Delta H) > -T(\Delta S)$

The standard Gibbs free energy of a reaction (ΔG°_{rxn}) is related to the equilibrium constant, K_{eq}, through the following equation:

$$\Delta G^\circ_{rxn} = -RT \ln(K_{eq})$$

The two Gibbs free energy equations can be combined and rearranged to:

$$\ln K_{eq} = -\frac{\Delta H^\circ_{rxn}}{R}\left(\frac{1}{T}\right) + \frac{\Delta S^\circ_{rxn}}{R}$$

which is the equation of the line when $\ln K$ is plotted on the y-axis and $\frac{1}{T}$ is plotted on the x-axis. The slope and the y-intercept can be used to find ΔH°_{rxn} and ΔS°_{rxn}, respectively.

➡ **Example**

What is the enthalpy of reaction based on the plot given?

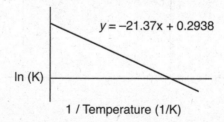

Solution

A plot of $\ln K$ vs. $\frac{1}{T}$ will result in a slope that equals $-\frac{\Delta H^\circ_{rxn}}{R}$. The slope of the graph is -21.37.

Set these two equal to each other and solve for ΔH°_{rxn}:

$$-21.37 = -\frac{\Delta H^\circ_{rxn}}{8.314\ \text{J/mol} \cdot \text{K}} \Rightarrow (-21.37)\left(\frac{-8.314\ \text{J}}{\text{mol} \cdot \text{K}}\right) = +177.7\ \frac{\text{J}}{\text{mol}}$$

Electrochemistry

24

BALANCING REDOX REACTIONS

Balancing redox (reduction-oxidation) reactions is based on balancing the number of electrons. Oxidation occurs when an atom loses electrons (LEO—lose electrons oxidation or OIL—oxidation is loss), and reduction occurs when an atom gains electrons (GER—gain electrons reduction or RIG—reduction is gain). This losing and gaining (or transferring) of electrons is what allows batteries to work. Since electrons have mass, the number of electrons gained and lost must be the same (law of conservation of mass). This is the basis for balancing redox reactions.

Oxidation numbers are assigned to elements to determine if it has lost electrons (becomes oxidized) or if it has gained electrons (becomes reduced). In general, the rules for assigning oxidation states IN ORDER are:

1. If the element is by itself, then the oxidation state is equal to the overall charge (zero if neutral or matches the charge of the ion).
2. Group I and group II metals have the same oxidation number as their charge.
3. F is -1.
4. O is usually -2.
5. H is $+1$, unless it is the most electronegative atom (i.e., LiH), then it is -1.
6. Assign the remaining elements where it balances out the oxidation states so it equals the overall charge on the compound or polyatomic ion.

➥ Example

How many electrons were lost/gained? Was the Zn oxidized or reduced?

$$Zn(s) + Cl_2(g) \rightarrow ZnCl_2(aq)$$

Solution

First, assign oxidation states to any element that is pure – Zn and Cl_2. Both are assigned oxidation states of 0 since both have an overall charge of 0. Second, assign oxidation states to elements in compounds, and typically the more electronegative atom is assigned first – $ZnCl_2$. Cl is more electronegative than Zn, so its oxidation state is equal to the charge Cl usually makes, which is -1. Since $ZnCl_2$ is a neutral compound, Zn must balance with the -1 charge on EACH Cl, making it have a $+2$ oxidation state. To determine if Zn was oxidized or reduced, use the acronyms to help (LEO/GER or OIL/RIG). Zn lost 2 electrons ($Zn^0 \rightarrow Zn^{2+}$), so it was oxidized.

➡ Example

Balance the following redox reaction under **basic** conditions:

$$NO_2^-(aq) + Al(s) \rightarrow NH_3(g) + AlO_2^-(aq)$$

Example: Balancing Redox Reactions Under Basic or Acidic Conditions

Question: Balance the following redox reaction under BASIC conditions	$NO_2^-(aq) + Al(s) \rightarrow NH_3(g) + AlO_2^-(aq)$
Assign oxidation numbers:	**Reactant side:** Assign Al first (elements by themselves, like Al, will have an oxidation state equal to the overall charge) Al = 0. Then, assign the O in the polyatomic ion because O is more electronegative than N, O = –2. This means N must have an oxidation state of +3 in order to match the overall charge of –1 $\left(NO_2^-\right)$. **Product side:** Assign H first because N can make multiple oxidation states, H = +1. This means N must be –3 to have an overall charge of 0 (NH_3). Next, assign O first because it is more electronegative than Al, O = –2, which means Al must be +3 in order to match the overall charge of –1 $\left(AlO_2^-\right)$.
Split reactions based on if the atom or compound is being oxidized or reduced:	N: +3 → –3: N gained 6 electrons, which means it was reduced: $$NO_2^-(aq) \rightarrow NH_3(g)$$ Al: 0 → +3: Al lost 3 electrons, which means it was oxidized: $$Al(s) \rightarrow AlO_2^-(aq)$$ O stayed at –2, which is why this was ignored when putting these half-reactions together. H was also ignored because it was only on one side of the equation. Therefore, the half-reactions were based on N and Al.
Balance the atoms in each half-reaction, except for O and H:	$$NO_2^-(aq) \rightarrow NH_3(g)$$ N is already balanced $$Al(s) \rightarrow AlO_2^-(aq)$$ Al is also already balanced
Balance O by adding water:	$$NO_2^-(aq) \rightarrow NH_3(g) + 2H_2O(l)$$ $$2H_2O(l) + Al(s) \rightarrow AlO_2^-(aq)$$

Balance H by adding H^+ ions: (this step still has to be done even under basic conditions. It will be fixed at the last step.)	$7H^+(aq) + NO_2^-(aq) \rightarrow NH_3(g) + 2H_2O(l)$ $2H_2O(l) + Al(s) \rightarrow AlO_2^-(aq) + 4H^+(aq)$
Balance charge using electrons:	$6e^- + 7H^+(aq) + NO_2^-(aq) \rightarrow NH_3(g) + 2H_2O(l)$ 6 electrons had to be added to the reactant side, so that the overall charge on the reactant side is zero. This then matches the overall charge of the product side. $2H_2O(l) + Al(s) \rightarrow AlO_2^-(aq) + 4H^+(aq) + 3e^-$ 3 electrons were added to the product side, so the overall charge on the product side matches the overall charge on the reactant side.
Balance number of electrons for each half-reaction:	$6e^- + 7H^+(aq) + NO_2^-(aq) \rightarrow NH_3(g) + 2H_2O(l)$ has 6 electrons, whereas: $2H_2O(l) + Al(s) \rightarrow AlO_2^-(aq) + 4H^+(aq) + 3e^-$ has 3 electrons. This means the bottom equation has to be multiplied by 2 to make each half-reaction have 6 electrons: $4H_2O(l) + 2Al(s) \rightarrow 2AlO_2^-(aq) + 8H^+(aq) + 6e^-$
Add the half-reactions together and simplify:	$6e^- + 7H^+(aq) + NO_2^-(aq) \rightarrow NH_3(g) + 2H_2O(l)$ $4H_2O(l) + 2Al(s) \rightarrow 2AlO^-_2(aq) + 8H^+(aq) + 6e^-$ = $6e^- + 7H^+(aq) + NO_2^-(aq) + 4H_2O(l) + 2Al(s) \rightarrow$ $NH_3(g) + 2H_2O(l) + 2AlO_2^-(aq) + 8H^+(aq) + 6e^-$ Then simplify: $NO_2^-(aq) + 2H_2O(l) + 2Al(s) \rightarrow NH_3(g) + 2AlO_2^-(aq) + H^+(aq)$
For basic conditions, one more step is required. For every H^+ present, add OH^- to *each* side.	$OH^-(aq) + NO_2^-(aq) + 2H_2O(l) + 2Al(s) \rightarrow$ $NH_3(g) + 2AlO_2^-(aq) + \underbrace{H^+(aq) + OH^-(aq)}$ combines to form $H_2O(l)$ Then simiplify: $OH^-(aq) + NO_2^-(aq) + H_2O(l) + 2Al(s) \rightarrow NH_3(g) + 2AlO_2(aq)$

BATTERIES: EXPERIMENTAL SETUP AND DEFINITIONS

Batteries are based on redox reactions, where the electric current is generated by the transfer of electrons. More specifically, electrochemical cells will have an anode and a cathode. Oxidation occurs at the anode, reduction occurs at the cathode, and a salt bridge connects the two to allow electron flow. When the flow of electrons is generated from a spontaneous reaction, this is called a **voltaic/galvanic cell**. An **electrolytic cell** is generated from a nonspontaneous reaction.

Electrons spontaneously flow from high potential energy to low potential energy, just like how a ball will fall down the stairs instead of up the stairs. The rate of electron flow is measured in amperes (A):

$$1\,A = 1\,C/s$$

where C is coulomb and s is seconds. Typically, the potential energy difference in batteries are measured in volts (V):

$$1\,V = 1\,J/C$$

The larger the potential energy, the more likely a reaction will proceed forward and the higher the volts. With voltaic/galvanic cells, the potential energy difference is called the **cell potential** (E_{cell}). If the cell potential is measured under standard conditions (1 M concentrations, 1 atm, 25°C), then this is the **standard cell potential** (E°_{cell}). The E°_{cell} can be measured from the standard electrode potentials:

$$E^\circ_{cell} = E^\circ_{cat} - E^\circ_{an}$$

where E°_{cat} is the cathode's potential and E°_{an} is the anode's potential. For a spontaneous reaction, E°_{cell} will be positive.

STANDARD HYDROGEN ELECTRODE AND STANDARD REDUCTION POTENTIALS

To assign electrode potentials, there had to be a standard electrode that the rest were based on. The standard hydrogen electrode (SHE) was selected as the standard where it was assigned to have a potential energy of zero:

$$2H^+(aq) + 2e^- \rightarrow H_2(g) \qquad E^\circ = 0$$

Anything that can be more easily reduced than hydrogen will have a positive E°, and anything that is harder to reduce than hydrogen will have a negative E°. For spontaneous reactions, the electrons will flow from high to low potential, or from more positive to less positive E°.

➡ Example _____

What is E°_{cell} for the following reaction?

$$Cu^{2+}(aq) + Zn(s) \rightarrow Cu(s) + Zn^{2+}(aq)$$

Half-reactions with cell potentials:

$$Cu^{2+}(aq) + 2e^- \rightarrow Cu(s) \qquad E^\circ = 0.34\,V$$

$$Zn^{2+}(aq) + 2e^- \rightarrow Zn(s) \qquad E^\circ = -0.76\,V$$

To calculate E_{cell}°, identify which is the cathode and which is the anode. The cathode will be the electrode with the higher electrode potential (Cu), and the anode will be the lower electrode potential (Zn). Plug the electrode potentials into the equation:

$$E_{cell}^{\circ} = E_{cat}^{\circ} - E_{an}^{\circ} = 0.34 - (-0.76) = 1.10$$

Therefore, $E_{cell}^{\circ} = +1.10$. If the half-reactions needed to be multiplied by a certain factor to match with the overall reaction, the electrode potential does NOT need to be multiplied.

BATTERIES: E_{cell}°, ΔG°, AND K_{eq}

There are now a few ways to calculate if a reaction is spontaneous or not, and they are all related to each other. For batteries, if E_{cell}° is positive, then it is a spontaneous reaction. For Gibb's free energy, a reaction is spontaneous if it has a negative ΔG. The relationship between ΔG° and E_{cell}° is:

$$\Delta G^{\circ} = -nFE_{cell}^{\circ}$$

where n is the number of moles of electrons transferred in the reaction, and F is Faraday's constant $\left(F = \dfrac{96{,}485 \text{ C}}{1 \text{ mol e}^-} \right)$. The relationship between K_{eq} and E_{cell}° is:

$$E_{cell}^{\circ} = \frac{0.0592 \text{ V}}{n} \log(K_{eq})$$

Recall that anything with a nought (°) is measured at standard conditions (25°C and 1 atm), which means K_{eq} was also measured at 25°C in order for this equation to be true. The relationship between ΔG° and K_{eq} is:

$$\Delta G^{\circ} = -RT \ln(K_{eq})$$

BATTERIES: NERNST EQUATION AND CALCULATING E_{cell}

If a cell potential (E_{cell}) was not measured under standard conditions, then it can be related to E_{cell}° through the Nernst equation:

$$E_{cell} = E_{cell}^{\circ} - \frac{0.0592 \text{ V}}{n} \log(Q)$$

where Q is the reaction quotient and is used when the reaction is not at equilibrium (K_{eq}).

NONSPONTANEOUS REACTIONS: ELECTROLYSIS

Electrolytic cells are used for nonspontaneous reactions. One example is the electrolysis of water:

$$2H_2O(l) \rightarrow 2H_2(g) + O_2(g)$$

where electric current is used to break water down into its gaseous substituents. Electrolysis is also used to convert metal oxides into pure metals. Since these reactions are nonspontaneous, E_{cell} will be negative. The spontaneous version of metals converted to metal oxides is called corrosion, i.e., iron rust.

Laboratory Skills

25

CARE AND USE OF LABORATORY APPARATUS

Laboratory instrumentation often requires preparation before using. Each piece of equipment is unique, but general care and use of laboratory apparatus can include washing, calibration, and maintenance. Some common examples include: balancing scales, thoroughly cleaning glassware, and calibrating pH probes.

PRECISION WITHIN GLASSWARE

Different types of laboratory glassware are used for different purposes. Beakers have limited utility for precise measurement of volumes but are useful for transferring liquids and mixing solutions. Graduated cylinders and volumetric glassware have higher precision in measuring volumes more accurately. Burets are often used in titrations and can give precise volume delivery. Information about the glassware is often printed on the side. The tolerance, or how precise a measurement can be made, is usually written as ± % or ± mL on the glassware. The smaller the number, the more precise the measurement.

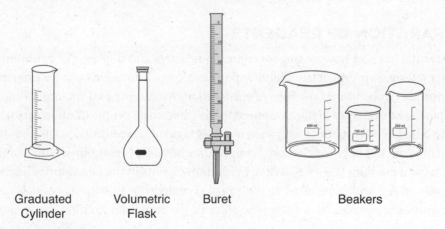

Graduated   Volumetric   Buret   Beakers
Cylinder   Flask

TYPES OF ERRORS

All experiments are prone to errors. Systematic errors shift all measurements in a fixed way so their mean value is displaced. This may be due to incorrect calibration of equipment, consistent improper use of equipment, or failure to properly account for environmental effects, such as temperature, pressure, or humidity.

Random errors fluctuate from one measurement to the next and yield results distributed about some mean value. They can occur for a variety of reasons, including lack of sensitivity and noise. Random errors displace measurements in an arbitrary direction, whereas systematic errors displace measurements in a single direction. Some systematic errors can be eliminated (or properly taken into account), but random errors are unavoidable.

DATA ANALYSIS

Once experimental data is collected, graphing can assist with data interpretation. Scatter plots are the most common way of plotting data and can have any type of linear or non-linear fit incorporated. The graph should be constructed with the independent variable on the x-axis and the dependent variable on the y-axis. For example, when plotting the data from a titration, the volume of acid or base added to a solution would be plotted on the x-axis, while the pH of the solution would be plotted on the y-axis. Graphs can be useful tools to interpret your data. In the example below of a titration, the inflection or steep part of the graph shows the endpoint of the titration.

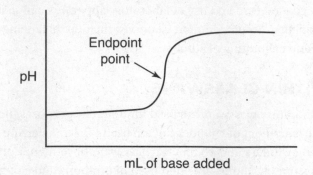

Titration curve. The inflection point is where the equivalence point occurs.
The moles of acid = moles of base at the equivalence point.

PREPARATION OF REAGENTS

It is essential to know how to prepare common reagents and dilutions of common reagents. In order to have reproducible, reliable experiments, stock solutions can be prepared. These solutions are concentrated versions of the "working" solutions and require dilutions before use. There are three types of dilutions used in the laboratory. Simple dilutions are when a unit volume of solute is combined with solvent to get needed concentration. Dilution factors are represented as (1:5) or "1 to 5," where 1 unit volume of solute is combined with 4 unit volumes of the solvent medium (1 + 4 = 5). When preparing reagents in the laboratory, chemicals must be measured out and transferred to their final container. To transfer chemicals completely, use quantitative transfer by washing the sides of the container holding the solute with the solvent in steps.

LAB SAFETY

Laboratory safety is essential to work in a safe and productive environment. Generally, you should be concerned about protecting yourself and your co-workers from cuts, chemical spills, inhalation of gases, and explosions. The rules and regulations will vary based on the types of experiments being performed and the equipment being used in a lab. You should consult a laboratory safety officer or person in charge of lab safety before you begin working in a new lab.

Personal Protective Equipment (PPE) are used to protect your body from laboratory chemical hazards. Typically, laboratory supervisors or safety officers will determine what PPE are appropriate in your laboratory and for the experiments that you are conducting. Basic PPE usually include: goggles/glasses, gloves, lab coats, ear protection, and closed-toed shoes.

Before commencing work, you should familiarize yourself with the location of safety showers, eyewash stations, and fire doors. Be prepared and familiarize yourself with laboratory instrumentation and chemicals prior to conducting an experiment. Any hazardous waste that is generated in the course of experiments must be handled and disposed of properly.

PART THREE

Organic Chemistry

PART THREE

Organic
Chemistry

Introduction

26

This review of the basic principles of organic chemistry is designed to closely follow the DAT content outline for this topic. In cases where the DAT content outline does not lead to a logical progression of basic organic chemistry concepts, there has been some reordering of the content to allow for a better flow of the review material. You should be prepared to study this review and its associated exercises, in conjunction with the DAT practice exams. Plan to study as much of this material as time allows prior to taking the actual DAT.

> It can't be overstated how important a *clear* understanding of general chemistry principles (as presented in this study guide) is for mastering the concepts associated with organic chemistry. Chemistry is chemistry—organic chemistry focuses on carbon-containing compounds, but the same principles that you learned in your first formal chemistry course apply. In many cases, just a basic knowledge of general chemistry will allow you to answer organic chemistry questions posed on the DAT.

Depending on the amount of time that has passed since you have completed your organic chemistry course work, significantly different levels of effort may be required before achieving the desired competence in this area. Those who have recently completed courses in organic chemistry or who are chemistry majors may find this task relatively easy. If it has been several years since you have studied organic chemistry, this task will obviously require more time and effort. Don't be discouraged if at first the material seems unfamiliar. By reviewing and practicing with this study guide, you can master the key areas needed to perform well in this DAT competency.

Bonding in Organic Compounds

27

Organic chemistry is the study of carbon-containing compounds. By far the most important bonding model for these molecular compounds is **covalent** bonding. In most cases carbon atoms are bonded to each other or the elements H, O, N, X (where X = F, Cl, Br, and I), and less commonly, S and P (these noncarbon atoms are also occasionally bonded to each other). There are also ionic bonding considerations in some organic compounds, but these interactions are not nearly as common. The shape (structure) of organic molecules is usually defined by the carbon-carbon covalent bond, making it the most important bonding scheme in organic chemistry.

You may remember that **covalent** bonding is defined as the sharing of two or more valence electrons between atoms. **Ionic** bonding involves the transfer of one or more valence electrons between atoms. The transfer of electrons between atoms creates oppositely charged ions (positively charged **cations** and negatively charged **anions**) that are attracted to each other. This is the mechanism of electrostatic bonding interactions (the oppositely charged ions stick together).

SIGMA (σ) AND PI (π) COVALENT BONDS

The **Valence Bond** theory is one approach to qualitatively predicting the length and strength of covalent bonds in molecular compounds. This theory is also useful in predicting the 3D shapes of molecules. It may be recalled that this model for bonding (originally postulated by the chemist Linus Pauling) involves three basic concepts:

1. Overlap of atomic orbitals containing unpaired valence electrons
2. Localization of valence electrons in the orbital overlap region between atoms (the bonding region)
3. The formation of hybrid orbitals from atomic orbitals to optimize orbital overlap between bonding atoms

The most important atomic orbitals in organic bond formation are the s and p. The s-orbital has a spherical shape and can hold two valence electrons of opposite spins. p-orbitals exist in sets of three (usually referred to as the p_x-, p_y-, and p_z-orbitals) due to the three ways the orbital can be oriented in 3D space and can hold a total of six valence electrons. These orbitals each have the approximate shape of a figure eight (see Figure 27.1 for 3D representations of these two orbital types).

An *s* Atomic Orbital   A *p* Atomic Orbital

Figure 27.1. The shapes and geometries of *s*-atomic and *p*-atomic orbitals

> The size, energy, shape, and orientation of atomic orbitals are defined by quantum mechanics (*Q* numbers *n*, *l*, and *m*$_l$), which treat electrons as if they have wave-like properties. Mathematical solutions to wave equations provide the basic orbital shapes. Note that *p*-orbitals have two lobes each with a different phase (see the different shading for each lobe in Figure 27.1) and a node between them where electron density is zero.

In some molecules atomic orbitals containing unpaired valence electrons overlap to form covalent bonds, but in most cases the geometry of atomic orbitals is not correct for optimum overlap (e.g., the greatest area of overlap to give the strongest, shortest bond). What usually happens to atomic orbitals to optimize orbital overlap is called orbital hybridization. This process is accomplished by mixing atomic *s*- and *p*-orbitals together in different proportions. The most common types of orbital hybridization in organic compounds are as follows:

1. The combination of an *s*-atomic and a *p*-atomic orbital to give *two sp*-hybrid orbitals
2. The combination of an *s*-atomic and two *p*-atomic orbitals to give *three sp*^{2}-hybrid orbitals
3. The combination of an *s*-atomic and three *p*-atomic orbitals to give *four sp*^{3}-hybrid orbitals

Note in the above examples that in the orbital hybridization process *the number of atomic orbitals combined is always equal to the number of hybrid orbitals formed*. Figure 27.2 shows the approximate shapes of the *sp*-hybrid, *sp*^{2}-hybrid, and *sp*^{3}-hybrid orbitals. It can be seen that although each of the hybrid orbitals is similar in shape, their lobes are proportionally different.

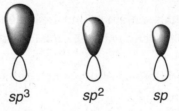

sp^3 *sp*^{2} *sp*

Figure 27.2. The shapes and relative sizes
of the *sp*^{3}-hybrid, *sp*^{2}-hybrid, and *sp*-hybrid orbitals

Orbital overlap between both *p*-atomic and hybrid orbitals can occur in *two* different orientations. The most common overlap orientation is end-to-end overlap between two *p*-atomic orbitals, a *p*-atomic orbital and a hybrid orbital, or two hybrid orbitals. Bonds that result from this kind of overlap are referred to as **sigma** (σ) bonds and form the bonding skeleton of organic compounds (called the sigma skeleton). The second kind of overlap is side-to-side overlap usually between two *p*-atomic orbitals in organic molecules. Bonds that result from this type of orbital overlap are called *pi* (π) bonds and *only* occur in conjunction with the formation of σ bonds. Figure 27.3 shows pictorial examples of these two kinds of orbital overlaps and the resulting bond types.

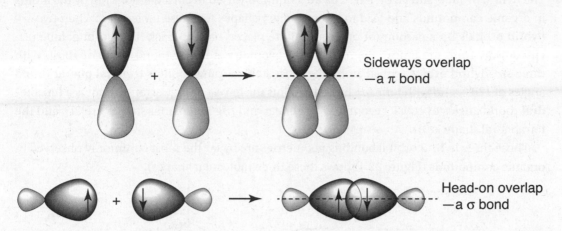

Figure 27.3. The formation of σ and π bonds by end-to-end and side-to-side orbital overlap

MULTIPLE BONDS IN MOLECULES

As you may recall, many organic molecular compounds contain multiple covalent bonding interactions—these are more commonly referred to as **multiple bonds**. A simplified bonding symbology is used to easily represent multiple bonds, which are actually combinations of σ and π bonds. A single line between bonding atoms implies a **single** σ bond. Two lines between bonding atoms imply a **double** bond consisting of both a σ and a π bond. Three lines between atoms imply a **triple** bond consisting of a single σ and two π bonds. The carbon-carbon bonds in the following compounds illustrate the use of this symbology: ethane, ethene (commonly called ethylene), and ethyne (commonly called acetylene). Recall that triple bonds are shorter and stronger than double bonds and double bonds are shorter and stronger than single bonds. In general, the shorter the bonding interaction between two atoms, the more energy it takes to break the bond (see Table 27.1 for a comparison of these carbon-carbon bond lengths and energies).

Table 27.1. The Lengths and Energies of Carbon-Carbon Covalent Bonds

$H_3C—CH_3$	$H_2C=CH_2$	$HC \equiv CH$
one σ bond	one σ bond and one π bond	one σ bond and two π bonds
(C—C single bond)	(C=C double bond)	(C≡C triple bond)
Length: 154 pm*	Length: 134 pm	Length: 121 pm
Energy: 356 kJ/mol	Energy: 598 kJ/mol	Energy: 813 kJ/mol

*1 pm = 10^{-12} m
(Data from Cotton, F. A., Wilkinson, G., and Gaus, P. L.,
Basic Inorganic Chemistry, 3rd ed. New York: Wiley, 1995; p. 12.)

MOLECULAR SHAPE THEORY

Valence Bond Molecular Shape Theory

The hybrid orbitals shown on page 202 are commonly used in covalent bonding by the atoms in organic compounds and lead to three primary shapes for these molecules. When two *sp*-hybrid orbitals on a carbon (or other atom) are placed back to back (large orbital lobe oriented away from the atom), the most stable geometry is **linear** (bond angle of 180°). With three *sp²*-hybrid orbitals on an atom, the most stable arrangement is **trigonal planar** (bond angles of 120°), and with four *sp³*-hybrid orbitals the lowest energy arrangement is a **tetrahedral** (bond angles of 109.5°) geometry. The linear and trigonal planar shapes are 2D, and the tetrahedral shape is 3D.

These three hybrid orbital bonding geometries are by far the most commonly observed in organic compounds (Figure 27.4 shows these three molecular shapes).

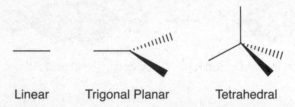

Linear   Trigonal Planar   Tetrahedral

Figure 27.4. The most common molecular geometries
for bonding atoms in organic compounds

Carbon atoms always use hybrid orbitals when forming bonds and the same is true for other atoms such as oxygen and nitrogen. In organic compounds hydrogen and halogen atoms almost always form single bonds. Thus their bonding orbitals are not hybridized during the bonding process (e.g., they use their unhybridized *s*-atomic and *p*-atomic orbitals to bond). To answer some DAT organic chemistry questions, it is necessary to predict the kind of hybrid orbitals the central atom in a molecule uses to form bonds and the resulting molecular shape.

The following example (see Figure 27.5) shows how the central carbon atom in methane (CH₄) "mixes" an *s*-atomic and three *p*-atomic orbitals to produce four *sp³*-hybrid orbitals.

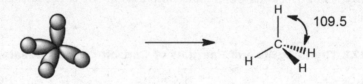

Figure 27.5. Four *sp³*-hybrid orbitals on the central carbon of
the methane molecule bonding with four 1*s*-hydrogen atomic
orbitals to make a tetrahedral shape (on the right)

Each of the four *sp³*-hybrid orbitals, centered on the carbon atom, is used to make a covalent bond with the *s*-atomic orbital from each of the four hydrogen atoms in the molecular formula. The resulting molecule has a tetrahedral shape with 109.5° bond angles. The graphic on the left of Figure 27.5 shows the approximate regions of orbital overlap in the methane molecule (between the carbon *sp³*-orbitals on the central carbon atom and the four hydrogen *s*-atomic orbitals). The graphic on the right shows a simplified 3D structural drawing of methane derived from the orbital overlap representation.

VALENCE SHELL ELECTRON PAIR REPULSION (VSEPR) MOLECULAR SHAPE THEORY

An alternative method for predicting the shapes of simple organic compounds is to use VSEPR theory. This approach uses a much-simplified explanation for molecular shapes and has advantages when there is limited time to look at the details of bond formation using an orbital overlap approach (e.g., valence bond theory).

This concept for predicting shapes as implied by its name involves electron pair repulsion between bonds in molecules. When a molecule has two bonds to a central atom, the geometry when the bonds are farthest apart from each other is a **linear** shape. This geometry minimizes electron-electron repulsion between the two bonding regions of the molecule and provides the greatest distance possible between the two covalent bonds (as also predicted by valence bond theory, the bond angle is 180°).

When a molecule has three bonds to a central atom the predicted geometry is trigonal planar with bond angles of 120°—again, as far apart as the bonds can get from each other. Four bonds to a central atom give a tetrahedral shape (bond angles of 109.5°), and so on. As stated earlier, linear, trigonal planar, and tetrahedral shapes are by far the most common for organic compound bonding centers.

VSEPR theory can be used to predict the type of hybridization that occurs in complex organic compound bonding centers and is the simplest approach for answering DAT questions of this type.

Use the following method to assign the bonding hybridization for carbon, oxygen, and nitrogen atoms in organic compounds:

1. Draw a valid Lewis skeletal structure (2D representation) of the compound—be sure not to break the octet rule.
2. Count the number of **electron groups** around each of the bonding centers in the molecule (e.g., each C, N, and O atom bonding center). An electron group is a single bond, a double bond, a triple bond, a nonbonding lone electron pair, or less commonly a single unpaired nonbonding electron. Each of these electron configurations is counted as *one and only one* electron group (they all count the same!).
3. Assign the bonding atom's hybridization based on the number of electron groups surrounding it. Bonding atoms with *two* electron groups are sp-hybridized, atoms with *three* electron groups are sp^2-hybridized, and atoms with *four* electron groups are sp^3-hybridized.

The following example illustrates the use of this procedure.

Assign the bonding hybridization to each of the C, O, and N atoms in the following Lewis formula (Structure 1):

(1)

Approach

Using the above procedure count the electron groups around each of the C, O, and N atoms and assign the hybridization.

Answer

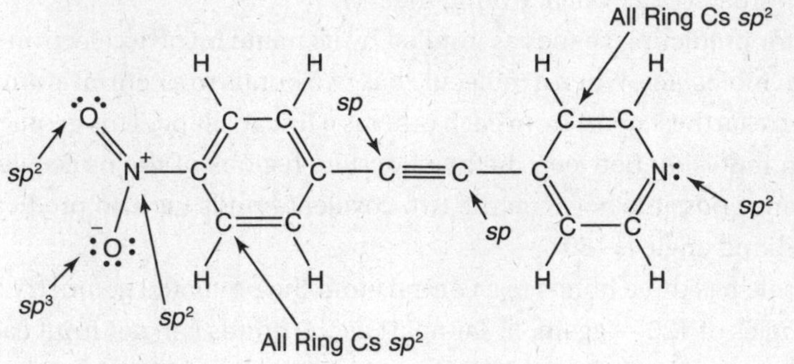

(2)

EXERCISE 1

Directions: Assign the correct orbital hybridization to the C, O, and N atoms in the following compounds. (Answers are on page 339.)

1.

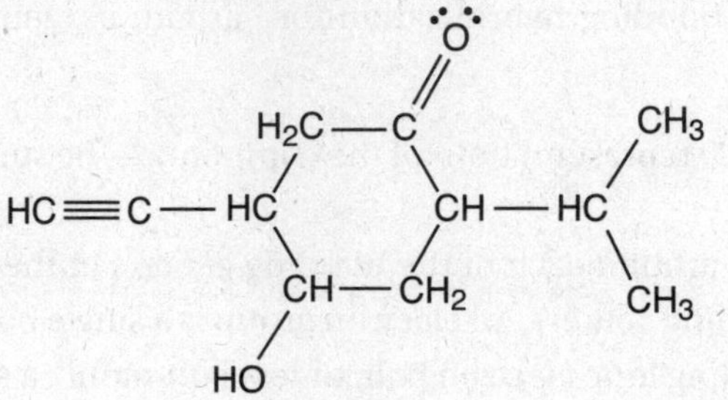

2.

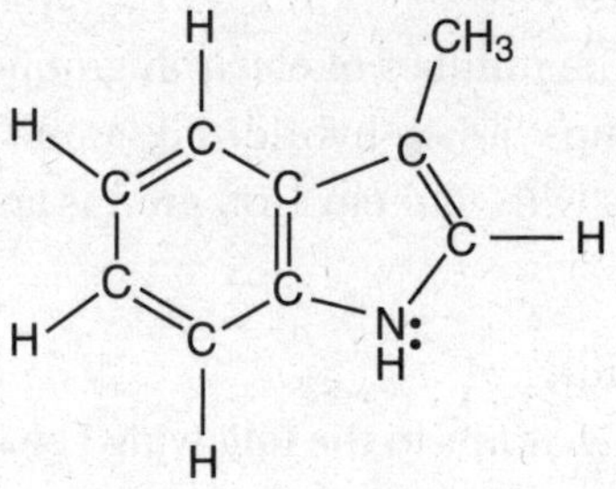

3.

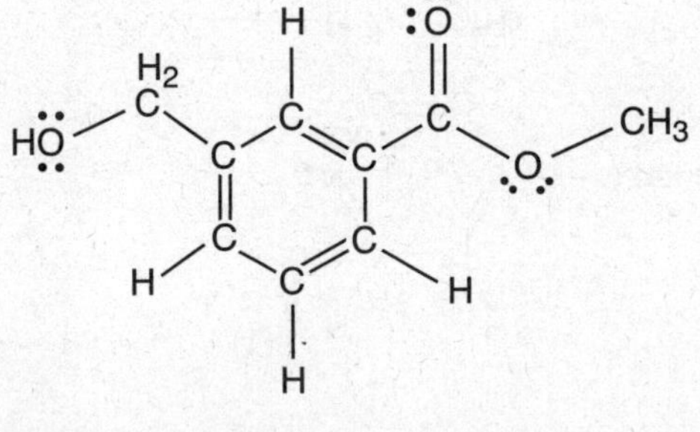

STRUCTURAL FORMULAS

There are several commonly used methods for showing the structures of most organic compound molecules on a 2D surface (such as a piece of paper, blackboard, or a computer screen).

A complete 2D representation showing all atoms, bonds, and nonbonding electrons in the molecule is called a **Lewis** formula. Shown below (Structure 3) is the Lewis formula for the alkyl compound normal hexane (C_6H_{14}).

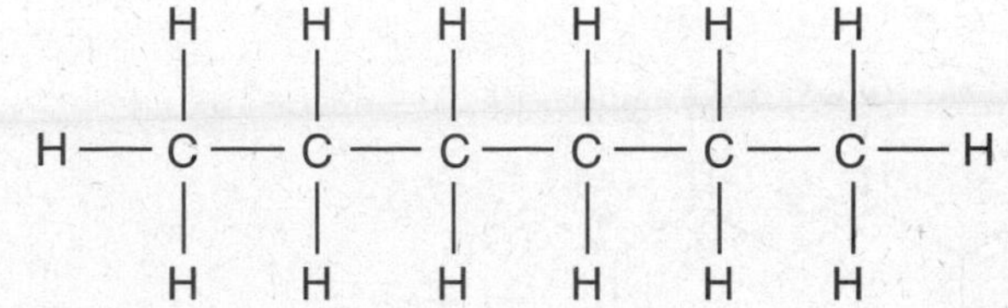

(3)

Another more abbreviated form referred to as "condensed" shows all the atoms in the structure, but only some or none of the bonds. The rest of the molecular structure implies the presence of the missing bonds. Shown below (Structure 4) is the condensed structure for normal hexane.

$$CH_3CH_2CH_2CH_2CH_2CH_3$$ (4)

> You should be familiar with the process for drawing 2D *Lewis* formulas. If you do not have a high degree of proficiency in this area, it is recommended that you practice drawing Lewis formulas using examples from a general chemistry text. Many DAT chemistry questions require a clear understanding of this procedure.

Yet another even more abbreviated form in common use is the Lewis *skeletal* structure, which is often rendered in 3D. In this case, only the covalent bond skeleton is shown. The presence of the carbon and hydrogen atoms associated with the compound is implied by the bonding scheme. Again, using the example of normal hexane, see the skeletal structure (Structure 5) shown below.

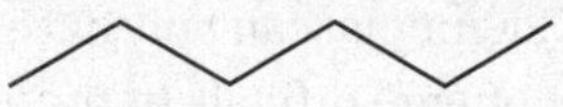

(5)

It may be recalled that when using skeletal structures to represent compounds, all non-carbon atoms, other than hydrogen, must be explicitly shown and it is best to also show all nonbonding electron pairs (also called "lone pairs"). The majority of this Organic Chemistry review will use skeletal structures to represent organic compound molecules.

EXERCISE 2

Directions: The following are some relatively simple examples of the use of Lewis skeletal structure nomenclature. If you are unfamiliar with this approach for showing molecular structures, it is recommended that you study these examples and attempt to draw a complete Lewis formula for each that matches the skeletal structure. Be sure to include any missing nonbonding electrons (as in lone pairs) in your Lewis formula. If at first you don't succeed, keep trying until the Lewis formula contains exactly the same number and types of atoms as indicated in the skeletal structure. (Answers are on page 340.)

1.

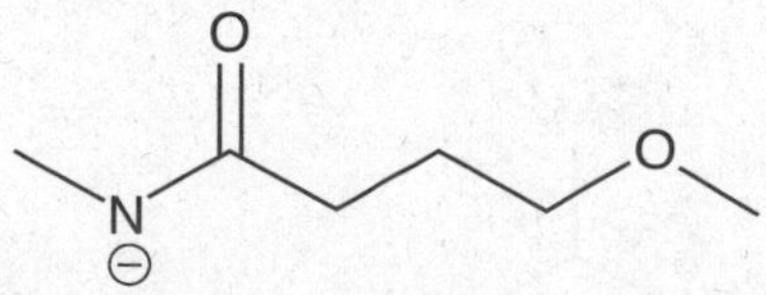

2.

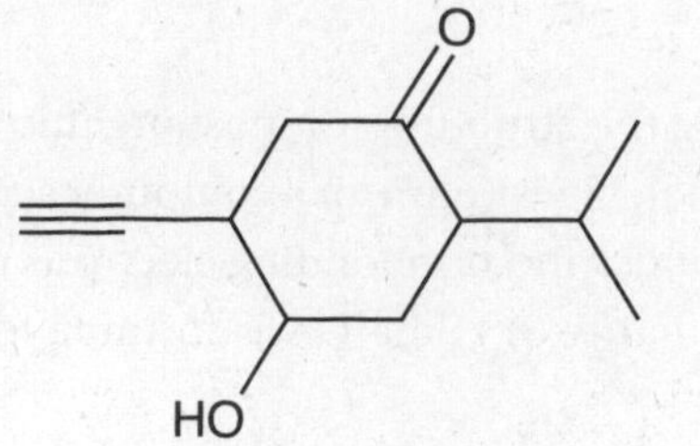

3.

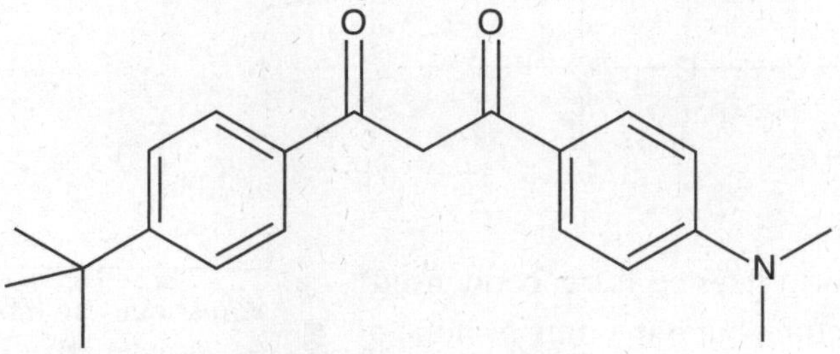

RESONANCE FORMS OF ORGANIC COMPOUNDS

In many cases more than one valid skeletal structure can be drawn for a given molecular formula. Unless a basic rule (like the *octet rule*) has been broken, any possible skeletal structure for a molecular formula is correct; however, it may not be the best (best is defined as the electron arrangement that gives the molecule the lowest possible potential energy—in other words it will be the most stable).

> The *octet rule* comes from Lewis bonding theory and states that period two elements (as designated by the Periodic Table of Elements) can only have eight valence electrons around their nuclei and no more. The low-energy orbitals of these elements (the $2s$ and $2p$) can hold up to eight electrons and once filled there are no other accessible orbitals to hold electrons. Period one elements, such as hydrogen, can have only two valence electrons around their nuclei, but elements in period three and higher can have eight or *more* and don't follow the octet rule.

When a given formula has several valid skeletal structures (called **resonance** forms), they can be combined (mixed together) to give a **hybrid**. It is usually not possible to represent a resonance hybrid very accurately by drawing it (sometimes textbooks try this), so instead all the resonance forms that contribute to the hybrid must be shown—this is a weakness of the theory on which skeletal structures are based (formally referred to as **Lewis Bonding Theory**). One simple skeletal structure can't represent the "true" electronic nature of the real molecule—in theory the hybrid best represents the real molecule. The process of drawing resonance forms of molecules is often referred to as **electron pushing**. Curved arrows are used to show the movement of electrons from a bonding or nonbonding region in the molecule to another. See the following example (Structure 6):

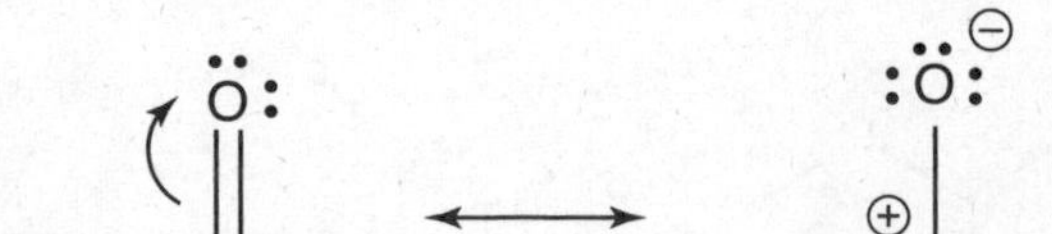

(6)

In this example, a pair of bonding π electrons are being moved from between the carbon-oxygen bond to the more electronegative oxygen atom in the structure. Double-headed arrows are used to show the transition from one resonance form to another. This type of double-headed arrow should *only* be used when drawing resonance forms of a molecule. As with all representations of molecular structures based on Lewis theory, only the *valence* electrons associated with the molecule are considered in the resonance scheme.

Some basic guidelines for drawing resonance forms of organic molecules follow.

1. Only lone pair and π-bonding electrons may be moved.
2. Under no circumstances can σ bonds be broken (the σ skeleton of the molecule must remain the same).
3. The "octet rule" as defined by Lewis bonding theory cannot be violated.
4. When given a neutral skeletal structure, start by creating charge separation between the two bonding atoms by moving a pair of π electrons between the atoms to the more electronegative atom (this will usually work if a π bond is present in the molecule). This will result in two atoms bonded to each other with equal and opposite formal charges (see Structure 6 in the earlier example).
5. If the given skeletal structure is a cation, push electron density (a lone pair of electrons or a pair of π-bonding electrons) toward the positive charge (don't break the octet rule).
6. If the given skeletal structure is an anion, push electron density (a lone pair of electrons or a pair of π-bonding electrons) away from the negative charge (again, don't break the octet rule).

Often one or two of the resonance forms will contribute more character (the more stable the form, the more it contributes) to the hybrid and some forms may contribute very little. The "best" skeletal structure will be the resonance form that contributes the most to the hybrid and will have the *lowest* potential energy. **Formal charge calculations** can be used to determine the best resonance form of the skeletal structure for a given molecular formula. The following equation can be used to calculate the formal charge of each atom of interest in a skeletal structure:

$$\text{Formal Charge}_{\text{atom}} = \text{Element's Group \#} - (\text{\# of bonds} + \text{\# of unshared } e^{-s})$$

Note: The species' total charge (usually zero unless it's an ion) must be the same as the sum of the formal charges of all the atoms in the molecule or ion. Also, recall that the element's Group # can be found on the Periodic Table of Elements.

The following example illustrates the process of drawing the important resonance forms and determining which is the most stable (lowest in energy) for simple organic molecular compounds.

Given the following skeletal Lewis formula (Structure 7), draw the important resonance forms. Which one is the lowest energy form?

> **GUIDELINES FOR FORMAL CHARGES ON ATOMS FOR A GIVEN LEWIS FORMULA**
>
> - Charges closest to zero are preferred.
> - The absolute value of nonzero charges should be as small as possible.
> - Negative charges should be on the most electronegative atoms.

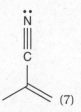

(7)

Approach

The given compound molecule is neutral; so begin by pushing a pair of bonding π electrons between the C–N triple bond onto the more electronegative N atom. This will give a new resonance form with charge separation. Next, look for other lone pairs or π electron pairs that can be moved without breaking the octet rule.

Answer

Shown below are the only three important resonance forms for the given molecule (Structure 7—note the use of curved arrows to show electron movement).

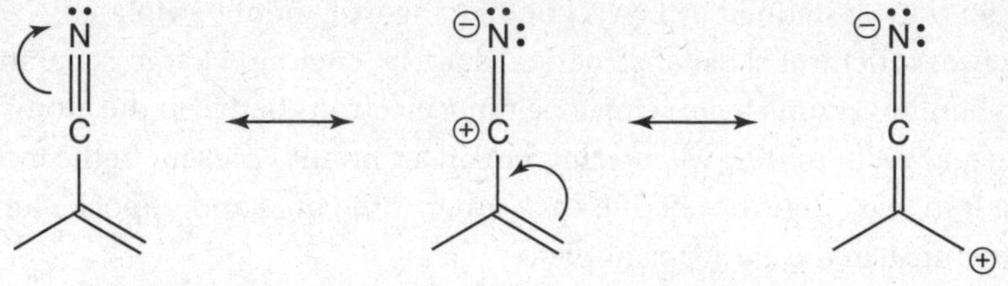

The first resonance form is the most important (lowest in energy) because its C and N atoms all have zero formal charges. When starting with a neutral molecule, this will usually be the case. Also note how charge is *conserved* throughout the process. If the starting molecule is neutral, its other resonance forms (even if they have formal charges) must also be neutral.

EXERCISE 3

Directions: Draw the important resonance forms of the following organic molecules given their skeletal Lewis formulas. (Answers are on page 340.)

1.

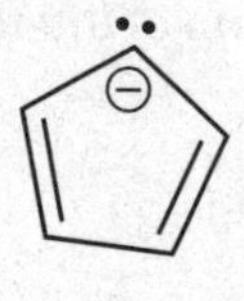

2.

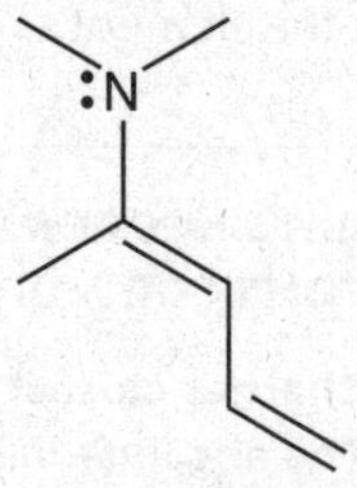

3.

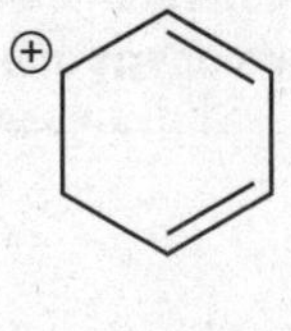

ORGANIC COMPOUND ISOMERISM

Chemical **isomers** are different compounds that have the same molecular formula. They fall into three basic categories.

1. **STRUCTURAL ISOMERS:** Also known as **constitutional** isomers, they have the same molecular formulas but differ in the way atoms in the molecule are bonded (connected) to each other.
2. **STEREOISOMERS:** Have the same molecular formula and connectivity but differ in the way their atoms are arranged in space. Stereoisomers can't be interconverted by σ (single) bond rotation.
3. **CONFORMER:** Also known as **conformational** isomers, they have the same molecular formula and connectivity but temporarily differ due to rotation about σ bonds in the molecule. Conformational isomers are actually the same compound because different conformations can be interconverted by σ bond rotation to produce identical conformers. The most common examples of this type of isomerism are based on **alkane** (single-bond saturated hydrocarbons) molecules. Conformers of alkanes are discussed in the *Alkanes* section (page 225) of this review.

A review of past DAT exams shows that questions on chemical isomers are quite common. To answer these questions you need to have a good understanding of all *three* types of isomerism.

Structural Isomers

Structural isomers are possible for organic compounds with relatively simple molecular formulas. In general the more atoms a compound is composed of the more structural isomers are possible. The simplest examples of this phenomenon are seen in alkanes and discussed in more detail in the *Alkanes* section (page 225) of this review. Other examples can include almost any category of organic compound. Figure 27.6 shows all the possible structural isomers for the molecular formula C_2H_4O. The use of skeletal Lewis structures is usually the fastest way to determine and depict all the structural isomers for a given molecular formula.

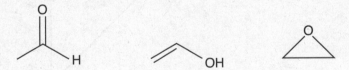

Figure 27.6. Three structural isomers for the molecular formula C_2H_4O

EXERCISE 4

Directions: Draw, using skeletal structures, all the possible structural isomers for the molecular formula $C_2H_6O_2$. (Hint: You should find five isomers.) (Answers are on page 341.)

Stereoisomers

Stereoisomers of organic compounds fall into two categories:

1. **ENANTIOMERS:** Compounds that are nonsuperimposable mirror images of each other. This type of stereoisomer always comes in pairs, which are sometimes referred to as the left- and right-handed isomers of the compound.

2. **DIASTEREOMERS:** Compounds that are non-mirror-image stereoisomers of each other. This category includes all forms of stereoisomerism except enantiomers.

In order for a compound to exist as an enantiomer it must be **chiral**. The Greek term chiral literally means handedness, as in a right and a left version of something. Human hands are often used to explain this concept as it relates to nonsuperimposable mirror-image isomers. Right and left hands reflect into each other, but can't be fully superimposed on each other. This same property is exhibited by enantiomers. They have handedness and are mirror images of each other, but can't be superimposed, as can be seen in Figure 27.7. This example shows conclusively how there are *two* ways to arrange four *different* groups around a tetrahedral molecular center.

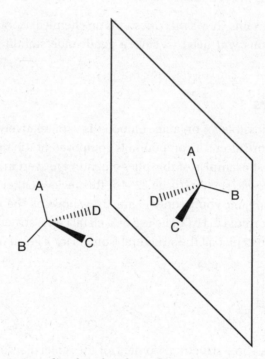

Figure 27.7. Two generalized molecules reflecting in a mirror plane—they are mirror images of each other, but are not superimposable, so they are chiral

You may remember struggling with this concept when first studying organic chemistry. It should be noted that a detailed understanding of the concept of chirality is not necessary to answer most of the questions related to this topic on the DAT. If the details of this idea are a little fuzzy, don't worry. Chiral compounds can be easily identified using one simple rule. They must contain at least one **chirality center**. A chirality center in organic compounds is a carbon atom that is sp^3-hybridized (tetrahedral shape) and has four *different* atoms or groups of atoms attached to it. Figure 27.8 shows a pair of enantiomers. They are nonsuperimposable mirror images of each other and both contain a single chirality center as designated by an asterisk.

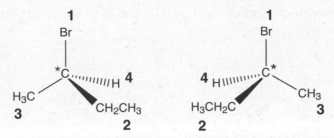

Figure 27.8. A pair of enantiomers containing one chirality center

Chiral molecules often contain more than one chirality center. The number of stereoisomers possible for a given compound is: **Stereoisomers = 2^n**, where n is the number of chirality centers present in the molecule. If the compound has one chirality center, it will have *two* stereoisomers. Compounds with two centers may exhibit up to *four* stereoisomers and those with three can have up to *eight*. As one can see, the number of possible isomers grows very rapidly as the number of chirality centers increases. Finding all the chirality centers in a given compound can be a bit challenging and takes some practice. This is particularly true when the compound contains a number of carbon rings as found in many naturally occurring organic compounds. These compounds are often isolated from plants and animals and contain both many rings and chirality centers. Shown below is an anti-inflammatory steroid molecule. Each of the chirality centers in this molecule is identified with an asterisk. As can be seen, the molecule (Structure 8) has a total of seven chirality centers so it can exhibit up to 128 stereoisomers. Questions of this type are common on the DAT.

(8)

You should practice identifying chirality centers in other similarly complex molecules. For examples, consult your favorite organic chemistry text.

Because large numbers of stereoisomers are possible for compounds with even a few chirality centers, it is necessary to use a special nomenclature system to clearly indicate which isomer is being named, studied, or referred to (as in a research paper or textbook). This procedure involves assigning the absolute configuration of the chirality center(s) using an **R** or **S** prefix (usually included in the compound's name). Each of the four groups bonded to the chiral carbon in the chirality center is assigned a priority (1, 2, 3, or 4). The lowest priority group (4) is positioned behind the chiral carbon,

> To find the chirality centers, look for *sp³*-hybridized carbons with four *different* groups attached. When the chirality center is in a ring, follow all the bonds away from the chiral carbon in all directions and look for differences between the attachments. Don't forget that skeletal structures don't show hydrogen atoms. You may want to draw them in.

leaving the remaining higher priority groups (1, 2, and 3) in a trigonal planar configuration (see the procedure in Figure 27.9).

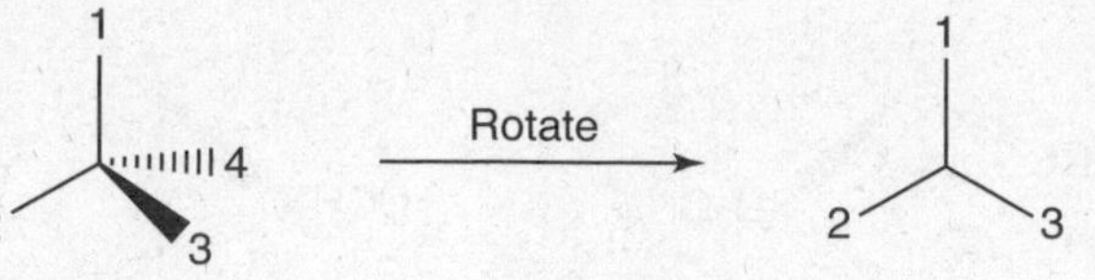

Figure 27.9. Converting a tetrahedral chirality center into a flat trigonal planar shape

If the group's priorities around the chiral carbon are 1 to 2 to 3 (highest to lowest priority) in a *clockwise* direction, then the center is designated *R*. If the group's priorities around the chiral carbon are *counterclockwise*, then the center is designated *S* (as in the example in Figure 27.9).

> The C-I-P method of prioritization is named after the chemists who first developed it and has several applications in organic chemistry.

The prioritization process for the groups attached to the chiral carbon in the chirality center use the Cahn-Ingold-Prelog (C-I-P) protocol.

This system compares the atomic numbers of the atoms bonded directly to the chiral carbon in the chirality center. The atom with the highest atomic number is assigned the highest priority (1). The atom with the next highest atomic number is second priority (2), and so on, until all four atoms attached to chirality center carbon are given priorities. If two or more of the attachments are groups of atoms (e.g., an organic functional group), the atomic numbers of the atoms in the groups bonded first to the chirality center carbon are compared and given priorities as above, but what if two or more of the atoms bonded to the chiral carbon are the same (as in the case where two of the groups have carbon atoms bonded directly to the chirality center carbon)? In this instance, which is common, one moves to the next atoms (in the above example, these would be the next atoms bonded to the two carbons attached to the carbon chirality center) in the attached groups and compares their atomic numbers. The one with the higher atomic number is assigned the higher priority. If the atoms at this level are the same (say two carbons again), move to the next atoms in the groups until a *difference* (the first point of difference decides the priority) is found, and the atom at this point with the higher atomic number gets the higher priority just as before. The following example shows how to assign the *R* and *S* configuration to chirality centers using the C-I-P system.

Designate the chirality centers for the pair of enantiomers shown in Figure 27.6 as *R* or *S*.

Approach

First, assign the priorities (using the C-I-P protocol) to each of the groups bonded to the chiral carbon in each chirality center of the molecules shown in Figure 27.8 (see Structures 9 and 10 below).

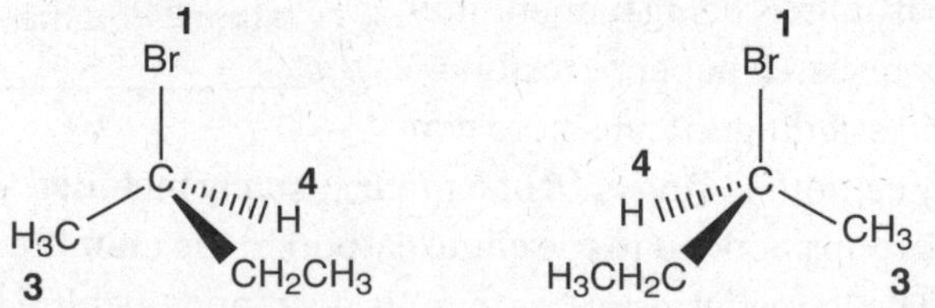

(9, 10)

Next, conceptually turn each of the molecules so that the lowest priority group (in this case it's an H atom for both structures) is hidden behind the carbon at the center of the chirality center. This will leave the remaining three groups in a planar configuration around the chirality center's chiral carbon.

Finally, observe the direction (clockwise or counterclockwise) when going from the highest priority group to the lowest priority group around the chirality center.

Clockwise (*R*) Counterclockwise (*S*)

The direction of the priorities (highest to lowest) for the molecule on the left is clockwise. Its chirality center is designated *R* and the direction for the one on the right is counterclockwise, so its chirality center is designated *S*.

(9, 10)

Practice this procedure so you can correctly assign the *R* and *S* designations to chirality centers when this type of question is encountered on the DAT. The example provided is relatively simple partly because of the way the two stereoisomers are drawn. Note that the lowest priority group (the hydrogen atom) was already positioned so that it was behind the chirality center carbon. Stereoisomer molecules will not always be drawn this way. Sometimes the molecule will be drawn with the lowest priority group in front of the chirality center carbon or to the side. In these cases, you will have to conceptually rotate the molecule until the lowest priority group is behind the chirality center carbon, leaving the higher priority groups in front. One approach to simplifying this situation is to rotate the molecule so that the lowest priority group is projecting from the *front* of the chirality center and prioritize the remaining groups as usual. This process assigns the *opposite* stereochemical configuration from the molecule's actual configuration. So, for example, if the center is assigned an *R* configuration using this method, remember to reverse this to *S* to reflect the actual configuration.

The following exercise will give you a chance to test your skill in assigning *R* and *S* configurations to chirality centers using the above process.

> You can see that the *R* enantiomer is the mirror image of the *S* enantiomer, and when they are placed directly opposite each other as in the example (Structures 9 and 10), the isomers reflect into each other.

EXERCISE 5

Directions: Designate the chirality centers in the following molecules as *R* or *S*.

Note that there may be more than one chirality center present in a given molecule. (Answers are on page 341.)

1.

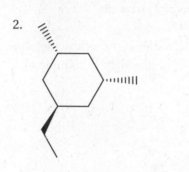

2.

3.

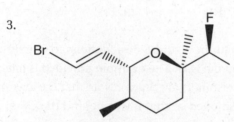

The physical and chemical properties of enantiomers are exactly the same except for two areas. When plane-polarized light is passed through a solution of a *pure* enantiomer, it will rotate the light in a specific direction and a specific number of degrees. A solution of its pure mirror image (the other enantiomer) will rotate the same light in the opposite direction the same number of degrees. This phenomenon is known as **optical activity** and is a property of any pure chiral stereoisomer. Stereoisomers that rotate light to the right (clockwise) are referred to as **dextrorotatory** [often labeled in the compound's name as **d** or (+)] and those that rotate light to the left (counterclockwise) are called **laevorotatory** [**l** or (−)].

When equal molar amounts of two enantiomers are made into a solution and plane-polarized light is passed through the sample, there is *no* optical rotation—that is, the sample is optically inactive. A sample with equal amounts of two enantiomers is called a **racemic mixture** or a **racemate** and is *always* optically inactive.

The other area where the properties of enantiomers differ is in their interaction with other chiral media. Enantiomers often exhibit different reaction rates with other chiral molecules. This again has to do with the handedness of the enantiomer. One pure enantiomer may geometrically fit together better with another chiral molecule and thus produce a reaction transition state, which is of lower energy. The other pure enantiomer may not have the right geometry to easily interact with this same chiral molecule. The rate of the reaction between the chiral molecule and the better-fitting enantiomer will be faster and in some cases *much* faster. This situation is similar to someone trying to put a left-handed glove on his or her right hand. No matter how hard the person tries, the glove will never fit as well on the right hand as it does on the left hand. The property of handedness can sometimes be used to separate mixtures of enantiomers from each other. Large biological molecules such as enzymes, which are chiral, usually have a preference for only one enantiomer (it fits better in their active site) and will use only that enantiomer in reactions it catalyzes, leaving the other enantiomer (the preferred enantiomer's mirror image) unreacted and unchanged.

> Recall that enzymes are complex chiral biological molecules that increase the speed of reactions in all living organisms—they act as catalysts. They are essential to life. In recent years, organic chemists have isolated many kinds of enzymes from plants and animals, and they are now regularly used to catalyze reactions in the laboratory and industry. One of the prime uses for these processes is the separation of mixtures of enantiomers. This application is particularly important in the pharmaceutical industry.

As stated earlier, **diastereomers** are stereoisomers that are not mirror images of each other. These isomers are also not superimposable on each other like enantiomers. Many different types of diastereomeric relationships between molecules are possible. In order for a chiral compound to be a diastereomer, it must contain at least two chirality centers. Such a compound can exist as up to four stereoisomers. Using the *R* and *S* configuration nomenclature explained on page 213, the four possible isomers are *RR*, *SS*, *SR*, and *RS*. The stereochemical relationship between these isomers is as follows. The *RR* and *SS* isomers are a pair of enantiomers and so are the *SR* and *RS* isomers (in both cases the two chirality centers in these isomers reflect into each other). Note that, for example, the *RR* and *SR* isomers are not a pair of enantiomers because both of their chirality centers do not reflect into each other. Since this pair of stereoisomer's isomers are not mirror images of each other, they are **diastereomers**. Figure 27.10 shows two compounds that contain two chirality centers each and exhibit this type of isomerism.

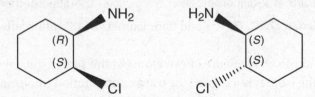

Figure 27.10. Two nonsuperimposable stereoisomers that are diastereomers

As can be seen by the chirality center configurations assigned to these two molecules (left molecule *R*, *S* and the right molecule *S*, *S*), they are stereoisomers of each other but not mirror images. There is a special kind of chiral diastereomer that is called a **meso** compound. A meso compound, like all chiral diastereomers, must contain at least two chirality centers, but in this case, it also must have plane of symmetry that allows one side of the molecule to reflect into the opposite side (see the example in Figure 27.11).

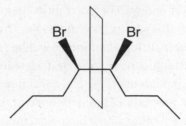

Figure 27.11. An example of a meso diastereomer. It contains two chirality centers that directly reflect into each other as shown by the mirror plane.

This kind of molecule, although this may be confusing, is a mirror image of itself—again one side of the molecule reflects exactly into the other side and is thus optically inactive.

There is another type of diastereomer that is not a chiral compound, and instead of having two chirality centers it has two *sp*²-hybridized carbon atoms adjacent to each other. This kind of organic compound is called an **alkene** and contains one or more carbon-carbon double bonds. As explained earlier in this section ("Multiple Bonds in Molecules"), carbon-carbon double bonds in organic molecules consist of one σ bond and one π bond. As you may remember, free rotation is possible about carbon-carbon single (σ) bonds but not carbon-carbon double bonds. Because of the side-to-side overlap of the *p*-atomic orbitals that form the π part of the double bond, rotation is very restricted. Rotation about a carbon-carbon double bond requires enough energy to *break* the π part of the bond and does not happen under ambient conditions. Due to the rigid nature of the carbon-carbon double bond, groups attached to either side of the bond are fixed in space and can't interact with each other. This property of the double bond leads to what are sometimes called cis/trans stereoisomers. Figure 27.12 shows a pair of cis/trans isomers.

trans-1,2-difluoroethene   *cis*-1,2-difluoroethene

Figure 27.12. The cis and trans isomers of 1,2-difluroethene

As can be seen in the above figure, if two atoms of the same type are on *opposite* sides of the double bond, the isomer is assigned the **trans** configuration (molecule on the left). If two atoms of the same type are on the *same* side of the double bond, the isomer is assigned the **cis** configuration (molecule on the right). As with the *R* and *S* designations for chirality centers, cis and trans designations appear as prefixes in the compound names.

You may wonder why cis and trans isomers are referred to as diastereomers. If you study the structures for a moment, you will see that the only difference between the left and right molecule shown in Figure 27.12 is the way the atoms are arranged in space. The connectivity is the same and so are their molecular formulas. Thus cis and trans isomers are stereoisomers, but there is one more observation to make. Are the two molecules nonsuperimposable mirror images of each other? The answer is no. So, if the two molecules aren't enantiomers and are non-mirror-image stereoisomers of each other, then they must be diastereomers!

There is another type of nomenclature that is used to distinguish these types of diastereomers from each other. The designations are similar to cis and trans and refer to the two forms as *E* and *Z*.

This approach to designating the configuration of these kinds of isomers is most commonly used when there are *no* like groups attached to the double bond, but it can be used to indicate the stereochemistry of any alkene. As with the *R* and *S* designations discussed earlier, the procedure for assigning *E* or *Z* to a specific stereoisomer involves the use of the C-I-P prioritization rules. The following example shows you how to specify the *E* and *Z* configurations of alkene stereoisomers.

Designate the alkene stereoisomer shown below (Structure 11) as *E* or *Z*.

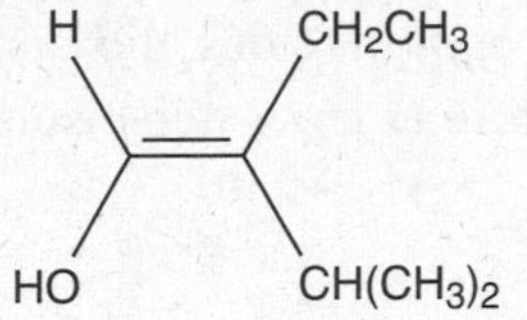

H   CH₂CH₃

HO   CH(CH₃)₂   (11)

Approach

Divide the given molecule into two parts by cutting the horizontal double bond in half. Below is the left side of the molecule after being segmented.

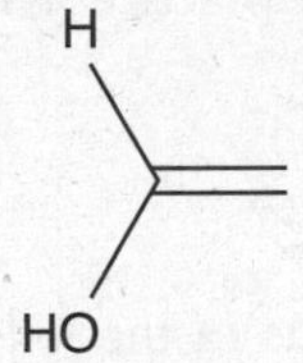

H

HO

Next, use the C-I-P rules to prioritize the groups as either first (1) or second (2). In this case, the two atoms attached directly to the double bond are oxygen and hydrogen. Since oxygen has the higher atomic number, it gets first priority and hydrogen second. See the result shown below.

2nd
H

HO
1st

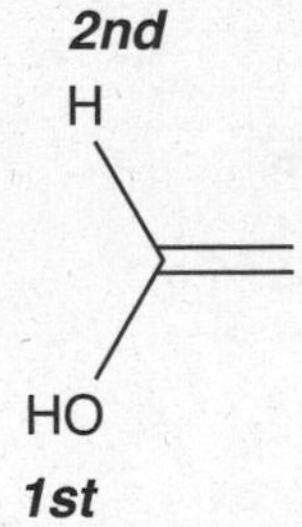

The groups attached to the right side of the molecule are prioritized in exactly the same way. See the result shown below.

2nd
CH₂CH₃

CH(CH₃)₂
1st

TIP

E is from the German word *entgegen*, which means "opposite," and *Z* is from the German word *zusammen*, which means "together."

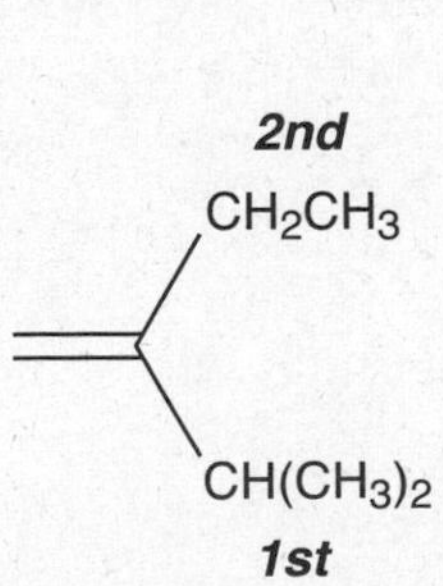

Now put the molecule back together (see below).

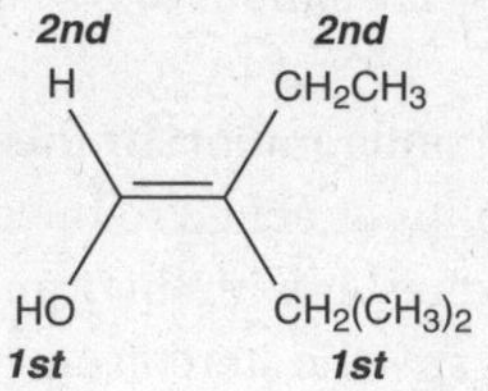

(11)

Answer

If the two first priority groups attached to the double bond are on the *same* side, the isomer is designated as *Z*, and if they are on *opposite* sides, the isomer is designated as *E*. In this case, they are on the same side, so Structure 11 is a *Z* stereoisomer (shown below).

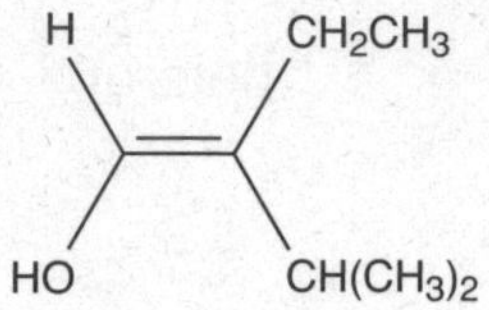

(11)

Z isomer

The following exercise will help you practice assigning *E* and *Z* designations to alkene stereoisomers.

EXERCISE 6

Directions: Designate the double bonds in the following alkene stereoisomers as *E* or *Z*. (Answers are on page 341.)

TIP

Remember skeletal structures of molecules don't show hydrogens, and in this case for simplicity, nonbonding electron pairs are not shown!

1.

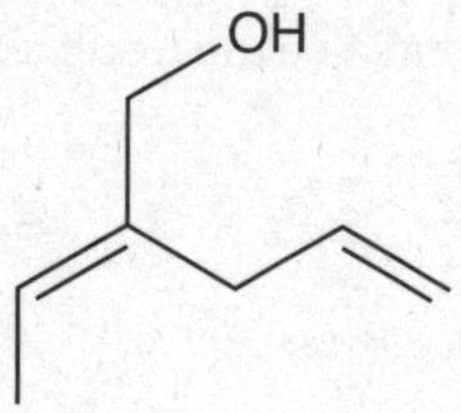

2.

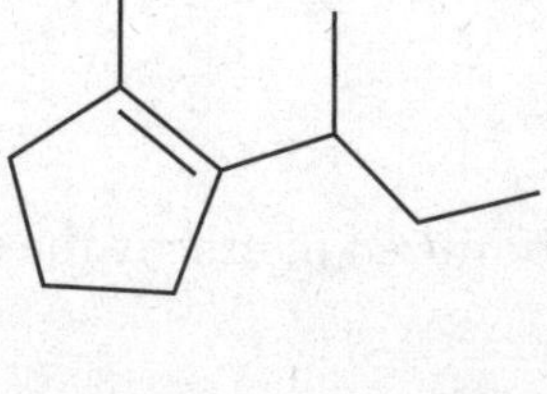

3.

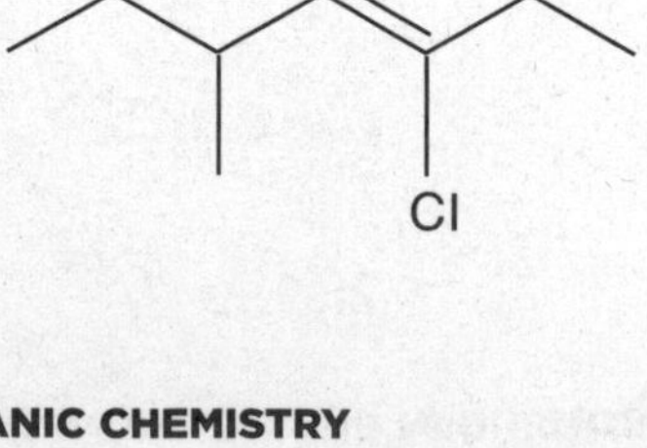

Organic Compound Functional Groups

28

DEFINING A FUNCTIONAL GROUP

What is a functional group in the context of organic chemistry?

A **functional group** is an atom or group of atoms with specific chemical and physical properties. The functional group is often the reactive portion of the molecule. There are approximately 25 functional groups that are commonly found in organic compounds. Compounds often contain more than one.

TABLE OF IMPORTANT FUNCTIONAL GROUPS

Table 28.1 shows the most commonly encountered functional groups on the DAT. You should be quite familiar with these groups and be able to identify them in complex molecules.

Table 28.1 Organic Compound Functional Groups

Hydrocarbon Functional Groups*

alkene   alkyne   or   aryl (phenyl as a substituent)

* By definition alkane hydrocarbons contain no functional groups

Heteroatom Functional Groups (may contain O, N, S, and/or X = F, Cl, Br, or I)

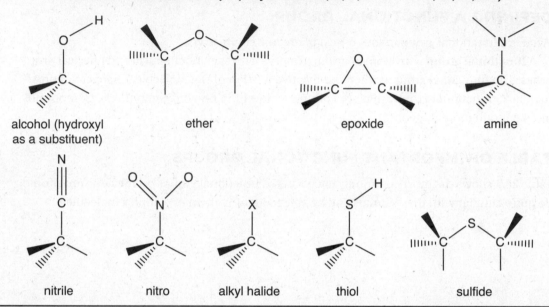

alcohol (hydroxyl as a substituent)   ether   epoxide   amine

nitrile   nitro   alkyl halide   thiol   sulfide

Carbonyl (C=O) Containing Functional Groups

aldehyde   ketone   carboxylic acid   ester

amide   anhydride   acid halide

EXERCISE 7

Directions: Identify and label all of the functional groups in each of the following molecules. (Answers are on page 342.)

1.

2.

3.

Alkanes 29

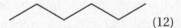

WHAT IS AN ALKANE?

Alkanes are organic compounds that contain only the elements hydrogen and carbon and are part of a larger class of compounds referred to as hydrocarbons.

Because the DAT is weighted toward knowledge and concepts related to hydrocarbons, these compounds will be emphasized in this review. Alkanes have the general molecular formula C_NH_{2N+2}, where N is a positive whole number integer. Alkanes are often referred to as *saturated* hydrocarbons because they contain the maximum number of hydrogen atoms possible for their molecular structures (they are saturated with hydrogen).

NOMENCLATURE OF ALKANES

Structural Representations of Alkane Molecules

The topic of representing the structures of organic molecules in 2D and 3D has been previously discussed in this review (see *Bonding in Organic Compounds* on page 201). The structures of hydrocarbons are easily represented by skeletal nomenclature (only the σ-bonding skeleton of the molecule is shown and elemental symbols for hydrogen and carbon atoms are omitted), and this will be the most common way these molecules are shown in this section. As a reminder, the skeletal structure of normal hexane (Structure 12), a common alkane, is shown below.

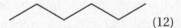 (12)

Abbreviated IUPAC Rules for Naming Alkanes

A detailed understanding of the nomenclature associated with *all* types of organic compounds is not necessary for you to do well on organic chemistry related DAT questions. If you are required to specifically recognize the name of a compound, it will most probably be an alkane or some other kind of hydrocarbon. As such, you should be familiar with the specific naming rules for hydrocarbons.

The naming of alkanes can be divided into two categories of compounds: **normal** or open-chain structures and **cyclic** structures.

NAMING NORMAL (OPEN-CHAIN) ALKANES

The most important factor in correctly naming normal alkanes is identifying the longest and most branched carbon chain (the principal chain) in the compound's molecular structure. Once this is determined, it provides the base name for the compound using a Greek prefix (in most cases)—indicating the number of carbon atoms in the principal chain followed by the letters "ane" for alk*ane*. The principal chain prefixes for up to ten carbons are as follows: meth-, eth-, prop-, but-, pent-, hex-, hept-, oct-, non-, and dec-. The first four can be remembered by this mnemonic device: "**mom eats peanut butter**" (**m**eth-, **e**th-, **p**rop-, and **b**ut-).

Small carbon branches (called alkyl substituents) attached to the principal chain are named and numbered so as to give the lowest set of attachment numbers possible. When writing the final compound name, substituents attached to the principal chain are listed in alphabetical order in front of the base name with their respective attachment numbers shown first. A list of the most common alkyl substituent IUPAC names along with their structures is shown in Table 29.1.

Table 29.1. Common Alkyl Substituents

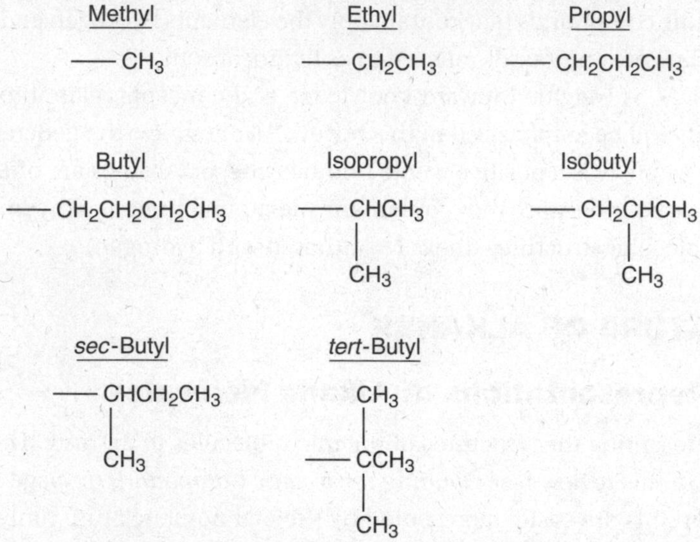

Methyl	Ethyl	Propyl
—— CH_3	—— CH_2CH_3	—— $CH_2CH_2CH_3$

Butyl	Isopropyl	Isobutyl
—— $CH_2CH_2CH_2CH_3$	—— $CHCH_3$ | CH_3	—— CH_2CHCH_3 | CH_3

sec-Butyl	*tert*-Butyl
—— $CHCH_2CH_3$ | CH_3	CH_3 | —— CCH_3 | CH_3

NAMING CYCLIC ALKANES

When naming cyclic alkanes (e.g., those that have a closed-ring structure), there are two additional considerations. First, the prefix "cyclo-" must be added to the compound's principal chain name, as in "cyclohexane" for a cyclic six-membered ring. Second, depending on how the compound's structure is represented, the *stereochemistry* (see *Bonding in Organic Compounds* on page 201) of the substance may need to be indicated in the name. The term *stereochemistry* refers to the 3D arrangement of two or more substituents attached to the ring. In this review, only the case where there are two substituents will be considered. When drawing cyclic structures, a *solid* shaded wedge-shaped bond indicates the substituent is attached to the top side of a ring. A *dashed* or *dotted* bond indicates the substituent is on the bottom side of a ring. When two substituents are on the same side of the ring, their stereochemistry is specified as **cis**. When two substituents are on opposite sides of the ring (top and bottom), they are designated as **trans**. The structure (13) shown below is an example of a 3D rendering of a *trans*-1,3-dimethyl substituted cyclopentane (note the five-membered ring).

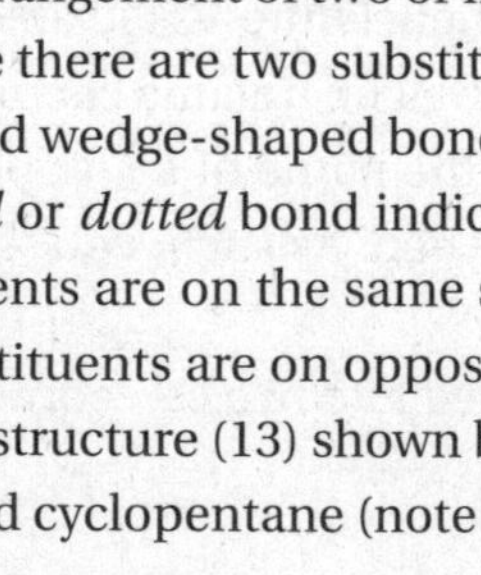

(13)

The cis/trans nomenclature used to indicate the stereochemistry associated with cyclic hydrocarbons shouldn't be confused with the nomenclature used to indicate the stereochemistry of *alkenes*, which is sometimes also called cis/trans. For more on the stereochemistry of alkenes see the *Bonding in Organic Compounds* section on page 201.

To indicate the specific stereochemistry for a cyclic alkane the prefix *cis-* or *trans-* is placed at the very beginning of the full name. The following 2D structures (14 and 15) and their associated names provide examples of the use of cis and trans nomenclature for cyclic alkanes:

cis-1,3-dimethylcyclopentane   *trans*-1,3-dimethylcyclopentane   (14, 15)

A summary of the IUPAC rules for naming alkanes is given in Table 29.2.

Table 29.2. IUPAC Nomenclature for Alkanes

(Summary of Rules)

1. Find the longest chain in the compound.[a,b]
2. Name each substituent group that is attached to the principal chain.
3. Alphabetize the substituent groups (methyl, ethyl, propyl, etc.—see Table 29.1 as needed).[c]
4. Number the principal chain from the end that gives the smallest number at the first point of difference.
5. Name the principal chain using the Greek prefix that corresponds to the number of carbons it contains and assign numbers to each substituent.

[a]If two chains are of the same length, choose the most branched as the principal.
[b]If the compound is cyclic, add the prefix *cyclo* to the parent chain name. If stereochemistry is indicated, use the terms *cis* and *trans*.
[c]Note: The prefixes *sec-* and *tert-* are not used in alphabetization.

It should also be noted that chirality centers may be present in hydrocarbon molecules. If the stereochemistry of these centers is shown in the structural formula (usually with wedge- and dash-shaped bonds) of the molecule, the absolute configuration is also shown in the name. The chirality center designation (*R* or *S*—see the *Bonding in Organic Compounds* section on page 201 for details on determining chirality center assignments) is written first followed by the number of carbons in the chirality center of the principal chain. This information usually follows cis/trans designations

Since all organic chemistry questions on the DAT are multiple choice, don't worry too much about the order of stereochemical data in the names of compounds. The correct answer should be fairly obvious if the test taker can recall the basics of alkane naming and stereochemical assignments (e.g., cis/trans and *R/S*).

for cyclic compounds—although the cis/trans designation is often omitted from the name when the compound's stereochemistry is specified.

By far the best approach for learning to name any organic compound is lots of practice.

EXERCISE 8

Directions: Use the rules in Table 29.2 on page 227 to name the following alkane structural formulas. (Answers are on page 343.)

1.

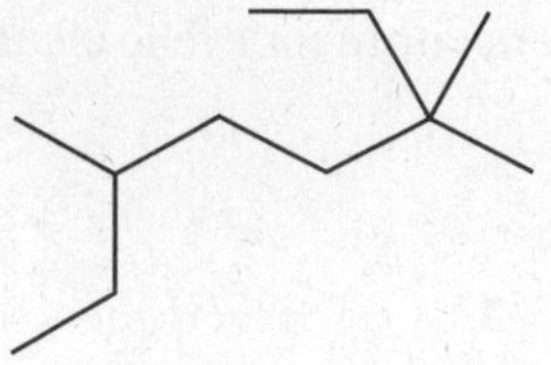

2.

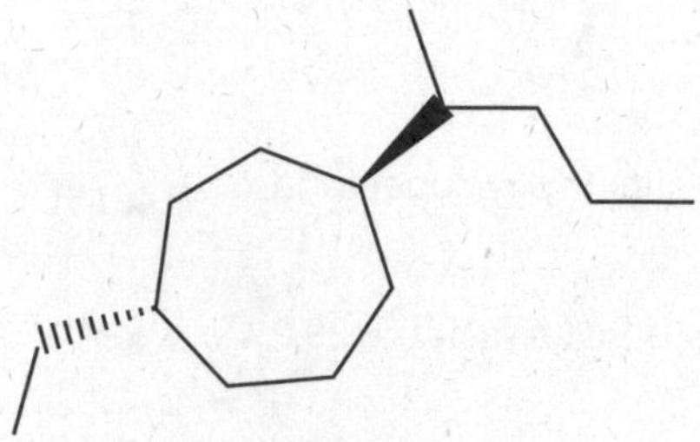

3.

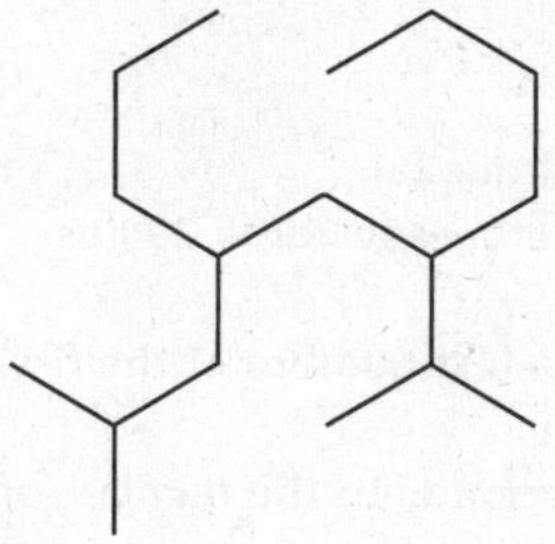

PROPERTIES AND USES OF ALKANES

Most alkanes (as well as other hydrocarbons) are derived from petroleum through a procedure referred to as "cracking" or refining, which involves a form of distillation. This process yields both straight-chained (normal) and branched alkanes.

The melting and boiling points of normal alkanes show a very regular increase in temperature as the number of carbons in their chains increase. This trend is directly associated with a rise in the dispersion forces (the weakest of the intermolecular forces) between the molecules as their molar masses increase. Greater numbers of electrons in the larger alkanes are more easily polarized, leading to stronger attractive forces and higher boiling points. See Figure 29.1 on page 229 for a graphical representation of this trend.

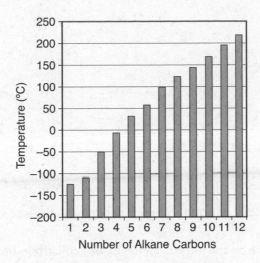

Figure 29.1. Alkane boiling points

Because the elements hydrogen and carbon which make up alkanes have relatively similar electronegativities, the magnitudes of dipole moments in their covalent bonds are low. This makes the molecules very nonpolar—one of the alkanes' most unusual properties. The alkane carbon chains are "coated" with weakly polarized hydrogen atoms, which make them hydrophobic. This along with their relatively low densities generally prevents them from mixing with water and instead hydrocarbon molecules agglomerate and float on top as oily films.

The most common uses of alkanes are as fuels, solvents, and precursors for the synthesis of more complex molecules. The only current source, for the foreseeable future, of the complex array of hydrocarbons used in today's society is *petroleum*.

As with most organic compounds, alkanes can exist in different isomeric forms. You may recall from the *Bonding in Organic Compounds* section on page 201 that isomers have the same molecular formulas but differ in the way their atoms are bonded to each other (constitutional isomers) or are arranged in space (stereoisomers). Any alkane with a molecular formula having four or more carbon atoms can exhibit constitutional isomerism. Both normal butane and isobutane have the same molecular formula but different molecular structures. The structures (in skeletal format) of these two alkanes are shown below (Structures 16 and 17). As the number of carbons in alkanes increases, the number of possible conformational isomers grows rapidly. For an alkane with 20 carbons, there are 366,319 possible constitutional isomers.

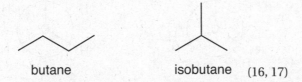

butane   isobutane   (16, 17)

Another related topic often studied in conjunction with simple alkanes is **conformational analysis**—a kind of temporary structural isomerism. Because the σ bonds in the skeletons of alkanes have the freedom of rotation, there are many different ways that the various parts of the molecule can move relative to each other. The simple two-carbon alkane, ethane, can be used to illustrate this point. Figure 29.2 shows two different conformational structures of ethane (these representations are sometimes called sawhorse forms and the length of the carbon-carbon bond has been exaggerated to provide prospective).

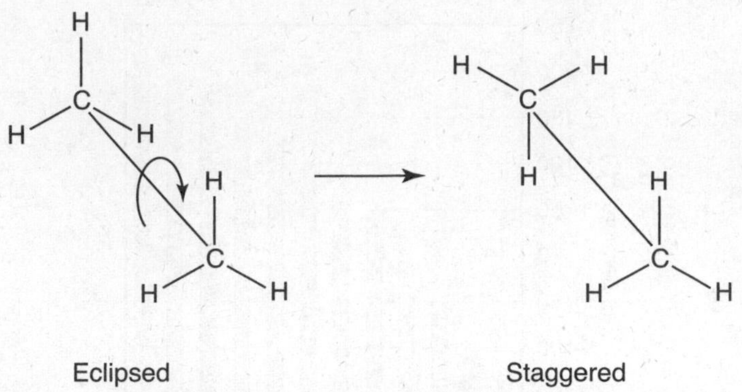

Eclipsed   Staggered

Figure 29.2. The most important conformations of ethane

Note that the structure on the left has all the hydrogen-carbon bonds on each of the two ethane carbons aligned relative to each other. This conformation of ethane is called **eclipsed**. In the structure on the right, the position of the carbon in the background (the one toward the top of the figure) has moved relative to the same carbon in the structure on the left. This change was made by allowing a 180° rotation about the σ carbon-carbon bond in the molecule and results in a new conformation called **staggered**. These two **conformers** of ethane have different stabilities (energies) and because of **torsional strain** in the eclipsed form, the staggered form is lower in energy. There are obviously other possible conformations of ethane depending on the degree of rotation about its carbon-carbon bond, but the two that differ most in energy and thus are the most important are staggered and eclipsed.

> There are three different kinds of strain associated with the various conformers of organic compounds. **Torsional** strain is caused by electron-electron repulsion between eclipsed bonds. **Steric** strain occurs when two groups of atoms (for example, two methyl groups) are too close to each other and try to occupy the same space. The larger the interacting groups, the higher the steric strain. The third kind of strain is called **angle** or **ring** strain and is discussed in detail under the topic of cyclic alkanes later in this section.

If you look carefully along the axis of the carbon-carbon bonds (align your eye with the carbon in the foreground and look up along the bond) in the two structures shown in Figure 29.2, you will discover another way to visualize the eclipsed and staggered conformations of ethane. These new representations are called **Newman projections** and are shown in Figure 29.3.

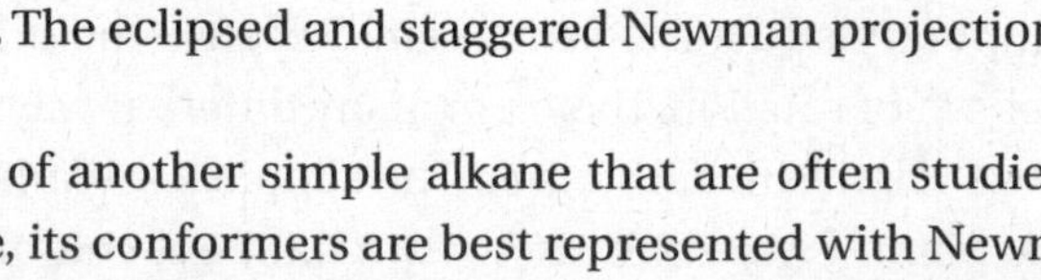

Eclipsed   Staggered

Figure 29.3. The eclipsed and staggered Newman projections of ethane

The conformations of another simple alkane that are often studied are those of normal butane. As with ethane, its conformers are best represented with Newman projections. If you look along the bond axis of carbons 2 and 3 in the butane structural formula in Figure 29.4 (left eclipsed sawhorse form), the eclipsed Newman projection (on the right) can be visualized.

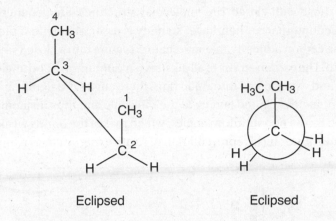

Eclipsed   Eclipsed

Figure 29.4. An eclipsed conformation of butane
(sawhorse on the left and Newman on the right)

Figure 29.5 shows all the important conformations of butane using Newman projections along with their relative energies. Each of the conformations is successively generated (going from left to right) by fixing the position of the butane molecule's *second* carbon (see Figure 29.4) and allowing carbon *three* to rotate about the C_2–C_3 bond axis. Each new conformation is generated by a C_2–C_3 bond rotation of 60°. As might be expected from the ethane example, Figure 29.5 clearly illustrates how the various *staggered* conformations (bottom of the figure) of butane are lower in energy than the less-stable *eclipsed* forms (top of the figure).

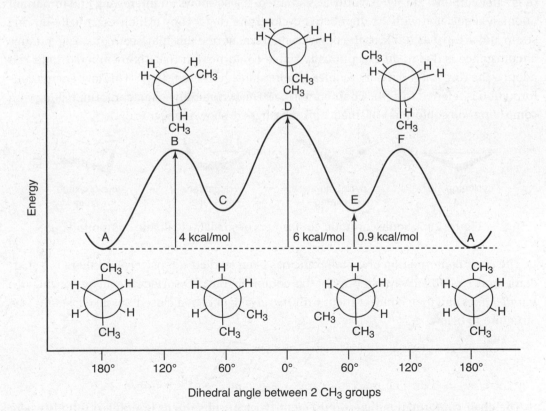

Figure 29.5. The relative energies of the conformations of butane

TIP

The reference to the dihedral angle on the x-axis of the graph in Figure 29.5 is related to the angle between the two terminal methyl groups of butane in the Newman projections.

Cycloalkanes, those with closed-ring molecular structures, are generally less stable than their open-chain counterparts. Their lower stability is associated with a property called **ring strain**. Forcing the carbon atoms in an open-chain structure into a closed ring causes this kind of molecular strain. The carbon atoms of all alkanes have optimum bond angles of 109.5° (those of a tetrahedron) and when forced into small rings these angles are significantly distorted. This causes an inherent increase in the energy of the molecule and thus instability (atomic orbital overlap is reduced by the nonoptimum angles, which makes the bonds weaker).

Figure 29.6 shows a graphical representation of relative ring strain as a function of ring size.

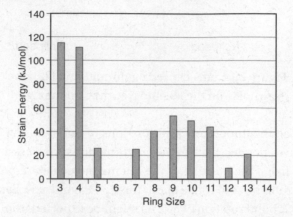

Figure 29.6. Cycloalkane ring strain energies

It clearly shows that small rings are particularly strained and that large rings (those with 12 or greater carbons) are significantly less strained. It also shows an interesting and important anomaly associated with six-membered cycloalkane rings. They exhibit essentially no ring strain and are just as stable as the open-chain form. At first this may seem puzzling, but this circumstance is due to an exceptionally stable conformation that six-membered rings can adopt—the ring is not flat but assumes a more stable puckered shape. This low-energy conformation is referred to as the **chair** conformer. The cyclohexane chair conformer along with some common conformers of smaller alkane rings are shown in Figure 29.7.

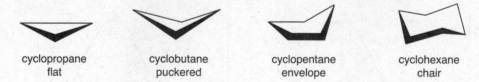

cyclopropane flat   cyclobutane puckered   cyclopentane envelope   cyclohexane chair

Figure 29.7. Some common conformers of small cycloalkane compounds

The chair conformation of cyclohexane has been studied extensively and there is a standard, more simplified way to represent this conformer on a 2D surface. Begin by drawing *two parallel lines* and then connect them with *two zigzag lines* in a closed box-like fashion—see Structure 18 below.

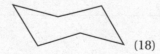

(18)

The chair conformation has two different types of substituent bonding positions where hydrogens or other substituents are attached to the ring. These two bond types are referred to as **axial** (these bonds extend directly above and below the ring) and **equatorial** (these bonds are oriented at approximately 45° angles around the equator of the ring). Both of these two types of bonds occur on each carbon in the six-membered ring, so for any chair conformation there are always six axial and six equatorial bonds. The chair conformation shown on the left below shows only the axial bonds, and the one on the right only shows the equatorial bonds (Structures 19 and 20), so they can easily be distinguished from each other.

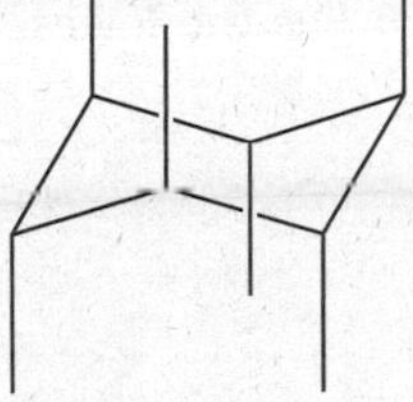

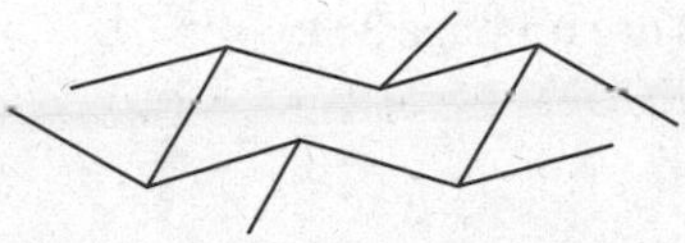

(19, 20)

Structure 21 below shows both the axial and equatorial bonds present on the cyclohexane ring with hydrogens attached—the complete structure (molecular formula C_6H_{12}).

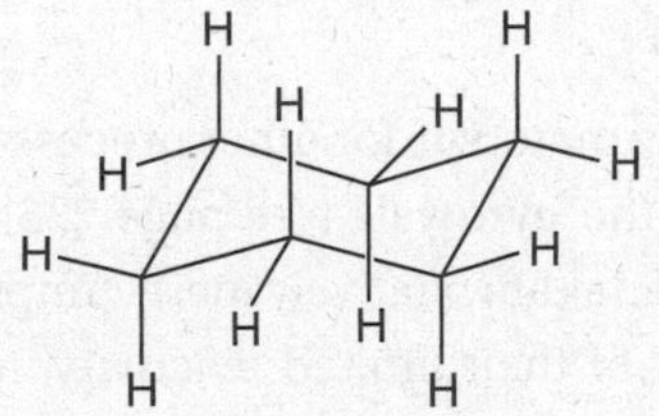

(21)

At room temperature the two possible chair conformations are in a 1:1 equilibrium ratio with each other as show in Figure 29.8.

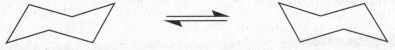

Figure 29.8. The left and right chair conformations of cyclohexane in equilibrium

Just like open-chain alkanes, cyclohexane can have substituents other than hydrogen attached to the ring. In general, these larger substituents (more bulky than hydrogen) are more stable in the equatorial position than in the axial. The equatorial position provides more "room" and thus a less crowded conformation with lower energy. Structures 22 and 23 show a methyl substituent in the axial and equatorial positions, respectively. The equatorial methyl is clearly further removed from the rest of the ring and less crowded. The conformation with the methyl group in the equatorial position is greatly favored over the conformation with the methyl group axial at equilibrium and will predominate.

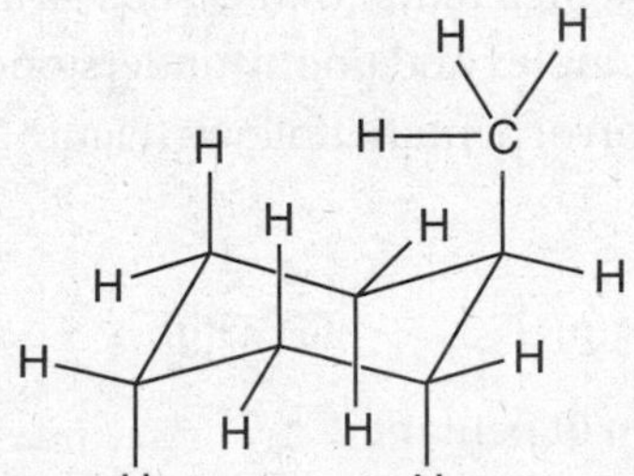

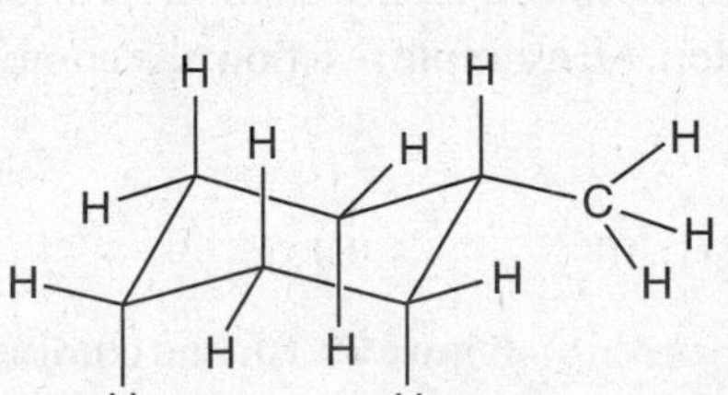

(22, 23)

It should be noted that when there are two or more substituents attached to a cyclohexane ring, if possible, the larger groups will occupy the equatorial positions and this conformation will be favored at equilibrium.

EXERCISE 9

Given the following 2D structure for *trans*-1-chloro-3-ethylcyclohexane, draw the 3D chair conformation that will predominate at equilibrium (the one that has the lowest potential energy). (Answers are on page 343.)

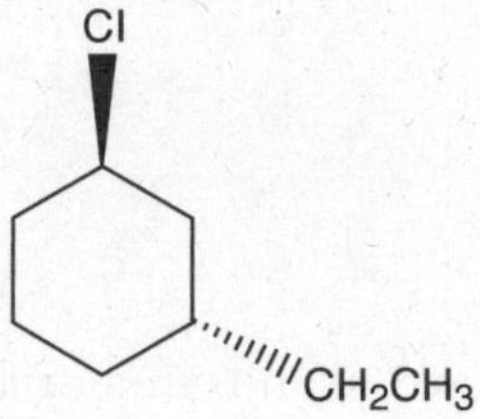

ALKANE REACTIONS

Simple alkanes used as starting materials for other processes are not synthesized directly, but they are usually obtained by the **pyrolysis** (see page 235) of larger, more complex alkanes obtained from petroleum. Alkanes are relatively inert compounds and do not undergo chemical changes easily. As a result of their limited reactivity, many low-boiling alkanes such as pentane, hexane, heptane, and octane make excellent solvents (media) for conducting synthetic organic reactions. There are few synthetically useful reactions that use alkanes as starting materials, but their **combustion** reactions are of immense commercial importance. One other alkane reaction commonly studied in organic chemistry courses is **halogenation**. This reaction has appeared on the DAT.

Alkane Combustion

When alkanes are combined with excess oxygen under the right conditions, they are completely oxidized to carbon dioxide and water products (see the general reaction shown in Figure 29.9).

$$C_NH_{2N+2} \quad + \quad O_2(g) \quad \rightarrow \quad NCO_2(g) \quad + \quad (N+1)\,H_2O(g) + \Delta$$

Figure 29.9. General combustion reaction for alkanes

This reaction is extremely exothermic and, as a result, large amounts of heat (Δ) are released into the surroundings. This makes alkanes excellent fuels for heating structures associated with human habitation where a constant temperature is desired. They are also ideal for use in the internal combustion engines. The process requires a high temperature, such as a flame or spark, for its initiation, and the mechanism is a very complex and poorly understood free-radical chain reaction. An example reaction, the combustion of pentane, follows (Figure 29.10).

$$C_5H_{12}(l) \quad + \quad 8O_2(g) \quad \overset{\Delta}{\rightarrow} \quad 5CO_2(g) \quad + \quad 6H_2O(g)$$

Figure 29.10. The combustion of pentane

Halogenation

The halogenation of alkanes using chlorine or bromine catalyzed by UV radiation or high temperatures (250–400°C) transforms these compounds into chloroalkanes or bromoalkanes. In some cases, fluorine can also be used in this process, but it is usually too reactive. Regardless of the alkane and halogen reactants used in the process, it almost always produces a mixture (often complex) of **haloalkane** products. This limitation significantly reduces the reaction's usefulness as a tool in organic compound synthesis. The general reaction for this process follows (Figure 29.11).

$$\underset{\displaystyle |}{\overset{\displaystyle |}{-C-}}H \;+\; X_2 \;\xrightarrow{\text{hv or }\Delta}\; \underset{\displaystyle |}{\overset{\displaystyle |}{-C-}}X \;+\; H-X$$

X is Cl or Br and rarely F.

Figure 29.11. Free-radical halogenation of alkanes

The halogenation of alkanes is one of the most-studied reactions in organic chemistry and has provided much insight into the particulars of free-radical reaction mechanisms. As can be seen from the general reaction above, halogen atoms in this process replace hydrogen atoms (a substitution process). Depending on the position of a hydrogen atom in the alkane structure, its reactivity toward substitution by halogen atoms varies considerably, with some hydrogens being very reactive and others less so. This spectrum of hydrogen atom reactivities toward replacement by halogen atoms leads to the mixtures of haloalkane products cited above. In general, hydrogens attached to *more* substituted carbon atoms (2° and 3° carbons) are more reactive to halogen substitution.

Pyrolysis of Alkanes

Decomposing chemical compounds by heating them to high temperatures is referred to as pyrolysis. The pyrolysis of alkanes found in petroleum is known as **thermal cracking**. This process involves the passing of mixtures of alkanes through a long metal column, which has been heated to a high temperature, sometimes by superheated steam. High molar mass alkanes are converted into smaller alkanes, alkenes, and some hydrogen gas. The major product produced by this process is ethylene gas, which is the precursor for the production of the economically important thermoplastic **polyethylene**.

Despite the importance of ethylene, most cracking operations are used to produce fuels. This type of pyrolysis is referred to as **catalytic cracking**. High-boiling hydrocarbon fractions from oil are forced into contact with fine silica-alumina particles at high temperatures (450–550°C) and slightly higher than atmospheric pressure. This method yields alkanes and alkenes that are highly branched and valuable in the formulation of gasoline. Many of the reaction mechanisms associated with these processes are believed to be free-radical in nature, but their complexities are beyond the scope of this review.

Unsaturated Hydrocarbons

30

Compounds consisting of only hydrogen and carbon that contain less than the maximum number of allowable hydrogen atoms are referred to as **unsaturated** hydrocarbons. There are three categories of unsaturated hydrocarbons:

- **Alkenes**—general formula of C_NH_{2N}
- **Alkynes**—general formula of C_NH_{2N-2}
- **Aromatic** compounds*

*It should be noted that **aromatic compounds** might not be in the strictest sense true hydrocarbons because they often contain atoms other than hydrogen and carbon. Nonetheless, they are usually classified as unsaturated hydrocarbons because they contain multiple bonded carbon atoms that are sp^2-hybridized.

Sites of unsaturation in molecules can be carbon double bonds, triple bonds, or rings. In general the degree, N, to which a hydrocarbon compound is unsaturated relative to an alkane (classified as **saturated**) can be calculated for the formula C_nH_m using the following equation:

$$N = \frac{1}{2}(2n + 2 - m)$$

ALKENES

The Alkene Functional Group

As indicated earlier in the *Unsaturated Hydrocarbons* introduction, an alkene is a hydrocarbon with the general molecular formula C_NH_{2N}, where **N** is a positive whole number integer. Alkenes are classified as **unsaturated** because they contain (one or more) **carbon-carbon double-bond** functional groups. The term *olefin* is sometimes used as a synonym for alkene when referring to these compounds.

You may recall from the *Bonding in Organic Compounds* topic on page 201 that the carbon-carbon double-bond functional group that characterizes alkenes consists of one σ and one π bond. The σ bond is formed by the end-to-end overlap between two sp^2-hybridized carbon atom orbitals and is cylindrically symmetric with free rotation. The π bond is formed by the side-to-side overlap between two unhybridized *p*-orbitals. Rotation about this σ part of the double bond is very restricted and requires enough energy to break the bond. This does not happen under ambient conditions. The alkene functional group is generally shown as a simplified carbon-carbon double bond in skeletal format. (See Structure 24, where R can be a hydrogen atom, alkyl substituent, another functional group, or a heteroatom.)

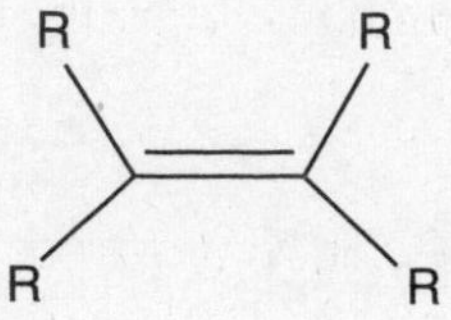

(24)

As discussed in the earlier in *Bonding in Organic Compounds* topic (see *Organic Compound Isomerism* on page 211), restricted rotation makes the formation of stereoisomer relationships between alkenes possible. These pairs of diastereomers can be designated as cis and trans or more generally *E* and *Z*.

Naming Alkenes

The procedure for naming alkenes is very similar to that of alkanes (for a review of this procedure see the **Alkane** topic in the chapter review). The alkene functional group is a carbon-carbon double bond. Note the change in the suffix from "**-ane**" for alkanes to "**-ene**" for these compounds.

STEP 1 The principal chain from which the alkene molecule's root name is derived must be the longest chain that contains the double bond. *Find* the longest continuous carbon chain containing the double bond.

STEP 2 The position of the double bond in the principal chain must be given the lowest number possible, without regard to other substituents that may be present. This determines the direction in which the principal chain is numbered. Under current IUPAC guidelines the number indicating the position of the first carbon in the double bond is placed *directly* before the "ene" suffix.

STEP 3 If the stereochemistry around the double bond is shown in the structural formula, the specific configuration must be shown in the name (cis/trans or *E*/*Z*). See the section on *Organic Compound Isomerism* for the details of these assignments.

Study the following alkene Structure (25) and associated name as an example:

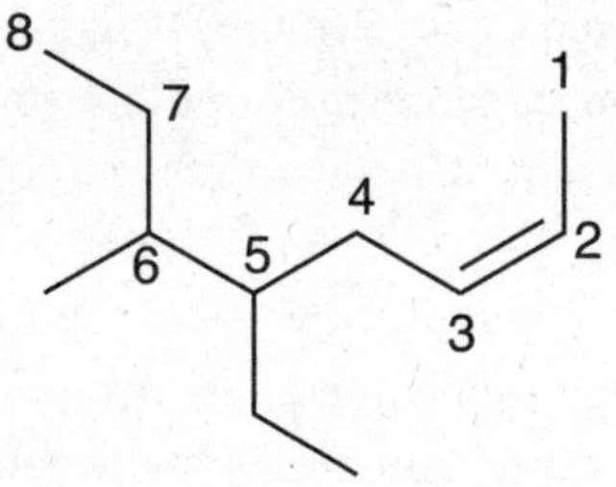

(*Z*)-5-ethyl-6-methyloct-2-ene

(25)

Notice how the longest carbon chain (eight carbons) containing the double bond (beginning in the 2 position) leads to the root name "oct-2-ene." Note that this compound contains two chirality centers (carbons 5 and 6). Since their stereochemistry is not defined in the given structure (1), their configurations are not included in the name. Another point you should be aware of is that more than one double bond may be present in an alkene. Greek prefixes are used to indicate the number of double bonds (*diene* means two double bonds, *triene* means three, *tetraene* means four, and so on).

EXERCISE 10

Directions: Using the guidelines shown on page 238, provide the best name for the following compound (note that stereochemistry for chirality centers is shown for this Structure (26). (Answers are on page 344.)

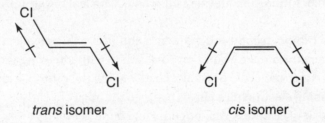

(26)

Alkene Physical Properties and Uses

The π character of alkene carbon-carbon double bonds makes these compounds more polarizable, and as such, they tend to have slightly higher melting and boiling points than their saturated hydrocarbon (alkanes) counterparts. Due to symmetry, trans alkene isomers are usually less polar than cis isomers. As shown in Figure 30.1, dipole moments in the trans isomer tend to cancel each other—leaving no net dipole moment. Those in a cis isomer tend to add together.

Figure 30.1. Dipole moments in the cis and trans isomers of 1,2 dichloroethene

Two factors tend to predict the stability of alkenes. First, for steric strain reasons trans isomers tend to have lower heats of combustion than cis isomers and second, the more substituted (more alkyl attachments to the double-bond sp^2-carbons) an alkene is, the more stable it is. This second factor is due to hyperconjugation—the donation of electron density into sp^2-orbitals. This is an inductive effect.

Alkenes are ubiquitous in nature and are produced in large quantities from petroleum for a variety of industrial uses including as precursors for economically important synthetic polymers (e.g., polyethylene).

Alkene Synthesis

Alkenes are most commonly prepared by **elimination** reactions. Two elimination reactions that are important for the DAT are **dehydration of alcohols** and **dehydrohalogenation** of alkyl halides. The product of both of these reactions is an alkene. Figure 30.2 shows the general reaction schemes for these processes.

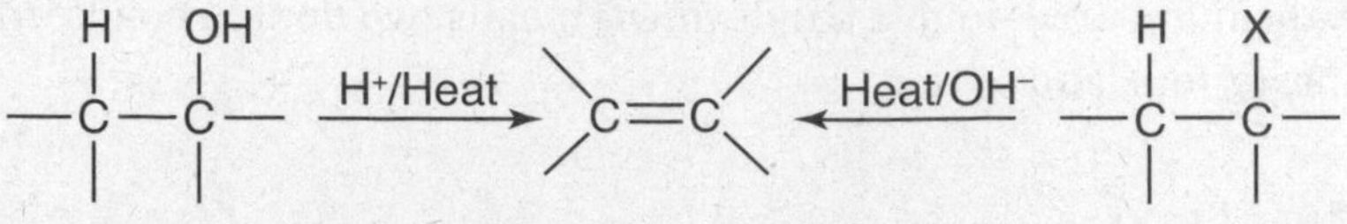

Figure 30.2. Elimination reactions commonly used to prepare alkenes

There are two commonly accepted mechanisms for alkene-forming elimination reactions:

- **Monomolecular Elimination (E1)** and
- **Bimolecular Elimination (E2)**

E1 reactions exhibit first-order kinetics and consist of a two-step process. The first step, which is rate-determining, involves the formation of an intermediate **carbocation** (R–C+) resulting from the loss of a leaving group (usually a water molecule or halogen anion). In the second step, the loss of a proton (usually under basic conditions) adjacent to the carbocation leads to the alkene product. Elimination reactions of this type are not usually very synthetically useful because they often produce mixtures of alkene and substitution products. Figure 30.3 shows the mechanistic steps of this process.

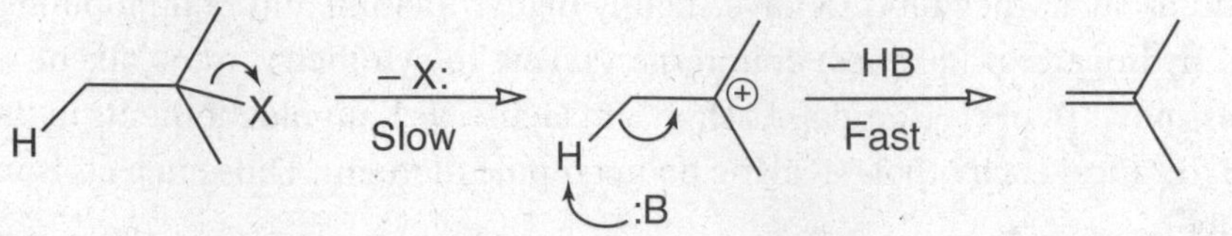

Figure 30.3. E1 reaction mechanism, where *X* is a leaving group, and :B is a base

E2 reactions exhibit second-order kinetics and occur in a single step. In this process, a proton is abstracted from a carbon next to a carbon with a **leaving group** (as with E1 reactions, usually a water molecule or a halogen anion). As the proton is abstracted (by a strong base) the remaining electron pair moves between the adjacent carbon and the leaving group departs with a pair of electrons. An *anti*periplanar bond geometry (almost coplanar) between the reactive proton and leaving group stabilizes the transition state of this process and can significantly increase the reaction's rate. The net outcome of this concerted process is the formation of a double bond—an alkene product. Because this reaction proceeds without the formation of an intermediate carbocation, there is less chance of a product mixture. Even in this case, depending on the starting compound's structure, a mixture of alkenes is possible. From a stereochemical perspective, trans products, due to their lower energy, are favored over cis products. Figure 30.4 shows the mechanism of this process.

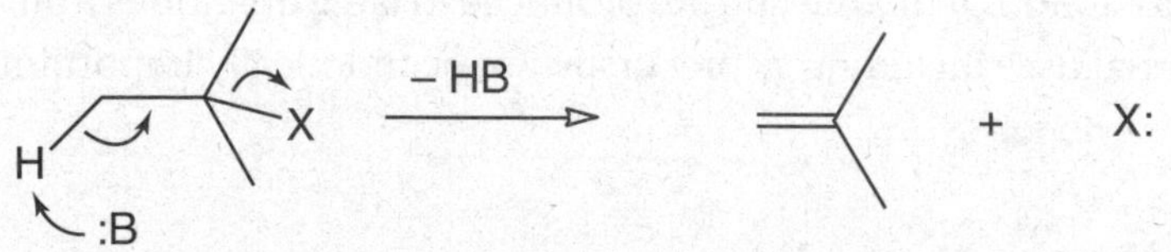

Figure 30.4. E2 reaction mechanism, where *X* is a leaving group and :B is a base

Reactions with heat and basic conditions proceed almost exclusively through E2 (usually desirable). If there is more than one β-carbon with a reactive proton next to the leaving group of the substrate, a mixture of alkenes usually results. The process is regioselective and in most cases the more substituted alkene (lower in energy) will predominate—this is known as "Zaitsev's rule." This outcome is illustrated by the real reaction example shown in Figure 30.5.

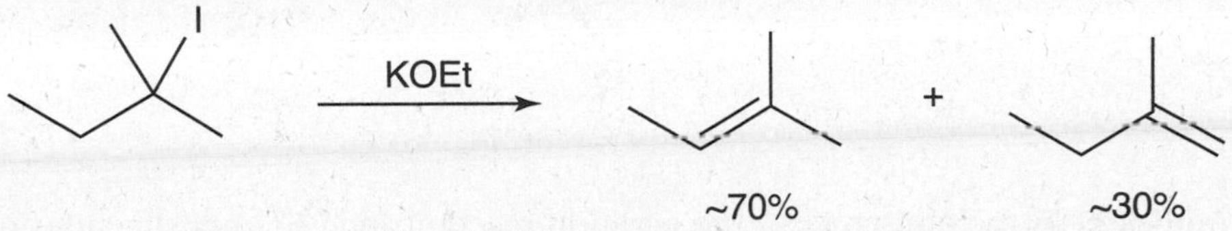

Figure 30.5. An elimination reaction that produces a mixture of E2 products

In general, heat and acidic conditions (such as the dehydration of alcohols) will produce an E1 product often mixed to some degree with other products (not desirable). When reactions proceed through an E1 mechanism, the major elimination product is almost always the *more-substituted* alkene (the Zaitsev product). Be familiar with both of these elimination reaction mechanisms.

EXERCISE 11

Directions: Provide the most likely major product(s) for the elimination reaction shown in Figure 30.6. (Answer is on page 344.)

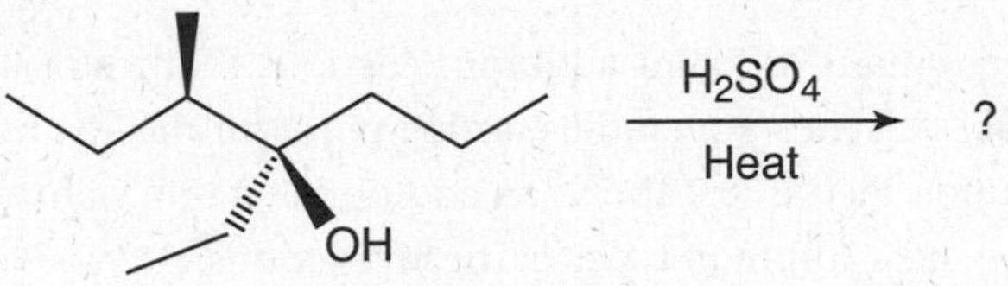

Figure 30.6. Elimination reaction exercise

Alkene Reactions

The alkene functional group can be transformed by the appropriate reagents and reaction conditions into many types of synthetically important functional groups. The most commonly encountered alkene reactions seen on the DAT are outlined below.

ALKENE ADDITION REACTIONS

The π portion of the alkene double bond can act as a nucleophile (a species that's attracted to the nucleus of an atom) attracting electrophiles, which use the π electrons to form σ bonds and thus "add" to the alkene functional group.

Addition Reaction Stereochemistry Terms

Syn Addition: In the syn process, the addition reactants add to the same side of the alkene double or alkyne triple bond. Structure 27 shows a generalized syn addition product, where *X* and *Y* are the addition reactants.

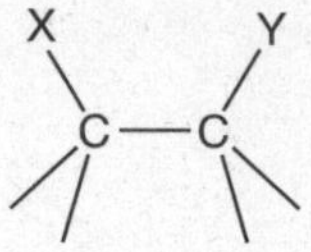

(27)

Anti Addition: In the anti process, the addition reactants add to opposite sides of the double or triple bond. Structure 28 shows a generalized anti addition product, where *X* and *Y* are the addition reactants.

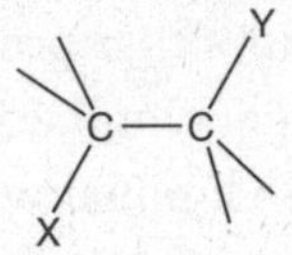

(28)

Don't confuse the terms *syn* and *anti*, which refer to reaction mechanism processes, with *cis* and *trans*, which refer to a pair of alkene stereoisomers and more specifically a pair of diastereomers.

Alkenes can undergo many different addition reactions that result in many types of new compounds. This makes alkenes a versatile starting point for the synthesis of more complex and valuable compounds. Figure 30.7 shows an addition reaction web, which provides generalized examples of the most common types of these reactions.

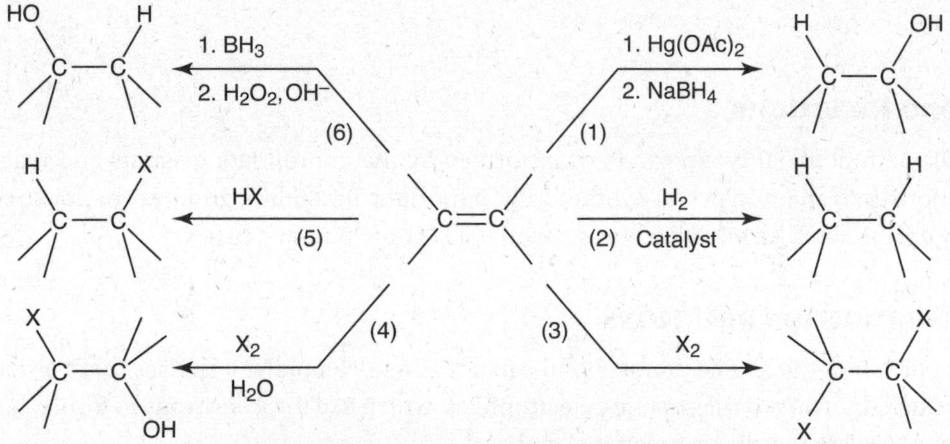

Figure 30.7. Alkene addition reaction web

A side note about the "Reaction Webs" used in this review: In most reaction web diagrams, the reactants and products have been generalized to represent the most common form of the reaction. Usually only the main product is shown. There are often additional products that are not shown because they are minor or not essential to understanding the reaction's outcome.

Alcohols (see Figure 30.7 proceeding in a clockwise direction) can be prepared by either reaction 1 [oxymercuration – mercury acetate ($Hg(OAc)_2$) followed by sodium borohydride ($NaBH_4$) reduction] or reaction 6 [borane (BH_3) followed by basic hydrogen peroxide (H_2O_2)].

MARKOVNIKOV'S RULE

Vladimir Markovnikov was a Russian chemist who discovered a predictable pattern for addition reactions involving carbocation intermediates. **"Mark's" rule** refers to the addition of a reactant (e.g., halide anion, hydroxyl anion, etc.) to the more substituted carbon in the double bond of an alkene. Different reaction conditions allow a chemist to add reactants in either Mark or non-Mark orientation to an alkene double bond. In Figure 30.7, reaction 1 results in **Markovnikov addition** of water and reaction 6, **non-Markovnikov syn addition** of water. The two methods are complementary. In Figure 30.8, the outcomes of both processes are shown with real reaction examples.

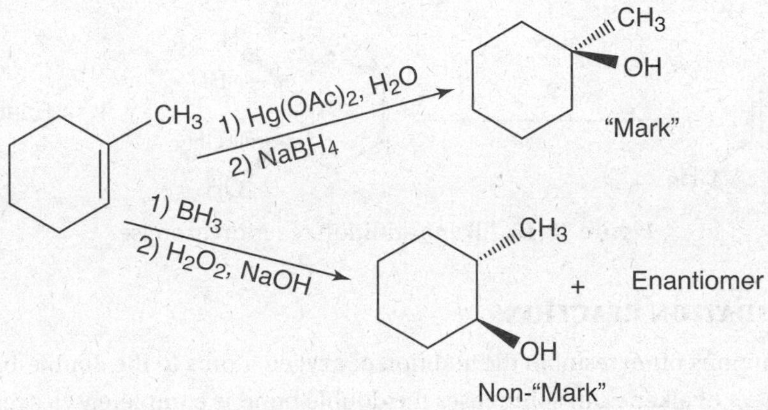

Figure 30.8. Markovnikov and non-Markovnikov addition of water to an alkene

In reaction 2, the addition of H_2 gas is catalyzed by a supported transition metal (e.g., Pt, Pd, Ni, Rh, etc.) in a syn stereochemical fashion. The product is an **alkane**.

Reactions 3 [addition of a halogen (X_2, where X = Cl or Br) to give a **1,2-dihalide**] and 4 (addition of aqueous halogen to give a **1,2-halohydrin**) proceed by the same mechanism, the first step of which is the formation of a **halonium ion** intermediate (Structure 29 shown below).

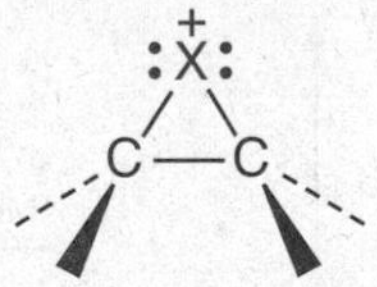

(29)

It can be seen from the halonium ion's structure that one side of the carbon-carbon bond is blocked by a halogen cation (X+), thus nucleophilic addition of either X– (reaction 3) or H_2O (reaction 4) can occur from only one side. This results in an *anti* stereochemical addition for both reactions.

Alkyl halides (also called haloalkanes) can be synthesized using reaction 5. The starting alkene is treated with a **halo acid** (HCl or HBr) in an organic solvent (often an ether). The reaction mechanism involves the protonation of the double bond of the alkene by the acid to form a carbocation intermediate (C+). This is followed by nucleophilic addition of a halide anion ($X-$). Addition of HX follows Markovnikov's rule. Because a carbocation intermediate is involved in the transformation, rearrangements to lower-energy carbocations can lead to product mixtures. The reaction mechanism for this process is shown in Figure 30.9.

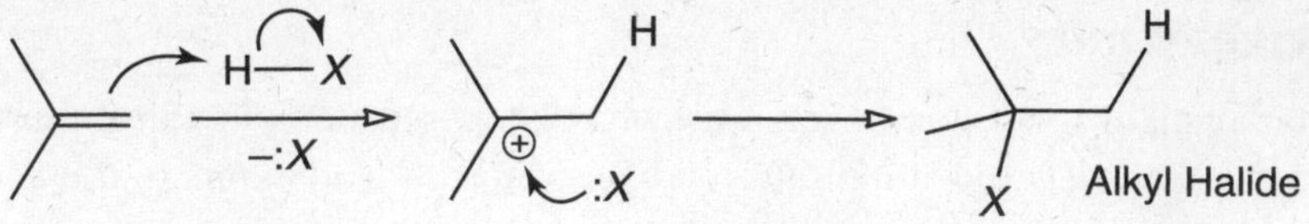

Figure 30.9. Mechanism for the hydrohalogenation of an alkene, where X is Br or Cl

EXERCISE 12

Given the following transformation, provide the best set of reagents/conditions that would most likely produce the products shown in Figure 30.10. (Answer is on page 345.)

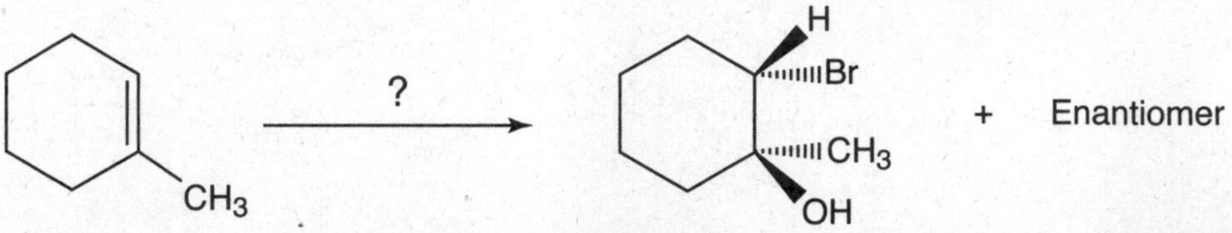

Figure 30.10. Alkene addition reaction exercise

ALKENE OXIDATION REACTIONS

Oxidation reactions often result in the addition of oxygen atoms to the double-bond carbons (sp^2-hybridized) of alkenes. In some cases the double bond is completely cleaved in the process. Technically, the bonding of any electronegative element's atoms to carbon is considered "oxidation," but many of the reactions shown in the earlier alkene web (Figure 30.7) are not generally classified this way. Figure 30.11 shows those reactions that are commonly considered alkene oxidations.

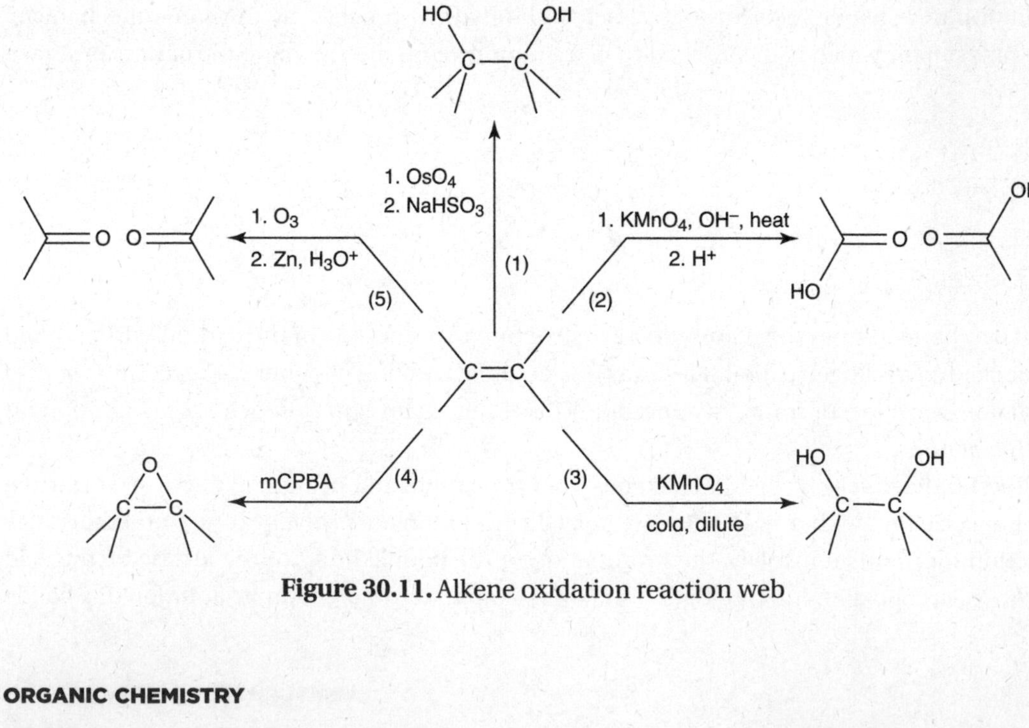

Figure 30.11. Alkene oxidation reaction web

Starting with reaction 1 (Figure 30.11, proceeding in a clockwise direction), an alkene can first be treated with osmium tetroxide (OsO_4) to produce a cyclic osmate, which is then cleaved by addition of aqueous sodium bisulfite ($NaHSO_3$). The reaction proceeds by **syn** addition to produce a **diol**. This procedure has some drawbacks related to the expense and toxicity of osmium tetroxide.

In reaction 2, treatment of an alkene with hot, basic, potassium permanganate ($KMnO_4$) followed by acid results in cleavage of the double bond and the formation of two **carboxylic acid** fragments. If the alkene is symmetric, the fragments are the same and a single carboxylic acid product is produced. If the alkene is asymmetric, two different carboxylic acids are formed, which may be difficult to separate. Cleavage of tetrasubstituted double bonds results in **ketones** (similar to reaction 5 discussed below) and the carbon at the end of *terminal* alkenes is lost as carbon dioxide (CO_2) gas under these conditions. This reaction outcome is illustrated in Figure 30.12.

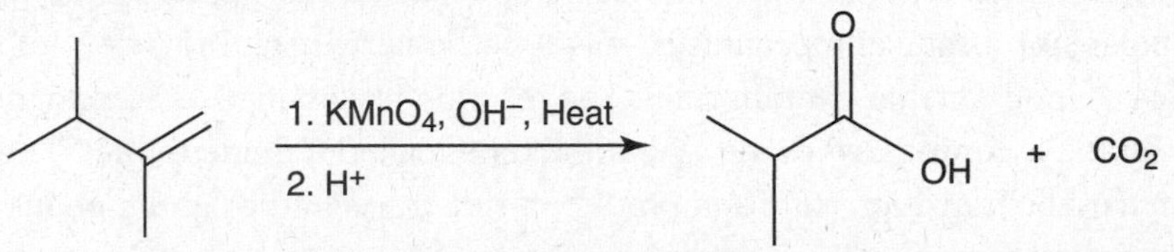

Figure 30.12. Oxidative cleavage of a terminal alkene
by hot, basic, potassium permanganate

Reaction 3 is similar to reaction 2 except that the oxidative conditions are much milder and the product produced is a diol with a *syn* addition orientation.

Epoxides (also called oxiranes) are produced when alkenes are reacted with peroxycarboxylic acids. In reaction 4, *m*-chloroperoxybenzoic acid (mCPBA) is used to affect such an oxidation. Another commonly used reagent for this process is peroxyacetic acid (PAA).

Ozonolysis of an alkene is shown in reaction 5. This oxidative process results in the cleavage of the double bond and the formation of carbonyl compounds—either **ketones** or **aldehydes** depending on the alkene's structure. First, the alkene is reacted with ozone to form a molozonide that isomerizes to an ozonide intermediate that is reduced with acidic zinc to produce ketone or aldehyde products. Figure 30.13 shows a real reaction example of this procedure.

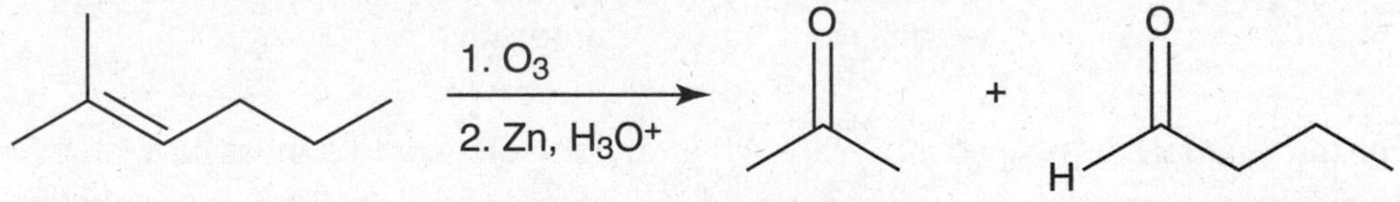

Figure 30.13. Formation of a ketone and an aldehyde by ozonolysis of an alkene

EXERCISE 13

Directions: Provide the reactant that would likely produce the product shown in Figure 30.14 using the given reagents/conditions. (Answer is on page 345.)

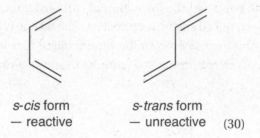

Figure 30.14. Alkene oxidation reaction exercise

THE DIELS-ALDER REACTION

The Diels-Alder reaction (a name reaction) is an unusual addition process that proceeds by neither a polar nor a radical mechanism. It is a particularly useful reaction for synthesizing organic compounds that contain rings. The reaction is classified as a cycloaddition and involves reacting a **conjugated diene** with an **alkene** (called a **dieneophile**). These species combine in a cyclic transition state and produce a ring through the simultaneous formation of two carbon-carbon bonds. The mechanism of this process is termed **pericyclic** because the reaction product is produced in a single concerted step by the cyclic redistribution of bonding electrons.

The diene in the reaction must be able to assume a conformation that allows both of its double bonds to align on the same side of their connecting sigma bond (see Structure 30 below, which shows the aligned and unaligned forms). The reactive conformation is sometimes referred to as the *s*-cis form. If the diene has large terminal substituents, the *s*-cis conformation can be unstable (high energy) and its lower-energy *s*-trans form may predominate. Such dienes react slowly or not at all with the dieneophile.

s-cis form
— reactive

s-trans form
— unreactive   (30)

For the reaction to proceed at a reasonable rate, the dieneophile must have an electron withdrawing group or groups attached to its double-bond carbons. The withdrawing species is usually some kind of carbonyl-containing functional group (for example, aldehyde, ketone, ester, carboxylic acid, etc.), although other polarizing groups can be used.

Another aspect of the Diels-Alder reaction is that it forms a *predominant* product when stereoisomer formation is possible. Thus the reaction is considered to be *stereoselective* (see Exercise 14 on page 247). Figure 30.15 shows a generalized scheme for the Diels-Alder reaction for the formation of a six-membered ring.

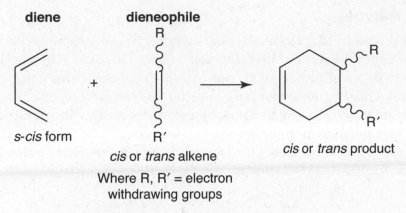

Figure 30.15. A generalized Diels-Alder reaction

This process can also be used to synthesize rings of other sizes, commonly five-membered rings and bicyclic compounds.

EXERCISE 14

Directions: Provide the major product for the reaction shown in Figure 30.16. Hint: Stereochemistry will be a factor for successfully predicting the major product for this process. (Answer is on page 346.)

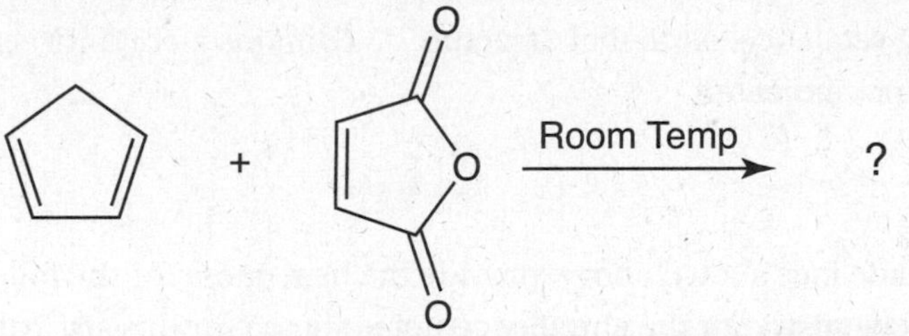

Figure 30.16. Diels-Alder reaction exercise

ALKYNES

The Alkyne Functional Group

As indicated earlier in the *Unsaturated Hydrocarbons* section on page 237, an alkyne is a hydrocarbon with the general molecular formula C_NH_{2N-2}, where N is a positive whole number integer. Alkynes are classified as **unsaturated** because they contain (one or more) **carbon-carbon triple-bond** functional groups.

As discussed in the *Bonding in Organic Compounds* topic of this review, the carbon-carbon triple-bond functional group that characterizes alkynes consists of one σ bond resulting from the orbital overlap of two *sp*-hybridized carbon atoms and two π bonds resulting from the side-to-side overlap of *two* sets of *p*-atomic orbitals. The bonding interactions of the two sets of *p*-orbitals are perpendicular to each other. The alkyne functional group is generally shown as a simplified carbon-carbon triple bond in skeletal format—see Structure 31 below, where *R* can be a hydrogen atom, alkyl substituent, another functional group, or a heteroatom.

$$R \!-\!\!-\! C \equiv C \!-\!\!-\! R \qquad (31)$$

Naming Alkynes

The naming process for alkynes is almost identical to that for naming alkenes—for a refresher on this process see the *Naming Alkenes* section on page 238 of this review. When naming alkynes the suffix "*-ane*" is changed to "*-yne.*" The principal chain from which the alkyne's name is derived must be the *longest* in the molecule that contains the triple bond. Multiple triple bonds are indicated, as with alkenes, by using Greek prefixes (diyne, triyne, tetrayne, etc.). Since the carbons in the triple bonds are *sp*-hybridized, these functional groups don't exhibit any stereochemical isomerism and this makes the naming process easier. The following Structure (32) illustrates these points.

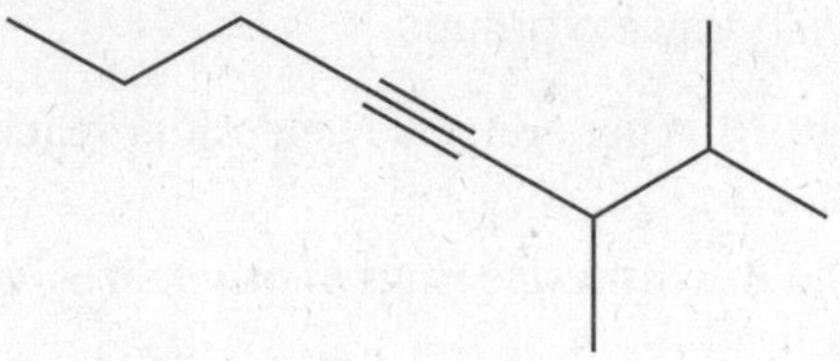

2,3-dimethyloct-4-yne   (32)

Notice that the longest continuous carbon chain is eight carbons long (oct-) and that, just as with alkenes, the position of the first carbon in the triple bond must appear in the name (oct-4-yne). Also note that the eight-carbon chain must be numbered from *right* to *left* in this case to give the first methyl substituent the lowest possible number (2)—this leads to the 2,3-dimethyl numbering sequence. Note that Structure 32 contains a chirality center, but its configuration (*R* or *S*) is not indicated.

EXERCISE 15

Directions: Using the guidelines shown above, provide the best name for the following compound. Note that stereochemistry for the chirality center is shown for this structure. (Answer is on page 347.)

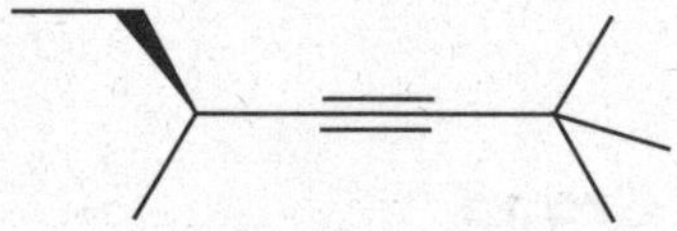

Alkyne Physical Properties and Uses

Alkynes have physical properties similar to alkanes and alkenes except they are a little more polar due to their even more polarizable triple bonds. This results in somewhat higher melting and boiling points relative to similar-sized hydrocarbons. Alkyne dipole moments are relatively small, but their solutions can still be slightly polar. The hydrogens of terminal alkynes are slightly acidic ($pK_a \sim 25$) and as discussed later under this topic these compounds can be deprotonated by very strong bases such as sodium amide.

The common name for the simplest alkyne is acetylene (C_2H_2). Acetylene is a flammable gas, which when mixed with oxygen gas, is used in metal-cutting torches. Other simple alkynes are often used as precursors for the synthesis of more complex compounds with many applications, such as the manufacturing of pharmaceuticals.

Alkyne Reactions

As with alkenes the alkyne functional group is reactive and can undergo many types of chemical transformations—important examples of these reactions follow.

SYNTHESIS REACTIONS

There are only a few practical ways to synthesize alkynes, and even the available methods require harsh conditions and often produce low product yields. One approach is dehydrohalogenation of **vicinal** (side-by-side) dihalides. Figure 30.17 shows this elimination reaction.

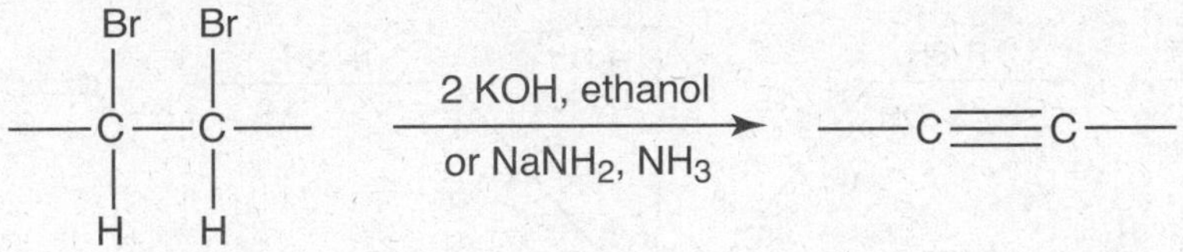

Figure 30.17. Preparation of an alkyne by dehydrohalogenation

If possible, it is better to start with a simple alkyne and further derivatize it. Using a *very strong base* such as sodium amide ($NaNH_2$), terminal alkynes can be deprotonated to produce salts of an acetylide anion.

> Protons attached to *sp*-hybridized carbons in a triple bond (H-C≡C-) are slightly acidic (pK_a ~ 25). The resulting acetylide anion is stabilized by the high *s*-orbital character (50%) of the carbon carrying the negative charge (-C≡C:-).

The salt of the acetylide anion isn't generally isolated, but it immediately reacts with a primary alkyl halide (RCH_2–*X*, where *X* = Cl, Br, and I) to produce an internal alkyne. If acetylene (H–C≡C–H) is used to prepare the acetylide ion, it can be alkylated to produce a terminal alkyne. This process is one of the most important methods available for *forming carbon-carbon bonds.* Figure 30.18 shows the general reaction scheme for this procedure.

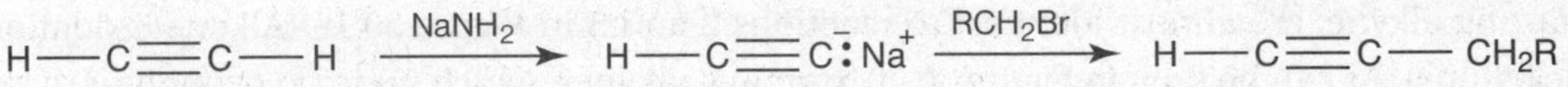

Figure 30.18. Synthesis of an internal alkyne by acetylide ion alkylation

ADDITION REACTIONS

As with alkenes, alkynes undergo a number of different *addition reactions* to produce new categories of organic compounds. Figure 30.19 shows an addition reaction web that includes the most common examples.

In Figure 30.19, reductive addition to produce **alkanes** and **alkenes** can be accomplished using reactions 1, 2, and 3. Reaction of an alkyne with excess H_2 and a standard transition metal catalyst (Pt, Pd, Ni, Rh, etc.) produces an alkane by ***syn*** addition. A *trans*-alkene is produced by treating an alkyne with Li metal in liquid ammonia (NH_3) and a *cis*-alkene by reaction of an alkyne with one equivalent of H_2 and **Lindlar's catalyst**.

> **TIP**
> **Recall that Lindlar's catalyst is a "poisoned" Pd metal catalyst that is less active than the standard version.**

Alkyl halides are produced from alkynes by reactions 4 and 5. Alkynes reacted with excess halogen (X_2, where *X* = Cl, Br, and I) result in tetrahalides (reaction 4). Those reacted with excess haloacid (HCl or HBr) in an organic solvent produce **geminal** (attached to the same carbon atom) **dihalides** (reaction 5).

As with alkenes, hydroboration/oxidation of alkynes produces **carbonyl compounds**. Terminal alkynes produce **aldehydes**—see reaction 6. Because alkynes have *two* π bonds, it is possible for two molecules of BH$_3$ to add across the triple bond, leading to undesirable side products. To prevent this issue, sterically hindered borane reagents such as disiamylborane and 9-BBN are used for these reactions. Alkynes can also be hydrated by using acid and a mercuric sulfate catalyst. This process produces **ketones** (reaction 7). Terminal alkynes give methyl ketones and internal alkynes can give a *mixture* of ketones, which limits the reaction's utility.

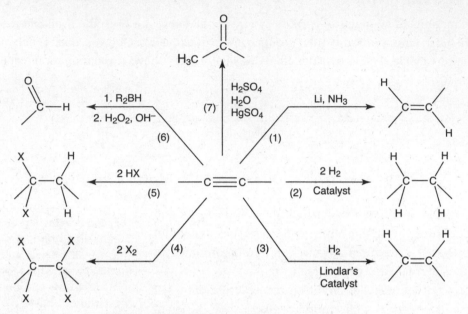

Figure 30.19. Alkyne addition reaction web

OXIDATION REACTIONS

Strong oxidizing agents (potassium permanganate/base or ozone) lead to the cleavage of alkyne triple bonds and the formation of **carboxylic acids**. These reactions, except for the starting alkyne, are almost identical to reactions 2 and 5 in Figure 30.19 (Alkene Oxidation Reactions). As can be seen in Figure 30.20, terminal alkynes, which undergo ozonolysis, have their carbon chains shortened by one carbon atom—which is lost as a molecule of carbon dioxide (CO_2). The above processes may require more heat and time to completely cleave the very strong triple bond and product yields are often lower.

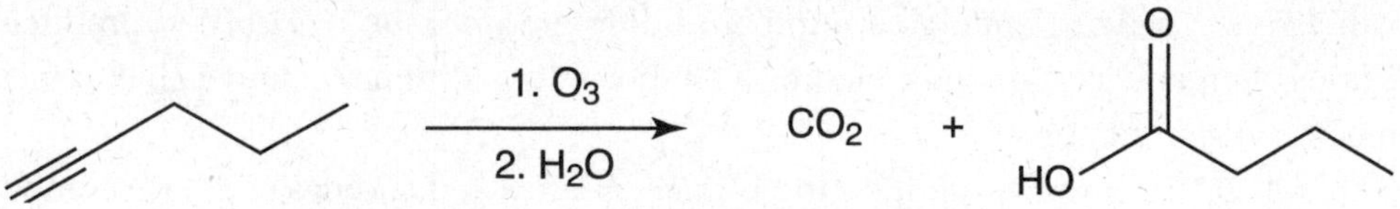

$$\xrightarrow[\text{2. H}_2\text{O}]{\text{1. O}_3}$$

$$CO_2 \quad + \quad$$

Figure 30.20. Ozonolysis of a terminal alkyne

EXERCISE 16

Directions: Provide the most likely major product(s) for the reaction shown in Figure 30.21. (Answer is on page 347.)

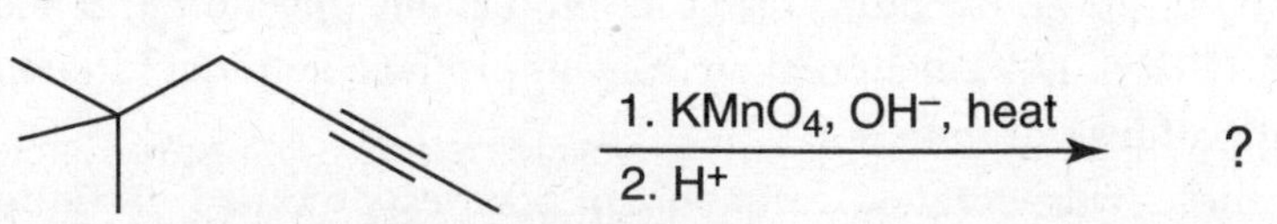

$$\xrightarrow[\text{2. H}^+]{\text{1. KMnO}_4,\ \text{OH}^-,\ \text{heat}} \quad ?$$

Figure 30.21. Alkyne addition reaction exercise

AROMATIC COMPOUNDS

The Arene (Benzene) Functional Group and Other Aromatic Molecules

The term *aromatic* originally referred to the olfactory response that some "fragrant" organic compounds elicit, but today it describes a special group of compounds that follow **Huclek's rule**. This rule states that in order for a compound to be aromatic it must possess **$4n + 2\pi$ electrons** (where **n** is a positive whole integer). These compounds can have 2, 6, 10, 14, etc. π electrons. In addition to this criterion, the compound's π bonding system must be *cyclic*, *conjugated* (the double bonds must alternate with single bonds), and in a *planar* conformation. All types of compounds (neutral, anions, and cations) that meet all of these criteria are unusually stable and considered to be "aromatic" (examples are shown in Figure 30.22). Fully conjugated single-ring π systems are called **annulenes**.

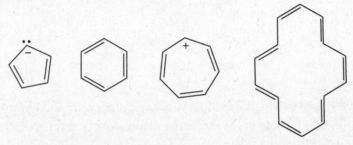

Figure 30.22. Some examples of aromatic compounds

What are termed **antiaromatic** compounds can also exist. They have *$4n$ π electrons* and their π systems are planar and conjugated like aromatic compounds. These compounds are usually, due to their high energy, quite reactive. Some examples are shown in Figure 30.23.

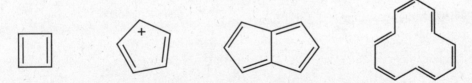

Figure 30.23. Some examples of antiaromatic compounds

Physical Properties and Uses of Aromatic Compounds

From a physical standpoint, aromatic compounds have properties similar to other hydrocarbons, but their chemical properties are quite different. These molecules are *unusually* stable because of their planar shapes, side-to-side *p*-orbital overlap (resulting in π-bonding interactions), and electron delocalization. In general, aromatic compounds are not reactive toward addition processes, unlike other unsaturated hydrocarbons. All types of aromatic compounds occur naturally and many thousands of different aromatic molecules have been produced synthetically.

Naming Arene Compounds

The parent molecule for many aromatic compounds is called **benzene**, which has the molecular formula C_6H_6. As such, the majority of aromatic compounds can be considered derivatives of benzene—this class of compounds is generally referred to as **arenes**.

It should also be noted that in the case of arene compounds the base functional group, benzene, contains only carbon and hydrogen atoms, and therefore, it is a true hydrocarbon. In many cases derivatives of benzene (and other aromatic compounds), including examples in this review, contain atoms such as oxygen, nitrogen, and halogens (F, Cl, Br, and I). These compounds have been grouped in with benzene even though they are not true hydrocarbons.

The **arene** (also referred to as benzene) functional group consists of a six-membered carbon ring with three alternating carbon-carbon double bonds (remember the arene ring's hydrogens are not shown—Structures 33, 34, 35, 36, 37 below). There are many IUPAC-accepted common names for monosubstituted arenes. You should be familiar with the names and structures of the following substances (Structures 33, 34, 35, 36, 37):

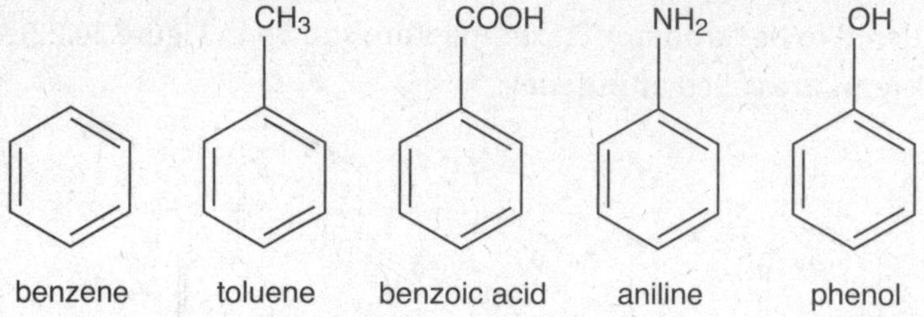

benzene   toluene   benzoic acid   aniline   phenol   (33, 34, 35, 36, 37)

It's also worth the time to become familiar with a few **polycyclic** and **heterocyclic** aromatic compounds. You should be able to recognize the names and structures of the following substances (Structures 38, 39, 40, 41, 42):

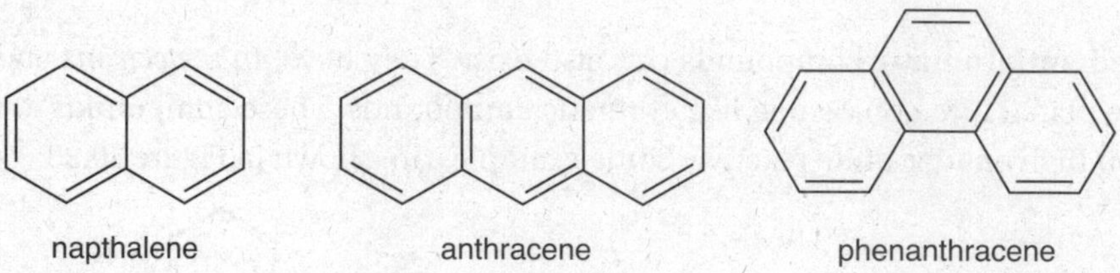

napthalene   anthracene   phenanthracene   (38, 39, 40)

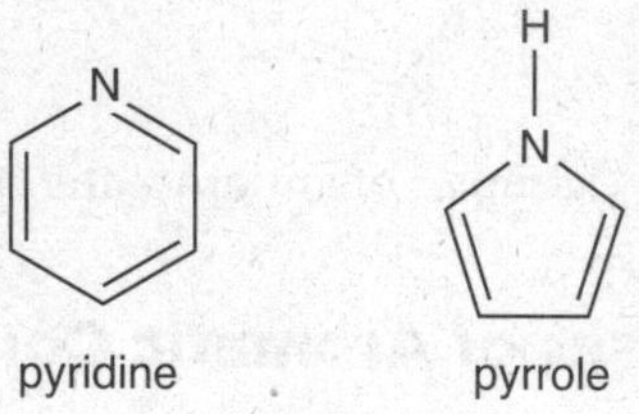

pyridine   pyrrole   (41, 42)

The process for naming **disubstituted** aromatic compounds uses a simple terminology to indicate the relative positions of the two groups on the arene ring. If the groups attached to arene ring carbons are immediately *next to each* other, the configuration is called *ortho* (abbreviated in names as "*o*"). If they are attached to ring carbons with **one unsubstituted carbon in between**, the configuration is referred to as *meta* (abbreviated as "*m*"), and if the groups are attached to ring carbons **straight across** from each other, the substitution pattern is called *para* (abbreviated as "*p*"). The following constitutional isomers of dichlorobenzene illustrate the use of this naming process (Structures 43, 44, 45). When there are two different substituents on the ring, they are listed in alphabetical order.

Aromatic compounds with *more than two* substituents are named using a numbering system similar to that for cycloalkanes to indicate where substituents are on the arene ring.

Although not particularly difficult to learn, it's unlikely that you will be required to answer questions on the DAT that use this naming procedure.

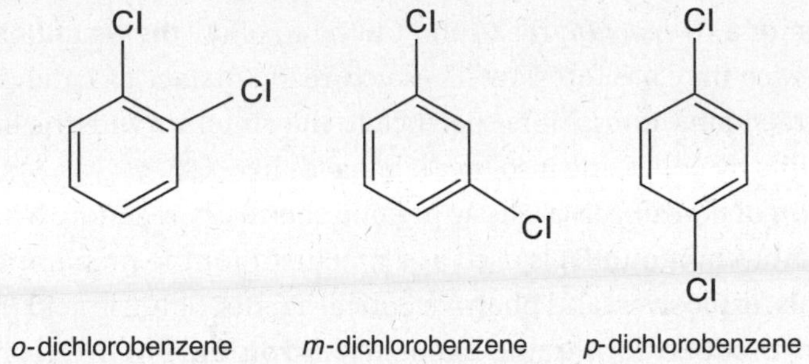

o-dichlorobenzene   m-dichlorobenzene   p-dichlorobenzene   (43, 44, 45)

EXERCISE 17

Directions: Using the guidelines described on pages 251–252, provide the correct name for the following compound. (Answer is on page 347.)

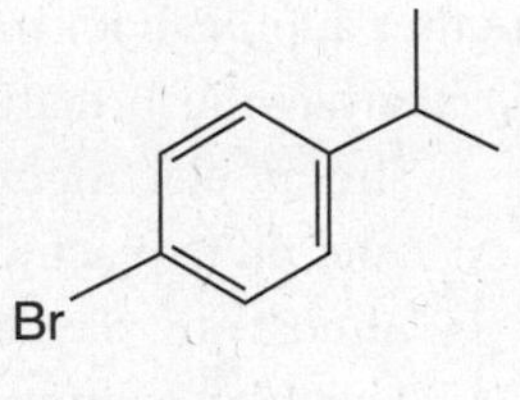

Reactions of the Benzene Ring

SUBSTITUTION REACTIONS

Unlike unsaturated hydrocarbons, the most important reactions of simple arene compounds are not addition reactions but **substitution** reactions. The double bonds in the benzene ring are unreactive toward addition except under very special conditions. Instead, because of the ring's *high π electron density*, it acts as an electron donor and thus attracts and reacts with electron-deficient species (commonly referred to as **electrophiles**). Figure 30.24 shows a substitution reaction web for benzene that includes the most common examples.

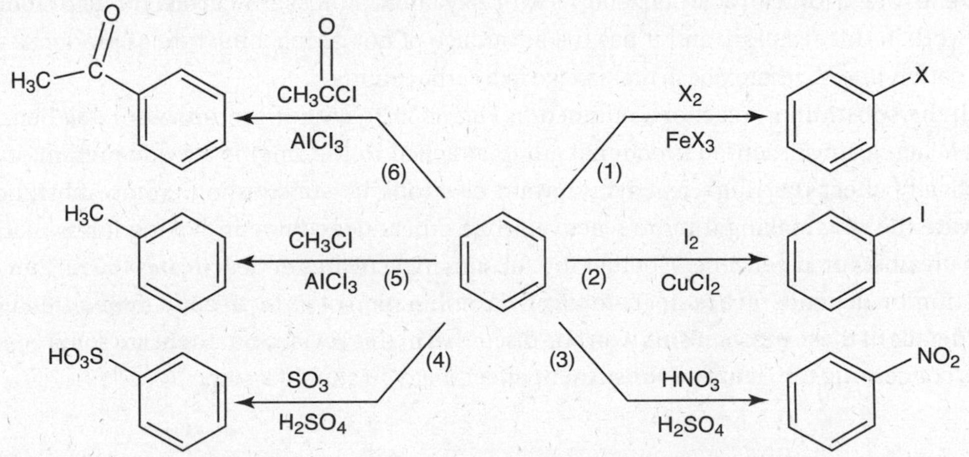

Figure 30.24. Benzene substitution reaction web

As can be seen from Figure 30.24, many different functional groups can be attached to the benzene ring using substitution reactions. **Halogenated benzene** compounds can be prepared by using reactions 1 and 2, where X in reaction 1 is either Cl or Br. Note that these reactions require the addition of a *co-reactant* (FeX_3 and $CuCl_2$) to allow the reaction to proceed at a practical rate, otherwise they are too slow. These co-reactants act as catalysts and significantly improve these reactions' rates. More specifically, they interact with the halogen and make it a better electrophile by polarizing it so that it behaves like X+.

Reaction 3, the nitration of benzene, is a classic organic chemistry reaction. **Nitrobenzene** (and other nitrated aromatic compounds) is used as a precursor for the preparation of many other important chemicals, explosives, and pharmaceutical agents. Sulfuric acid (H_2SO_4) and nitric acid (HNO_3) react to produce the nitrating agent, the **nitronium ion** (NO_2+) in this reaction, a good electrophile.

Sulfonation of benzene is shown in reaction 4. This is an historically important reaction, because **aromatic sulfonic acids** were once used to prepare dyes and "sulfa drugs." Here sulfur trioxide (SO_3) and sulfuric acid (the mixture is referred to as fuming sulfuric acid) react to form HSO_3+, which is the sulfonating electrophile.

Reaction 5 is a name reaction, **Friedel-Crafts alkylation**, and is a very important method for synthesizing alkyl benzenes (another approach for making C–C bonds). In the example shown, aluminum trichloride ($AlCl_3$) catalyzes the formation of CH_3+ (a carbocation, another strong electrophile) from chloromethane, which goes on to react with the electron-rich benzene ring. Almost any alkyl halide can be used in this reaction, making it very versatile. If there is already another functional group attached to the benzene ring, in many cases the reaction fails. Another limitation involves the formation of a carbocation (R–C+) intermediate. Carbocations, depending on their structures, can *rearrange* to form new, more stable (lower energy) carbocations. When this happens, the reaction produces what can be a hard-to-separate mixture of alkyl benzenes.

> Many reactions in organic chemistry are named after their discoverers. Thus the alkylation reaction (reaction 5) described in Figure 30.24 is named after chemists **Friedel** and **Crafts**. There are numerous "name reactions" that you will encounter in this review. Knowing the names of these reactions is a helpful memory aid.

The last reaction, 6, shown in Figure 30.24, was developed by the same chemists as reaction 5 and is called **Friedel-Crafts acylation**. In this variation of the alkylation reaction, the electrophile is R–+C=O, an acyl cation, which like the carbocations in reaction 5, react with the benzene ring to form an acyl benzene. As with alkylation, almost any **carboxylic acid chloride** will work in this reaction, and it has the advantage of not giving a mixture of products—the acyl cation intermediate doesn't rearrange like carbocations.

All the substitution reactions outlined in Figure 30.24 are for the *unsubstituted* benzene ring. When a substituent (a functional group attached to the ring) is already present, it can drastically affect the ring's reactivity toward electrophilic substitution. Some substituents **activate** the ring making it more reactive, while others **deactivate** it making it less reactive than unsubstituted benzene. Whether the substituent activates or deactivates the ring toward substitution depends on a rather complicated combination of *inductive* and *resonance* effects. The details of these mechanisms won't be discussed in this review, but there are some general rules concerning the **benzene substituent effect** that you should know.

Substituents that **activate** benzene toward substitution generally direct the incoming electrophile to the *ortho* and *para* ring positions relative to the group already present. Functional groups that fall into this category include:

- –R, –OR, –OH, –OC=OR, –NHC=OR, –NH$_2$, and NR$_2$ (where *R* is an alkyl group)

> Unfortunately, as is usually the case, there is an exception to these hard, fast rules. Halogen ring substituents (–F, –Cl, –Br, and –I) are **deactivating**, but direct the electrophile to *ortho/para* ring positions.

Substituents that **deactivate** the benzene ring always direct the incoming electrophile to the *meta* ring position relative to the group already present. Functional groups in this category include:

- –C=OOH, –C=OOR, –C=OR, –C=OH, –NO$_2$, and –SO$_3$H (where *R* is an alkyl group)

➡ Example

The following example illustrates the use of the above substituent effect rules. Given the following acylation reaction of phenol (Figure 30.25), predict the major product(s).

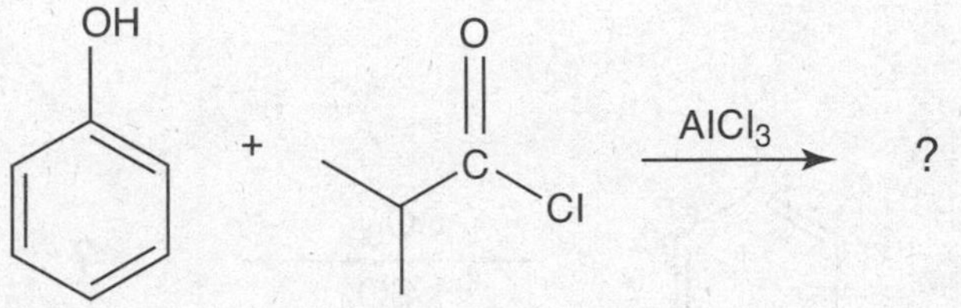

Figure 30.25. Acylation of phenol example reaction

Solution

The –OH group of phenol is an activating, ortho/para director. Thus there are two major products (see Figure 30.26):

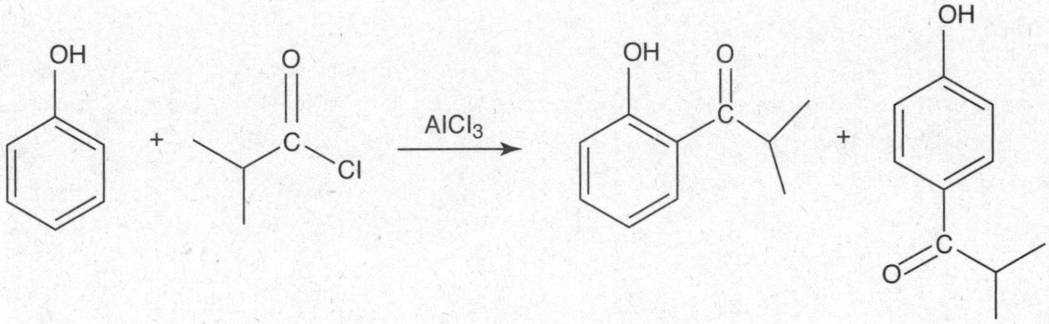

Figure 30.26. Major acylation products of phenol

AN IMPORTANT ADDITION REACTION

Even though the benzene ring is normally unreactive toward addition, there is one important addition reaction you should know—the addition of hydrogen to the double bonds of the benzene ring. This process requires elevated temperature/pressure and a powerful hydrogenation catalyst (finely divided rhodium metal supported on carbon—Rh/C is often used). This reaction, shown in Figure 30.27, reduces the benzene ring to **cyclohexane**.

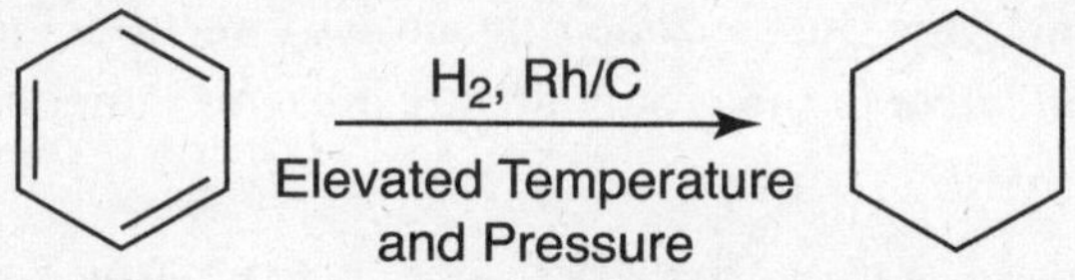

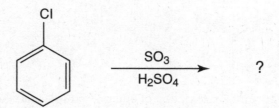

Figure 30.27. Metal (Rh) catalyzed addition of hydrogen gas (H_2) to benzene

EXERCISE 18

Directions: Given the following sulfonation reaction of chlorobenzene (see Figure 30.28), predict the major product(s). (Answers are on page 347.)

Figure 30.28. Sulfonation reaction exercise

Oxygen Functional Group Compounds

31

There are a number of important categories of organic compounds that contain the element oxygen. Many DAT questions require knowledge of the physical properties, synthesis, and reactions of this broad range of molecules. This chapter focuses on compounds with oxygen-containing functional groups.

The DAT topic outline for organic chemistry specifically refers to the following categories of oxygen-containing compounds (functional group name and associated general formula of each follows):

ALCOHOLS: contain a **hydroxyl** group bonded to an alkyl (or aryl) group

ETHERS: contain an **oxygen atom** bonded to two alkyl (aryl) groups

ALDEHYDES: contain a **carbonyl** group bonded to a hydrogen atom and an alkyl (or aryl) group

KETONES: contain a **carbonyl** group bonded to two alkyl (and/or aryl) groups

CARBOXYLIC ACIDS: contain a **hydroxyl** group bonded to a **carbonyl carbon group**

CARBOXYLIC ACID DERIVATIVES: all contain a **carbonyl** group along with various other **hetero atoms** bonded to the carbonyl carbon (e.g., oxygen, chlorine, and nitrogen)

You should be aware that many questions that involve these types of compounds appear on the exam. Pretty much any one of these molecules can be converted into any of the others, often by a single reaction step. It can be a bit challenging to keep the chemical reactions of all these compounds in one's head because there are so many. As advised in earlier parts of this book, look for general reaction patterns and prepare a unique set of flash cards for reactions associated with each functional group.

ALCOHOLS AND ETHERS

The Hydroxyl Functional Group

Alcohols and **phenols** (aromatic alcohols) are defined by their **hydroxyl** functional groups. More specifically, alcohols have hydroxyl groups bonded to sp^3-carbons and phenols to sp^2-carbons of arene (benzene) rings. They can all be thought of as **derivatives of the water molecule**, where one of its *hydrogens* has been replaced with **carbon**. Figure 31.1 shows generalized structural examples of these two types of compounds.

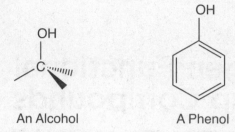

An Alcohol   A Phenol

Figure 31.1. The generalized structures of an alcohol and a phenol

Naming Alcohols

Alcohols are named using IUPAC rules by replacing the *-e* suffix of **alkane** with the suffix *-ol.* For example, **methane** becomes **methanol** and **ethane** becomes **ethanol**. For more complex alcohols, you must identify the longest carbon chain (principal chain) containing the carbon with the hydroxyl group, and its position in the chain must be given the lowest possible number. Small **alkyl groups** on the principal chain must be **named and numbered**. The root name of the alcohol is derived from the principal chain. The following Structure (46) illustrates the naming process (which is very similar to the naming of hydrocarbons).

4-ethyl-6-methyl-2-heptanol

(46)

You can see that the longest continuous chain (principal chain) with an attached hydroxyl group is **seven-carbons** (numbered chain), thus the root name for this compound is **heptanol**. The carbon with the attached hydroxyl group is given the lowest number (2) which defines the numbers for the **ethyl** (4) and **methyl** (6) substituents which are listed in the name in alphabetical order. Note that Structure 46 contains two chirality centers, but their configuration (*R* or *S*) is not indicated.

Alcohols that are commonly used in industry, domestic settings, and have a very long history are often named using the word **alcohol** as the root—non-IUPAC nomenclature. Examples are methyl and ethyl alcohol. Also the term **diol** is commonly used to refer to compounds that have two hydroxyl groups (often directly adjacent to each other). Phenols are named in the same way as substituted benzene compounds. The root name for this class of compounds is always **phenol**. For example, **m-chlorophenol** has a **chloro** group attached to the phenol ring in the **meta** position—see Structure 47 below.

OH

Cl   (47)

EXERCISE 19

Using the guidelines on page 258, provide the correct name for the following compound. (Note that stereochemistry for the chirality center is shown for this structure. (Answer is on page 348.)

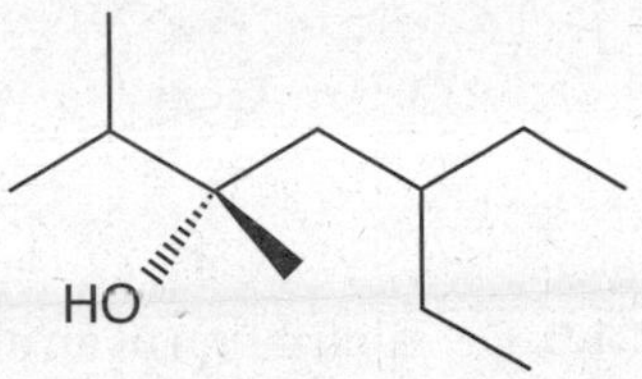

Properties and Uses

Because of the presence of the highly electronegative oxygen atom in alcohols, the hydroxyl functional group is very **polarized**. It is in fact so polarized that, like water, alcohols are capable of forming **hydrogen bonds** with themselves, other alcohols, carboxylic acids, amines, and water. Alcohols up to about four or five carbons are so polar that they are miscible with water, unlike the majority of organic compounds. When the alkyl part of alcohol molecules is larger, they no longer dissolve in water and behave more like hydrocarbons. Figure 31.2 shows a generalized scheme for hydrogen bonding between two alcohol molecules.

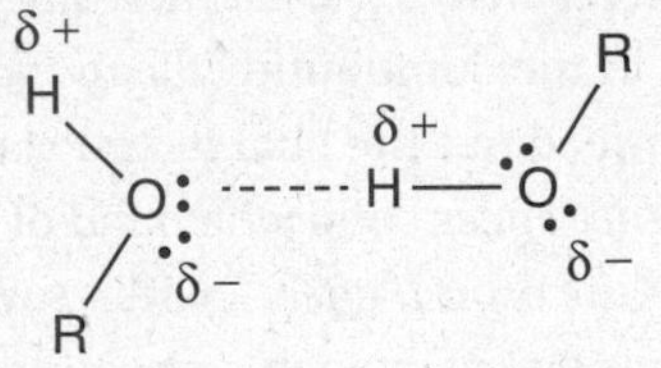

Figure 31.2. A hydrogen bond interaction between
two highly polarized alcohol molecules

Remember, the **intermolecular attractive force** known as **hydrogen bonding** can occur only between molecules where a hydrogen atom is attached to a highly electronegative atom. These atoms include **oxygen**, **nitrogen**, and **fluorine**. This kind of bonding is possible in these cases because the hydrogen's single electron is essentially "stripped" away from its nucleus when attached to a highly electronegative atom. The remaining almost "bare" proton carries a highly positive charge and is very electrophilic. Hydrogen bonding is one of the strongest intermolecular forces (forces between molecules) and extremely important in many organic and biological reaction processes.

Hydrogens attached to the oxygens of hydroxyl groups in alcohols have another special property in addition to being capable of hydrogen bonding. They are more *acidic* relative to the hydrogens attached to many other functional groups with pK_a's ranging from ~15.5 (approximately the pK_a of water) to 18.0 for alcohols with many branched alkyl groups. As you may recall, simple alkyl group branches attached to a carbon are electron donating, an inductive effect. If a carbon with a hydroxyl group has several alkyl groups attached to it, their electron-donating effect will destabilize the anion (referred to as an **alkoxide**) formed when the hydroxyl proton is lost. This makes the protons of hydroxyl groups in highly branched alcohols less acidic. Figure 31.3 provides a pictorial diagram of the destabilizing electron-donating effect of alkyl groups (denoted as "R" in the figure) on an alkoxide anion.

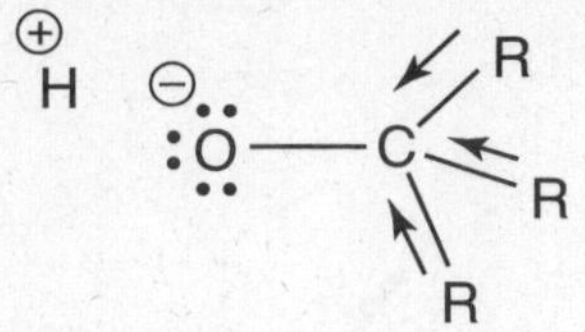

Figure 31.3. Destabilization of an alkoxide anion by alkyl group electron donation

Note: The diagram arrows imply electron flow toward the oxygen anion from the R groups (where R is any alkyl group—in this case there are three alkyl groups attached to the carbon bearing the negatively charged oxygen atom.) The oxygen anion is destabilized by the presence of alkyl groups and thus the species is less likely to lose its hydroxyl proton (the group is shown in its ionized state).

Remember, the term **acid** refers to a species that can *donate protons* (H^+ *ions*). There are several factors that determine acidity of a compound. These include what kind of atom the hydrogen is attached to (*the element effect*), if there are electron-donating or electron-withdrawing atoms or groups in the compound (*the inductive effect*), if other resonance forms of the compound can spread out the charge and stabilize an anion resulting from the loss of a proton (*the resonance effect*), and what kind of orbital hybridization the atom bearing the acidic proton has (*the orbital effect*). Often several of these effects may be at play at the same time in a compound. In such a situation they can be additive, making a hydrogen either very acidic or very nonacidic or they may counter each other, resulting in a less dramatic effect on acidity. You should also recall that the relative acidity of hydrogens can be quantified by using pK_a's (a base 10 log scale of the deprotonation/protonation equilibrium constant K_a). Remember, *the lower the* pK_a of a given acid, *the more acidic* or easily ionized it is.

Alcohols, because they have so many familiar applications, are well known by most of the general public who simply refer to all these compounds as "alcohol." Methanol and ethanol are two of the most important of all industrial chemicals and are used widely as solvents, in drug formulation and synthesis, polymer synthesis, as gasoline additives, and in foods/beverages. Ethanol is of course the "active ingredient" in all alcoholic beverages.

Alcohol Synthesis and Reactions

SYNTHESIS

There are several commonly used approaches to the synthesis of alcohols and phenols. Alkenes can be converted to alcohols using *addition* reactions. These processes have already been covered under the *Alkenes* section—refer to this section for the details of these reactions.

Another technique is the use of *substitution* reactions. These reactions are classified by their mechanisms in a way analogous to the elimination reactions (E1 and E2) covered under the *Alkenes* section. The most important thing for the synthesis of alcohols is **bimolecular nucleophilic substitution (S$_N$2)**. These reactions are effective for the preparation of alcohols from primary (1°) and secondary (2°) alkyl halides when reacted with a hydroxide base (e.g., sodium or potassium hydroxide). Highly branched alkyl halides usually give elimination products and produce low alcohol yields. Figure 31.4 shows the generalized mechanism for these reactions.

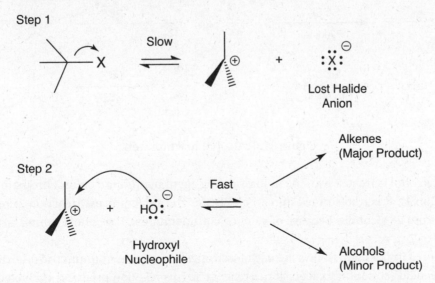

R—X	HO:⊖	[HO----R----X]	HO—R	:X:⊖
Alkyl Halide	Hydroxyl Nucleophile	Transition State	Alcohol Product	Lost Halide Anion

Figure 31.4. The S$_N$2 reaction mechanism where R–X is a 1° or 2° alkyl halide

As can be seen in Figure 31.4, the term bimolecular substitution comes from the fact that *two* separate reactants (the substrate and the nucleophile) must come together to form the transition state, which then leads to the loss of a halide anion and the alcohol product (note that counter ions not involved in the reaction process shown in Figure 31.4 have been omitted). These reactions exhibit **second-order kinetics**, which supports the bimolecular mechanism. Factors that affect the rate and yield of these reactions include the identity of the "leaving" halide atom (generally bromine and iodine are the best halogen leaving atoms), the reaction solvent (polar aprotic solvents that can't hydrogen bond are best), and the structure of the alkyl halide substrate (1°, are better than 2°, and 3° usually don't work). Because a nucleophilic attack occurs on the side of the carbon opposite to the side with the leaving group (called "back side" attack), if a chirality center is present, its stereochemistry will be *inverted* as a new bond forms and the leaving group bond breaks.

Unimolecular nucleophilic substitution (S$_N$1) reactions can be used to produce alcohol products, but have the drawback of usually producing low yields. When branched alkyl halide substrates are reacted with hydroxide bases in polar protic solvents (solvents that can hydrogen bond), elimination products (alkenes) usually dominate with low alcohol yields. Figure 31.5 shows the general two-step mechanism for these processes.

Step 1

Slow

+ :X:⊖

Lost Halide Anion

Step 2

Fast

+ HO:⊖

Hydroxyl Nucleophile

Alkenes (Major Product)

Alcohols (Minor Product)

Figure 31.5. The S$_N$1 reaction mechanism

The first step of the mechanism involves the spontaneous loss of a halide anion (X–) and formation of an intermediate *carbocation* (see Figure 31.4). Because this step is slow, it determines the rate of the reaction and as such these processes typically exhibit *first-order kinetics*. In the second step, which is fast, the carbocation intermediate reacts with a hydroxide anion to form either alkenes (if the anion acts as a base and abstracts a proton from the carbocation) or alcohols (if the anion acts as a nucleophile and attacks the carbocation directly as shown in Figure 31.5). As indicated earlier, this process (S_N1) is usually not a good way to prepare alcohols, but this substitution mechanism regularly shows up in DAT questions. You should be familiar with both substitution mechanisms.

Other common methods for synthesizing alcohols are the reduction of carbonyl compounds and the reaction of carbonyl compounds with organometallic reagents, both of which are types of *addition reactions*. These processes are discussed later in this review under the reactions of *Aldehydes and Ketones* and *Carboxylic Acids*. Phenols are synthesized in the same way as other benzene derivatives (see the *Aromatic Compounds* section on page 251) using electrophilic substitution reactions. It should be recalled that the hydroxyl group is *activating* (makes the benzene ring more reactive to substitution) and *metal/para directing* when attached to the benzene ring.

HYDROXYL FUNCTIONAL GROUP REACTIONS

The reactions of alcohols are quite varied with some of the most important falling into the category of oxidation. You should recall that this was also an important reaction category for unsaturated hydrocarbons. On the other hand, elimination of water (H_2O) from alcohols can be used to prepare alkenes, technically a reduction reaction. Figure 31.6 shows a generalized reaction web for some of the most important reactions of alcohols.

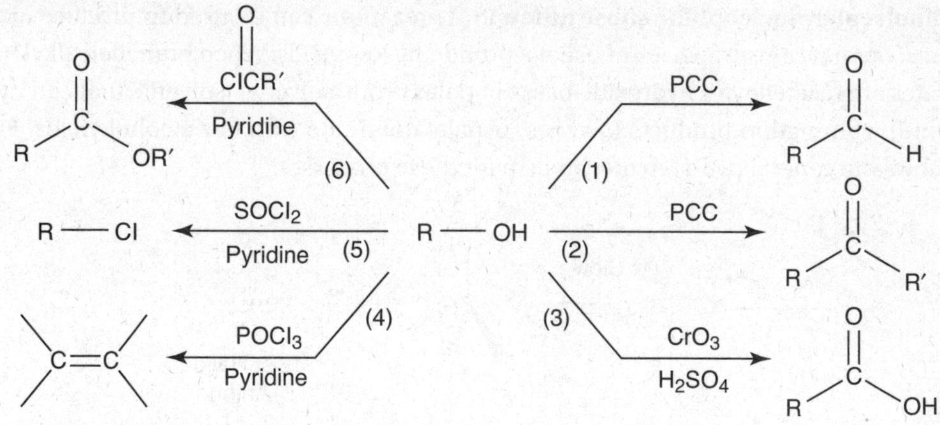

Figure 31.6. Alcohol reaction web

If a 1° alcohol is treated with the mild oxidizing agent pyridinium chlorochromate (PCC—see reaction 1), it is transformed into an **aldehyde**. The same process (reaction 2) produces **ketones** from 2° alcohols. Because of valence considerations, 3° alcohols *cannot* be directly oxidized.

Reaction 3 in the figure shows the use of a stronger oxidizer, chromium trioxide, dissolved in sulfuric acid (commonly called "Jones reagent"). This reaction produces **carboxylic acids** from 1° alcohols, but the harsh conditions often produce low yields. This reaction gives

ketones from 2° alcohols. Primary alcohols can also be oxidized to carboxylic acids by reaction with potassium permanganate (KMnO$_4$).

There are several ways to dehydrate alcohols to prepare **alkenes**. Reactions using strong aqueous acid and heat can sometimes be used, but because of the formation of an intermediate *carbocation,* this approach often produces mixtures of alkenes (see the *Alkenes* section). A better, milder approach uses phosphorus oxychloride (POCl$_3$) in the basic solvent pyridine (see reaction 4). This reaction proceeds by an S$_N$2 mechanism and thus avoids the problematic formation of carbocations.

Alcohols can be transformed into **alkyl halides** using S$_N$2 reactions. As with the formation of alcohols from alkyl halides (the reverse process discussed earlier in this section), 1° alcohols are better than 2° alcohols, and 3° alcohols usually don't work. The limitation in all these reactions is that the hydroxide anion (–OH) is a very poor leaving group. This problem can be overcome by transforming it into a much better leaving group using the reagent *p*-toluenesulfonyl chloride (commonly referred to as *tosyl chloride*). Figure 31.7 shows the generalized reaction of an alcohol with this compound followed by a reaction with a nucleophile—in this case a halide anion (X–).

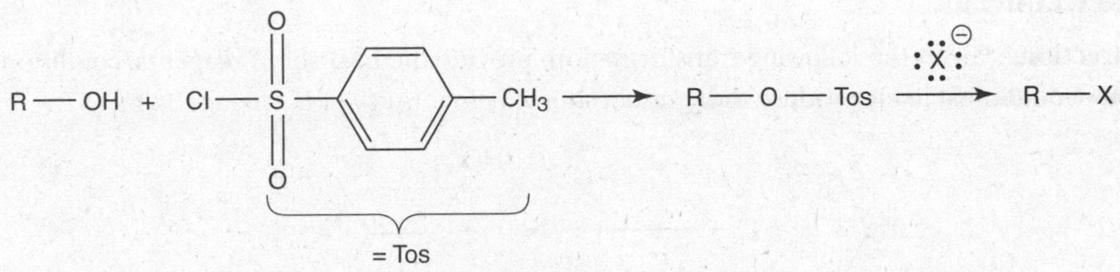

Figure 31.7. Preparation of an alkyl halide from an alcohol using tosyl chloride

Note: The alcohol must be 1° or 2° and *X* may be Cl, Br, or I. The R–O–Tos intermediate shown is commonly referred to as a "tosylate."

Reaction 5 in Figure 31.6 shows another reagent, thionyl chloride (SOCl$_2$), that is valuable for the specific preparation of **alkyl chlorides** from 1° and 2° alcohols. This reaction forms an intermediate "inorganic ester" (a chlorosulfite) which undergoes an S$_N$2 process when the R group is attacked by a chloride anion. The reaction usually produces alkyl chlorides in excellent yield. **Alkyl bromides** can be prepared by an analogous reaction by treating 1° and 2° alcohols with phosphorus tribromide (PBr$_3$), also an S$_N$2 reaction.

Reaction 6 shows one of the general procedures for making an **ester** from an alcohol. This approach uses an acid chloride that reacts with an alcohol in a basic solvent, such as pyridine, to form an ester (a carbonyl compound that will be discussed later in this review). The pyridine solvent traps hydrogen chloride gas, which is formed as a side product during the reaction.

As you can see, the alcohol hydroxyl group is a reaction center for a variety of reagents commonly used in organic synthesis schemes. There are occasions when it is desirable to leave the hydroxyl group unchanged during the transformation of other functional groups present in a molecule. This can be accomplished by first using a technique that "protects" the hydroxyl group—that is, a reaction that changes the hydroxyl group into an unreactive species that can later be reversed when other reactions have been completed. The net process leaves the hydroxyl group unchanged. One of the most common methods of alcohol protection is a reaction with chlorotrimethylsilane. This process produces a trimethylsilyl (TMS) ether, which is inert to oxidizing agents, reducing agents, and organometallic addition reagents. Figure 31.8 shows the generalized protect/deprotect reactions of an alcohol using chloro-TMS (protection) and acid (deprotection). Note that triethyl amine is used as a solvent in the protection step to capture HCl gas—a byproduct of the reaction.

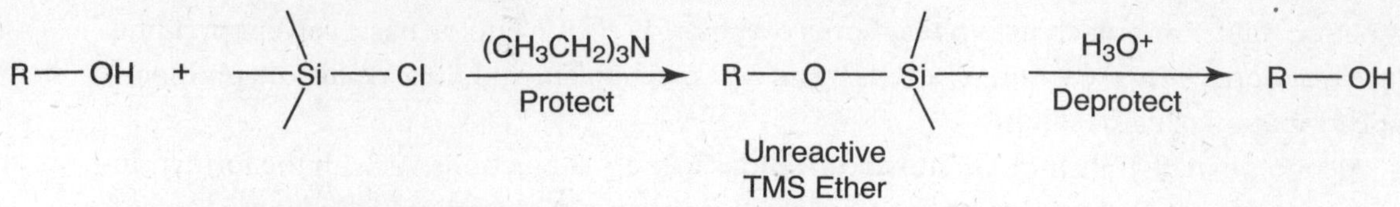

$$R-OH \ + \ \overset{|}{\underset{|}{Si}}-Cl \ \xrightarrow[\text{Protect}]{(CH_3CH_2)_3N} \ R-O-\overset{/}{\underset{\backslash}{Si}}- \ \xrightarrow[\text{Deprotect}]{H_3O^+} \ R-OH$$

Unreactive
TMS Ether

Figure 31.8. The protection/deprotection of an alcohol hydroxyl group

The TMS protecting group can be easily removed by reacting the TMS ether with aqueous acid as shown in Figure 31.8. Note that the alcohol is regenerated in this step [the TMS ether is converted into a TMS alcohol (TMS–OH) byproduct that is not shown in the figure].

EXERCISE 20

Directions: Given the following transformation, provide the best set of reagents/conditions that would most likely produce the product shown below. (Answer is on page 348.)

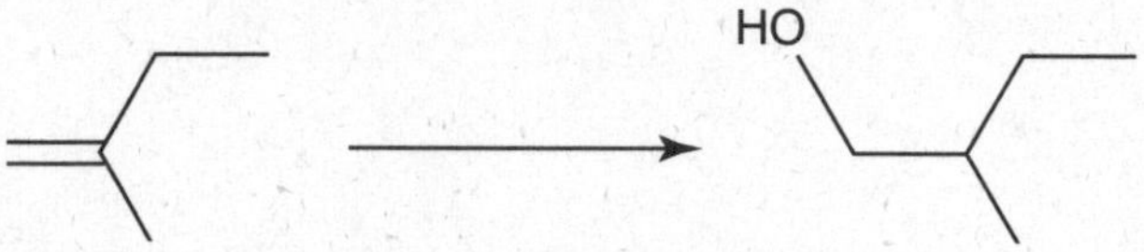

The Ether Functional Group

Ethers, as with alcohols, can be thought of as *derivatives of the water molecule* where both of its *hydrogens* have been replaced with *carbon*. The carbon-containing groups can be alkyl, aryl, or less commonly vinyl. Figure 31.9 shows the generalized structure of the ether functional group.

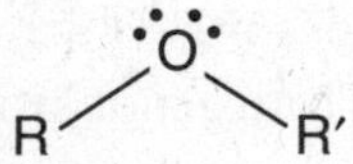

Figure 31.9. The generalized ether functional group

Ethers can be symmetric where both carbon-containing groups are the same (in Figure 31.9, R = R′) or asymmetric where the attached carbon groups are different (in Figure 31.9, R ≠ R′).

Naming Ethers

There are two IUPAC-accepted ways of naming ethers.

BY ALPHABETIZING ATTACHED R GROUPS

In this approach each R group is identified by a common name and placed alphabetically in front of the principal name "ether." Structures 48 and 49 along with their names illustrate this method.

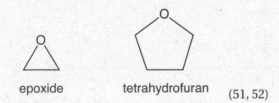

ethyl methyl ether   sec-butyl ethyl ether   (48, 49)

Note that both of these structures (48 and 49) are examples of asymmetric ethers. If the two R groups are identical, the Greek prefix "di" is used in the name—for example, "dimethyl ether," where both R groups are methyl groups.

DESIGNATING THE SMALLER R AS AN ALKOXY SUBSTITUENT

Here, the smaller of the R groups (assuming it's an alkyl group) is named as an alkoxy substituent and the larger group is the principal name. Structure 50 along with its name shows how this method is used.

o-methoxytoluene   (50)

This method is usually used for more complex ethers and is less likely to be encountered on the DAT.

For cyclic ethers there are yet two other types of nomenclature, which won't be discussed in this review. There are common names for three- and five-membered cyclic ethers you should know. **Epoxides** are three-membered cyclic ethers and **tetrahydrofuran** (often used as a solvent) is a five-membered cyclic ether (see Structures 51 and 52 below).

epoxide   tetrahydrofuran   (51, 52)

EXERCISE 21

Using the guidelines on page 264, provide an IUPAC-accepted name for the following compound (note that stereochemistry for the chirality centers is shown for this structure). (Answer is on page 348.)

Ether Physical Properties and Uses

Because ethers, unlike alcohols, cannot function as hydrogen bond donors, they can't form hydrogen bonds with each other. This makes their boiling points much lower than similar-sized alcohols. Due to their bent shapes and highly electronegative oxygen atoms, ethers are significantly more polar (they exhibit dipole-dipole attractions) than alkanes and thus exhibit higher boiling points—dimethyl ether boils at ~ –25°C and propane at ~ –42°C.

One of the common uses of ethers is as solvents for organic chemistry reactions. Three properties make them ideal for this application:

1. They are relatively inert to many reagents/reaction conditions used for organic synthesis.
2. They dissolve a wide range of organic compounds.
3. Many ethers have relatively low boiling points, which makes them easy to remove once a reaction is complete.

Ether Synthesis and Reactions

ETHER SYNTHESIS

The most important commercial ether is diethyl ether, which is prepared in large quantities by acid-catalyzed dehydration of ethanol. This industrial process, which is believed to involve an S_N2 mechanism, has drawbacks for preparing other types of ethers. It only gives good yields with primary alcohols and it can only be used to prepare symmetric ethers. This process also proceeds through an S_N2 mechanism. Another much more versatile reaction process for preparing all types of ethers is the **Williamson ether synthesis**.

This reaction involves two steps. In the first step, a very strong base (usually NaH) is used to deprotonate an alcohol to form an alkoxide anion or in the case of phenol a phenoxide anion. Next, in the second step, the anion acts as a nucleophile and attacks an alkyl halide in S_N2 fashion to produce an ether. Figure 31.10 shows a summary of the process.

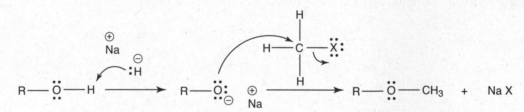

Figure 31.10. The generalized mechanism of the Williamson ether synthesis

This technique is often used to prepare asymmetric ethers. Because the second step in the process proceeds by S_N2, for the best results the alkyl halide must generally be primary (in Figure 31.10 a methyl halide is used as an example) due to steric considerations—the combination of the strongly basic nucleophile and a branched alkyl halide produces mostly elimination products. When designing the synthesis of an asymmetric ether, this issue must be taken into consideration as illustrated in Figure 31.11 (the synthesis of *tert*-butyl methyl ether).

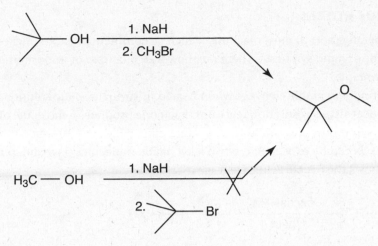

Figure 31.11. Two possible pathways for the synthesis of *tert*-butyl methyl ether

In reference to Figure 31.11, the upper pathway works and as noted with an X, the lower one doesn't (the tertiary alkyl halide is too sterically hindered).

A third way to synthesize ethers is by alkoxymercuration-demercuration. This procedure is similar to oxymercuration-demercuration process discussed in the *Alkenes* section (reaction 1 in Figure 30.7) for the preparation of alcohols. Instead of adding water in Markovnikov fashion to an alkene, this technique adds an alcohol (also with Markovnikov regiochemistry) to produce an ether.

EPOXIDE SYNTHESIS

Epoxides (also called oxiranes) are produced when alkenes are reacted with peroxycarboxylic acids. Meta-chloroperoxybenzoic acid (mCPBA) is used to affect this oxidation. Another commonly used reagent for this process is peroxyacetic acid (PAA)—see reaction 4 in Figure 30.7 of the *Alkenes* section. If the alkene reactant is a cis isomer, a cis epoxide is formed, and if the alkene is trans, a trans epoxide is formed.

Halohydrins can also be used to synthesize epoxides. The reaction proceeds through an intramolecular S_N2 mechanism. An alkene is first converted to a halohydrin (discussed in more detail in the *Alkenes* section), which is then reacted with a base to give the epoxide. Figure 31.12 shows a summary of this two-step process.

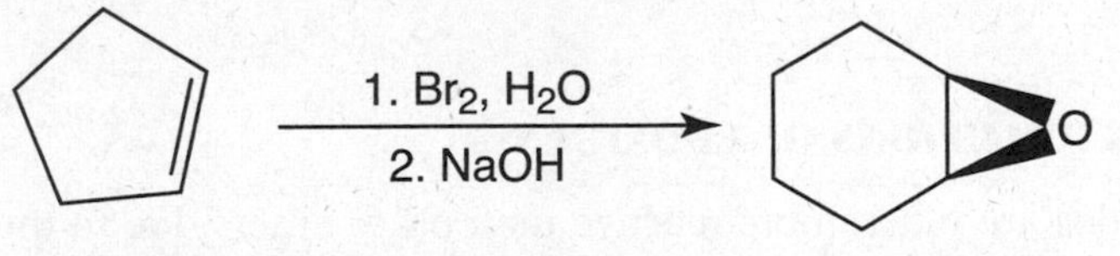

Figure 31.12. Epoxide synthesis from a halohydrin

EXERCISE 22

Propose a viable synthesis for the following ether. (Answer is on page 348.)

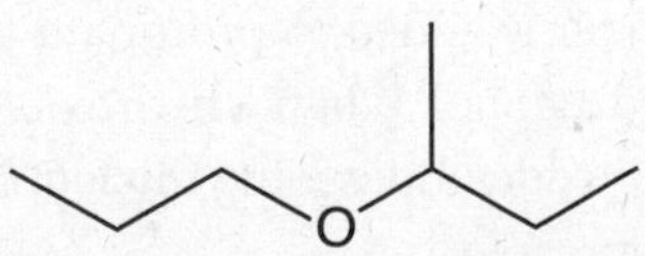

REACTIONS OF ETHERS

Ethers are generally inert to most reactions, which as commented earlier makes them effective solvents for organic synthesis. There are, however, a couple of important exceptions to this general principle.

Ethers can undergo **acidic cleavage** when heated in strongly acidic solution. The process involves two successive substitution reactions. Each one produces a molecule of alkyl halide. If the ether is symmetric, two moles of the same alkyl halide are produced. If the ether is asymmetric, as would be expected, the two alkyl halide molecules have different structures. Figure 31.13 shows the overall acidic cleavage reaction.

$$R-O-R' \xrightarrow[\text{heat}]{\text{excess HX}} R-X \ + \ R'-X \ + \ H_2O$$

Figure 31.13. Acidic cleavage of an asymmetric ether

When an alkyl phenyl ether is reacted under these conditions, the products are *phenol* and an alkyl halide.

Exposing alkyl ethers to atmospheric oxygen results in the slow formation of **hydroperoxides**—this process is called **auto-oxidation** and proceeds through a free-radical mechanism (Figure 31.14).

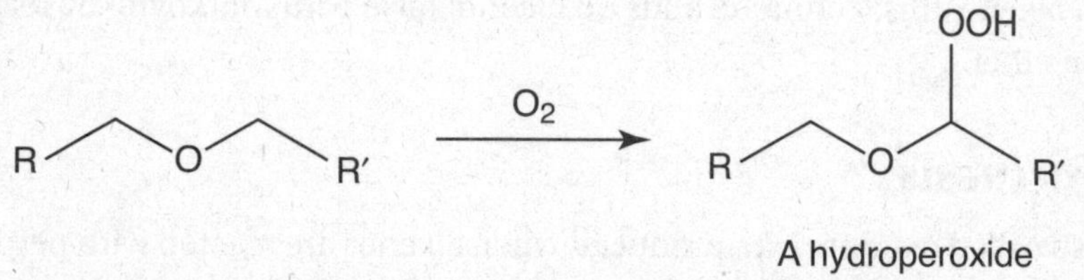

A hydroperoxide

Figure 31.14. The auto-oxidation of a generalized alkyl ether

The slow buildup of peroxides is just about inevitable when ethers are stored for long periods, but the process can be slowed by lowering the storage temperature and preventing exposure to light. Hydroperoxides are unstable and are particularly sensitive to heat. Before heating an ether (i.e., during a distillation), it should always be tested for the presence of peroxides. Many dangerous explosions (ethers are generally very flammable to begin with) have occurred during ether distillations and other operations involving heat due to peroxide contamination.

RING-OPENING REACTIONS OF EPOXIDES

In general, epoxides are much more reactive than other ethers due to their strained three-membered ring system. This makes them susceptible to ring openings by both acids and bases.

When a base has *strong* nucleophilic character, the ring opening occurs through an S_N2 mechanism and the nucleophile attacks the *less*-substituted carbon (less sterically hindered) in the epoxide ring. If an attack takes place at a chirality center, inversion of the stereochemistry occurs. In a second step, water is added to protonate the alkoxide anion—the result is always some kind of a substituted alcohol. When a hydroxide anion is the nucleophile, a 1,2-diol is produced. A generalized epoxide undergoing nucleophilic attack and subsequent protonation by water is shown in Figure 31.15.

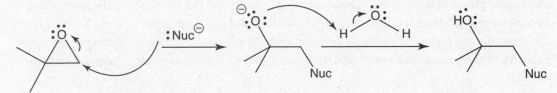

Figure 31.15. Nucleophilic ring opening of a generalized epoxide

Typical nucleophilic anions used in these reactions include: hydroxide, alkoxide, cyanide, sulfide, hydride (from a reducing agent), and the Grignard reagent. Obviously, many types of 1,2-substituted alcohols can be produced through these types of reactions.

Acid-catalyzed opening of epoxide rings is another approach to making substituted alcohols. In these processes the order of protonation is reversed relative to nucleophilic ring opening—it happens first and is then followed by nucleophilic attack (see the example reaction in Figure 31.16).

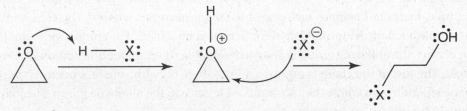

Figure 31.16. Acid-catalyzed ring opening of an epoxide

In the above example (Figure 31.16), the nucleophile is a halide anion and produces a halo-alcohol. If dilute aqueous acid is used (water is the nucleophile), a 1,2-diol is the product.

EXERCISE 23

Directions: Provide the most likely major product(s) for the epoxide reaction shown in Figure 31.17. (Answer is on page 349.)

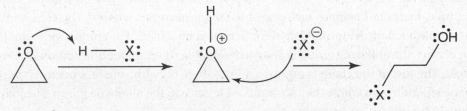

Figure 31.17. Epoxide ring-opening exercise

ALDEHYDES AND KETONES

The Aldehyde and Ketone Functional Groups

Aldehydes and **ketones** belong to the family of **carbonyl**-containing compounds. The carbonyl group consists of a carbon-oxygen double bond (C=O) and has already been referred to numerous times in this review. Both aldehydes and ketones contain the *carbonyl* group. They are some of the most numerous compounds in terms of naturally occurring and synthetic organic compounds on Earth. They can be thought of as being similar in structure to alkenes where both carbons in the double bond are *sp²*-hybridized—in this case both the carbon and the oxygen atoms in the carbonyl double bond are also sp^2-hybridized. Just as the alkene functional group undergoes addition reactions, so does the carbonyl group. Figure 31.18 shows the structures of formaldehyde and acetone (two of the most commonly produced and used industrial chemicals in the world) and the generalized structures of an aldehyde and a ketone.

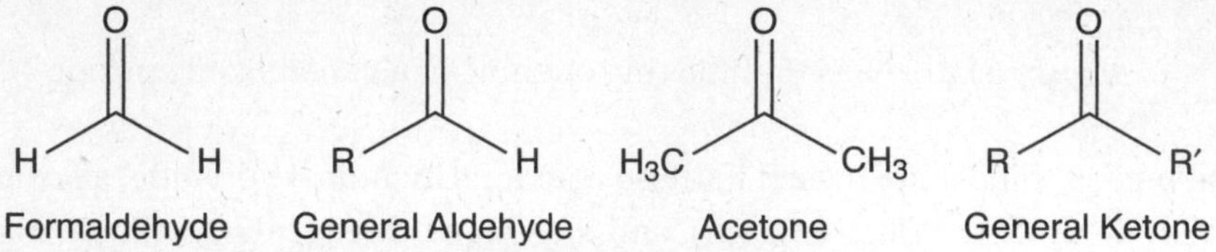

| Formaldehyde | General Aldehyde | Acetone | General Ketone |

Figure 31.18. Formaldehyde and acetone and the general structures of aldehydes and ketones

Naming Aldehydes and Ketones

Aldehydes are named using IUPAC rules by replacing the *-e* suffix of *alkane* with the suffix *-al*. For example, *methane* becomes *methanal* and *ethane* becomes *ethanal*. The common name for the simplest aldehyde, formaldehyde, is accepted by IUPAC. For compounds with longer carbon chains, the aldehyde group is always designated the number one carbon (it has to be terminal). The rest of the chain is numbered from there on with substituents receiving these numbers depending on where they are attached relative to the aldehyde group. The following Structure (53) provides an example.

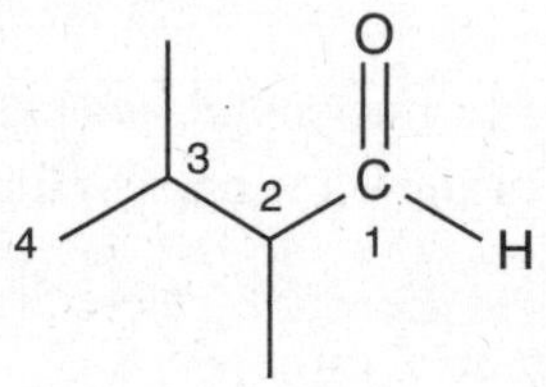

2,3-dimethylbutanal   (53)

The longest chain containing the aldehyde group is four carbons and thus the root name of the compound is *butanal* (the compound also has two attached *methyl* substituents at positions *2* and *3* along the chain). The compound contains a chirality center, but its stereochemistry is not defined, so its designation (*R* or *S*) is not included in the name. When it is necessary to refer to the aldehyde group as a substituent, the prefix *formyl-* is used.

Ketones are named using IUPAC rules by replacing the *-e* suffix of *alkane* with the suffix *-one*. For example, **propane** (the smallest carbon chain that can be a ketone) becomes **propanone** and **butane** becomes **butanone**. The principal chain is the longest chain that contains the ketone group and is numbered from the end nearest the carbonyl carbon. The following Structure (54) provides an example.

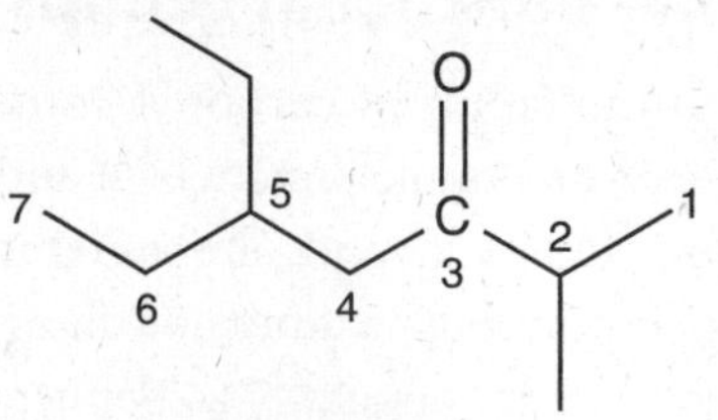

5-ethyl-2-methylheptan-3-one   (54)

The longest chain containing the ketone group is seven carbons and thus the root name of the compound is *heptanone* with the carbonyl group in the *3* position (the compound also has an *ethyl* and a *methyl* group attached to the principal chain in the *2* and *5* positions, respectively). When it is necessary to refer to the ketone group as a substituent, the prefix *oxo-* is used.

EXERCISE 24

Directions: Using the guidelines on page 270, provide the correct name for the following compound (note that the stereochemistry for the chirality center is shown for this structure above). (Answers are on page 349.)

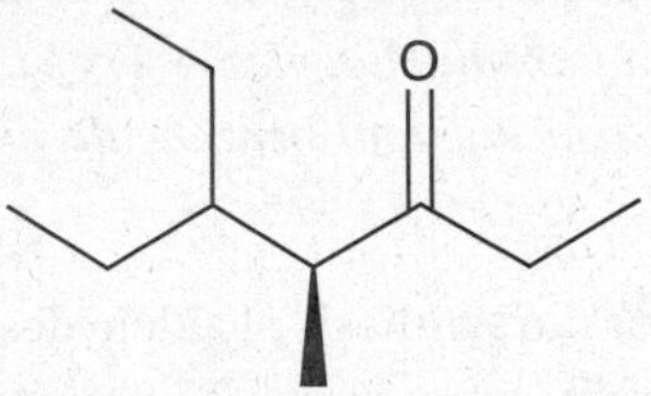

Properties and Uses

The carbon-oxygen double bond, the carbonyl group, to a major extent defines the physical and chemical properties of aldehydes and ketones. The carbonyl group, because it contains oxygen, is highly polarized. Most of the group's electron density resides at the oxygen end (which carries a partial negative charge) with the carbon end being electron deficient with a partial positive charge. The generalized carbonyl Structure (55) shown below illustrates this property.

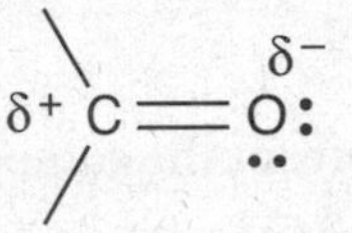

(55)

As a result of the polarized carbonyl group, aldehydes and ketones have elevated boiling points relative to similar alkanes and alkenes. This is due to dipole-dipole intermolecular attractive forces between these molecules. They are not capable of true hydrogen bonding, but the partially negatively charged oxygen in the carbonyl can act as a hydrogen acceptor with molecules such as water and alcohols that can hydrogen bond.

From a physical chemical perspective, the carbonyl group gives aldehydes and ketones special properties. The positively charged carbon acts as an electrophile and reacts with the same kinds of nucleophiles already covered in this review. Conversely the negatively charged oxygen has, as might be expected, nucleophilic properties and reacts with electrophiles. Another carbonyl affect is that the hydrogens on carbons directly adjacent to its carbon (called the α **position**) are slightly acidic (pK_a ~ 17–19) and can be removed by a strong base. This phenomenon is important in the synthesis of more complex carbonyl-group-containing compounds and will be discussed later in this review. As stated earlier, aldehydes and ketones are some of the most numerous organic compounds known to exist and are used for everything from solvents and over-the-counter drugs to home building materials.

Synthesis and Reactions of Aldehydes and Ketones

This review has already discussed several of the best methods for preparing aldehydes and ketones. Recall the following reactions:

- Oxidation of *primary alcohols* → gives *aldehydes* (see page 262)
- Oxidation of *secondary alcohols* → gives *ketones* (see page 262)
- Oxidative cleavage of *alkenes* with at least one vinylic hydrogen → gives *aldehydes* (see pages 244 and 245)
- Oxidative cleavage of *alkenes* with no vinylic hydrogens → gives *ketones* (see pages 244 and 245)
- Hydroboration/oxidation of *terminal alkynes* → gives *aldehydes* (see page 250)
- Acid-catalyzed hydration of *terminal alkynes* → gives *methyl ketones* (see page 250)
- Friedel-Crafts acylation of *benzene and benzene derivatives* → gives *aromatic ketones* (see page 253)

Another valuable technique for the synthesis of aldehydes on a laboratory scale is the *partial reduction of esters* (another kind of carbonyl compound discussed later in the review) by treatment with the reagent diisobutylaluminum hydride (DIBAH). Figure 31.19 provides a generalized example of this synthetic process.

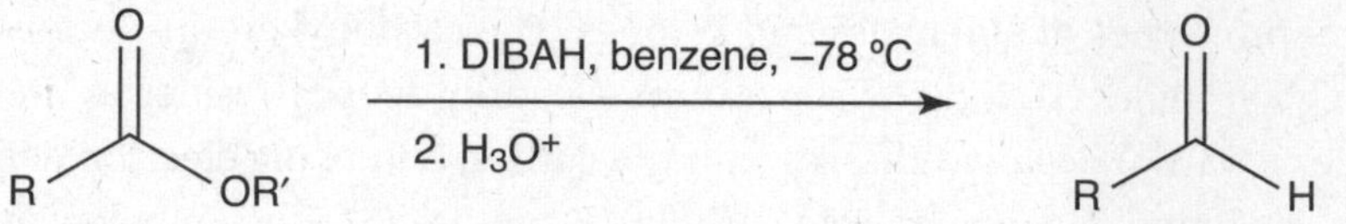

Figure 31.19. A method for the preparation of aldehydes from esters

EXERCISE 25

Directions: Propose a viable synthetic route for the compound shown below starting with any alkyne of your choice. (Answer is on page 349.)

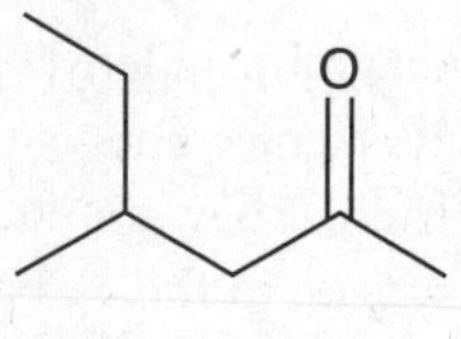

The most important reactions of aldehydes and ketones fall into three categories:

- Nucleophilic addition (which includes reduction reactions)
- Enolate ion reactions
- Oxidation

Nucleophilic addition involves an attack at the partially positive carbon (an electron-deficient reaction center or "electrophile") in the carbonyl group by a myriad of neutral and negatively charged nucleophiles. These reactions produce all sorts of new valuable functional groups that can be retained in the molecule or transformed to yet other groups. The general mechanistic scheme for this large group of processes is shown in Figure 31.20.

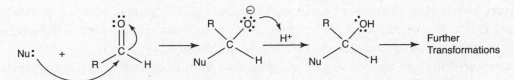

Figure 31.20. Nucleophilic addition to the carbonyl functional group

The nucleophile shown in Figure 31.20 is neutral, but it can also have a formal negative charge. In many cases, the hydroxyl group shown in the **third species** (left to right) of the figure is lost (often as water) and only the functional group associated with the nucleophile remains. As implied, this species then often undergoes further changes, which produce the target product. The starting compound shown in the scheme is an **aldehyde**, but exactly the same sort of process takes place with **ketones**.

> Because of less steric hindrance at the carbon of the carbonyl group, *aldehydes* (have only one large group attached) are generally *more reactive than ketones*. Another factor that makes aldehydes more reactive is that their carbonyl groups are more polarized than those of ketones. This makes the carbon in the carbonyl group more *positive* and thus more attractive to nucleophiles.

Figure 31.21 shows a nucleophilic addition reaction web that includes many of the most important examples of this reaction type. Note that the molecule at the center of the reaction web is generalized and can represent either an **aldehyde** or a **ketone**.

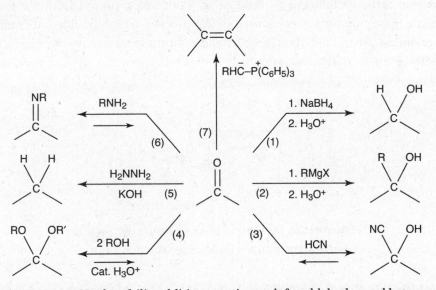

Figure 31.21. Nucleophilic addition reaction web for aldehydes and ketones

In reaction 1, the use of a **hydride donor** (in this case sodium borohydride—$NaBH_4$, with a proton source) leads to the formation of **alcohols** from **aldehydes** and **ketones**. Another commonly used reducing agent for this process is lithium aluminum hydride ($LiAlH_4$) followed by the addition of water, another proton source.

More complex alcohols can be produced from **aldehydes** and **ketones** (see reaction 2) by reaction with a **Grignard reagent** ($RMgX$, where X is usually Cl or Br). This reaction begins with the positively charged Mg ion complexing with the partly negatively charged carbonyl oxygen. This further polarizes the carbonyl bond and makes its carbon more susceptible to attack by the R:⁻ nucleophile of the Grignard reagent. Aqueous acid is added in the second step to protonate the intermediate anion and give an alcohol.

Cyanohydrins (see reaction 3) can be synthesized from *aldehydes* and *ketones* by treatment with the acid HCN. Because the reaction is reversible, the addition of a small amount of base to generate a little CN⁻ anion greatly increases the rate of this process. The intermediate formed by nucleophilic attack by the CN⁻ anion on the carbon atom in the carbonyl group is protonated by the acidic HCN to give the final product.

When two equivalents of an alcohol in the presence of a catalytic amount of acid (the process is reversible) are reacted with an *aldehyde* or *ketone*, an **acetal** or **ketal** (in the case of a ketone—see reaction 4) is produced. The nucleophilic addition of the first equivalent of alcohol initially produces a hydroxy ether called a **hemiacetal (himiketal)**. The mechanism involves an initial protonation of the carbonyl oxygen and two subsequent nucleophilic attacks by alcohol molecules on its carbon. Loss of water and a proton leads to the formation of the *acetal (ketal)*.

Reaction 5 is called the **Wolff-Kishner** reaction and is a convenient method for changing carbonyl groups into a CH_2. In this process, the carbonyl is first reacted with hydrazine, H_2NNH_2, to form a *hydrazone* intermediate which when heated loses nitrogen gas (N_2) to form an **alkane**. The protons needed to form the CH_2 group come from the *reaction solvent*, which is usually dimethyl sulfoxide (DMSO).

Nucleophilic addition of *primary (1°) amines*, shown in reaction 6, to *ketones* and *aldehydes* yields products that are called **imines**. This reaction process proceeds much as the others outlined in Figure 31.21 with the amine nitrogen attacking the partially positively charged carbon of the carbonyl followed by the loss of water and a proton from the tetrahedral intermediate. If a *secondary amine* is used in this process, a slightly different compound is formed, **enamine** (a carbon-carbon double bond adjacent to an amine—see Figure 31.22 for a generalized example of this reaction).

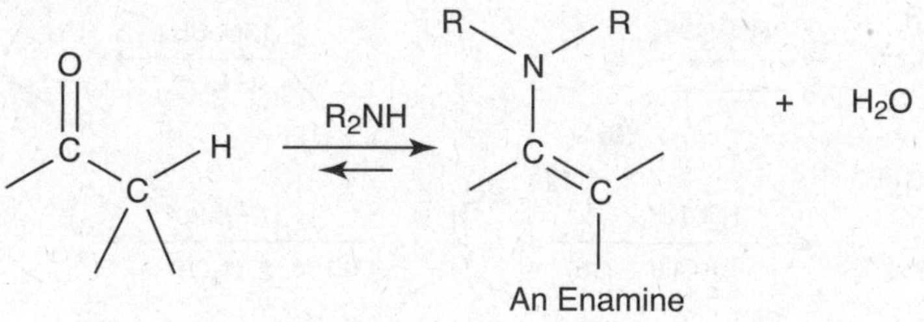

Figure 31.22. Formation of an enamine by reacting a secondary amine with an aldehyde or a ketone

The last reaction shown in Figure 31.21 (reaction 7) is another name reaction called the **Wittig** reaction. It is used to form **alkenes** by coupling the carbonyl carbon in aldehydes or ketones to another carbon provided by a phosphorus-containing reactant called an **ylide** $[R_2C=P(C_6H_5)_3$ is the generalized formula for a commonly used ylide]. Because the ylide is formed by an S_N2 process from an alkyl halide, methyl or primary alkyl halides are preferred for the preparation of the reagent. Nucleophilic attack at the carbon of the aldehyde or ketone carbonyl by the ylide carbon produces a meta-stable *four-membered ring* intermediate consisting of two joined carbons, an oxygen from the carbonyl, and the phosphorus atom of the ylide (see the generalized structure in Figure 31.23).

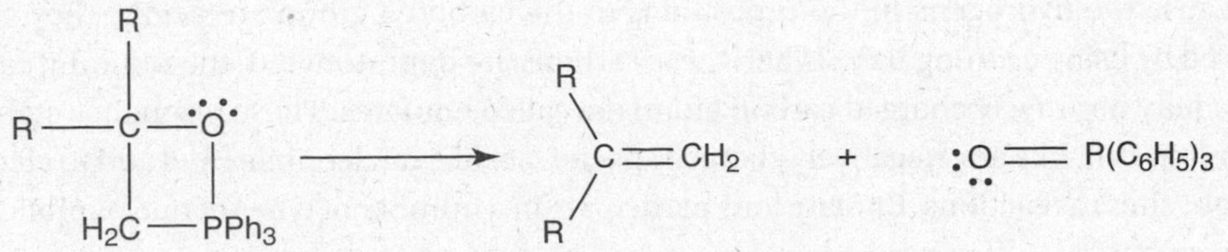

Figure 31.23. The formation of an alkene from a
four-membered ring intermediate of the Wittig reaction

This species spontaneously decomposes to give the *alkene* and triphenylphosphine oxide $[O=P(C_6H_5)_3]$—Figure 31.23. This reaction produces only a *single alkene structural isomer* and the carbon-carbon double bond is always where the carbonyl group was in the aldehyde or ketone. It does have the limitation of usually producing a mixture, if possible, of stereoisomers (*E* and *Z*).

EXERCISE 26

Directions: Propose a viable synthetic route for the compound shown below starting with cyclopentanone and any other reagents/small organic molecules needed. (Answer is on page 350.)

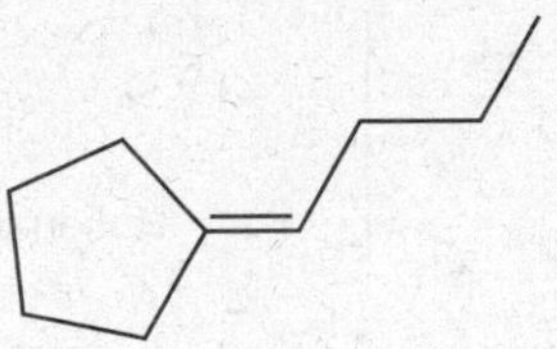

As stated earlier, the hydrogens on either side of the carbonyl groups of aldehydes and ketones (as well as some other carbonyl-containing functional groups) are slightly *acidic*. It is possible for one of these hydrogens to be transferred to the oxygen atom of the carbonyl group, resulting in another isomer called an **enol**. You may recall that all aldehydes and ketones with α carbons bearing a hydrogen atom are in equilibrium with tiny amounts of the enol form (about 0.0000001%). These two isomers, which differ only in the placement of a single proton, are called **tautomers**.

You should remember that the two **tautomers** associated with aldehydes and ketones are called the **keto** and the **enol** forms. The process of converting between these two isomers is called **enolization** (also referred to as "tautomerization"), with the equilibrium between the two greatly favoring the keto form. The generalized Structures (56 and 57) shown below illustrate the enolization equilibrium of aldehydes and ketones.

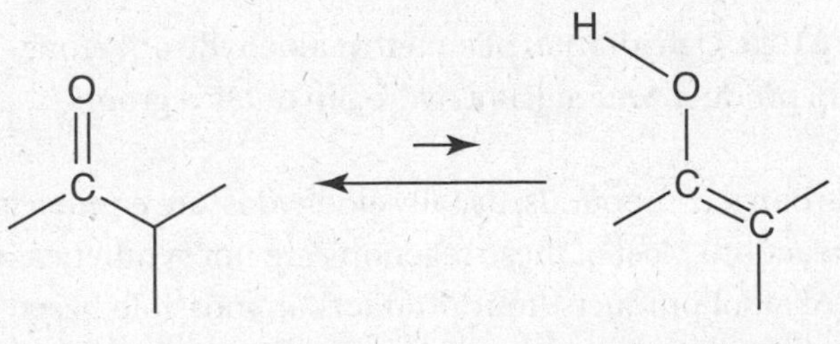

(56, 57)

Because the hydrogens in the α positions to the carbonyl group are acidic, they can be removed by using a strong base. When these carbons are deprotonated, the resulting carbanions (a fully negatively charged carbon atom) are called **enolates**. These resonance stabilized carbanions can, like any negatively charged species, act like nucleophiles and add to electron-deficient sites in reactions. **Enolate** ions participate in a number of types of nucleophilic addition reactions.

A classic enolate reaction of aldehydes and ketones is called the **aldol** (*ald* from aldehyde and *ol* from alcohol) **reaction**. In this reaction the enolate ion formed by abstraction of a proton by a base from the α carbon of an aldehyde or ketone goes on to attack the carbon of the carbonyl of a second aldehyde or ketone molecule. The product of the reaction is called an **aldol** and contains both a carbonyl group and an alcohol group β to the carbonyl. The generalized process of forming an "aldol" is shown in Figure 31.24. Because this reaction is an *equilibrium-driven process*, the yield of many condensate reactions is low, with aldehydes generally giving higher yields. The aldol product of the reaction can be dehydrated (caused to lose water) by heating in the presence of a base (referred to as a **condensation** reaction). This leads to the formation of an α, β **unsaturated aldehyde**, or **ketone** (see Figure 31.25).

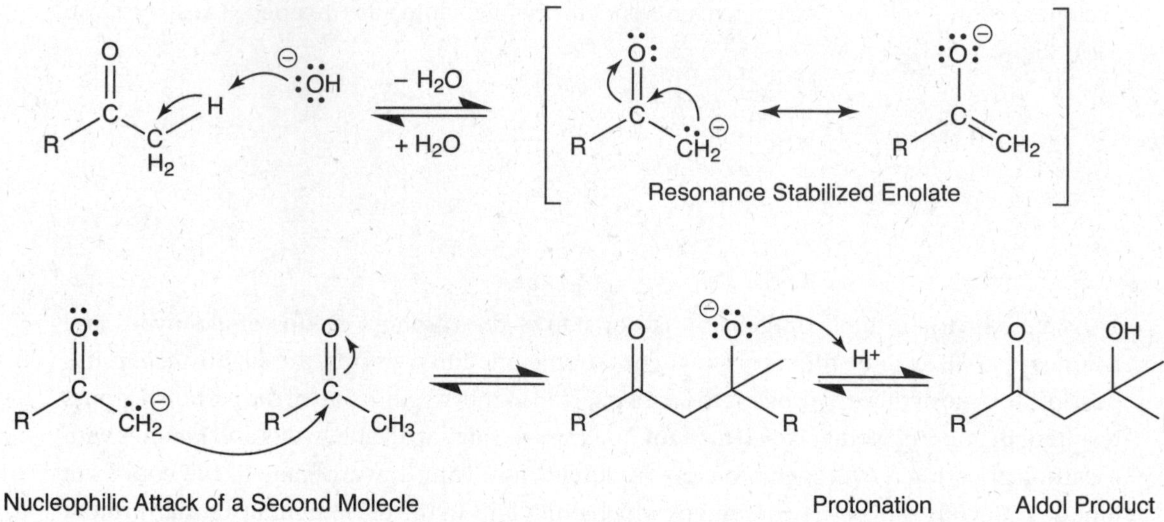

Resonance Stabilized Enolate

Nucleophilic Attack of a Second Molecle   Protonation   Aldol Product

Figure 31.24. The aldol reaction, where *R* is a hydrogen or alkyl group

Aldol Product   Dehydration Product

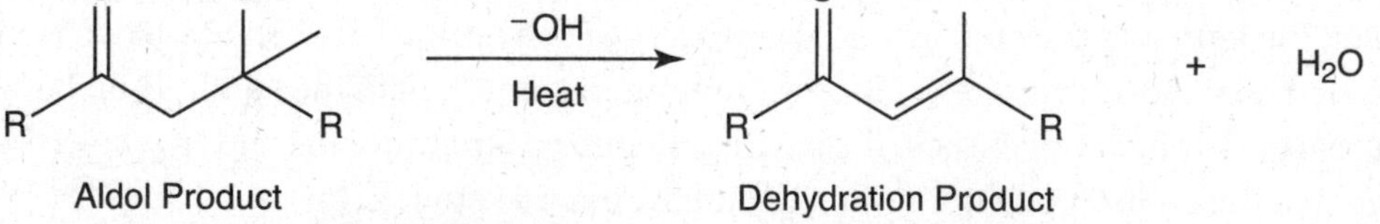

Figure 31.25. Dehydration of a methyl aldehyde or ketone
aldol product, where *R* is a hydrogen or alkyl group

When two different carbonyl compounds, usually aldehydes, are condensed, the process is termed a **crossed aldol** reaction. Most of these reactions are not synthetically useful because they produce a mixture of aldol products (four products are possible based on the ways the two aldehyde reactants can combine with each other). There are, however, cases where an enolate can be reacted with an aldehyde that has no α hydrogens (such as formaldehyde or benzaldehyde) and only one product is produced. **Intramolecular aldol** reactions using dicarbonyl compounds can be used to make five- and six-membered ring systems.

A variation of the aldol condensation reaction is the direct alkylation of *ketones*. In order to quantitatively convert the ketone reactant to an enolate, a strong hindered base is necessary. Lithium diisopropylamide (LDA) is commonly used to form the enolate, which then reacts with an alkyl substrate with a good leaving group (usually an alkyl halide) in an aprotic solvent, giving the alkylated product (see Figure 31.26). It can be seen that this is clearly an S_N2 reaction. *Aldehyde* substrates almost always give poor yields of the alkylated products because they tend to condense with themselves (see the aldol reaction in Figure 31.24) instead of reacting with the alkyl halide.

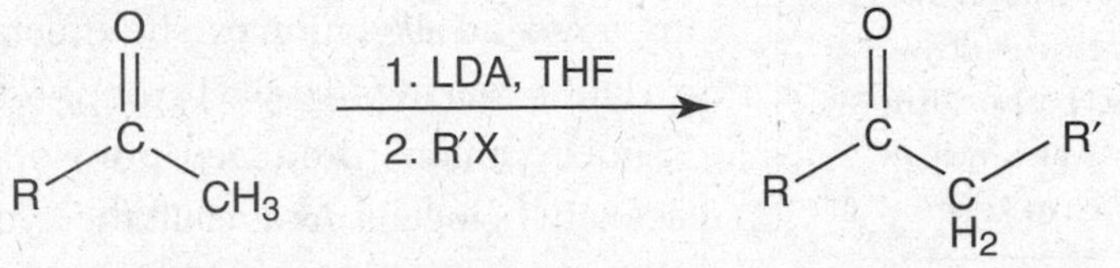

Figure 31.26. Direct alkylation of ketone α carbons

Note that X is usually I in this reaction.

Carbons with hydrogens α to *two* carbonyl groups are particularly acidic ($pK_a \sim 9$), mostly because of resonance stabilization. Upon deprotonation by a base, the resulting enolate can spread out its negative charge over both carbonyls. Structure 58 shows a pictorial representation of the charge delocalization process.

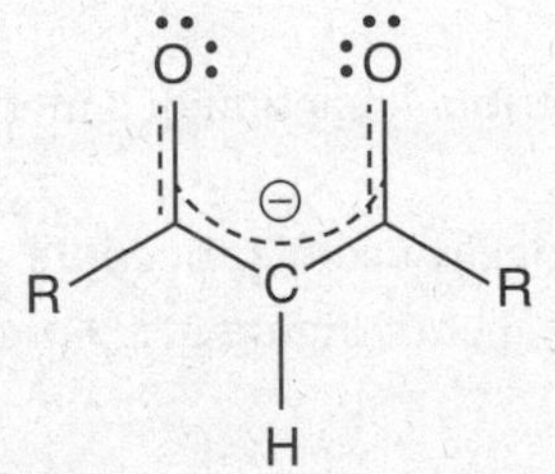

(58)

Several alkalation reactions take advantage of the high acidity of these special protons since a simple base such as sodium hydroxide (NaOH) can be used to form enolates from them. The most important of these alkylation processes uses a *ketoester* commonly called *ethyl acetoacetate* (see Figure 31.27) and is referred to as the **acetoacetic ester synthesis**. This reaction process consists of three basic steps. First is the formation of an enolate by reaction of a base with ethyl acetoacetate. Second, the enolate is reacted with a primary alkyl halide (RX, where *X* is usually Br or I) in S_N2 fashion. Third, the alkylated ketoester is treated with aqueous HCl at an elevated temperature, which results in the *hydrolysis* of the ester functional group (a reaction covered later under *Carboxylic Acid Derivatives* on page 284) followed by *decarboxylation* (loss of CO_2—this reaction is discussed under *Carboxylic Acids* on page 283) of the ketoacid. The final product is a **methyl ketone** with an alkyl group attached to its carbonyl carbon. Figure 31.27 shows a summary of the overall reaction.

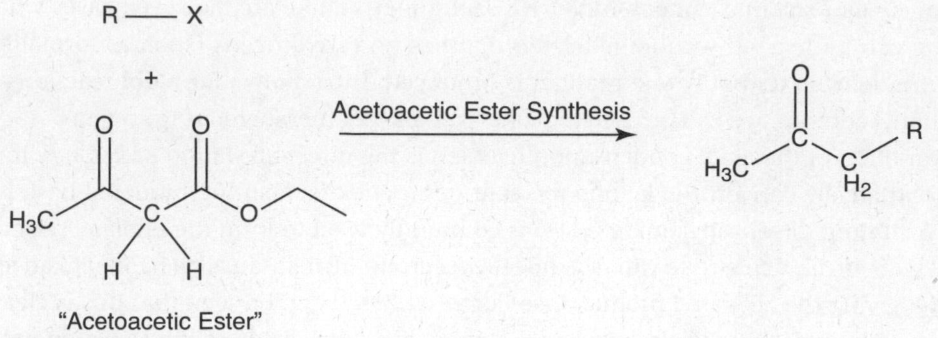

Figure 31.27. The acetoacetic ester synthesis used for the alkylation of ketones

When the halogen used is *iodine* (I_2) this process produces "iodoform" (HCI_3), which is a yellow-colored precipitate that can be used to confirm the presence of a methyl ketone. Other kinds of ketones don't give a positive "iodoform test."

If desired, because the ketoester has two acidic protons, a second alkylation can be effected prior to decarboxylation placing *two* alkyl groups α to the carbonyl.

Enolate anions produced from *methyl ketones* can react with halogens. As a result the hydrogens α to their carbonyls are replaced with halogen atoms (usually Br or I). If an excess amount of the halogen is used in the reaction, all the hydrogens are replaced and a **haloform** (HCX_3) product is produced, which is a good leaving group. The starting methyl ketone is converted into a carboxylate salt. This transformation, known as the **haloform reaction**, is shown in Figure 31.28.

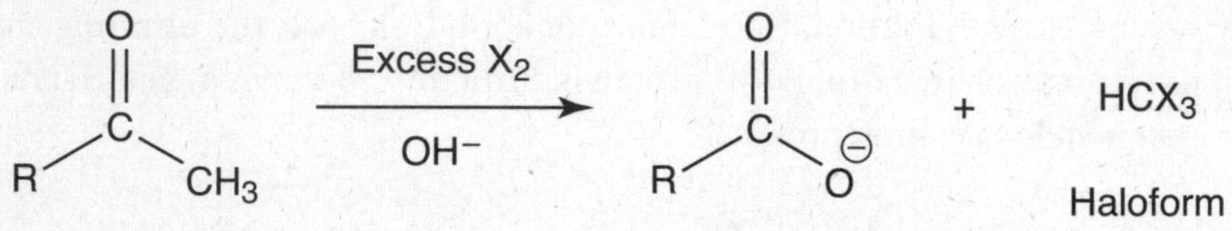

Figure 31.28. The haloform reaction—reaction of a methyl ketone with excess X_2

Although not a particularly synthetically useful procedure, *aldehydes* are easily oxidized to **carboxylic acids** using a number of reagents. Figure 31.29 provides a generalized example of this process.

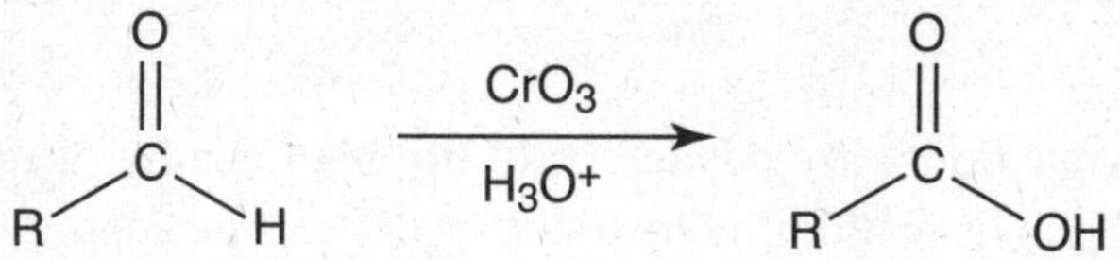

Figure 31.29. Oxidation of aldehydes to carboxylic acids

EXERCISE 27

Directions: Provide the most likely major product(s) for the reaction shown in Figure 31.30. (Answers are on page 350.)

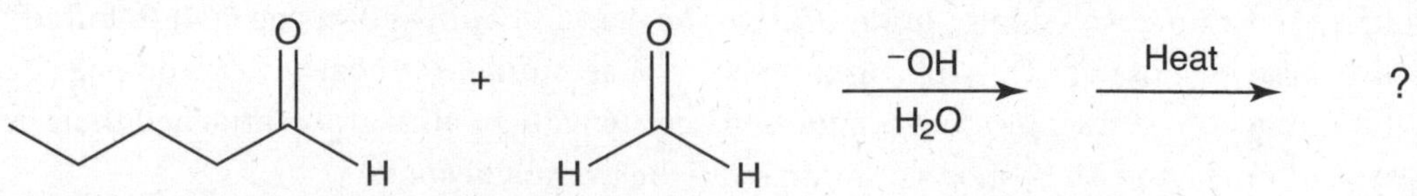

Figure 31.30. Aldol condensation reaction exercise

CARBOXYLIC ACIDS

The Carboxylic Acid Functional Group

Another member of the carbonyl-containing family of compounds are carboxylic acids. The molecules of these substances all contain what is called a **carboxyl functional** group. The atomic architecture of this group consists of a *hydroxyl* group attached to the carbon of a *carbonyl* group. These compounds are often referred to as "organic acids" and are one of the most important and numerous classes of naturally occurring organic molecules. Figure 31.31 shows a generalized structural formula for a carboxylic acid and two of the simplest varieties, **formic acid** and **acetic acid**.

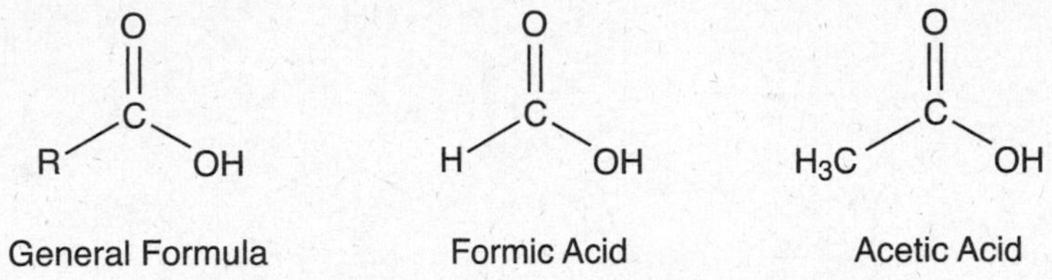

General Formula   Formic Acid   Acetic Acid

Figure 31.31. Some carboxylic acids

Naming Carboxylic Acids

There are two accepted forms of IUPAC nomenclature for carboxylic acids. The most commonly used of these involves replacing the *-e* suffix of the corresponding alkane with *-oic acid*. As with aldehydes, the carboxyl group is always terminal, so it is designated number 1 in the principal chain (the longest continuous carbon chain containing the carboxyl group) of the molecule. The following example (Structure 59) shows the IUPAC naming process for these compounds.

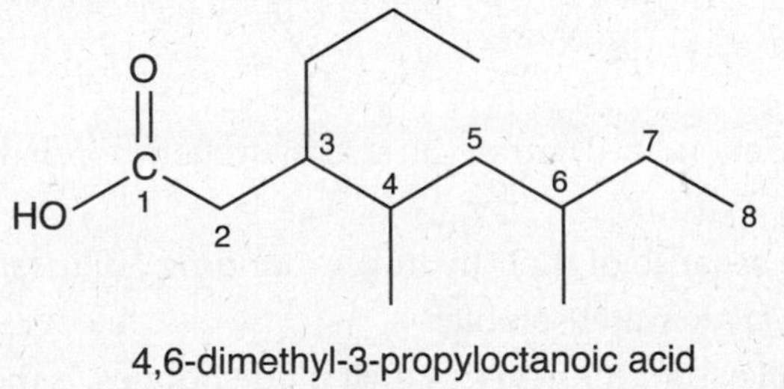

4,6-dimethyl-3-propyloctanoic acid   (59)

The principal chain in the compound contains eight carbons, so the root name for the compound is **octanoic acid**. The number assignments of the other substituents, two *methyl* groups at carbons 4 and 6 and a *propyl* group at carbon 3, are defined by the carboxyl group at carbon number 1 in the principal chain. Note that this example compound contains *several* chirality centers, but their stereochemistry is not defined and as such doesn't appear in the name.

Another approach is used if a compound has a carboxyl group bonded to a carbon ring. In these cases, the suffix *-carboxylic acid* is used. For example, a *cyclopentane ring* with a *carboxyl* group attached would be called *cyclopentanecarboxylic acid* (Structure 60).

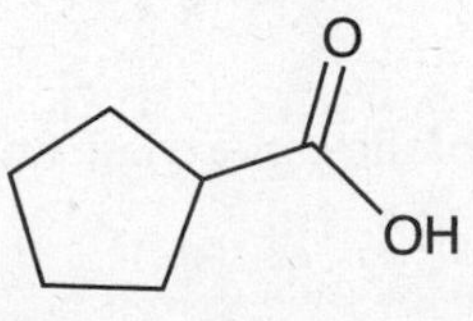

(60)

Because carboxylic acids were some of the first organic compounds to be isolated and characterized, they have many IUPAC-accepted common names. At a minimum, you should know the common name for methanoic acid (**formic acid**) and ethanoic acid (**acetic acid**). Both of these acids are shown in Figure 31.31.

EXERCISE 28

Using the guidelines on page 279, provide the best name for the following compound. Note that the stereochemistry for the chirality center is shown for this structure. (Answer is on page 350.)

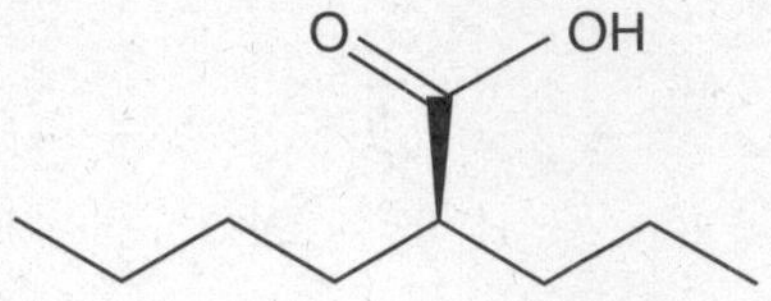

Properties and Uses

As with alcohols, carboxylic acids are capable of **hydrogen bonding** and, as such, have significantly higher boiling points than their corresponding alkanes. Most of these acids can also exist as hydrogen-bonded cyclic **dimers**, which is a particularly strong intermolecular interaction. This property makes the boiling points of carboxylic acids even higher than those of alcohols. Figure 31.32 shows how this interaction can occur between two acid molecules.

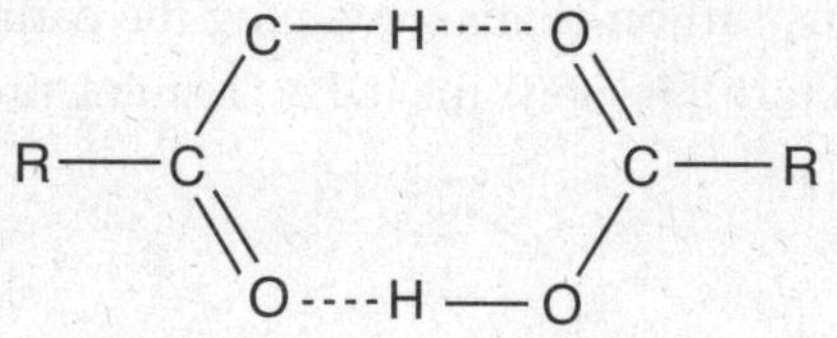

Figure 31.32. Generalized carboxylic acid hydrogen-bonded dimer

As might be expected, because of their hydrogen-bonding abilities, many of the smaller acids (less than six carbons) are water soluble.

The defining property of carboxylic acids, as their name implies, is their **high acidity**. Their acidic properties are largely due to the **resonance stabilization** of the carboxylate anion that is formed when its hydroxyl proton is lost. Figure 31.33 shows how the negative charge of the ion is delocalized over both oxygens of the carboxyl group.

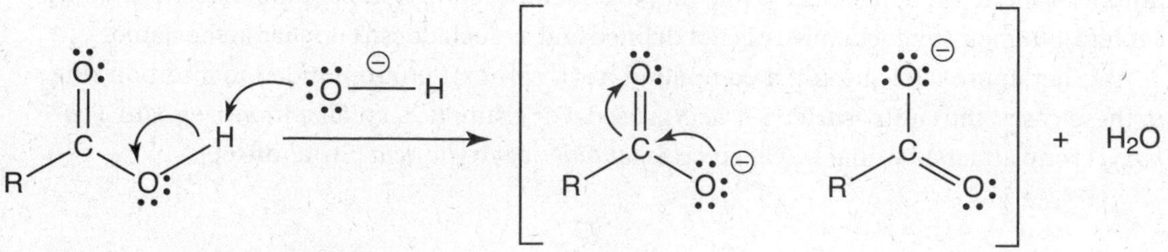

Figure 31.33. Delocalization of the carboxylate anion of a carboxylic acid

As Figure 31.33 illustrates, the carboxyl proton readily reacts with hydroxide bases to form water and the carboxylate anion (recall how similar this process is to enolate formation). The pK_a's of carboxylic acids that have small attached alkyl groups have a tight range of ~4.7–4.9 (for example, acetic acid's $pK_a = 4.75$). The carboxylate can be further stabilized by *electron withdrawing groups* attached at the α carbon position, resulting in a corresponding increase in acidity. For example, triflouroacetic acid (F_3CCOOH—note the three, highly electronegative fluorine atoms) has a $pK_a = 0.20$.

Reaction of carboxylic acids with hydroxide bases (e.g., NaOH or KOH) produces *metal carboxylate salts* (see Figure 31.33—the metal cation is not shown) that are quite soluble in water because of their ionic character. This behavior can be used to purify acids by using a basic aqueous solution (the base reacts with the acid to form a salt) to extract them from an organic phase followed by acidification of the aqueous extract. The crude "free acid" often precipitates from the acidic solution and can then be collected by filtration for further purification (see the *Separation and Purification* section). As with other carbonyl-containing compounds, the hydrogens α to the carbonyl of carboxylic acids are also acidic and notably more acidic ($pK_a \sim 10$) in β-dicarboxilic acids (also called 1,3-dicarboxilic acids). Abstraction of a proton from the carbon between the two carboxyl groups of these compounds produces an anion that is stabilized not only by *resonance* but also by the electron withdrawing effects of *both carboxyl groups*. 1,3-Ketoacids, organic compounds that contain both a carboxyl group and a ketone group, exhibit similar α hydrogen acidity.

Benzoic acid ($pK_a = 4.2$—Structure 35), a benzene ring with an attached carboxyl group, is the *simplest aromatic carboxylic acid*. *Deactivating* groups attached to its aromatic ring tend to *increase* benzoic acid's acidity because of their electron withdrawing properties. *Activating* groups (which are electron donating) make it *less* acidic.

TIP

Remember the terms *activating* and *deactivating* benzene ring substituents from the *Aromatic Compounds* section of this review. For a list of these groups, see page 251.

Synthesis and Reactions of Carboxylic Acids

SYNTHESIS

Many of the most common techniques used to prepare carboxylic acids have already been covered in earlier sections of this review. You may recall the following:

- Oxidation of *alcohols* → gives *carboxylic acids* (see page 262)
- Oxidation of *aldehydes* → gives *carboxylic acids* (see page 278)
- Oxidative cleavage of *alkenes* → gives *carboxylic acids* (see page 244)
- Oxidative cleavage of *alkynes* → gives *carboxylic acids* (see page 250)

Two additional processes can also be used to synthesize carboxylic acids. One involves the hydrolysis of the nitrile functional group ($-C\equiv N$). This method provides a path for converting alkyl halides into carboxylic acids. Figure 31.34 outlines the general approach for achieving this transformation.

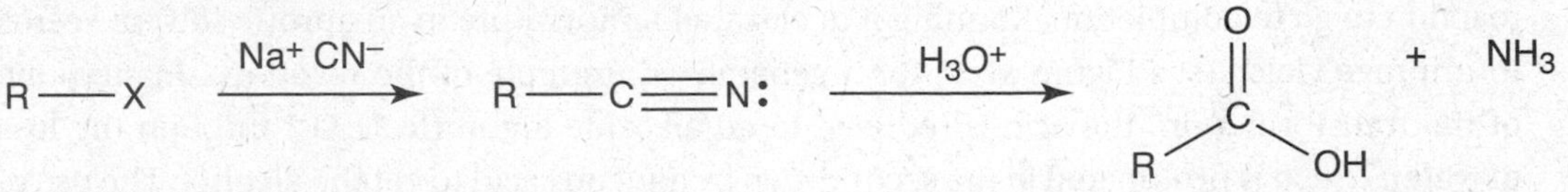

Figure 31.34. Preparation of carboxylic acids forms primary and secondary alkyl halides

As seen in the figure, an alkyl halide can be readily converted into a nitrile by S_N2 reaction with a nucleophilic cyanide anion (CN^- in this case is provided by the sodium cyanide salt). The resulting nitrile is then hydrolyzed by treatment with aqueous acid. A byproduct of the reaction is ammonia gas. This procedure, because it involves an S_N2 mechanism to make the nitrile, works best for *primary alkyl halides,* although some secondary substrates also give good yields. It is not a good method for converting *tertiary alkyl halides* to acids because of competing elimination reactions.

The **Grignard reagents** is another approach that can be used to convert **tertiary alkyl halides** to carboxylic acids. Figure 31.35 shows the general process for this reaction, which uses carbon dioxide gas as the carboxyl source.

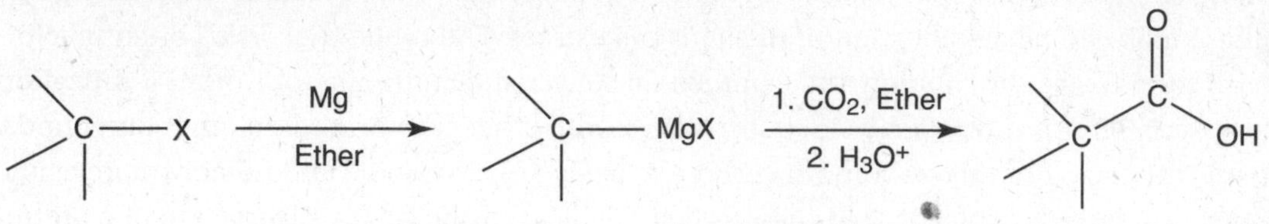

Figure 31.35. Conversion of tertiary alkyl halides to carboxylic acids

EXERCISE 29

Directions: Propose a viable synthetic route for the compound shown below starting with the alkyl halide of your choice and other reagents/small organic compounds as needed. (Answer is on page 351.)

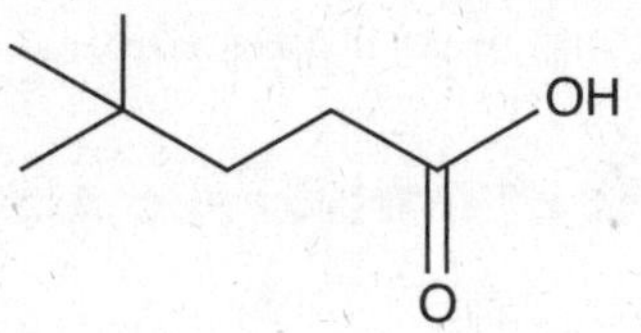

REACTIONS

Like most carbonyl-containing compounds, carboxylic acids under certain conditions may undergo nucleophilic substitution. A few of the substitution reactions already covered for aldehydes and ketones are applicable to carboxylic acids because the hydroxyl of the acid's carboxyl is a poor leaving group. With a few exceptions, the hydroxyl group must be converted into a better leaving group before reactions of this type are practical. Except for **esterification** (see page 283), these types of carboxylic acid reactions will be covered later in this review under *Carboxylic Acid Derivatives* (see page 284).

A couple of reactions that are directly applicable to carboxylic acids follow. One is the *reduction,* using lithium aluminum hydride ($LiAlH_4$) or borane (BH_3), of **carboxylic acids** to primary alcohols. Because of the high oxidation state of the acid, it can be difficult to get this reaction to go to completion. Running it at elevated temperature in an aprotic solvent seems to improve yields (see Figure 31.36 for a generalized example of the reaction). In step one of the transformation, the acid is reduced to an alkoxide anion (RCH_2O^-) through the loss of water, which is protonated in the second step by aqueous acid to get the alcohol. The use of BH_3 in this reaction improves the rate, and it is a more selective reducing reagent.

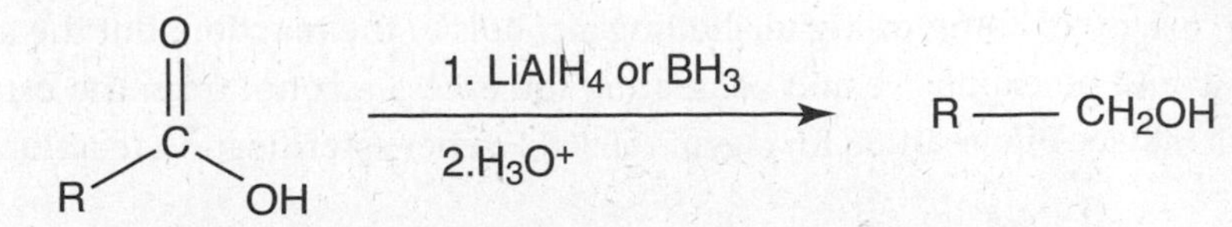

Figure 31.36. Reduction of a carboxylic acid to a primary alcohol

Decarboxylation of carboxylic acids (a type of **elimination** reaction) was already mentioned in the discussion on the **acetoacetic ester synthesis**. This is not a general reaction of carboxylic acids, but it is unique to 1,3-dicarbonyl compounds (those compounds that contain two carbonyl functional groups, one of which is a carboxylic acid, separated by one carbon atom—often a β-keto acid). Upon heating, these types of carboxylic acids lose their carboxyl groups as **carbon dioxide** (CO_2) **gas**. The mechanism of this process involves a cyclic conformation, and this accounts for the need for a second carbonyl group β to the carbonyl group of the acid. Figure 31.37 shows the decarboxylation reaction mechanism.

> Recall that *reducing agents* should be thought of as contributing the nucleophilic hydride anion ($H^{·-}$), which attacks the partially positively charged carbon of the carbonyl group in, for example, a carboxylic acid. As with almost all reduction reaction processes in organic chemistry, the overall result is the addition of hydrogen atoms to the reacting substrate's active site.

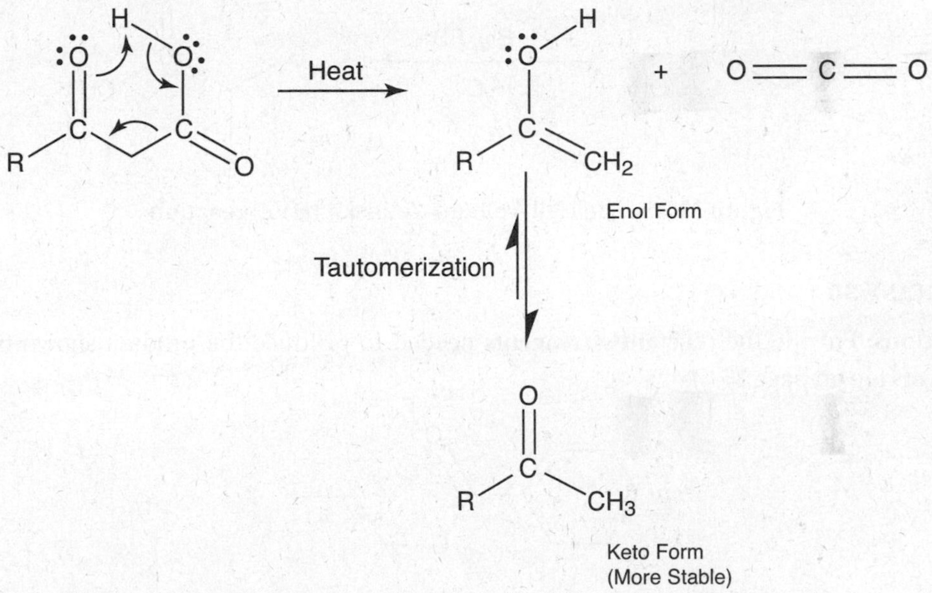

Figure 31.37. The decarboxylation mechanism of a β-keto acid

Esterification is another important reaction of carboxylic acids. There are a number of methods used to prepare **esters** from acids, and they all involve reaction with an *alcohol*. One of these procedures was shown earlier in Figure 31.6, the Alcohol Reaction Web reaction 6 (page 262). This process involves first converting a carboxylic acid into an acid chloride (a very reactive carbonyl compound discussed later in the review under *Carboxylic Acids Derivatives* on page 284), which is then reacted with an *alcohol* to produce an **ester**.

Another method, known as **Fischer esterification**, forms **esters** by heating carboxylic acids in an alcohol solvent with a catalytic amount of acid (only a few drops are needed). This reaction gives good yields but is effectively limited to producing methyl, ethyl, propyl, and butyl esters because their corresponding alcohols must be used as **solvents** in the process. It would be possible to use more complex higher-boiling alcohols in the reaction, but the large quantity required would be expensive and separating the excess alcohol from the ester product would be difficult (see Figure 31.38 for a generalized Fischer esterification reaction).

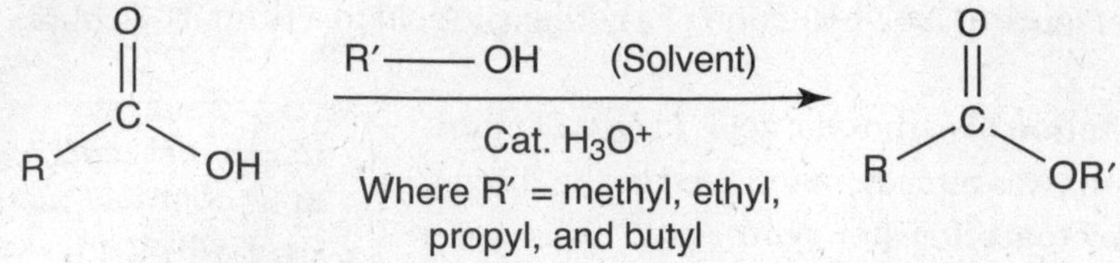

Figure 31.38. The Fischer esterification reaction

As indicated earlier, the hydrogens on carbons α to the carbonyl group of carboxylic acids are slightly acidic and can theoretically be abstracted by a strong base. Unfortunately, these carboxylic acids do not enolize sufficiently for them to be effective nucleophiles, so they don't generally undergo the same enolate nucleophile reactions observed with aldehydes and ketones. There is however a way to **brominate** the α carbon of carboxylic acids known as the **Hell-Volhard-Zelinskii (HVZ) reaction**. Figure 31.39 provides an example of this reaction.

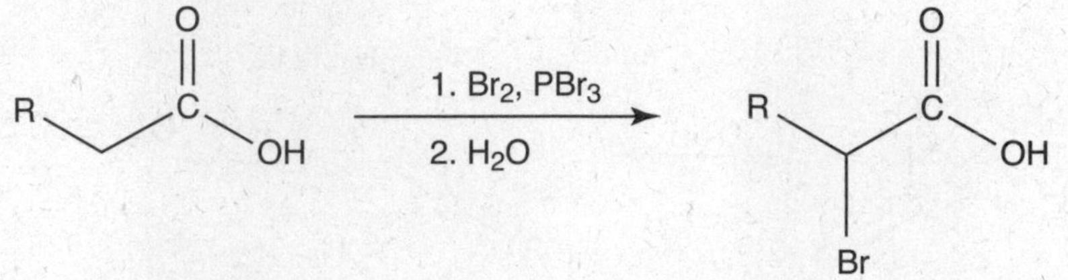

Figure 31.39. The Hell-Volhard-Zelinskii (HVZ) reaction

EXERCISE 30

Directions: Provide the reactant(s)/reagents needed to produce the product shown below. (Answers are on page 351.)

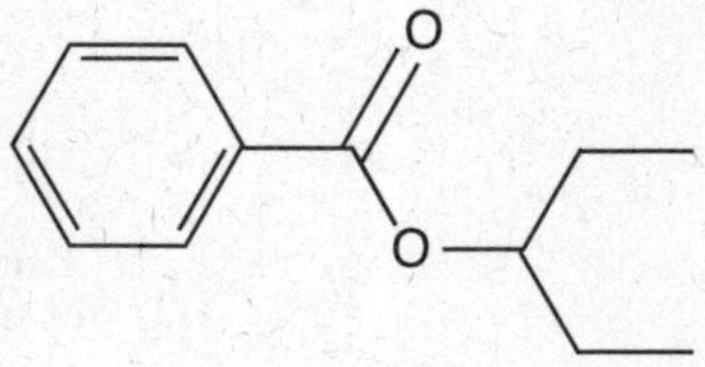

CARBOXYLIC ACID DERIVATIVES

Carboxylic Acid Derivative Functional Groups

Carboxylic acids can be converted into a number of important derivatives, some of which have already been discussed in this review. Many of these substances are important intermediates in the synthesis of more complex organic compounds. The structures and names of the most common of these compounds (along with the structure of carboxylic acids for reference) are shown in Figure 31.40. They are listed from left to right in order of increasing reactivity to nucleophilic substitution at the carbonyl carbon.

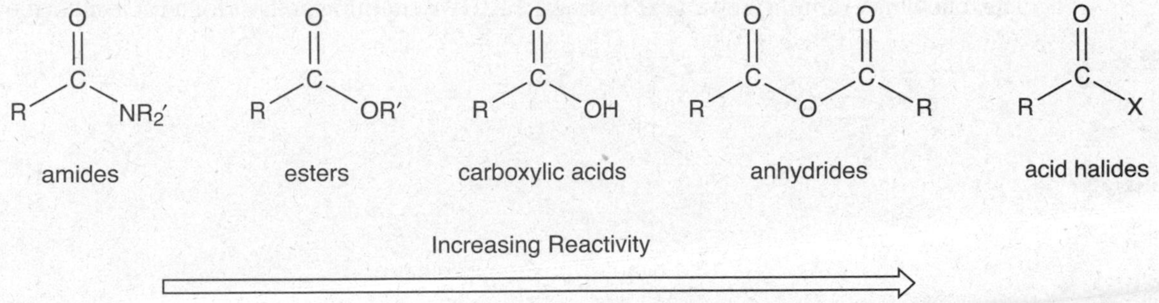

Figure 31.40. Common carboxylic acid derivatives

All carboxylic acid derivatives can undergo nucleophilic attack at the carbonyl carbon depending on the reaction conditions. The order of reactivity outlined in Figure 31.40 can be explained on the basis of the tendency of the group attached to the carbonyl carbon (shown on the right side of each structure in the figure) to "leave." The *better* the leaving group, the more reactive the compound to nucleophilic substitution. As a leaving group is lost, it typically becomes an *anion*. The lower the pK_a of the leaving group's conjugate acid, the more stable its anion will be. For example, the conjugate acid of an acid chloride's leaving group, the *chloride anion*, is HCl, which is extremely acidic ($pK_a \sim -7$). The chloride anion leaving group is quite stable without its proton. Thus, acid chlorides are very reactive toward nucleophilic substitution reactions. The pK_a of an amide's leaving group, an *amine*, is ~40, which makes its anion ($NR'_2{}^-$) very unstable. It is a poor leaving group because of its basic character. Amides are the least reactive toward nucleophilic substitution.

The generalized mechanism for nucleophilic substitution reactions of carboxylic acid derivatives is shown in Figure 31.41. This process starts out with nucleophilic attack at the carbonyl carbon (where Z is the carboxylic acid derivative's leaving group) and results in a new carbonyl-containing product.

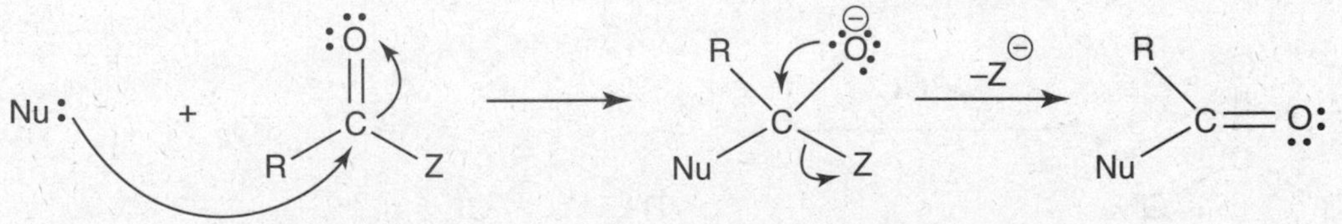

Figure 31.41. Generalized nucleophilic substitution mechanism for carboxylic acid derivatives

Note the loss of Z, the leaving group of the carboxylic acid derivative. As with other similar mechanisms, the nucleophile (Nu:) may be neutral or negatively charged but must have an available lone electron pair.

> In some substitution reactions, run under acidic conditions, the protonation of the oxygen carbonyl makes the carbonyl carbon more susceptible to nucleophilic attack. These conditions make the reaction rates of less reactive derivatives, such as amides, faster.

Acid Halides

NAMING ACID HALIDES

Acid halides (also called acyl halides) are named under the IUPAC system by changing the *-ic acid* suffix of the parent carboxylic acid to *-yl halide*. By far the most common type of acid halide you are likely to encounter on the DAT is an *acid chloride*.

TIP

Acid bromides
and iodides
exist but are
rarely referred
to in general
organic chemistry
studies.

The following example (Structure 61) shows the IUPAC naming process for an acid chloride.

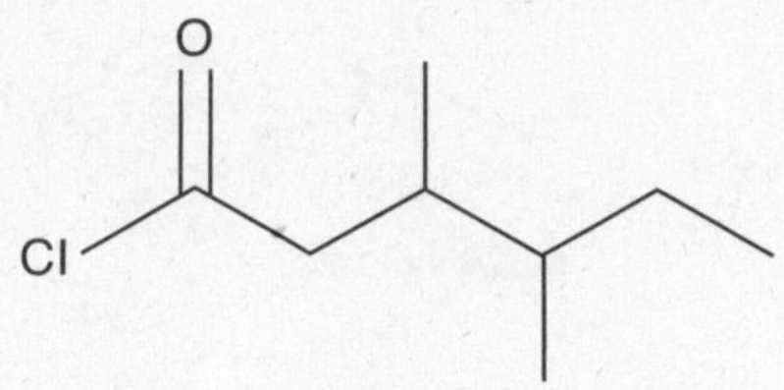

3,4-dimethylhexanoyl chloride (61)

The longest carbon chain terminated by the acid chloride group (six carbons including the carbonyl carbon) gives the root name **hexanoyl chloride**. The number assignments of substituents, two **methyl** groups at carbons 3 and 4, are defined by the carbonyl group at carbon number *1* in the principal chain. The example Structure (61) contains two chirality centers, but their stereochemistry is not defined, so the name doesn't contain any assignments (*R/S*) for these centers.

PROPERTIES AND USES OF ACID HALIDES

Acid halides are very reactive and highly susceptible to hydrolysis. They must be protected from contact with sources of water such as humid air. The primary use of these substances is as intermediates in the synthesis of more complex organic compounds.

SYNTHESIS AND REACTIONS OF ACID CHLORIDES

The standard way to synthesize acid chlorides is the treatment of a carboxylic acid with the reagent thionyl chloride ($SOCl_2$). The reaction is usually run in a basic solvent such as pyridine, which captures hydrogen chloride gas, a byproduct of the process (see Figure 31.42). The reaction proceeds by an S_N2 type mechanism. Other types of acid halides can be synthesized by similar procedures.

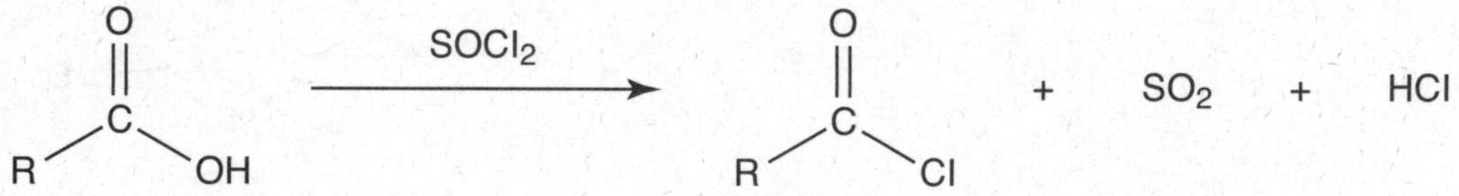

Figure 31.42. The preparation of acid chlorides from carboxylic acids

As commented earlier, organic chemists usually use acid chlorides to produce new, more functionalized compounds. For the reaction of an **alcohol** and an **acid chloride** to prepare an **ester**, see Figure 31.6, reaction 6 (page 262). Like the preparation procedure for acid chlorides just discussed above, these reactions produce HCl as a byproduct and are run in a basic solvent to capture it. This is often the most efficient way to produce an ester, and the reaction yields are high.

Another important reaction involving an acid chloride already discussed in this review is **Friedel-Crafts Acylation**, which is used to make **alkyl aryl ketones**. For a generalized example of this transformation, see Figure 30.24, reaction 6 (page 253). It should be recalled that this procedure involves the generation of an *acylium ion* (R–+C=O) by reaction of an acid chloride with a Lewis acid such as $AlCl_3$. The acylium ion reacts with the substrate through an electrophilic aromatic substitution mechanism.

Figure 31.43 shows a reaction web that includes three additional reactions that involve acid chlorides.

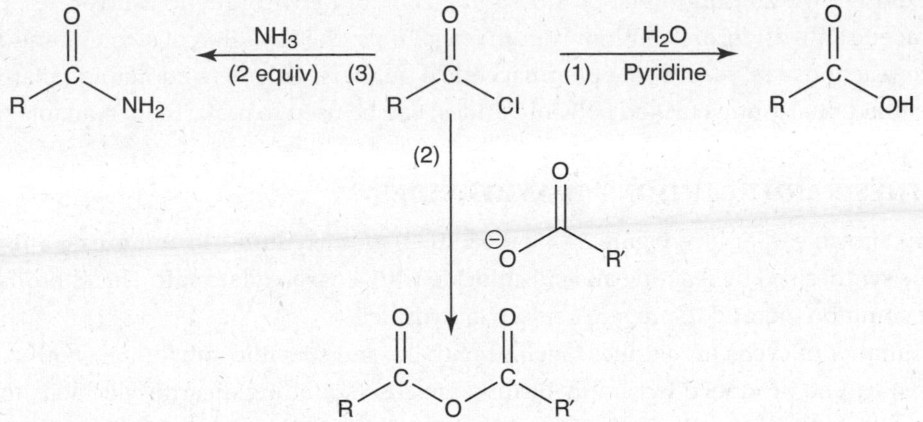

Figure 31.43. Acid chloride reaction web

Reaction 1 in Figure 31.43 shows the hydrolysis of an **acid chloride** to produce a **carboxylic acid**. The basic solvent pyridine reacts with HCl evolved in process to form a **pyridinium hydrochloride salt** (not shown).

Anhydrides are formed when an **acid chloride** is reacted with a **carboxylate salt** (see reaction 2 in Figure 31.43—only the carboxylate anion is shown). The carboxylate anion acts as a nucleophile attacking the acid chloride carbonyl carbon. The chloro group leaves as an anion as the anhydride product is formed.

A variety of **amides** can be synthesized by reacting **acid chlorides** with **ammonia** (NH_3 – see Reaction 3) or primary and secondary amines. **Two equivalents** of the basic nitrogen reactant must be used. One equivalent acts as a nucleophile attacking the acid chloride carbonyl carbon. The other acts as a base and reacts with the HCl byproduct produced in the reaction to form an **ammonium chloride salt** (the salt is not shown in the reaction diagram). Primary, secondary, and tertiary amides can be prepared using this approach.

Anhydrides

NAMING ANHYDRIDES

Anhydrides come in two forms, symmetrical and mixed. **Symmetric** anhydrides are named using the IUPAC system by replacing the **acid** suffix of the parent carboxylic acid with the term **anhydride**. **Mixed** anhydrides, which are produced from two different carboxylic acids, are named by **alphabetizing the names of both acids** and replacing the suffix **acid** with **anhydride**. The following simple Structures (62 and 63) illustrate both of these IUPAC naming rules.

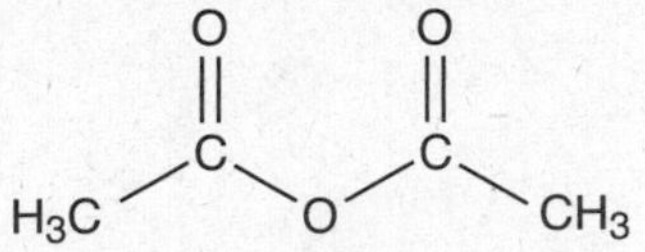

acetic anhydride   (62) 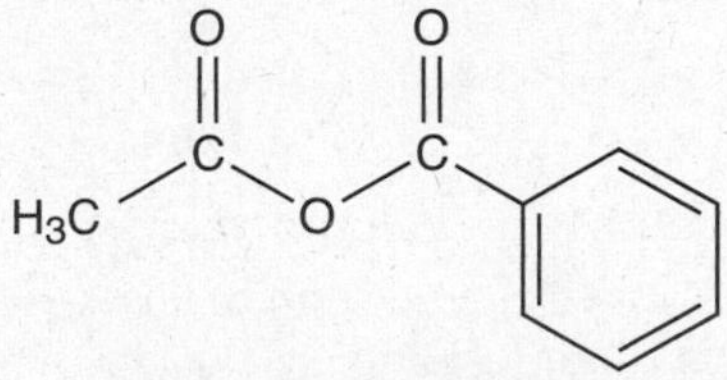   acetic benzoic anhydride   (63)

PROPERTIES AND USES OF ANHYDRIDES

Similar to acid chlorides, although less reactive, anhydrides are easily hydrolyzed when they are exposed to water and must be stored in a cool, dry environment. Anhydrides, particularly acetic anhydride, are commonly used reagents for the acylation of alcohols and amines. These reactions are used in the pharmaceutical industry. Polymers containing many anhydride functional groups (called polyanhydrides) can be used to make biodegradable plastics.

SYNTHESIS AND REACTIONS OF ANHYDRIDES

As was shown earlier (see Figure 31.43, reaction 2), both **symmetric** and **mixed anhydrides** can be synthesized by reacting an **acid chloride** with a **carboxylate salt**. This is probably the most common method to prepare a mixed anhydride.

A number of cyclic anhydrides (such as phthalic and succinic anhydride—both common names) can be produced by simply heating the corresponding dicarboxylic acids to a high temperature, which results in the loss of water (a dehydration process). Under these conditions, five- and six-membered anhydride rings are formed. Figure 31.44 shows an example of this reaction.

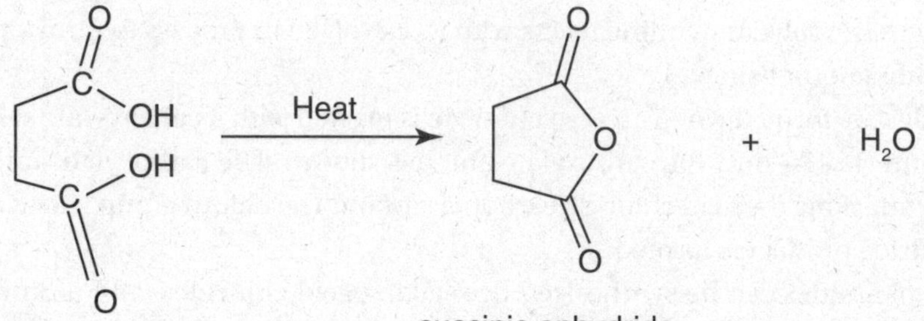

succinic anhydride

Figure 31.44. The thermal synthesis of a cyclic anhydride (succinic anhydride)

In this example succinic acid (common name) is converted to succinic anhydride (common name).

The important reactions for anhydrides are similar to those for acid halides. Figure 31.45 shows a reaction web that includes some reactions that involve anhydrides (note the similarity to Figure 31.43).

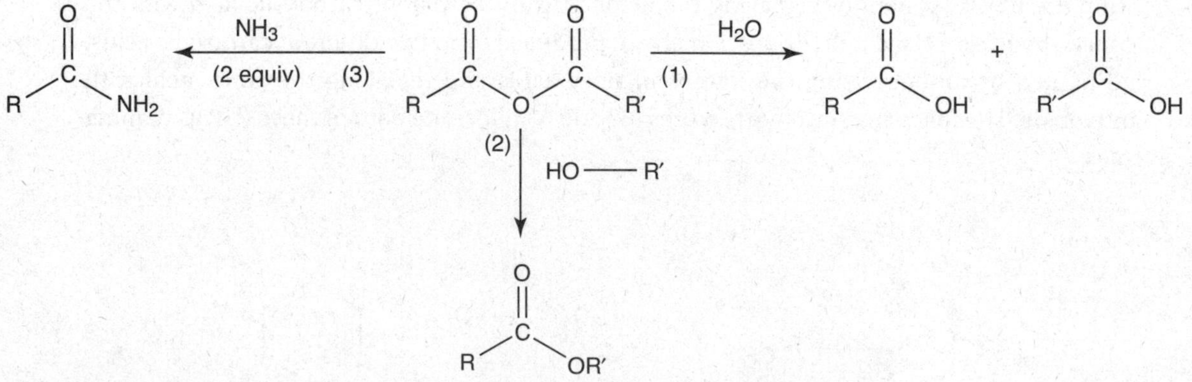

Figure 31.45. Reaction web for anhydrides

Reaction 1 shows the **hydrolysis** of an anhydride to produce a **carboxylic acid**. If the anhydride is **symmetric** (when R = R′), two moles of the same acid will be produced. If a **mixed** anhydride is used (R ≠ R′), a 1:1 mixture of the two parent carboxylic acids will result. Because separating the mixture can be difficult, this is generally not a good way to make a carboxylic acid.

In reaction 2, an **anhydride** is reacted with an **alcohol** to prepare an **ester**. This is yet another approach to synthesizing an ester but can have drawbacks because one mole of a carboxylic acid byproduct (not shown in the figure) is produced for every mole of the ester. Separating the acid from the ester may not be easy.

As with acid chlorides, **amides** can be prepared (see reaction 3) by treating an **anhydride** with two moles of **ammonia or a primary or secondary amine**. Just as with acid chlorides, two moles of the nucleophile are required because one mole of ammonium carboxylate salt is produced as a byproduct (not shown in the figure).

Anhydrides can also be used in place of acid chlorides for **Friedel-Crafts Acylation** reactions (see Figure 30.24, reaction 6, page 253).

Esters

NAMING ESTERS

For IUPAC naming purposes, esters are thought of as being derived from the dehydration product of an **alcohol** reacting with a **carboxylic acid**. The part contributed to the ester from the **alcohol** comes first in the name and is often just an **alkyl** group. The part contributed from the **carboxylic acid** appears second in the name and is referred to as an **acyl** group (R–C=O). This group is named by changing the **-ic acid** suffix of the carboxylic acid to the suffix **-ate**. For example, an ester produced by combining **ethanol** and **acetic acid** would be named "ethyl" (from the ethanol) "acetate" (from the acetic acid). Structure 64 shows another example of this naming procedure. Cyclic esters are referred to as **lactones**.

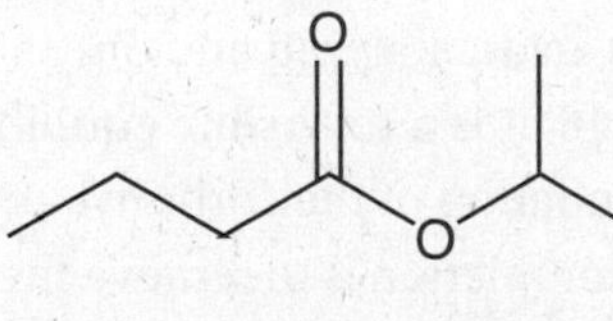

isopropyl butyrate

(64)

PROPERTIES AND USES OF ESTERS

Esters, like other carboxylic acid derivatives, can undergo hydrolysis reactions but are much less reactive with water than acid halides and anhydrides. Under normal ambient conditions, esters are fairly stable, and the low-boiling ones, like **ethyl acetate**, can be used as solvents for a variety of applications. These solvents are fairly polar due to the oxygen atoms in their structures. There are many naturally occurring esters that have very pleasant odors, which are found in the flowers and the fruits of plants.

SYNTHESIS AND REACTIONS OF ESTERS

A number of methods for making esters have already been covered in this review. Recall that esters can be prepared by:

- Reaction of an *acid chloride* and an *alcohol* (Figure 31.6, reaction 6, page 262)
- Reaction of an *anhydride* and an *alcohol* (Figure 31.45, reaction 2, page 288)
- The *Fischer Esterification* process (Figure 31.38, page 284)

All of these methods, as well as other less-known procedures, have their merits and drawbacks depending on the specific synthetic application. Many factors must be considered before selecting the most appropriate technique.

The most common reactions involving esters are *hydrolysis*, transforming them to *amides*, and a process called *transesterification*, which makes a *new* ester from a starting ester substrate. Figure 31.46 shows generalized examples of all these reactions.

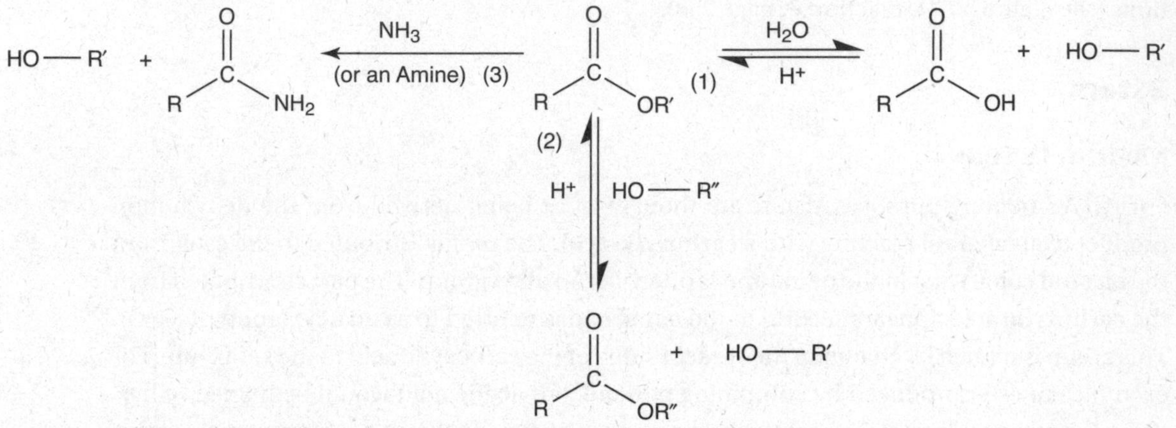

Figure 31.46. Ester reaction web

Hydrolysis of esters can be carried out under either acidic (see Figure 31.46, reaction 1) or basic conditions. The acidic process is acid-catalyzed and only a few drops of added acid are needed, but as indicated in Figure 31.46, it is a reversible equilibrium process. The first step of the reaction mechanism is the protonation of the carbonyl's oxygen. One way to force the reaction toward the product side and completion is to remove the alcohol product as it is produced. Another approach, which is usually easier but may have other limitations, is to use a large excess of water, which is the nucleophile in the reaction.

Remember that according to the Le Châtelier principle, when a reaction's equilibrium is disturbed, the reaction will adjust its equilibrium position to compensate for the change. Adding a large quantity of a reactant to the reaction process will shift the reaction's equilibrium to the right (product side). Removing a reaction product will also shift the process to the right toward the product side.

When ester hydrolysis is conducted under basic conditions it *is not base-catalyzed* and a full equivalent of base is required. The reaction product is a **carboxylate salt**. This approach is historically very old and is referred to as **saponification**. It has been used for thousands of years in soap-making to hydrolyze triacylglycerols (the primary components of animal fats) to produce *fatty acid salts* and *glycerol* (1,2,3-propanetriol). Fatty acid salts produced in this manner have long aliphatic carbon chains attached to the polar carboxylate salt group (see Structure 65—note: the metal counter ion from the base, also commonly called lye, isn't shown). These substances possess both *polar* and *nonpolar* properties in the same molecule. This makes them ideal for cleaning applications.

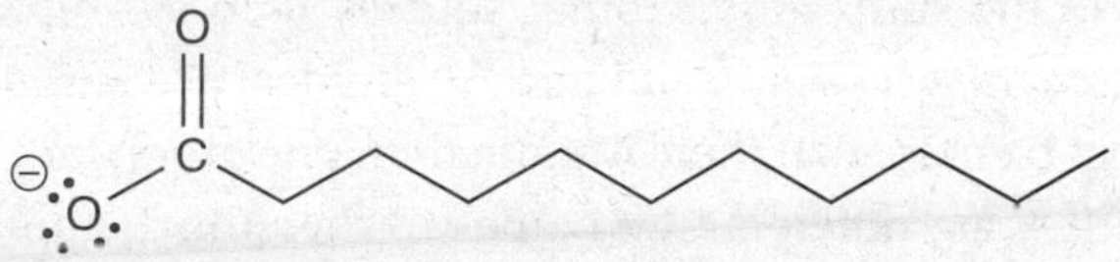

(65)

Acid-catalyzed transesterification (see reaction 2 in Figure 31.46) involves the use of *alcohols as nucleophiles* to attack an ester substrate's carbonyl carbon. This results in the loss of the ester's alkoxy group and the addition of a new one provided by the alcohol nucleophile. The starting ester is *transformed* into a new ester. Like acid-catalyzed hydrolysis of esters, this reaction is a reversible equilibrium process, and a large excess of the alcohol nucleophile must be used for the reaction to be successful.

As with other carboxylic acid derivatives, esters can be transformed into **amides** (reaction 3 in Figure 31.46). By using ammonia or primary or tertiary amines as the nucleophile, many different kinds of amides can be produced. The alkoxy leaving group of the ester produces a full equivalent of alcohol if the reaction is taken to completion. Because esters are not particularly reactive, elevated temperatures are usually required to increase this reaction's rate.

Other reactions involving esters already discussed in this review include the partial reduction of an *ester* to an *aldehyde* using DIBAH (see Figure 31.19, page 272) and the *Acetoacetic Ester Synthesis* used for the alkylation of ketones (see Figure 31.27, page 278). Another ester-related enolate reaction is called the *Claisen condensation*. Figure 31.47 shows an example of this process. A starting ester with at least two α protons must be used to favor the product equilibrium position of the reaction.

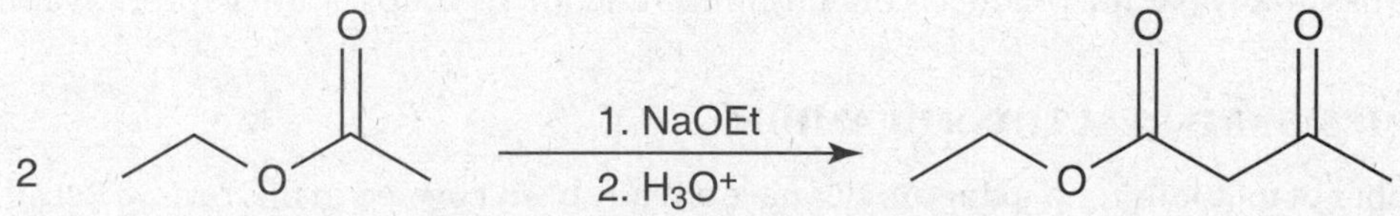

Figure 31.47. The Claisen condensation

To avoid *transesterification* side reactions, the condensation must be carried out with an alkoxide base that matches the alcohol side of the ester reactant (see Figure 31.47—because ethyl acetate is the reactant, ethoxide *must* be used as the base). As with aldol reactions, *intramolecular* Claisen condensation can occur. These reactions use a diester and favor the formation of five- and six-membered rings (this process is sometimes called a *Dieckmann cyclization*).

Reduction of esters (as with aldehydes and ketones) can be accomplished with lithium aluminum hydride ($LiAlH_4$) followed by water. There are a couple of differences—sodium borohydride doesn't work for this transformation, and when an ester is reduced, *two* alcohols are formed (one forms the acid side of the ester and one forms the alcohol side).

Amides

NAMING AMIDES

Amides are analogous to esters in that they contain two groups—an *amine* group and an *acyl* group. Primary amides are named by replacing the *-ic acid* suffix of the carboxylic acid contributing the acyl group to the suffix *amide* (other suffixes such as *–oic acid* and *–ylic acid* are treated the same way). With secondary and tertiary amides, alkyl groups attached to the amide nitrogen atom must be named. If there is more than one group and they are the same, the prefix *di-* is used. If they are different, the names of the groups appear in alphabetical order at the beginning of the complete IUPAC name. All groups attached to the amide nitrogen atom are given an *N-* prefix, which precedes the name of the alkyl group. Structure 66 shows an example of this naming process that uses all the rules. Cyclic amides are referred to as *lactams*.

N-ethyl-*N*-methylbutyramide (66)

PROPERTIES AND USES OF AMIDES

Amides are not easily hydrolyzed because the resulting amine anion is not a good leaving group—it's a relatively strong base compared to the other leaving groups discussed in this section. Primary and secondary amides are quite polar and are capable of intermolecular hydrogen bonding. As such, they have higher melting and boiling points than other comparable carboxylic acid derivatives, and they are often water soluble due to their hydrogen-bonding properties. Many natural products contain amide functional groups. Proteins are polyamides.

SYNTHESIS AND REACTIONS OF AMIDES

A number of methods for making amides have already been covered in this review. Recall that amides can be prepared by:

- Reaction of an *acid chloride* with NH_3 *or an amine* (primary or secondary) (see Figure 31.43, reaction 3, page 287)
- Reaction of an *anhydride* with NH_3 *or an amine* (primary or secondary) (see Figure 31.45, reaction 3, page 288)
- Reaction of an *ester* with NH_3 *or an amine* (primary or secondary) (see Figure 31.46, reaction 3, page 290)

Important reactions of amides include **hydrolysis** and a name reaction called the **Hofmann Rearrangement**.

As with esters, amides can be hydrolyzed under either acidic or basic conditions, but the processes must be considerably more strenuous. Under *acidic conditions*, the first step of the reaction mechanism involves protonation of the oxygen atom of the amide carbonyl carbon with water acting as a nucleophile (as with ester hydrolysis, a large excess of water must be used). The amine leaving group in this reaction ends up in a protonated ammonium salt form. Under basic conditions, the final products are a free amine and a carboxylate salt (the last step of the reaction mechanism is actually an acid-base reaction), again similar to basic ester hydrolysis (see below).

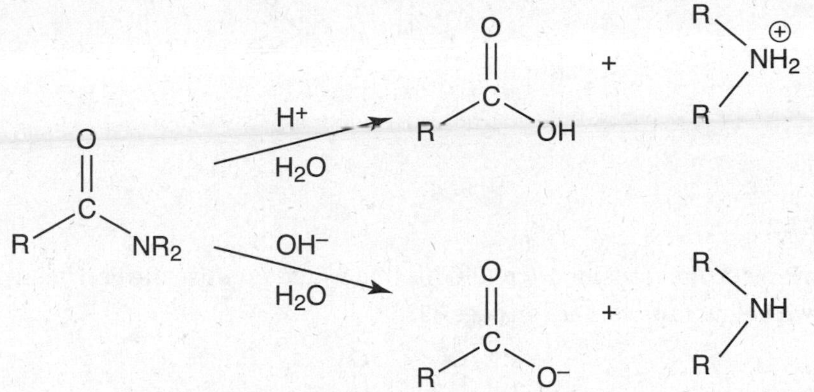

Figure 31.48. Amide hydrolysis reactions

The *Hofmann Rearrangement* transforms primary amides into **primary amines**. This reaction results in the formation of an *isocyanate* (R–N=C=O) intermediate, which is hydrolyzed by water to give an amine product with loss of the original carbonyl carbon as carbon dioxide (see Figure 31.49 for a generalized example of this reaction).

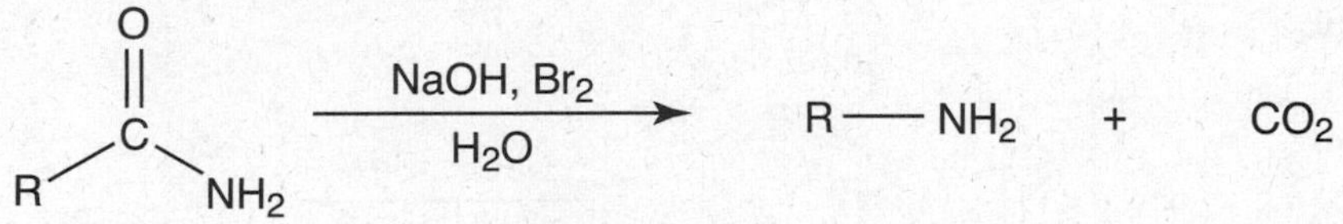

Figure 31.49. The Hofmann Rearrangement reaction

The base reagent deprotonates the primary amide nitrogen, which is then brominated by nucleophilic substitution. A second deprotonation of the bromoamide results in a bromoamide anion. The R– group attached to the amide carbonyl carbon then *migrates* over to bromoamide anion nitrogen, which leads to the formation of an *isocyanate*.

Reduction of amides with lithium aluminum hydride (LiAlH$_4$) followed by water produces amines. In this case no carbon atoms are lost, but the carbonyl oxygen is completely removed (see Figure 31.50 for an example of the process).

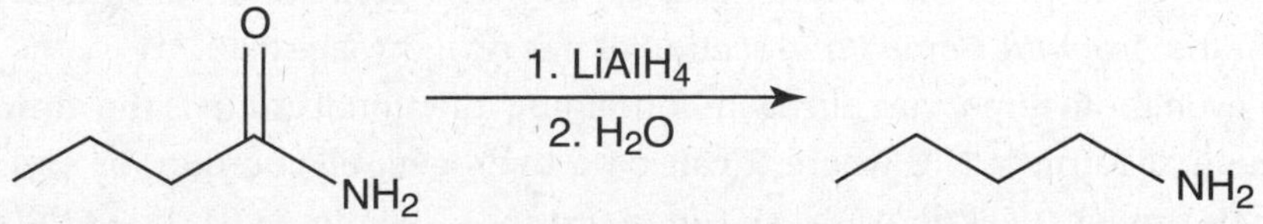

Figure31.50. Reduction of a primary amide to produce a primary amine

EXERCISE 31

Directions: Identify the *carboxylic acid* and *alcohol* that could be used to synthesize the following compound. (Answers are on page 351.)

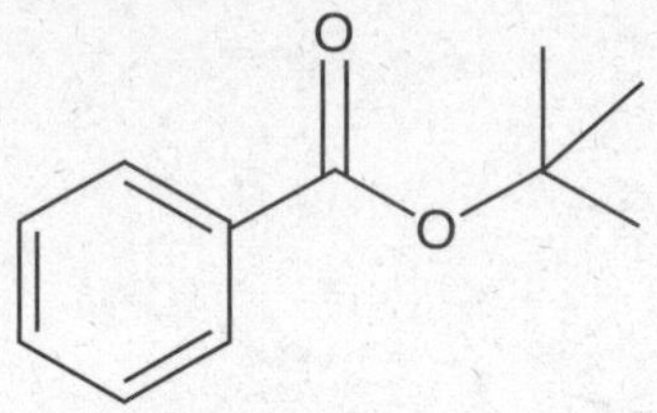

EXERCISE 32

Directions: Provide the reactant(s)/conditions that would produce the best yield of the compound shown below. (Answers are on page 352.)

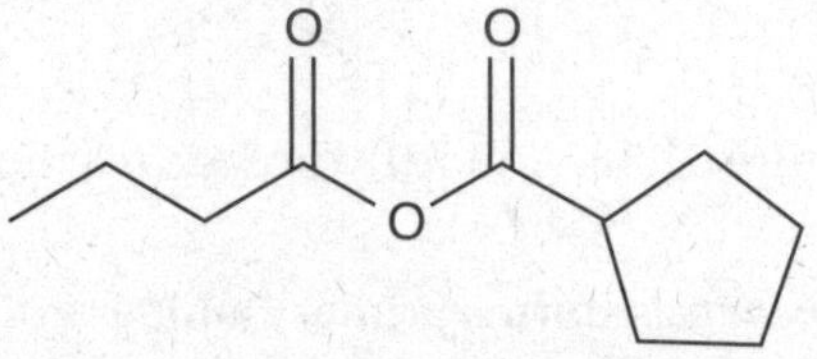

EXERCISE 33

Directions: Predict the major product(s) produced by the reaction shown below. (Answers are on page 352.)

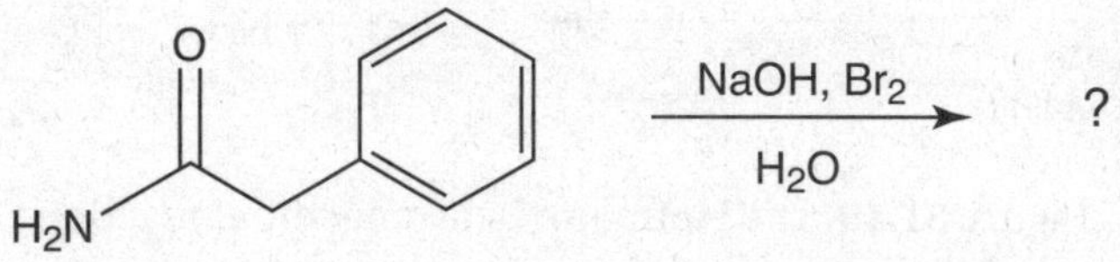

AMINES

The Amine Functional Group

Several types of nitrogen-containing organic compounds were discussed or referenced earlier in this review. The majority of these compounds were covered in the *Oxygen-Containing Functional Groups* sections. These nitrogen-containing compounds included cyanohydrins, imines, enamines, nitriles, isocyanates, and amides. The preparation of nitrobenzene was discussed in the *Aromatic Compounds* section of this review (page 000).

Another even more important nitrogen-containing functional group is the **amine**. Amines have the general formula NR_3, where R can be a hydrogen, alkyl group, or aryl group. All amines can be thought of as derivatives of *ammonia* (NH_3). Figure 31.51 shows the general 3D structure of an amine (approximately trigonal pyramidal) and example amine compounds, triethylamine (a commonly used solvent) and aniline (an arylamine).

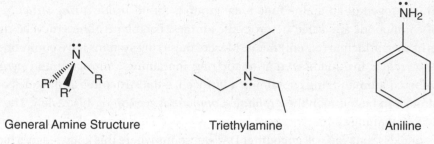

Figure 31.51. General amine structure and examples

As can be seen in the generalized amine structure shown above, substituents are attached to the *sp³* hybridized nitrogen atom by single covalent bonds resulting in an approximate tetrahedral geometry about the nitrogen. In their neutral form, amine nitrogens always have an associated *lone valence electron pair*. This feature of the amine structure plays an important part in the functional group's chemical properties. Amines are classified by the number of alkyl and/or aryl groups (Rs) attached to their nitrogen atoms: a **primary** amine has one R attached (RNH₂:); a **secondary** amine has two (R₂NH:); and a **tertiary** amine three (R₃N:). Note in Figure 31.51 that triethylamine is a tertiary alkyl amine and aniline (common name) is a primary aryl amine.

> A fourth group can also be bonded to the nitrogen atom using its lone electron pair. In this case the nitrogen must carry a formal positive charge (R_4N^+) and the species is called a **quaternary ammonium ion** (the counter ion is not shown in the formula).

Naming Amines

There are several ways using the IUPAC system of naming amines. For amines with simple *alkane* groups attached to the nitrogen atom, the final *-e* of the alkane name is changed to the suffix *-amine*. For example, an amine with an isopropane group attached to its nitrogen would be called *isopropanamine*. One with cyclohexane bonded to the nitrogen would be named *cyclohexanamine*. Alternatively, the suffix *amine* can simply be added to the *alkyl* substituent's name. For example, an amine with one isopropyl group attached to its nitrogen can be named *isopropylamine*. Secondary and tertiary amines where the alkyl groups are the same are named by adding the standard prefixes *di-* or *tri-* to the alkyl group name. See the compound *triethylamine* in Figure 31.51. If an amine functional group is a lower-priority substituent attached to a compound structure with higher-priority substituents, such as a carboxylic acid or alcohol functional group, the prefix *amino-* is added to the beginning of the name. Structure 67 shows an example of this naming approach.

4-aminohexanoic acid   (67)

Aryl amines are usually named as derivatives of aniline (see Figure 31.51), the simplest aromatic amine.

When the nitrogen of an amine functional group is found *inside a ring structure*, these types of compounds are called **heterocyclic amines**. Each type of heterocyclic ring system has its own principal (parent) name. Most of these ring systems have common names such as *pyrrole* (a five-membered aromatic ring containing a nitrogen) and *pyridine* (a six-membered aromatic ring containing a nitrogen)—the structures and names of these compounds can be found in the *Aromatic Compounds* section of this review. The details of the IUPAC naming system for these amines is beyond the scope of this review because it is very unlikely that you will encounter DAT questions where this knowledge is required.

EXERCISE 34

Directions: Using the guidelines shown on page 295, provide an unambiguous name for the following compound. Note that the stereochemistry for the chirality centers is shown for this structure. (Answer is on page 352.)

Properties and Uses of Amines

As commented earlier, simple amines have an approximate tetrahedral shape with a lone electron pair associated with the nitrogen atom. Because nitrogen is fairly electronegative (~3.0), amines are capable of forming *hydrogen bonds.* These bonds are not as strong as those formed by alcohols, carboxylic acids, and water because oxygen is more electronegative (~3.5). As such, ammonia and low molecular weight amines have boiling points that are higher than the corresponding alkanes but lower than similar alcohols. Like alcohols, again because they can hydrogen bond, amines having *less than five or six carbon atoms* in their structures are usually soluble in water. Because they can't hydrogen bond, tertiary amines generally have lower boiling points and are not water soluble.

> Remember, the *Brönsted-Lowry* definition of a base is that it is a **proton-accepting** species. In the case of amines they use their nitrogen lone pairs to form a bond with a proton, also known as a *hydrogen cation*. Also recall that neutral species that accept protons via a lone pair are called **Lewis** bases.

The most important chemical property of amines is that they can act as **weak bases** and are sometimes referred to as "organic bases." Figure 31.52 shows how the lone pair of an amine can accept a proton from a proton donor (an acid).

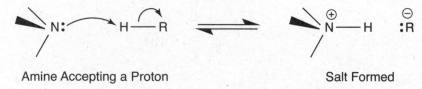

Amine Accepting a Proton   Salt Formed

Figure 31.52. An amine acting as a Lewis base

The result of the process shown in Figure 31.52 is the formation of a *quaternary ammonium salt*, described earlier in this section. Amines are more basic than oxygen-containing organic compounds (even though these compounds usually have multiple lone electron pairs) and water because the nitrogen atom with a lone pair is *less electronegative*. This makes the lone pairs of nitrogens in amines more *accessible* for bonding with protons since they are not held as tightly as in the case of oxygen lone pairs. It is very important to understand this simple point because it explains why amines are more basic than most other organic compounds. It also explains why amines are often good nucleophiles.

In general, because alkyl groups are electron donating, alkyl amines (pK_a's of their conjugate acids are ~10–11) are *stronger bases* than unsubstituted ammonia (pK_a of the ammonium ion is ~9). The effect of pushing electron density toward the nitrogen atom of the amine is to make it more willing to share its lone pair with a proton and thus a better proton acceptor—a stronger base. It also makes the nitrogen less willing to give up a proton for the same reason. Once protonated it helps stabilize the resulting positive charge as well.

Aryl amines are *less basic* than alkyl amines because the lone pair of the nitrogen can be delocalized over the aromatic ring, thus making it less available for bonding. Figure 31.53 shows this process for the aryl amine aniline (the pK_a of its ammonium ion is ~5).

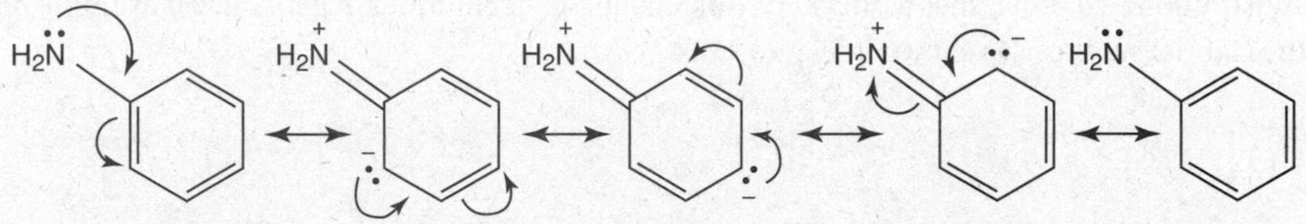

Figure 31.53. Delocalization of the nitrogen lone pair of aniline on the benzene ring

As might be expected, electron-donating groups attached to the aromatic ring of aryl amines make them more basic and electron-withdrawing groups make these compounds less basic.

Amines are used extensively in industry to prepare pharmaceuticals, pesticides, and fertilizers. A number of different kinds of *diamines* (these contain two amine functional groups) can be polymerized with various carboxylic acid derivatives to prepare polyamides, commonly known as *nylons*. Many different kinds of amines occur in nature, some of which are very biologically active. Examples of these include: atropine, nicotine, coline, adrenaline, mescaline, and morphine. Many naturally occurring amino acids (compounds that contain both amine and carboxylic acid function groups) are known and many others have been synthesized. Amino acids are the building blocks of *proteins*, which are polyamides.

EXERCISE 35

Directions: Order the following compounds from the weakest to strongest in basicity. (Answer is on page 352.)

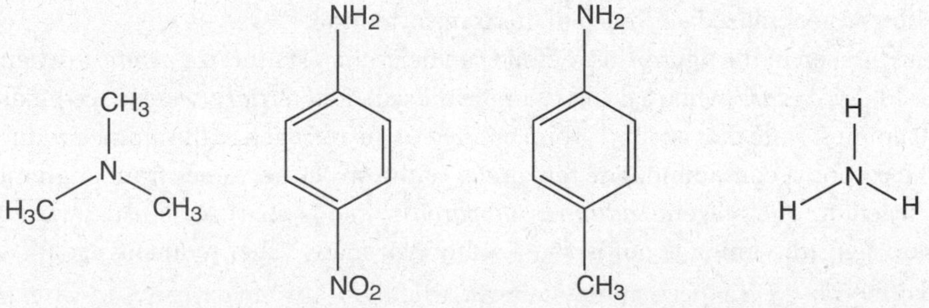

Synthesis and Reactions of Amines

There are numerous standard and innovative approaches to preparing amines. A couple of amine synthesis reactions were previously discussed in the *Oxygen-Containing Functional Groups* sections of this review. These involve the general hydrolysis of amides to give amines (see Figure 31.48, page 293) and the transformation of primary amides to primary amines, commonly referred to as the *Hofmann Rearrangement* (see Figure 31.49, page 293).

As indicated earlier, amines are often good nucleophiles, but standard S_N2 reaction processes (e.g., reaction of ammonia with a primary alkyl halide) to make more alkylate amines usually produce mixtures. Mixtures occur if ammonia, primary, or secondary amines are used because the reaction can't be stopped after just one or two substitutions. For each proton present on the amine nucleophile, a substitution is possible. Tertiary amine substrates produce *quaternary ammonium salt* products. If a **primary amine** is desired and the necessary amide substrate is available, the *Hofmann Rearrangement* can be used, but if this is not the case, a process called **Gabriel synthesis** can be used. This innovative approach uses what is effectively a blocked primary amine precursor, phthalimide, which prevents the multiple substitution reaction issues associated with regular S_N2 techniques. A generalized example of the Gabriel synthesis is shown in Figure 31.54.

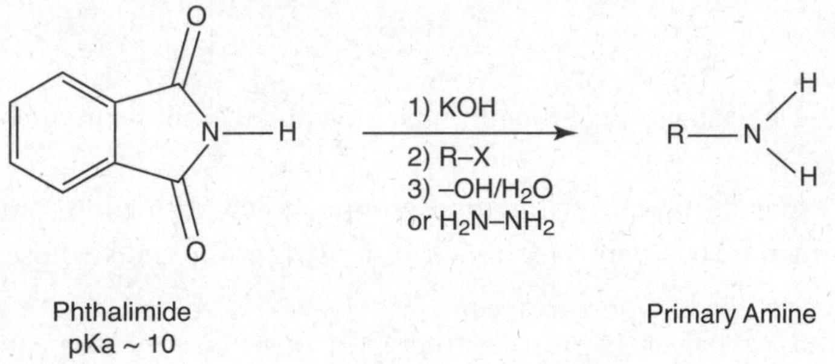

Phthalimide
pKa ~ 10

1) KOH
2) R–X
3) –OH/H₂O
or H₂N–NH₂

Primary Amine

Figure 31.54. The Gabriel synthesis, used to prepare primary amines

In the first step of the synthesis, the phthalimide acts as a very weak acid and is deprotonated by a base. The resonance stabilized phthalimide anion that forms is a good nucleophile, and attacks the alkyl halide in S_N2 fashion in the second step to form alkylated phthalimide. In the last step (step three in the figure), the alkylated imide is hydrolyzed with aqueous base to give a dicarboxylated byproduct (not shown in Figure 31.54) and the desired **primary amine** product. Alternatively, *hydrazine* can be used in the last step to remove the blocking group.

There are many approaches to the reduction of other functional groups that contain nitrogen to produce amines. One of the most important of these is the reduction of **imines**. This technique is referred to as **Reductive Amination** and is quite versatile because pretty much any *aldehyde* or *ketone* can be converted to an *imine* and then reduced to an *amine*. Figure 31.55 shows a generalized approach to this transformation.

As can be seen in the figure, this method can be used to synthesize *primary* (when ammonia is used), *secondary* (when a primary amine is used), and *tertiary* (when a secondary amine is used) amines. Note that an alkyl group bonded to the nitrogen of the amine product comes from the carbonyl compound. The remainder of the structure comes from ammonia or the amine reactant. The reagent *sodium cyanoborohydride* ($NaBH_3CN$) is usually used for the reduction step (the imine is not isolated), although many other reducing agents will work (e.g., H_2/Ni).

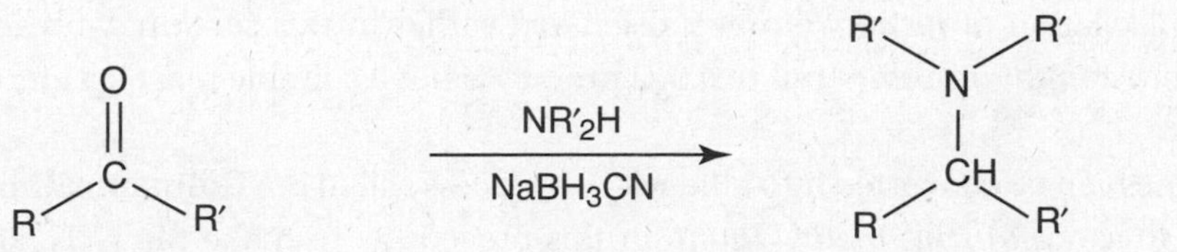

Ketone or Aldehyde
Where R is alkyl or aryl
and R′ is alkyl, aryl, or H

Amine Product
Where R is alkyl or aryl
and R′ is alkyl, aryl, or H

Figure 31.55. The preparation of primary, secondary, and tertiary amines by reductive amination

Other function groups that are often reduced to amines include **nitro** groups (see Figure 31.56), **nitriles** (see Figure 31.57), and **amides** (see Figure 31.58—this reaction was discussed earlier in the *Carboxylic Acid Derivatives* section on page 284).

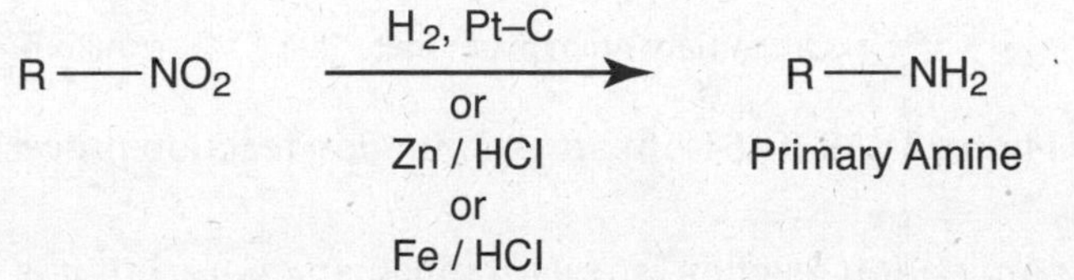

Figure 31.56. The reduction of nitro compounds to prepare primary amines

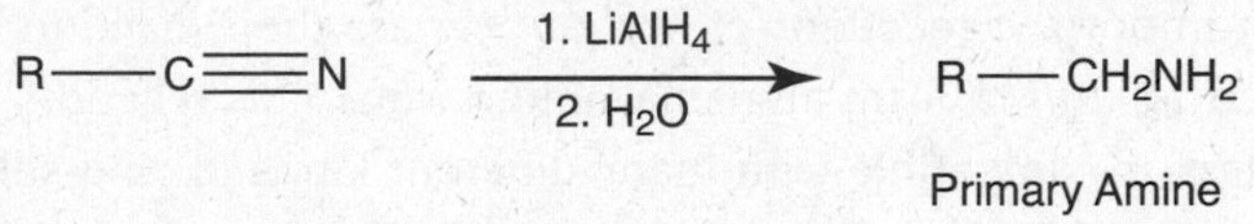

Figure 31.57. The reduction of nitrile compounds to prepare primary amines

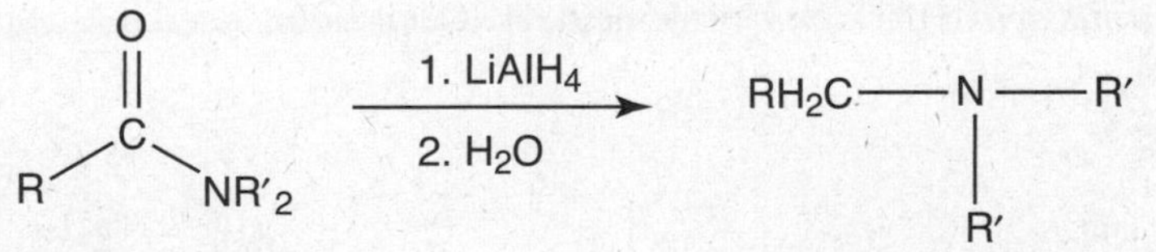

Amine
Where R is alkyl or aryl
and R′ is alkyl, aryl, or H

Amine Product
Where R is alkyl or aryl
and R′ is alkyl, aryl, or H

Figure 31.58. The reduction of amides to prepare primary, secondary, and tertiary amines

The reactions of amines, particularly aryl amines, are some of the most important synthetic tools in organic chemistry. The synthesis of **amides** from amines has already been covered in the *Carboxylic Acid Derivatives* section of this review. Recall that amides can be made by:

- Reaction of *ammonia or an amine* with an *acid chloride* (see Figure 31.43, reaction 3, page 287)
- Reaction of *ammonia or an amine* with an *anhydride* (see Figure 31.45, reaction 3, page 288)
- Reaction of *ammonia or an amine* with an *ester* (see Figure 31.46, reaction 3, page 290).

The alkylation of tertiary amines, discussed earlier in this section, works well to make *quaternary ammonium salts*, but this S_N2 process is not a suitable reaction for other kinds of amines.

Amines can be converted into **alkenes** by a process called the **Hofmann Elimination** (also referred to as *exhaustive methylation*). In this procedure, to make the NH_2^- anion a better leaving group the amine substrate is first reacted with *excess iodomethane* to produce a *quaternary ammonium salt*. This reaction is followed by heating the *salt* with silver oxide (Ag_2O), which acts as a base to effect an elimination that occurs by a concerted E2 mechanism. This step gives an *alkene*, water, and a trimethylamine byproduct. Figure 31.59 shows this two-step process for a primary amine substrate.

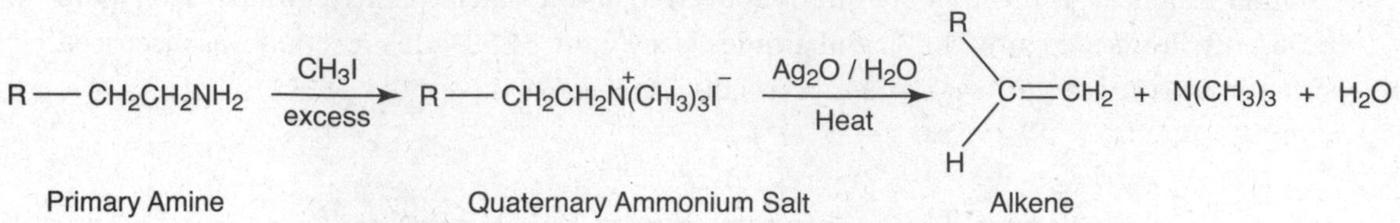

Figure 31.59. The Hofmann elimination reaction process

The Hofmann elimination reaction isn't used much anymore, but it is historically important because it was once used as a degradative tool to assist in determining the structures of naturally occurring amines.

By far the most important reactions of *aryl amines* are their reaction with **nitrous acid** (which is generated *in situ*) to form arenediazonium salts. This reaction, referred to as the **Sandmeyer reaction**, is compatible with many different kinds of ring-substituted anilines. Alkyldiazonium salts can also be prepared, but they are dangerously explosive and generally can't be isolated (see Figure 31.60 for the diazotization reaction of aniline). You should carefully note that *nitrous acid* (HNO_2) *not* nitric acid (HNO_3) is being used in this reaction.

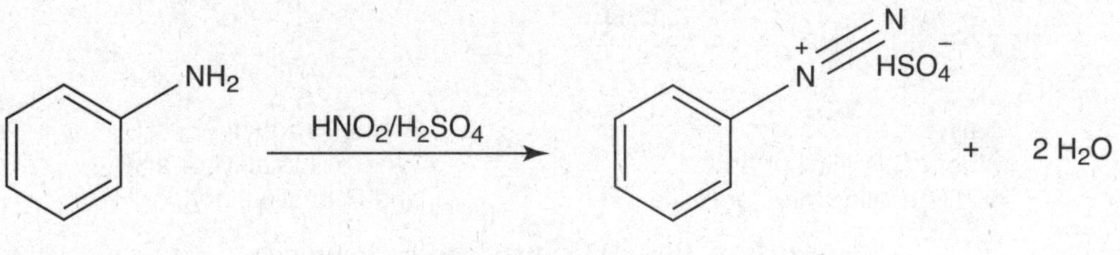

Figure 31.60. The diazotization of aniline

You may recall from past studies that the diazonio group ($N\equiv N$) can be replaced by nucleophiles to make *numerous* substituted aromatic compounds—that is why this reaction pathway is so important.

> The overall pathway of nitration of the aromatic ring → reduction of the nitro group to an amine → diazotization of the amine group → and substitution by an appropriate nucleophile is probably the most important method of aromatic substitution known.

Figure 31.61 shows the generalized reaction for the substitution of the diazonio group with a nucleophile (note the loss of the diazonio group as *nitrogen*).

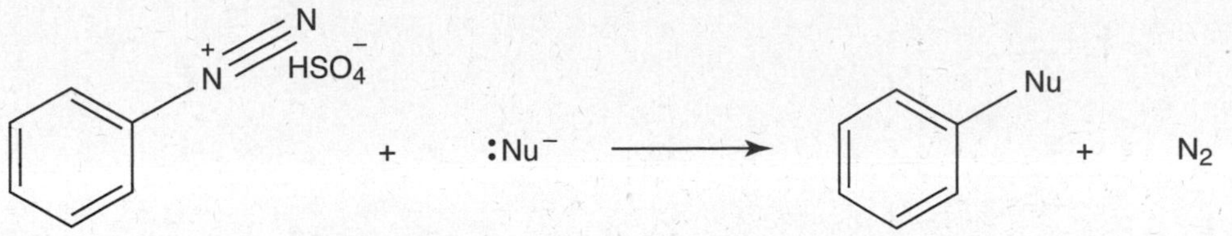

Figure 31.61. Nucleophilic replacement of the diazonio group of an arenediazonium salt

Figure 31.62 shows a generalized arenediazonium salt nucleophilic substitution reaction web.

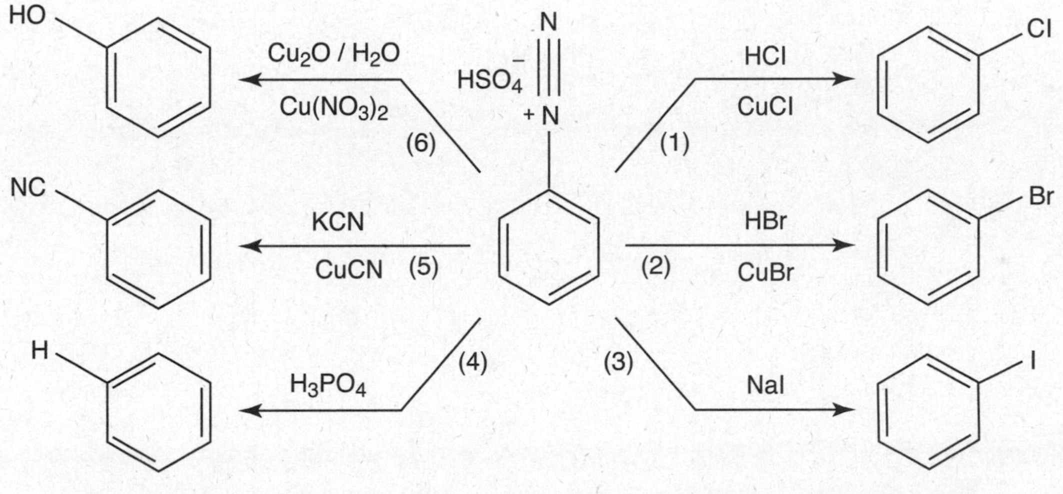

Figure 31.62. Nucleophilic substitution reaction web for arenediazonium salts

EXERCISE 36

Propose a viable synthetic route for the compound shown below starting with aniline and any other reagents/small organic molecules needed. (Answer is on page 353.)

Note that arenediazonium salts can be coupled to form **aromatic azo compounds (Ar–N=N–Ar′)**, which are sometimes brightly colored because of their extended conjugated π electron systems. Historically these compounds have been used extensively as *dyes*.

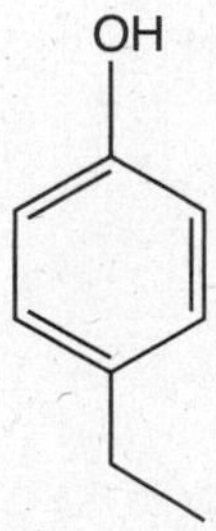

Organic Compound Characterization Techniques

32

In the history of the study of organic compounds, numerous approaches for the characterization of their molecular structures have been developed. When a chemist isolates or synthesizes an organic compound, he or she must have a reliable method for assigning a structure to the compound and eventually an IUPAC name. This is particularly important for safety, research, and legal (e.g., the patent application process) reasons if the compound has never been previously isolated or synthesized. The chemists must know the exact structure of the molecule they are dealing with.

The most powerful and efficient methods currently in use to characterize the structure of organic molecules involve spectrometric and absorption and emission spectroscopic techniques. These tools are quite sophisticated, and in the right hands, they can be used to quickly and confidently assign a structure to a relatively complex organic molecule. The most commonly used spectrometric technique in organic compound characterization is **Mass spectrometry (MS)**. It provides data related to the compound's molecular weight and structure. Its primary drawback is that it is destructive and results in the fragmentation of the sample molecules into many irretrievable pieces. This generally isn't a problem because extremely small samples can be used.

> The acronym **IUPAC** stands for the **International Union of Pure and Applied Chemistry.** Among other things, this union of chemists has developed and sanctioned a systematic method of nomenclature for chemical compounds. This method of naming compounds is the recognized international standard.

Absorption spectroscopy involves the detection and study of electromagnetic radiation absorbed by the organic molecule being characterized. The absorbed radiation can be from almost any area of the electromagnetic spectrum, but the most important areas for applications in organic chemistry (and DAT questions) are the **infrared (IR)**, **ultraviolet/visible (UV/VIS)**, and **radio-frequency (RF)** regions. As might be expected, **emission spectroscopy** involves the study of electromagnetic radiation emitted by the molecule being characterized. It is detected and interpreted to provide structural information. Figure 32.1 shows a schematic of the Electromagnetic Spectrum. The IR, UV/VIS, and RF regions are the most commonly used types of radiation for determining organic molecular structures.

Past DATs have had questions either directly or indirectly related to spectroscopic characterization concepts.

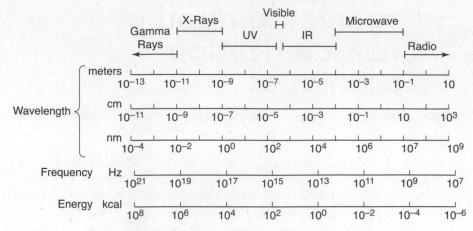

The Electromagnetic Spectrum

Figure 32.1. Wavelengths, frequencies, and energies
associated with the Electromagnetic Spectrum

An important fact often overlooked by those studying molecular characterization methods is that before a structure can be assigned to a compound, it needs to be relatively pure and in some cases very pure (>99.9%). There are numerous laboratory and industrial "separation" techniques for isolating and purifying organic compounds—some relatively simple and others quite complex and expensive. The *Separation and Purification* section of this review outlines some of these procedures.

MASS SPECTROMETRY

Mass spectrometry (MS) usually uses high-energy electrons (often in the form of a beam) to eject electrons from and break bonds in molecules. The technique is destructive and usually results in a significant level of molecular fragmentation—electron beam bombardment literally causes the exposed molecule to fall apart into pieces. Even though the molecule being studied absorbs/emits energy during the fragmentation process, neither the energy absorbed or emitted is measured or studied. As such, mass spectrometry is not considered to be a spectroscopic technique. Instead, this characterization procedure focuses on the detection of positively charged species resulting from the molecular fragmentation process.

The most important molecular characterization clues obtained from mass spectrometry are:

1. An estimate of the molecule's **mass** (its molecular weight in atomic mass units).
2. The molecule's **fragmentation pattern**, which is usually unique and can sometimes be matched to a database of known MS fragmentation patterns of tens of thousands of compounds. If a high confidence match is obtained with a compound in the database, the compounds are either identical or as a minimum very similar.

In many cases, just having an estimate of the molecule's molecular weight is reason enough to conduct a mass spectrometry experiment. This information along with **elemental analysis** data will usually allow the researcher to determine the molecule's molecular formula—an invaluable starting point for assigning its molecular structure.

Elemental analysis is used for determining the partial or complete chemical formula of a compound. Most commonly, it involves the complete combustion in air or oxygen of the substance and then quantifying the amount of elemental oxides produced. In the case of organic compounds, the carbon is converted to carbon dioxide and the hydrogen to water. From these, the percent carbon and percent hydrogen in the substance can be found. If oxygen is also present in the compound, its percentage can be estimated by the difference between the original compound's mass and the total masses of the carbon and hydrogen found. Similar mass balance procedures are used to estimate the percentages of other elements in the compound (e.g., nitrogen and halogens). With the percentages of the elements present and the molecular weight of the compound, a *molecular formula* can be proposed (the atomic masses of the number of carbons, hydrogens, oxygens, etc. proposed in the formula must add up to the molecular weight obtained from the compound's mass spectrum). Also note that one atomic mass unit (amu) is equal to 1.660×10^{-24} grams.

The first species formed during electron bombardment is a radical-cation (a positively charged ion with an odd number of electrons) and results from the ejection of a single electron from the analysis molecule. This radical cation is referred to as the **molecular ion** and is represented by $M^{+\cdot}$. Since the loss of a single electron from a molecule has essentially no effect on its mass, the $M^{+\cdot}$ represents the molecular weight of the original compound being studied. The $M^{+\cdot}$ is inherently unstable and once formed begins to spontaneously decompose into various fragments. Some of the fragments are cations or radical cations, which are sorted by mass using a strong magnetic field present inside the MS instrument. The magnetic field deflects the flight paths of positively charged species as a function of their mass—the paths of heavier ions are deflected less than light ones. Because of shorter flight paths, heaver ions reach the instrument's detector before lighter ones. Neutral fragments, such as radicals or uncharged molecules, do not interact with the magnetic field and are not detected by the instrument.

MS spectra are plotted with the amount of each cation (**relative intensity**) detected on the vertical axis vs. their masses (from lowest to highest) on the horizontal axis. More specifically the cation's masses are represented by their *mass-to-charge ratio* (*m/z*). The charges of the detected cation fragments are almost always +1 so their *m/z* ratio (mass/1) is an accurate measure of their true masses. Figure 32.2 shows a typical MS spectrum for the compound hexane.

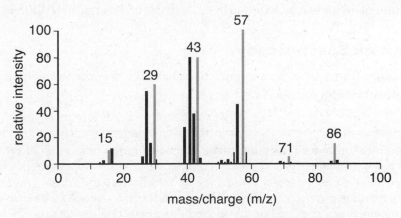

Figure 32.2. The mass spectrum of the alkane hexane

To prepare for DAT questions on this topic, there are three important features in most MS spectra that you should be familiar with. All of these can easily be found in the example spectrum shown in Figure 32.2. First look for the **base peak.** This will be the tallest peak (highest relative intensity) seen in the spectrum and represents the most stable cation fragment. This peak is automatically scaled to 100, and all the other spectrum peaks representing ions in lower abundance will be smaller. Next, find the molecular ion peak (the **M$^{+\cdot}$ peak**), which is usually the first significant peak (to the right of all the others) with the largest m/z in the spectrum. This peak represents the molecular weight of the compound. In the case of the example spectrum in Figure 32.2, the hexane's molecular weight is 86 amu. Because all organic compounds contain carbon, ~99% of which is the carbon-12 isotope, there is usually a much smaller peak in front of the **M$^{+\cdot}$** peak called the **M$^{+\cdot}$ + 1 peak** (this peak is one m/z unit higher than the **M$^{+\cdot}$** peak) which results from the presence of a small amount of carbon-13 isotope in the sample.

Other peaks with an m/z greater than the **M$^{+\cdot}$** + 1 peak are also sometimes present in the spectrum. These are often due to the presence of various halogen isotopes (such as ^{37}Cl and ^{81}Br) in the sample molecules.

> Note that a mass spectrometer detects the masses of individual molecules. As such, the whole-number atomic masses of the most common individual isotopes must be used to estimate the mass of the **M$^{+\cdot}$**. For example, the compound in Figure 32.2, hexane, has a whole-number mass of 86 [(6 C $\times$ 12 amu) + (14 H $\times$ 1 amu) = 86 amu].

The last feature you should pay attention to is the pattern of ion peaks shown in the spectrum. These peaks represent the *fragmentation pattern* of the molecular ion and are usually unique to the molecule being analyzed. Although an exact interpretation of the peak pattern isn't usually possible, it can provide clues as to the types of functional groups present in the sample's molecules. For example, if the **M$^{+\cdot}$** peak in a particular mass spectrum has an m/z of 113 and another nearby peak (to the left of the **M$^{+\cdot}$** peak) has an m/z of 78, one can conclude with good confidence that a chlorine atom (35 amu) was lost from the molecular ion and a chloro group must be present in the sample compound molecules. The presence of halogen in the compound's *elemental analysis* can be used to further support this assumption.

ABSORPTION SPECTROSCOPY

As mentioned earlier, the most important types of radiation absorption for characterizing common organic compounds are in the IR and UV/VIS regions of the electromagnetic spectrum. The most important of these techniques by far is IR spectroscopy, which will be given a detailed treatment in this review, followed by an overview of the topic of UV/VIS spectroscopy.

IR Absorption Spectroscopy

The data obtained from IR spectra is usually used to identify the *functional groups* associated with the compound being studied.

> You should recall from earlier studies that a **functional group** is an atom or group of atoms with specific chemical and physical properties. The functional group is often the reactive portion of the molecule. There are approximately 25 functional groups that are commonly found in organic compounds. Compounds often contain more than one and some many more. See the *Organic Compound Functional Groups*, Chapter 28 for a table of functional groups (Table 28.1, page 222).

This can often immediately tell chemists whether they are dealing with an alcohol, ketone, amine, or other common category of molecule. More complex spectra may indicate the presence of several different types of functional groups. Typically radiation from the middle of the infrared spectrum is employed in IR spectroscopy; the energies of photons within this region correspond to energy differences between vibrational states in covalently bonded molecules. Thus IR spectroscopy is also called *vibrational spectroscopy*. In accordance with quantum theory, these vibrational states are quantized and thus molecules will only absorb infrared photons with specific energies. When IR radiation is absorbed, the molecule will vibrate (with its atoms moving relative to each other as if attached by springs) at a faster rate. There are two types of vibrational modes—*stretches*, in which bond lengths change, and *bends*, in which bond angles change. Furthermore, there are two types of stretches—symmetric and asymmetric—and four types of bends—rocking, scissoring, wagging, and twisting.

Not all possible vibrational modes absorb infrared radiation, however; only those that change the dipole of the molecule during movement are "IR-active." Those modes that do not, e.g., the symmetric stretch of O=C=O along the axis of the molecule, are IR-inactive. Additional modes may be created when vibrations interact with each other or "couple" to form combination modes.

An IR spectrum is plotted as % transmittance vs. frequency but instead of using reciprocal time (e.g., s^{-1}), frequency is given in reciprocal wavelengths or **wavenumbers** (cm^{-1}). The relationships between wavenumber, wavelength (λ), and frequency (v) for electromagnetic radiation are as follows:

$$\text{wavenumber (in } cm^{-1}) = \frac{1}{\lambda \text{(in cm)}} = \frac{v \text{(in } s^{-1})}{c} \text{, where } c = 3.00 \times 10^{10} \text{ cm/s}$$

The typical wavenumber range used in IR spectroscopy is 4,000–400 cm^{-1} (corresponding to a wavelength range of 2.5×10^{-4} to 2.5×10^{-3} cm or 2.5 to 25 μm) and is usually plotted from highest to lowest frequency, thus the highest energy vibrations are to the left and the lowest are to the right. Figure 32.3 is the IR spectrum for formaldehyde, $H_2C=O$, and provides a good example of some of the most common types of bond vibrations found in the spectra of organic molecules. Note the stretching vibrations in the region above 1,400 cm^{-1} and the bending vibrations at wavenumbers below 1,400 cm^{-1}.

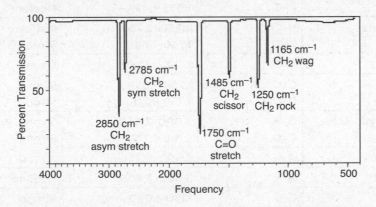

Figure 32.3. The IR absorption spectrum for formaldehyde

Since each vibrational state is further split into rotational and translational states, each absorption occurs over a range of frequencies rather than at just one; this causes both broadening of the absorption signal, which appears as a *band* rather than a peak, and the appearance of additional "structure" in the spectrum in the form of shoulder and side bands near more intense bands.

The intensity of bands is affected by three principal factors: *concentration* of the compound (which equally affects the intensity of all absorptions), *bond polarity* (the more polar the stronger the absorption), and the level of *asymmetry* in the molecule. In general, the more asymmetry between the bonds in a molecule, the stronger the absorption band will be, as predicted by quantum mechanics.

The frequencies of specific IR bands are affected by any factor, which affects vibrational energy. Stretching modes, which require more energy to excite, occur at higher energies and thus higher frequencies than bending modes. Also, the shorter and thus stronger the bonds involved in a vibration, the higher the energy and thus frequency of the absorption. Vibrational modes involving triple bonds are at higher frequencies than for double bonds, which are in turn at higher frequencies than for single bonds. Another important factor involves inductive effects; electron-withdrawing and conjugated substituents typically weaken adjacent bonds and thus lower their absorption frequencies. Yet another factor that must be considered is the presence of hydrogen bonding, which tends to broaden absorption bands for O–H and N–H stretches, especially in solutions or liquids in which fast hydrogen exchange is possible.

> A detailed understanding of the factors that affect absorption band shape, strength, and position is not necessary to answer most DAT IR spectroscopy questions. The most important thing you need to remember is the general position (in cm^{-1}) of the absorption bands for the most common kinds of bonds and functional groups found in organic compounds.

Table 32.1. Important Functional Group IR Absorption Bands

Functional Group	Bond Type	Band Position (cm^{-1})	Intensity
Alkanes	C–H	3,000–2,850	Strong
	C–C	~1,200	Weak
Alkenes	=C–H	3,095–3,010	Medium
	C=C	~1,650	Medium
Alkynes	≡C–H	~3,300	Medium
	C≡C	2,260–2,100	Medium
Aromatics	Ar–H	3,100–2,900	Weak
	C–C	1,625–1,425	Medium
Aldehydes	H–C=O	2,850–2,750	Medium
	C=O	1,740–1,690	Strong
Ketones	C=O	1,750–1,680	Strong
Esters	C=O	1,750–1,650	Strong
	O–C=O	1,350–1,200	Strong
Carboxylic Acids	O–H	3,000–2,500	Strong, Broad
	C=O	1,780–1,710	Strong
Alcohols	O–H	3,600–3,200	Strong, Broad
Amines	N–H	3,500–3,200	Medium
Ethers	C–O	1,150–1,050	Strong

In general, O–H, N–H, and C–H stretches are found between 3,700 and 2,700 cm^{-1}, multiple bond stretches (in roughly the order C≡N, C≡C, C=O, C=C, aromatic) between 2,300 and 1,400 cm^{-1}, single bond stretches between 1,600 and 1,300 cm^{-1} for N–O, and between 1,300 and

900 cm^{-1} for C–O, C–N, and C–C. In fact, the 4,000 to 1,300 cm^{-1} range is called the **functional group region** because bands within it are often well separated and relatively strong and thus easy to correlate to specific functional groups, although precise identification of a compound based solely on the bands in this frequency range is difficult. Table 32.1 shows the absorption band positions (in cm^{-1}) for the functional groups most often referenced in DAT questions. You should study Table 32.1 until you are very familiar with the approximate position of the referenced IR absorption bands *and* the functional groups they correspond to.

Most bending frequencies are found in the range from 1,400 cm^{-1} to 600 cm^{-1}; unfortunately, these overlap significantly with the stretching frequencies for single bonds and also with the frequencies for many of the combination vibrational modes mentioned above, quite often making this region of the spectrum too crowded and complicated to interpret. However, a band-for-band match within this frequency range between the IR spectra of a known compound and a sample of an unknown compound is strong proof that the two compounds are identical. Therefore this range is called the **fingerprint region**.

UV/VIS Absorption Spectroscopy

The applications of UV/VIS absorption spectroscopy in the characterization of organic compounds are quite specialized, and as such, the discussion on this topic will be brief. This type of absorption spectroscopy is used primarily to provide information about the **degree of unsaturation** and **conjugation** in organic compounds.

The terms **saturated** and **unsaturated** refer to the hydrogen atom content of organic compounds. Saturated compounds contain the maximum possible number of hydrogen atoms in their molecules. Unsaturated compounds contain fewer hydrogen atoms because they contain multiple bonds, rings, or other functional groups that reduce their possible hydrogen content. Any combination of multiple bonds, rings, and functional groups is possible in unsaturated compounds. The majority of organic compounds fall into the unsaturated category. The **degree of unsaturation (DU)** for most organic compounds can be calculated using the following formula:

$$DU = \frac{2C + 2 + N - (H + X)}{2}$$

C is the number of carbon atoms, N is the number of nitrogen atoms, H the number of hydrogen atoms, and X the number of halogen atoms in the compound. Any oxygen atoms in the formula can be ignored. If the molecular formula of a compound is known, its DU can be calculated (using the above formula) and used to estimate the number of possible multiple bonds and rings it contains. This information can be very valuable in ultimately determining its complete atomic structure.

Conjugation in unsaturated compounds refers to a specific arrangement of double bonds in the molecule. A compound is conjugated when its double bonds alternate with single bonds. Examples of *isolated* and *conjugated* double bonds are shown in the following structural formulas (68 and 69):

Isolated Double Bonds   Conjugated Double Bonds   (68, 69)

EXERCISE 37

Directions: Determine which of the compounds' given molecular formulas shown below have the *same* degree of unsaturation. (Answers are on page 353.)

$$C_3H_6 \qquad C_2Cl_6 \qquad C_5H_9N \qquad C_3H_5NO_2$$

The wavelength (represented by the Greek letter λ) of the radiation in this part of the electromagnetic spectrum is commonly reported in **nanometers (nm)**. More specifically, the area most important for molecular structure information is relatively narrow and ranges from ~200 nm to ~500 nm. This range starts in the near-ultraviolet region and overlaps into the violet/blue region of the visible part of the spectrum. The majority of unsaturated compounds absorb radiation in the 200 nm to 400 nm range, but a few absorb longer wavelength radiation in the visible region (rarely, even into the red, ~700 nm).

As discussed earlier, when an organic molecule is irradiated with electromagnetic energy, the radiation, depending on its wavelength, may be absorbed or it may pass though the compound. IR radiation absorbed by molecules causes their covalent bonds to vibrate (resulting in stretching and bending), but the energy of UV/VIS radiation is much higher and leads to a change in the molecule's electron configuration. In organic compounds containing double bonds, absorption of UV/VIS radiation energy results in the promotion of electrons from *bonding* molecular orbitals (ψ, referred to as ground state) to higher energy *antibonding* molecular orbitals (ψ^*, referred to as excited state) in the compound. The energy absorbed during this transition (which is called a $\pi \rightarrow \pi^*$ transition) is measured and interpreted to provide structural information about the molecule being irradiated. Other kinds of electron transitions can occur when radiation is absorbed if certain functional groups are present in the molecule. For example, if a carbon-oxygen double bond (called a carbonyl group) is present, an $n \rightarrow \pi^*$ (where n refers to a nonbonding molecular orbital) transition is observed. This transition involves the promotion of an electron from a ground state nonbonding molecular orbital to an excited state antibonding molecular orbital and requires less energy than a $\pi \rightarrow \pi^*$ transition.

A detailed discussion of *molecular orbital theory* is beyond the scope of this review, but you may recall from your general chemistry studies that this theory is yet another approach to explaining atom bonding in molecular compounds (the details of *valence bond theory* and VSEPR theory were discussed in the first section of this review).

In brief, when atomic orbitals are combined linearly (a mathematical operation), two kinds of molecular orbitals are usually produced—bonding and antibonding molecular orbitals (MOs). Another kind of MO that can be formed from a combination of atomic orbitals is referred to as a nonbonding MO. As might be expected, bonding MOs are lower in energy than the atomic orbitals they were derived from, and when occupied by electrons, they stabilize the bonding interaction. Antibonding MOs are higher in energy than the atomic orbitals from which they were formed, and when occupied by electrons, they destabilize the bonding interaction. For a bonding interaction between two or more atoms to be stable, there must be more electrons occupying bonding MOs than antibonding MOs. Nonbonding MOs neither stabilize nor destabilize the bonding interaction.

UV/VIS spectra of organic compounds are usually recorded by irradiating samples with continually increasing wavelengths of radiation (higher to lower energy). When the energy of the radiation is sufficient to promote an electron to a higher energy level, energy is absorbed and the absorption is observed as a positive peak (rather than a negative band as in IR spectroscopy) in the spectrum. Spectra are displayed with the wavelength in nanometers at the bottom of the graph and relative absorption (which is unit-less) along the left vertical axis. Figure 32.4 shows an example UV/VIS absorption spectrum of the compound isoprene.

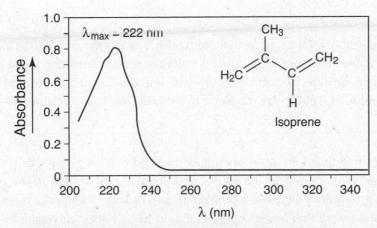

Figure 32.4. The UV/VIS absorption spectrum of isoprene

Unlike IR spectra of organic compounds, UV/VIS spectra generally have very few features. As seen in Figure 32.4, there is often only a single broad absorption peak, referred to as λ_{max}, observed in the spectrum. Spectra of other more complex molecules may show additional absorption peaks due to additional electron transitions. This can be seen in the UV/VIS absorption spectrum of a conjugated ketone (see Figure 32.5).

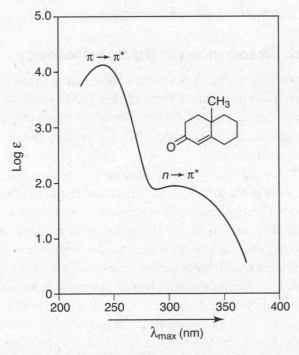

Figure 32.5. The UV/VIS absorption spectrum of a conjugated ketone

Note the two absorption peaks resulting from two different electron transitions, $\pi \to \pi^*$ and $n \to \pi^*$. Also note that this spectrum has been plotted using the log of the molar absorptivity (ε) for the vertical axis. This is an alternative to using absorption (A) and can make some spectra easier to interpret.

Remember, Beer's Law relates molar absorptivity (ε) to absorption (A). According to Beer's Law:

$$A = \varepsilon bc$$

c is the concentration of the sample in molarity (M), and b is the path length of the sample container. If the sample concentration and container remain constant, it can be seen that A is directly proportional to ε. Molar absorptivity is a measure of how strongly a molecule absorbs radiation at a particular wavelength and is unique to the compound being studied.

The degree of conjugation in an organic compound can be estimated from its UV/VIS spectrum. In general, the longer the conjugated double-bond system in the molecule, the lower the energy required for a $\pi \to \pi^*$ transition and thus the longer the wavelength of the energy absorbed (recall that lower energy radiation has a longer wavelength). Most λ max absorption peaks are found between 200 nm and 400 nm, but when the conjugation system is really long, as for example in the compound β-carotene (it has 11 conjugated double bonds and its $\lambda_{max} = 455$ nm), the λ_{max} absorption may fall in the visible part of the electromagnetic spectrum. Compounds with this characteristic UV/VIS spectrum appear "colored" to the human eye. The general rule for the length of a conjugation system is that for every conjugated double bond, the absorption energy wavelength is increased by approximately 30 nm to 40 nm. Additional isolated double bonds generally don't increase the absorption wavelength. The addition of alkyl (e.g., methyl, ethyl, propyl, etc.) groups to the conjugation system of the molecule adds about 5 nm to the wavelength's absorption.

Nuclear Magnetic Resonance (NMR) Spectroscopy

The most important spectroscopic tool currently available for the characterization of organic compounds is NMR spectroscopy. Several different types of NMR spectroscopy are commonly used for molecular characterization, but DAT questions involving this powerful technique have been confined to **proton (^{1}H)** and **carbon (^{13}C)**. As such, this review will focus primarily on these types of NMR spectroscopy.

As with IR and UV/VIS spectroscopy, NMR involves the detection (and presentation in the form of a spectrum) of absorbed radiation, specifically **radio frequency (RF)** radiation. Unlike other forms of absorption spectroscopy, NMR absorptions are not caused by energy changes of electrons, but instead they result from the absorption of RF radiation by the nuclei of the atoms in compounds being analyzed. Only certain atomic nuclei absorptions are suitable for NMR detection. The primary requirement for this procedure is that the nuclei being irradiated have what is referred to as **nuclear spin**. Not all atomic nuclei have this property, but those that do behave as if they are spinning about an axis. Because all nuclei are positively charged, those that spin create their own minute magnetic fields, which can interact with external magnetic fields. As it turns out, the nuclei of both hydrogen and carbon-13 atoms have the property of spin. This makes the use of this technique very valuable for the study of organic compounds since, to some extent, they always contain these two elements.

PROTON (^{1}H) NMR

Because the nucleus of the atom is all that is studied in this procedure, hydrogen atoms are often called "**protons**," and the absorption technique is called proton (^{1}H) NMR. In the absence of an external magnetic field, the spins of protons are randomly oriented, but when exposed to a strong external field, they each become aligned with it. Because each proton has its own magnetic field, there are two possible alignment orientations with the external field, either with it (parallel to) or against it (antiparallel to). Figure 32.6 shows a diagram of what this orientation process might look like when protons with randomly oriented spins are exposed to an external magnetic field.

Randomly oriented spinning protons
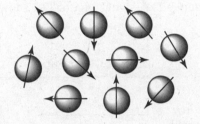

Spinning protons aligned *with* and *against* an external magnetic field (B_o)
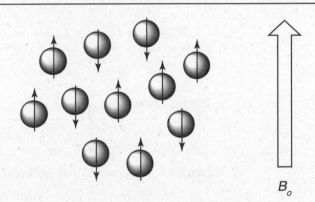

B_o

Figure 32.6. Alignment of protons with randomly oriented spins by an applied external magnetic field (B_o)

The energies of the two possible orientations are not the same. Protons aligned antiparallel to the external field are slightly higher in energy than those that are parallel. When a lower energy proton in the parallel state absorbs exactly the right amount of energy, supplied by RF radiation, it can be promoted into the higher energy antiparallel state. When this occurs, the proton is said to have **spin-flipped** and is in **resonance** with the applied RF radiation. This phenomenon is the basis for *nuclear magnetic resonance* spectroscopy—the energy absorbed by the proton is detected and represented as a peak in an NMR spectrum. The higher the strength of the applied magnetic field, the higher the frequency of the RF radiation required to flip the proton from the parallel spin state to the antiparallel spin state.

TIP

Be aware that in discussions related to ^{1}H NMR spectroscopy the terms "hydrogens" and "protons" are used interchangeably.

In the process of obtaining an NMR spectrum of a compound, the sample is placed inside the field of a super-conducting magnet (ranging in strength from about 4.7, to 21.6 tesla) and irradiated with RF radiation of various frequencies (ranging from ~200 to 920 MHz depending on the strength of the instrument's magnetic field). The energy absorbed (or emitted) by the various nuclei generally appears as sharp peaks in the spectrum.

The recorded NMR spectrum is plotted with the relative intensity of the RF absorption peaks on the vertical axis and the position of the absorption peaks on the horizontal axis. Peak positions (referred to as **chemical shift**) are plotted from high frequency (called downfield) to low frequency (called upfield) from *left to right*. NMR absorption peak positions are measured relative to a standard reference signal produced by **tetramethylsilane (TMS)** that is added to the analysis sample prior to performing the NMR experiment. The TMS absorption signal is arbitrarily assigned at 0 parts-per-million (ppm). Most NMR absorption signals are well downfield from the reference TMS signal. Figure 32.7 shows the basic layout of a ^{1}H and C NMR spectrum.

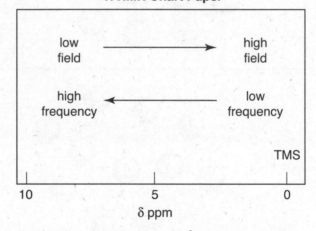

Figure 32.7. Basic format of a ^{1}H NMR spectrum

Chemical shift defines the position of NMR absorption signals and is measured in ppm according to the following equation:

$$\text{Chemical Shift} = \frac{\text{absorption peak position (in Hz) downfield from TMS}}{\text{frequuncy}(v) \text{ of the NMR spectrometer (in MHz)}}$$

It can be seen that the ratio of Hz/MHz (millions of Hz) leads to the parts-per-million unit system. The use of ppm units for the position of NMR absorption signals is called the δ scale.

Figure 32.8 shows a typical ^{1}H NMR spectrum for the compound ethanoic acid (commonly referred to as acetic acid, the active ingredient in vinegar).

The spectrum shows only two absorption peaks at ~2.1 ppm and 11.4 ppm. As indicated in the figure, the upfield peak (2.1 ppm) is due to energy absorbed by three protons attached to a carbon and the downfield peak arises from a proton attached to oxygen. Why do these absorptions appear in such different locations in the spectrum, and what basic compound characterization information does NMR spectroscopy provide?

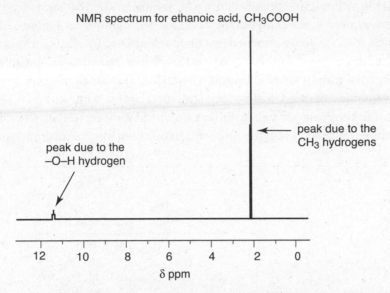

NMR spectrum for ethanoic acid, CH₃COOH

peak due to the —O–H hydrogen

peak due to the CH₃ hydrogens

δ ppm

Figure 32.8. ^{1}H NMR spectrum for ethanoic acid

NMR spectroscopic data provides the key information needed to map out the *carbon-hydrogen skeleton* of an organic compound. This carbon-hydrogen connectivity along with a little additional information (such as a molecular formula and possible functional groups present) is key to assigning a compound a complete structural formula. There are four key pieces of information that a proton NMR spectrum can provide:

ITEM 1: THE NUMBER OF ABSORPTION SIGNALS IN THE SPECTRUM

The number of signals that are observed in a ^{1}H NMR spectrum tells the analyst the number of different magnetic environments that the compound's protons (hydrogens) are experiencing. In other words, the number of signals seen in the spectrum indicates the number of magnetically nonequivalent protons in the molecule. If all the proton environments are exactly the same, then only one signal is observed, but this is relatively rare. In most cases, protons attached to different atoms in the compound have different magnetic characteristics. The example spectrum shown in Figure 32.8 shows two signals, which indicates two different "kinds" of protons are present in the ethanoic acid molecule.

ITEM 2: THE POSITION (CHEMICAL SHIFTS) OF THE SIGNALS IN THE SPECTRUM

Shielded and **deshielded** are terms used to categorize the different magnetic environments of protons. Shielded protons tend to have higher electron density around them and "feel" the external magnetic field of the spectrometer relatively less. These protons are usually, but not always, bonded to lower electronegative atoms, such as carbon, or are a significant distance from other more electronegative atoms, such as oxygen, nitrogen, or halogens in the compound. Signals associated with these kinds of protons are usually found upfield (closer to the TMS peak) at lower absorption frequencies. Deshielded protons have lower electron density around them and "feel" the external magnetic field of the spectrometer relatively more. They are usually either bonded directly to a significantly higher electronegative atom or near one in the molecule being analyzed. The signals from these protons appear downfield (farther away from the TMS peak) at high absorption frequencies.

Just by looking at a proton's chemical shift, it is possible to say what kind of atom it is either bonded to or very near in the compound's structure. For example, as Figure 32.8 shows, the absorption peak for a hydrogen attached to a highly electronegative oxygen atom in ethanoic acid is significantly further downfield (11.4 ppm) relative to the hydrogens attached to a much less electronegative carbon atom (2.1 ppm). The chemical shifts of protons in NMR spectra can provide valuable information about the structural connectivity and possible functional groups present in the molecule being studied. Figure 32.9 shows the relative chemical shift ranges for protons associated with the most commonly seen functional groups on the DAT.

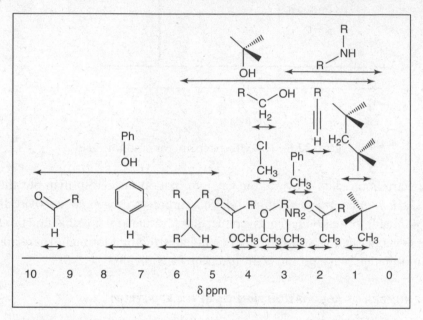

Figure 32.9. Relative chemical shifts of protons in ^{1}H NMR spectra

Note: Protons attached to alkene and arene functional groups are significantly less shielded (further downfield) than protons attached to most other types of carbon atoms. This is because of their interaction with the π bonding system in these functional groups.

ITEM 3: THE SPLITTING PATTERNS OF THE ABSORPTION SIGNALS

When a carbon with hydrogen substituents is bonded to one or more carbons with hydrogen substituents, the absorption (or emission) signals of the neighboring hydrogens are split into *groups of peaks*. The splitting is caused by the nonequivalent neighboring hydrogens' magnetic fields interacting with each other. If a hydrogen (or group of hydrogens) has no immediate neighbors, as can be seen in the spectrum of ethanoic acid (Figure 32.8), its absorption signal remains unsplit and it appears as a single peak or **singlet**. The hydrogens' magnetic fields in ethanoic acid are too far apart to "feel" each other. A detailed understanding of the signal splitting mechanism isn't needed to use information from splitting patterns presented in spectra encountered on the DAT.

In general, the number of peaks an absorption signal is split into is equal to the number of its neighboring hydrogens *plus one peak*. This is called the **"n + 1" splitting rule**, where *n* is the number of immediate neighboring hydrogen atoms the absorption signal in question interacts with. This splitting pattern leads to groups of peaks that are referred to as **doublets** (one neighboring hydrogen), **triplets** (two neighboring hydrogens), **quartets** (three neighboring hydrogens), **pentets** (four neighboring hydrogens), and **sextets** (five neighboring hydrogens). When a signal is split into more than six peaks, it is usually referred to as a **multiplet**.

Figure 32.10, the ^{1}H NMR spectrum of ethyl acetate, shows an example of the peak-splitting phenomenon described on page 316.

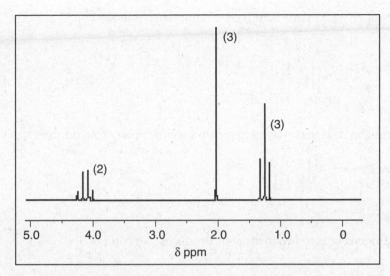

Figure 32.10. ^{1}H NMR spectrum for ethyl acetate

Note: The numbers in parentheses next to each peak group indicate the number of protons associated with each absorption signal in the spectrum.

Note the peak groups (from left to right) observed in the above spectrum—a quartet, a singlet, and a triplet. The annotated structural formula of ethyl acetate (Structure 70) shows how the molecule's protons interact with each other to produce this splitting pattern.

CH$_2$ next to carbon
with 3 attached Hs —
gives a quartet signal

CH$_3$ next to carbon
with no attached Hs —
gives a single peak

CH$_3$ next to carbon
with 2 attached Hs —
gives a triplet signal

(70)

As can be seen from the ethyl acetate example, the splitting patterns observed in NMR spectra can provide valuable information about the connectivity of the carbon skeleton and the number of hydrogens attached to each of the skeleton carbons. There are certain splitting patterns that are seen over and over again in ^{1}H NMR spectra. The ones most commonly seen in spectra encountered on the DAT are shown below. You should become familiar with these patterns and the structural information they provide.

1.

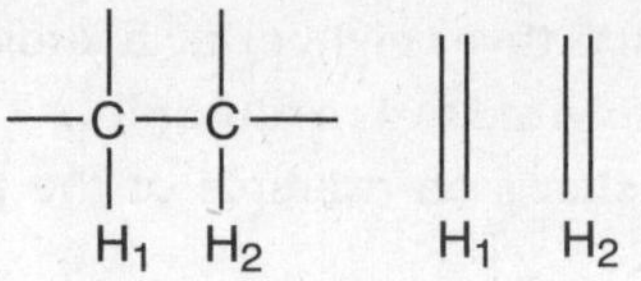

One hydrogen next to one hydrogen produces two doublets

2.

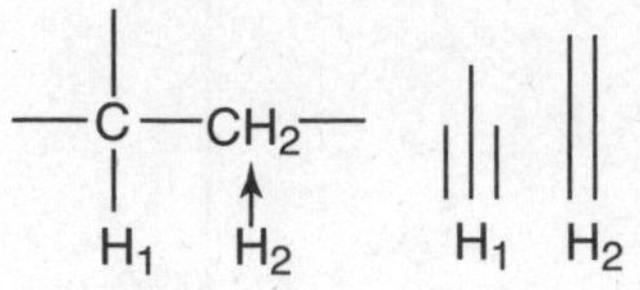

One hydrogen next to two hydrogens produces a triplet and a doublet

3.

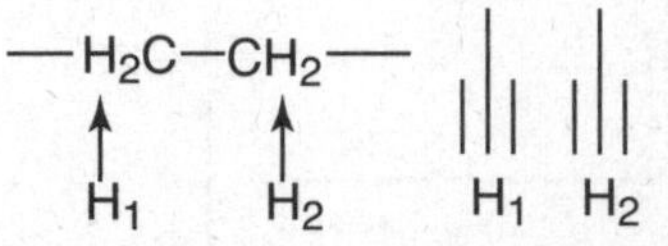

Two hydrogens next to two hydrogens produces two triplets

4.

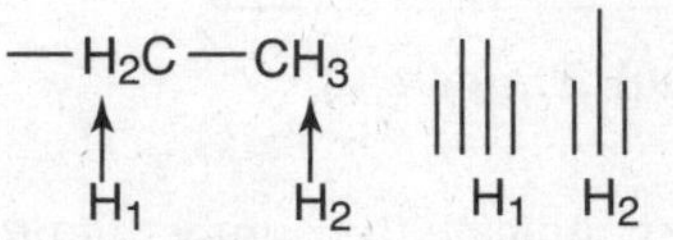

Two hydrogens next to three hydrogens produces a quartet and a triplet

5.

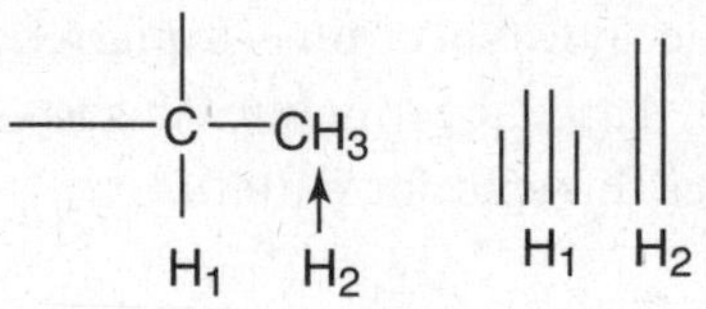

One hydrogen next to three hydrogens produces a quartet and a doublet

An additional important point about signal splitting has to do with hydrogens attached to elements significantly more electronegative than carbon. Generally, when protons are attached to atoms such as oxygen or nitrogen *their absorption signals are not split*. These proton signals appear as **singlets**, even if they are next to a carbon with hydrogen. The reason these proton signals are not split is rather complex. Being aware of this exception is important for the DAT, but a complete understanding of the mechanism is not.

ITEM 4: THE RELATIVE SIZE OF PROTON ABSORPTION SIGNALS

The relative area under the absorption signal (this includes all the peaks associated with the signal) in a ^1H NMR spectrum provides data about the relative ratios of the different kinds of protons present in the compound being analyzed. The relative area under each peak is measured in the form of an integral line (also called an integral trace), which is computer generated. The integral line is superimposed on top of the NMR spectrum and crosses over all the peak groups in steps from left to right. The height and number of peaks in a peak group correspond to the number of protons with the same approximate chemical shift. The heights of the steps of the integral trace are proportional to the area under the peak groups. Figure 32.11 shows an example ¹H NMR spectrum of the compound propanoic acid that includes the integrator trace. The spectrum shows three different peak groups indicating three different kinds of protons are present in the compound.

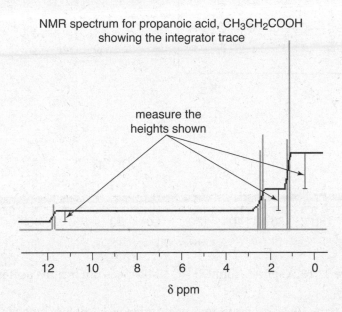

Figure 32.11. ¹H NMR spectrum of propanoic acid with signal integration

One can see from the relative heights of the bars in the figure that the ratios of the different kinds of protons (from left to right) in propanoic acid are 1:2:3. In this particular case, this ratio represents the *actual* number of different kinds of protons in the molecule: the –OOH group (1 proton), the –CH$_2$– group (2 protons), and the –CH$_3$ group (3 protons). This is often, but not always, the case. Sometimes the integral areas only provide the *relative* ratios of different kinds of protons in a compound.

CARBON (¹³C) NMR

As mentioned earlier, just as the nuclei of hydrogen atoms spin, so do the nuclei of the carbon-13 isotope atoms—this allows their transitions between parallel and antiparallel states relative to an external magnetic field to be detected and recorded.

The most valuable information provided by ¹³C NMR spectra is the number of magnetically unique carbon atoms in a compound. This can provide critical information about the carbon atom skeletal structure of a molecule. There is generally no coupled splitting between adjacent carbon atoms, but attached hydrogen atoms *do* split carbon atom signals. This phenomenon, as with ¹H NMR, can provide useful structural information, but it can also make coupled-splitting spectra complicated, so ¹³C NMR spectra are usually run in a *spin-decoupled* mode. This produces a spectrum of singlets where each peak represents a magnetically unique type of carbon.

A significant difference between ¹H NMR and ¹³C NMR spectra is the range of the chemical shifts of proton nuclei signals relative to carbon nuclei signals. The carbon range is much larger, running from the zero ppm at the TMS reference signal (upfield) to greater than 200 ppm downfield. A carbon spectrum can easily be distinguished from a proton spectrum by simply looking at the range of the peak shifts—in many cases it also makes carbon spectra easier to interpret due to greater spaces between signals. Figure 32.12 is an example ^{13}C NMR spectrum of the compound ethyl acetate.

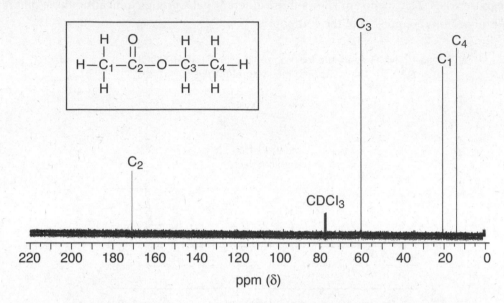

Figure 32.12. A spin-decoupled ^{13}C NMR spectrum of ethyl acetate

As can be seen in the above example, the spectrum consists of four singlet peaks—one for each of the unique carbon signals in the carbon backbone of the compound (the slightly split peak at ~77 ppm is from the deuterated chloroform solvent used to dilute the sample). A carbon signal's shift is related to its specific magnetic environment. A summary table (Table 32.2) of carbon nuclei shifts is provided below.

Table 32.2. Summary List of ^{13}C NMR Signal Chemical Shifts

Alkyl C Shifts	Approx. Position (ppm)	Hetero Atom C Shifts	Approx. Position (ppm)
R–CH$_3$	8–35	C–O	50–80
R2–CH$_2$	15–50	C–N	40–60
R3–CH	20–60	C–Cl	35–80
R4C	30–40	C–Br	25–65
Unsat. C Shifts		**Carbonyl C Shifts**	
≡C–	65–85	Amide C	165–175
=C–	100–150	Ester C	165–175
⬡–C	110–170	Carboxylic acid C	175–185
		Aldehyde C	190–200
		Ketone C	200–220

EXERCISE 38

Directions: Using the molecular formula and spectral data provided below, assign a plausible structural formula to this compound. The tabulated ^{13}C NMR data shows the chemical shift (in ppm relative to TMS) of each magnetically unique carbon in the molecule. (Answer is on page 353.)

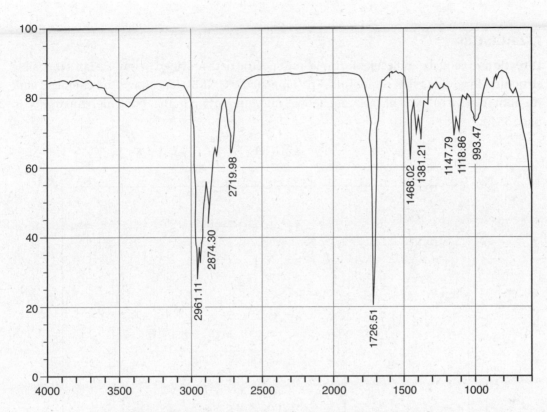

Figure 32.12. IR spectrum of the unknown compound

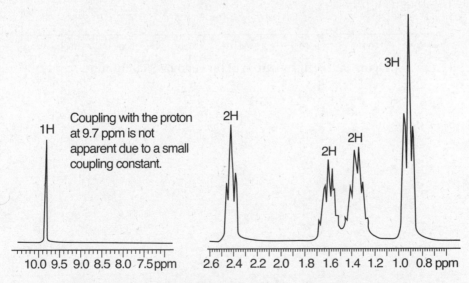

Figure 32.13. ^{1}H NMR spectrum of the unknown compound

Decoupled ^{13}C NMR data for the unknown compound

Peak	ppm
1	13.83
2	22.40
3	24.28
4	43.69
5	202.83

EXERCISE 39

Directions: Using the molecular formula and spectral data provided below, assign a plausible structural formula to this compound. The tabulated ^{13}C NMR data shows the chemical shift (in ppm relative to TMS) of each magnetically unique carbon in the molecule. (Answer is on page 354.)

$$C_6H_{14}O$$

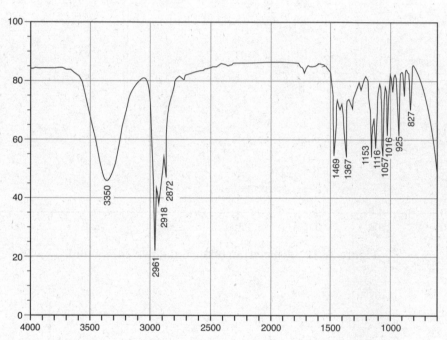

Figure 32.14. IR spectrum of the unknown compound

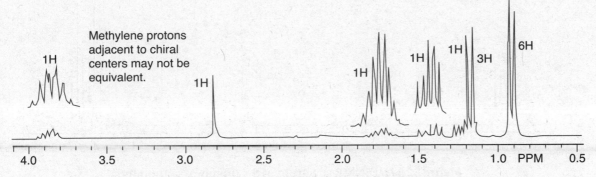

Figure 32.15. ^{1}H NMR spectrum of the unknown compound

Decoupled ^{13}C NMR data for the unknown compound

Peak	ppm
1	22.45
2	23.16
3	23.92
4	24.85
5	48.70
6	65.99

EXERCISE 40

Directions: Using the molecular formula and spectral data provided below, assign a plausible structural formula to this compound. The tabulated ^{13}C NMR data shows the chemical shift (in ppm relative to TMS) of each magnetically unique carbon in the molecule. (Answer is on page 354.)

$$C_5H_{10}O_2$$

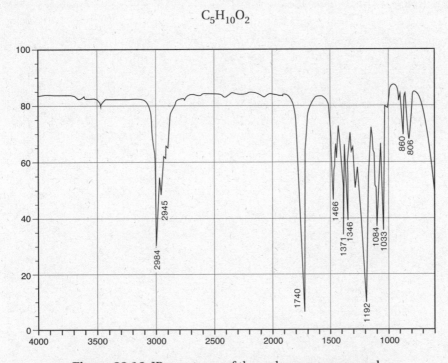

Figure 32.16. IR spectrum of the unknown compound

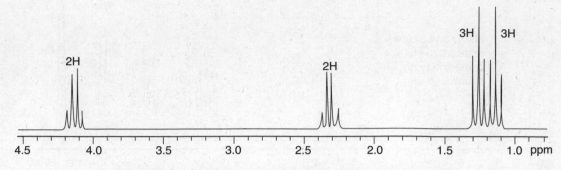

Figure 32.17. ^{1}H NMR spectrum of the unknown compound

Decoupled ^{13}C NMR data for the unknown compound

Peak	ppm
1	9.19
2	14.32
3	27.71
4	60.26
5	174.40

Separation and Purification Techniques

33

Before a compound can be fully characterized, used in a synthesis scheme, tested in a product or clinical trial, or patented, it must meet certain purity standards. Depending on the application, these standards may require an extremely pure substance (>99.9%) or something only relatively pure (~90.%). Regardless of the purity standard, organic chemists spend considerable time both devising and executing purification processes. All of these procedures and new ones that are constantly being developed depend on what is sometimes called "separation science"—the separation of the desired compound from the rest of the matrix. Depending on the source of the compound (a natural product from a plant or an animal or a synthetic compound designed and prepared by a chemist), its purification may require only a simple one-step procedure or for the unlucky chemist a much more sophisticated, time-consuming, and expensive technique.

Some of the most common separation processes referred to on the DAT are:

- Extraction
- Distillation (several kinds)
- Sublimation
- Recrystallization
- Filtration (several kinds)
- Chromatography

EXTRACTION

Extraction is the selective partitioning of a desired substance into a phase from which it can be easily removed. The process separates the substance from other components in the matrix and thus to some extent, depending on the situation, purifies it. There are several possible phase combinations for an extraction process (solid-liquid, liquid-liquid, gas-liquid, etc.), but by far the most common procedure used to isolate organic compounds is **liquid-liquid** extraction. You may recall performing this procedure numerous times in your organic chemistry laboratory classes.

The most critical factor in conducting a liquid-liquid extraction is the selection of the two liquid phases. In most cases, one liquid will be *water* and the other some low-boiling relatively nonpolar *organic solvent*, but the most important criterion for the procedure is that the two liquids must be **immiscible** (they mostly form separate layers, like oil and water, in the extraction vessel and can't dissolve into each other). Some other important criteria for liquids used in an extraction are:

- Neither liquid can react in a chemically irreversible way with the desired solute (the compound the chemist is trying to isolate).
- The extracting liquid added to the compound solution must have a higher affinity for the solute than the solvent it is dissolved in. The higher the affinity (referred to as the *partition coefficient*) of the extracting liquid the better.
- Once the solute has been partitioned into the higher affinity liquid (the extracting solvent), it must be relatively easy to remove the liquid (say, for example, by evaporation).

Liquid-liquid extractions are carried out using a special piece of laboratory glassware called a **separatory funnel**. These specially shaped funnels come in all sizes and have a ground glass/Teflon stopcock and ground glass/Teflon stopper. Figure 33.1 shows an example of this type of funnel as it appears in a laboratory setting.

> It may be recalled that the terms **miscible** and **immiscible** are used to refer to the solubility characteristics of a liquid in another liquid. *Miscible* means the two liquids are soluble in each other and form a single phase, like water and an alcohol. *Immiscible* means the two liquids are insoluble in each other and form two phases, like oil and water.

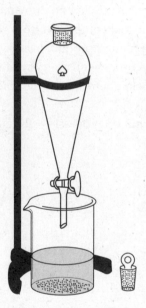

Figure 33.1. Standard separatory funnel supported on a ring stand

Note: The dark organic phase is being drained into a beaker leaving the colorless aqueous phase in the funnel. The ground glass stopper is used to seal the funnel while the contents are being shaken.

The use of a separatory funnel for extractions is straightforward. The user places the compound solution in the funnel and then adds an extracting solvent, making sure the two liquids form separate layers. Next, the funnel is sealed with a stopper (see Figure 33.1) and shaken for a period of time to allow the two liquid phases to comingle. After shaking, the liquid phases are allowed to separate. Finally the extracting liquid, which now hopefully contains the desired compound, is drained from the funnel and saved. Be careful to save the correct layer, and it's a good idea to save both layers until you are positive about which one has the product. Depending on the organic solvent used, the aqueous phase may be on the top (organic phase is more dense) or on the bottom (organic phase is less dense). More than one extraction with the extracting solvent is usually performed to make sure all the solute (desired compound) has been removed from the original solution. The extraction volumes are combined and the solvent is usually evaporated, leaving the isolated compound.

Separation of weak organic acids and bases from a reaction matrix is often accomplished by using liquid-liquid extraction. This process takes advantage of the fact that both of these classes of compounds can often be converted to water-soluble salts.

Figure 33.2 shows a flow chart of a procedure used to separate a carboxylic acid (in this case benzoic acid) from a neutral compound (naphthalene) by extracting (shaking in a separatory funnel) the organic phase (diethyl ether) with a dilute aqueous solution of sodium hydroxide. The details of carboxylic acid properties and reactions are covered under the *Oxygen-Containing Compounds* topic in this review.

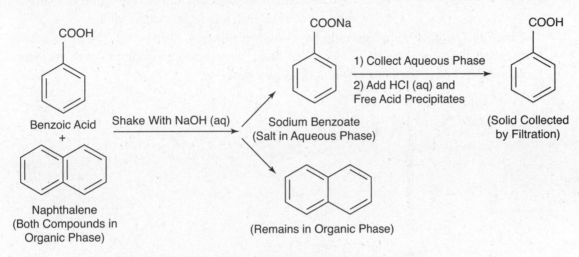

Figure 33.2. Separation of benzoic acid from naphthalene by aqueous sodium hydroxide extraction

As seen in the figure, benzoic acid reacts with aqueous sodium hydroxide (while being shaken in a separatory funnel) and is converted into the water-soluble salt, sodium benzoate. This salt migrates into the aqueous phase as the extraction procedure is conducted. The neutral naphthalene is unchanged and remains in the organic phase. The aqueous phase containing the sodium benzoate is collected and acidified to give a precipitate of the free benzoic acid, which is collected by filtration. A very similar scheme can be used to separate a weak organic base, such as an amine from a neutral compound, except that the amine is shaken with an aqueous solution of an acid (such as hydrochloric acid). The amine reacts with the acid to form a soluble salt, which as in the above example migrates into the aqueous phase. The free amine is isolated by adding a base to the collected aqueous phase.

An organic acid and organic base can also be separated from each other using the above principles. For practice, you may wish to devise a scheme for carrying out such a separation.

DISTILLATION

When separation of two or more *miscible* liquids from each other is required, some form of **distillation** is usually used. You may recall that distillation involves preferentially vaporizing a liquid (or liquids) with a high vapor pressure and then condensing the vapor back to a liquid so that it can be collected. Liquids with low boiling points vaporize at lower temperatures than those with high boiling points. The larger the difference between the liquids' boiling points, the easier they are to separate by this procedure. Depending on the difference of the volatilities of the liquids that require separation, different forms of distillation are used.

Simple Distillation

This technique is used to separate relatively low-boiling (<150°C) liquids that have large differences in boiling points. From experience, for this process to achieve a good separation between the two liquids, there must be at least a 30°C difference in their boiling points. This procedure can also be used to separate a liquid from nonvolatile impurities such as soluble salts and high molecular weight solutes.

Figure 33.3 shows a complete setup for a simple distillation. Note how all the components (distillation flask—also called still pot, still head, thermometer, condenser, and receiving flask) are attached to each other by ground glass joints.

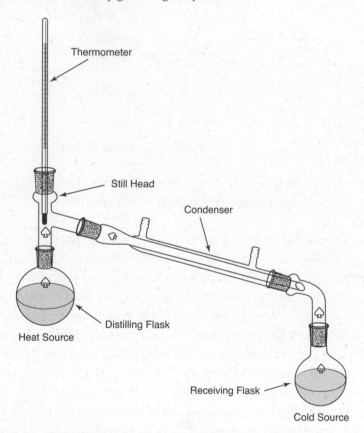

Figure 33.3. Glassware setup for a laboratory-scale simple distillation

The liquids to be separated are placed in the distilling flask and heated. When the lower boiling liquid's boiling point is reached, its vapors begin to travel through the still head until they reach the condenser (which is usually cooled by tap water) where its cold surface recondenses them into a liquid. The liquid flows down the angled condenser by gravity, eventually dripping into the receiving flask (usually cooled in an ice bath). As long as the boiling temperature of the liquid, as verified by the thermometer, remains relatively constant, it can be assumed that the liquid being collected is pure.

Vacuum Distillation

This procedure is very similar to simple distillation, but it is specifically used for separation of liquids that boil above 150°C. Under ambient conditions, such liquids must be heated to high temperatures before they begin to vaporize. In many cases, they are heat sensitive, and instead of vaporizing, they decompose before they begin to boil. If the pressure is lowered by a vacuum source, the liquids' vapor pressures increase, and they boil at lower temperatures. The lower the pressure, the lower they boil. Lower boiling points can prevent heat-induced decomposition. This type of distillation, like simple distillation, requires a boiling point difference between the liquids being separated of at least 30°C.

The only difference in the glassware setup for this type of still is the addition of a side-arm connector to the adaptor between the condenser and the receiving flask (see Figure 32.3). Figure 32.4 shows an example of this type of vacuum adaptor.

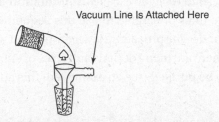

Figure 32.4. Vacuum adaptor for low-pressure distillations

Fractional Distillations

This type of distillation can separate liquids with boiling points that are closer to each other than 30°C. Sophisticated setups can separate liquids that boil as close to each other as a couple of degrees. For this procedure, the basic still remains the same, except a **fractionating column** is placed between the still head and the distilling flask. This setup is designed to force the vapor mixture from the distilling flask to condense and revaporize over and over again as it rises through the fractionating column. Each condensing-revaporizing cycle results in a slight enrichment in the proportion of the lower boiling liquid in the vapor phase. If the column is efficient, by the time the vapor mixture reaches its top, it is composed almost exclusively of the lower boiling component. Thus the close boiling liquids are separated from each other. Figure 33.5 shows an example of a fractionating column used for fractional distillations.

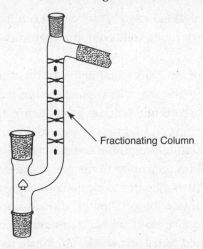

Figure 33.5. A fractionating column used for fractional distillations

There are a number of different kinds of fractionating columns. The one shown in Figure 33.5 has small glass protrusions, which extend from the wall of the column into the interior. These tiny glass "fingers" serve as condensing sites as the vapor mixture rises through the column. Other fractionating columns are simple glass tubes that have been filled with high surface area materials such as copper wool, glass beads, or even coarse glass wool. The components of the mixture being distilled that have relatively *narrow*-boiling ranges (a maximum of one or two degrees) are collected using a different receiving flask for each one. These different collections are called **fractions**. Although the procedure is a little tricky, it is also possible to perform a **fractional vacuum** distillation to separate high-boiling liquids with boiling points that are close to each other.

SUBLIMATION

The process of converting a solid to a gas is called **sublimation** and from a gas to a solid is called **deposition**. It is sometimes preferable to use this sequence of phase changes for the purification of solid compounds. The procedure is accomplished with a special piece of glassware called a **sublimator**. There are many designs and sizes of sublimators depending on the type and quantity of solid to be purified (see an example of this apparatus in Figure 33.6).

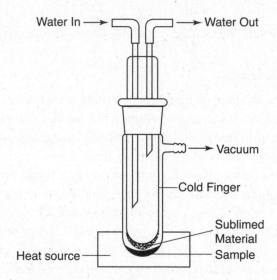

Figure 33.6. Example of a simple sublimator
for performing solid compound purifications

When the vapor pressure of a solid is equal to the ambient pressure, it will begin to sublime, just as a liquid begins to boil when its vapor pressure reaches ambient pressure. The transformation is very endothermic and requires a significant amount of energy. The conditions required for the phase change, solid to gas, are usually low pressure and heat applied directly to the sample. As the crude compound is carefully heated (it must *not* be allowed to melt) under vacuum, the solid is converted to the gas phase one molecular layer at a time. The gas phase of the sample then migrates to a cold surface (usually some kind of glass projection called a "cold finger" inside the sublimator) directly above the solid sample where it is deposited as a *purified* solid. The "cold finger's" temperature can be adjusted as needed by varying the cooling media (cold water or a low-temperature recirculating cooling bath—for lower temperatures the finger can be filled with a dry ice/acetone slurry).

As the process occurs, *volatile* impurities are removed by the vacuum system and *non-volatile* impurities remain in the solid phase in the bottom of the sublimator. To recover the purified sample, the sublimator is first allowed to cool (the cold finger should also be allowed to reach ambient temperature to prevent any moisture condensation) and then carefully opened to the atmosphere (or an inert gas) to reach ambient pressure. The cold finger is then removed from the top of the system and the purified solid sample collected. Great care must be taken when removing the deposition "finger" so that none of the purified compound falls back into the bottom of the sublimator where it may become contaminated. This technique is often the best way to purify solid compounds with high melting points.

RECRYSTALLIZATION AND FILTRATION

An easy and effective way to purify solid organic compounds is to **recrystallize** them. This separation process relies on the fact that *as the temperature of a solvent increases, the solubility of a solute increases.* Likewise, as the temperature of a solvent decreases, the solubility of a solute decreases.

Purification by recrystallization involves taking an impure (or "crude") solid compound, dispersing it in a cold or room-temperature solvent contained in a beaker, and then heating the mixture until a solution is formed. The hot solution is then sometimes poured through filter paper (referred to as a *hot filtration*) to remove any insoluble impurities. The resulting clear solution can be further heated if necessary to make sure it remains completely homogeneous. Next, the beaker is covered/insolated and the hot solution allowed to very slowly cool to room temperature. As the solution cools, the solubility of the compound being purified decreases and at some point, assuming too much solvent wasn't used, begins to fall out of solution as a pure crystalline solid. In general the slower the solution cools, the larger the resulting crystals. Large crystals of the compound are desirable because they are easier to collect and often higher in purity. In most cases the impurities, which were a minor portion of the original crude compound, remain in solution. Thus the compound is purified by selective solubility—the pure compound being less soluble and the impurities being more soluble. Choosing the correct recrystallizing solvent is critical for achieving this balance. In order to maximize the recovery of the "recrystallized" compound, the mixture is usually cooled below room temperature using an ice bath or other cold source. This further reduces the solubility of the compound, which facilitates additional crystal formation. Once crystallization is deemed complete, the crystals are typically collected by either **gravity** or **vacuum filtration**.

Figure 33.7 shows what the cooled recrystallized compound might look like prior to filtration.

TIP

There are a few exceptions to this rule involving ionic compounds, but it almost always holds true for organic compounds.

TIP

These two types of filtration are discussed in more detail later on in this section.

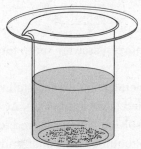

Figure 33.7. Recrystallized compound ready for collection

Note: The beaker is covered with a watch glass to provide insulation, which facilitates slower cooling of the solution—note the newly formed crystals on the bottom of the beaker.

As indicated earlier, the most important factor in achieving a good recrystallization result is solvent selection. The balance between the compound's solubility in the hot solvent and its solubility at lower temperatures has to be just right. Often, as with chromatography separations (discussed at the end of this section), a solvent system composed of two or more solvents is used. The most common systems involve dissolving the compound to be purified in a fairly polar solvent first and then adding small amounts of a nonpolar solvent until the compound just begins to come out of solution. This tipping point is apparent when the mixture begins to become slightly cloudy. Next, the mixture is heated until completely clear and a slow cooling process started. The reverse system where the dissolving solvent is nonpolar and small amounts of a polar solvent are added is also commonly employed.

The second most important factor is deciding how *much* of the solvent system to use. Usually less is better. One of the most common errors novice recrystallizers make is using too much solvent. The first part of the process works in that the compound to be purified completely dissolves, but no matter how long or low the solution is cooled, no crystals ever form. Reheating the mixture and boiling off some of the excess solvent can correct this oversight, but this wastes solvent and can even be hazardous if the solvent is extremely flammable. A better approach is to use less solvent and more heat (without boiling) and add a little more solvent as needed to completely dissolve the crude compound.

Pure compound crystals formed during recrystallization are typically collected by filtration. If they aren't extremely fine, vacuum filtration is the best choice. This approach uses a Buchner funnel and filtration flask. There are a number of different designs for these pieces of equipment (which we won't go into), but the setup must have a side-arm connector which can be attached to a vacuum source—thus the term "vacuum" filtration. Figure 33.8 shows an all-glass vacuum filtration system.

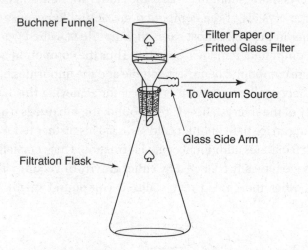

Figure 33.8. Laboratory glassware setup for vacuum filtration

The compound crystals are suspended in the recrystallization solvent and poured into the Buchner funnel and vacuum applied (see Figure 33.8). As the pressure in the filtration flask is lowered by the vacuum source, solvent (often referred to as the **filtrate**) is pulled through the porous Buchner funnel (some require filter paper and others have a fritted glass filter), leaving behind the solid crystals. The crystals are usually washed with pure cold solvent to remove any surface impurities. Here again, it is almost always better to be conservative with the amount of solvent used to wash the crystals. Too much solvent will often dissolve some of the desired compound lowering the recovery yield.

If the crystals are very small, like a fine powder, the pores of the filter paper or fritted glass filter, depending on the type of Buchner funnel being used, may become clogged when vacuum is applied. In this situation, it is best to use *gravity filtration*, which uses large pieces of filter paper with a lot of surface area that are less prone to be clogged. The folded or fluted filter paper is inserted into a regular glass funnel. As the name implies, the solvent slowly flows through the filter paper under gravity into a receiving flask, leaving the crystals behind. Figure 33.9 shows the glassware for this simple setup. As with vacuum filtration, the collected compound crystals should be washed with cold solvent and allowed to dry as the final step.

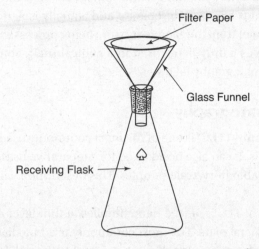

Figure 33.9. Glassware setup for gravity filtration

CHROMATOGRAPHY

The most advanced methodology currently available for separating mixtures of substances is a large collection of techniques referred to as **chromatography**.

This separation process is used on a daily basis in laboratory and industrial settings around the world. There are literally hundreds if not thousands of different kinds of chromatography with entire journals devoted to the use and development of new methods. This shouldn't be intimidating, because regardless of the variety and complexity of the various chromatographic methods, they all share two key features.

To affect the separation process, a sample (usually a mixture of compounds) is introduced to what is referred to as a **stationary phase**. The stationary phase can take many forms depending on the type of chromatography method, but it is a media of some type (e.g., paper, silica gel, a viscous oil, etc.) for which the components of the sample mixture have an affinity— to some degree they all stick to it. The sample mixture clinging to the stationary phase is exposed to a **mobile phase**, usually a liquid or a gas. The mobile phase moves through the stationary phase carrying the sample components with it. This process is termed **elution**. Depending on the affinity (how hard it sticks) of each component for the stationary phase, it moves at a different rate as the mobile phase carries it along. The *lower* the component's affinity for the stationary phase, the *faster* it moves as it is carried by the mobile phase. The *higher* the component's affinity, the *slower* it moves. The key separation mechanism that allows the process to work is that all the components of the sample mixture have *slightly different affinities* for the stationary phase. Thus, over time as the mobile phase moves through the stationary phase, the mixture components are separated because they all move at different rates.

TIP

The term *chromatography* literally means "graph of colors" because its earliest use by German chemists was to separate/ isolate plant pigments.

Depending on the specific type of chromatography, factors that affect the mechanism described on page 333 can be complex, but the basic principles of the sample interacting with a stationary and mobile phase to achieve separation are the same. Based on the desired applications there are generally two categories of chromatography:

- Those that are used for *analytical* analysis, and
- Those that are used for *preparative* purposes.

The analytical methods are used to provide data about the sample mixture, such as the number and relative amounts of its components and sometimes even the identity of the components. Preparative methods are used to separate and actually isolate components (in some cases on an industrial scale) from the sample mixture being processed so their properties can be further studied (such as a drug being used in a clinical trial). Some examples of each of these categories of chromatography follow.

Analytical Chromatography

Thin-layer chromatography (TLC) is one of the most commonly used types of chromatography for analytical analysis. It can also be adapted for preparative uses, but it is generally limited to producing small laboratory-scale samples. This description will focus on its analytical application.

The stationary phase of TLC is, as the name implies, a thin layer of media that is coated onto a glass, plastic, or metal plate. The most commonly used medias are silica gel and alumina. These are highly polar materials and result in a "polar phase" TLC plate. The more polar an analite, the more strongly it interacts with the polar phase on the plate and the slower it moves with the system's mobile phase. There are other media that are also used to prepare nonpolar or "reverse phase" TLC plates, but these are not as commonly used for organic compound separations. The mobile phase for this technique is a solvent system—usually a mixture of two or more slightly polar and nonpolar organic solvents.

The sample mixture (usually in solution phase) is placed near the bottom of the TLC plate (called the **origin**) as a small curricular spot using a very thin glass capillary tube (see Figure 33.10 for an example of a TLC plate with sample spots).

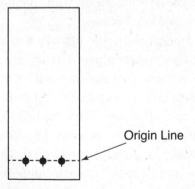

Figure 33.10. TLC plate with sample spots on origin line

The plate is allowed to dry and is then put into a sealed elution chamber containing a small amount of the solvent system (a few millimeters in the bottom of the container). As soon as the plate (the stationary phase) makes contact with the solvent (the mobile phase) at the bottom of the chamber, it begins to move up the plate by capillary action. A faint line that is formed by the moving solvent is referred to as the **solvent front**. As the solvent moves up the plate, the sample mixture components begin to separate (based on their affinity for the plate media) into individual spots. Figure 33.11 shows a simulated "time-lapse" view of this process. In this example, the sample mixture contains three different components (three separate spots can be seen on the plate).

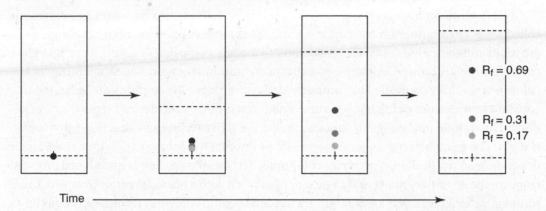

Figure 33.11. Simulated time-lapse view of the solvent front moving up a TLC plate

Note: The lower dotted line represents the sample *origin* line and the upper dotted line the *solvent front*. Observe how the solvent front moves up the plate and the sample component spots get more separated over time.

When the solvent front nears the top of the TLC plate, it is removed from the elution chamber, the position of the front marked (a pencil should be used), and the solvent allowed to evaporate. There are a number of ways to visualize the component spots. Sometimes they absorb light in the visible part of the spectrum and they appear colored to the human eye, making them easy to see. More often, they absorb in the UV region of the spectrum and can't be seen. To visualize these spots, the plate is irradiated with UV radiation from a "black light" which makes them glow violet or blue-violet.

If desired, the position of the component spots can be quantified using **retention factor** (R_f) calculations where:

$$R_f = \frac{\text{Distance Spot Moved from the Origin}}{\text{Distance Solvent Front Moved from the Origin}}$$

Distances used to calculate R_fs are usually measured in centimeters; thus, these length units cancel in the calculation and R_fs are unit-less. It should be noted that R_f values are always less than or equal to *one* ($R_f \leq 1$). You can see how an R_f greater than one wouldn't make sense because this would require one of the component spots to "jump" over the solvent front, which is carrying it. There are tabulated R_f values for specific compounds in reference books that can be compared to those calculated for lab experiments. This may allow the identification of some sample components, but the comparison is only valid if the reference R_fs and the experiment R_fs were obtained under identical experimental conditions. The TLC

A typical TLC plate is between 10 and 15 cm in length, and it can take 15 to 20 minutes for the solvent front to reach near the top of the plate. Theoretically, the longer the plate, the greater the possible separation between the sample mixture components spots, but there are practical considerations that limit the length of TLC plates.

plate to the far right in Figure 33.11 shows the R_fs (from bottom to top of plate R_fs = 0.17, 0.31, and 0.69) for the component spots for the simulated sample mixture elution.

Other common types of chromatography used for analytical analysis include **paper chromatography** and **gas-liquid chromatography (GLC)**. Paper chromatography is very similar to, but less effective than, TLC. Instead of a media-coated plate, a strip of heavy porous paper is used for the stationary phase. A solvent system moves up the paper by capillary action, separating the components of the sample similar to TLC.

GLC is a more sophisticated and sensitive procedure that involves the use of an instrument called a **gas chromatogram (GC)**. In this case, the stationary phase is often (although there are many different kinds) a viscous silicon oil that coats the inside of a long, very thin glass column, which is housed inside the gas chromatogram instrument. The temperature of the column is carefully controlled by computer-defined settings. The column can be heated to a constant temperature or the temperature varied depending on the desired separation conditions. The mobile phase for this process, unlike the other techniques described previously, is a *gas*. The gas, often helium or nitrogen, flows through the column at various rates, again depending on the desired experiment conditions. The sample mixture is introduced onto the column (the stationary phase) either neat or in solution with a heated syringe. Only very small samples (microgram levels are enough) are needed for good analytical results. As the gas flows through the heated column, it forces the vaporized sample mixture into contact with the oil coating on the interior of the column. Different components of the mixture have different affinities for the oil coating (as well as different boiling points) and move though the column at different rates, resulting in separation. As the mixture components exit the column, they are detected by various types of sensors depending on the instrument setup. Once detected, the components appear as peaks of varying heights on a computer screen. The chromatogram gives information about not only the *number of components* in the mixture but also the relative *amount* of each. A significant limitation of this type of chromatography is that the sample components must be fairly volatile to make it through the instrument column. High molecular weight compounds cannot generally be analyzed by this procedure because they decompose prior to vaporizing. Figure 33.12 shows a schematic of a very basic instrument used for GLC experiments.

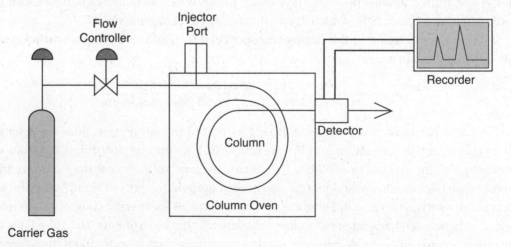

Figure 33.12. Schematic of a simple gas chromatograph used for GLC experiments

Preparative Chromatography

Most forms of preparative chromatography involve the use of media-packed columns. As with other forms of chromatography, there is a myriad of different kinds of media that can serve as the stationary phase, but the most commonly used for organic compounds are silica gel and alumina. As with TLC, these media produce a very polar stationary phase.

In its simplest form, a long glass or quartz column with one open end and a stopcock valve with a fritted glass filter (a plug of glass wool can also be used to retain the packing media) at the other end is packed with media. Figure 33.13 shows an example of such a column.

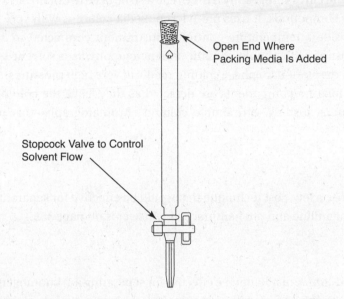

Open End Where
Packing Media Is Added

Stopcock Valve to Control
Solvent Flow

Figure 33.13. Glass/quartz column used for holding packing media

The packing process can be done either dry or wet (the column is first filled with a solvent and then the media added) depending on the type of media being used. A few centimeters of sand are usually added to the top of the media column to stabilize it. Following packing, the stopcock is opened and a solvent system (the mobile phase) is carefully added to the top of the column until it is freely flowing out the open valve at the bottom. Once a few volumes of solvent have flowed through the column, the solvent level is allowed to drop until it is just below the sand layer at the top of the column and the stopcock is closed. The column can't be allowed to run dry because this can cause the tightly packed media to "crack" and create fissures. This can greatly degrade the column's separation ability. The last step of the setup is to introduce the sample mixture to be separated onto the sand layer at the top of the column. This must be done carefully so as not to disturb the packed media. Typically, if the sample is a liquid, it is placed on the sand neat. If it is a solid, a very concentrated solution can be used. Once the sample has settled a centimeter or so into the sand, the stopcock is opened and small amounts of the solvent system are carefully added until the column is full. Some columns have a glass bulb, which can be attached to the top of the column, so it can hold large volumes of solvent; otherwise, the user must continually add new solvent and never let the level drop below the sand.

The separation process occurs as the solvent system (the mobile phase) flows through the tightly packed media (the stationary phase) carrying the sample mixture. It is sometimes possible to see bands of different colors form, corresponding to different components of the mixture. Being able to see colored bands, as with colored spots for TLC, is the exception. If a quartz column is employed, it will allow UV radiation to pass and violet glowing bands can be seen if the lab is darkened and the column is illuminated with a powerful black light. Either way, as the component bands reach the bottom of the column, they flow out and are collected as *solution fractions* (sample components dissolved in the mobile phase). After all the desired fractions are collected, the solvent is evaporated from each one to yield a pure sample of each component. Pure multi-gram or even larger quantities of each component can be obtained this way.

An automated type of packed column chromatography similar to GLC called **high-performance liquid chromatography (HPLC)** can also be used to obtain fairly large quantities of hard-to-purify compounds. It uses pre-packed media columns with very high separation ability housed inside a temperature-controlled instrument connected to a computer. The mobile phase, just as with simple column chromatography, is a solvent system, which is pumped through the stationary phase column media at very high pressures.

The various mixture components are detected as they leave the column and collected as solution fractions just as with simple column chromatograph—this process is often automated.

TIP

At one time, this technique was referred to as *high-pressure liquid chromatography*, but the term isn't used much anymore.

EXERCISE 41

Directions: Propose a low-cost technique that would be effective for separating a large quantity of a mixture of aniline and phenanthracene. (Answer is on page 355.)

EXERCISE 42

Directions: Would *simple* distillation be effective for separating a 1:1 homogeneous mixture of benzene and ethyl acetate? (You will need to look up the boiling points of these compounds.) (Answer is on page 355.)

Answers to Practice Exercises

34

EXERCISE 1 (PAGE 206)

1.

2.

3.

1.

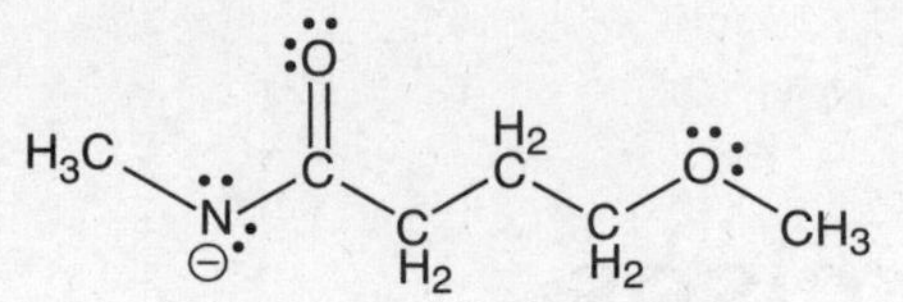

2.

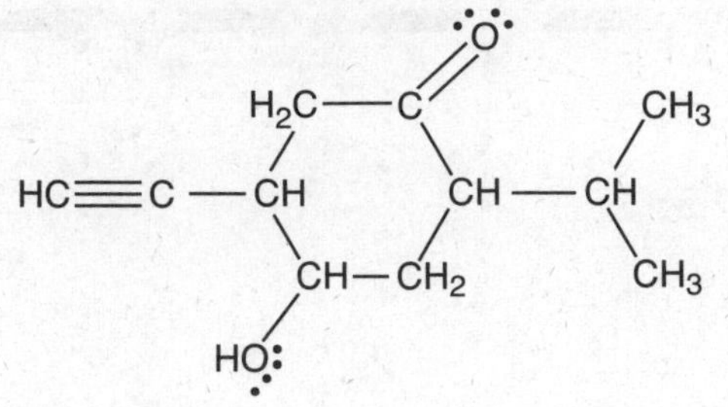

3.

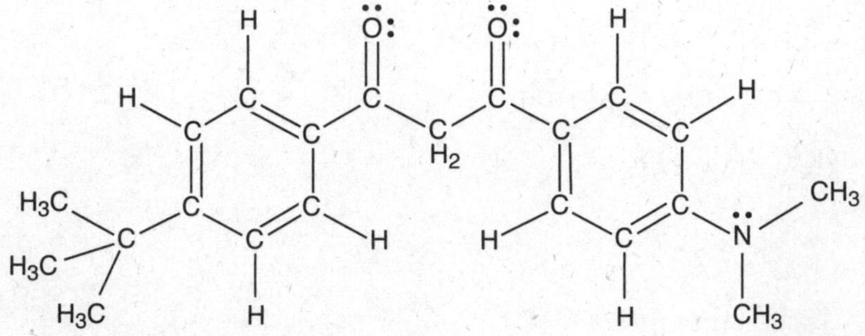

EXERCISE 3 (PAGE 210)

1.

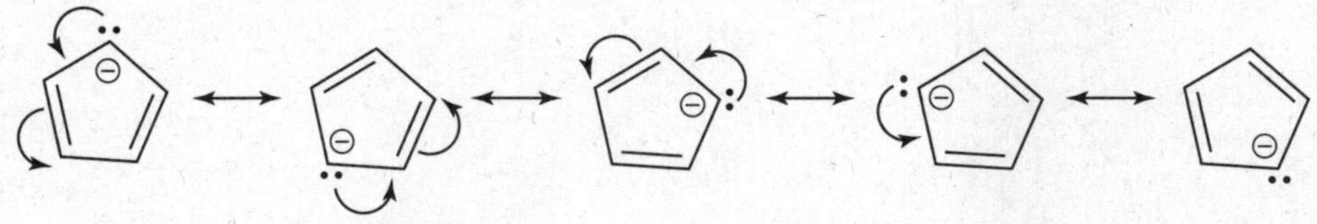

2.

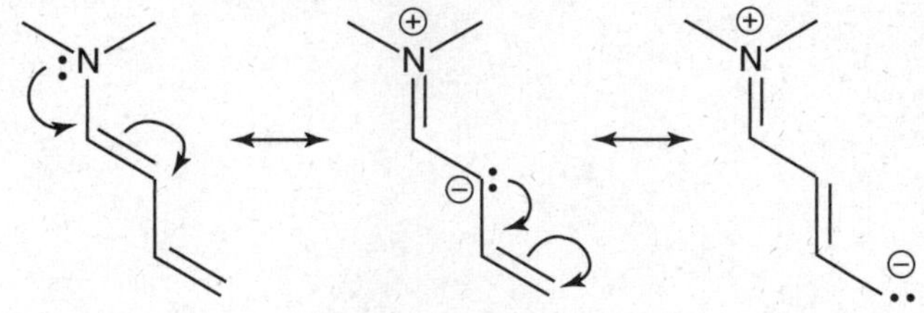

3.

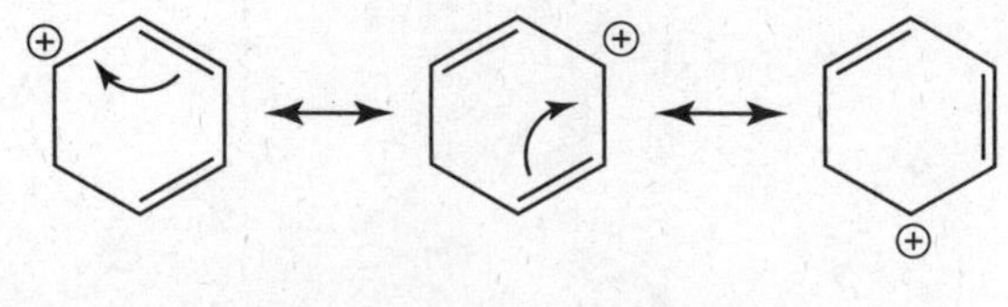

EXERCISE 4 (PAGE 211)

The following are possible structural isomers for molecular formula: $C_2H_6O_2$

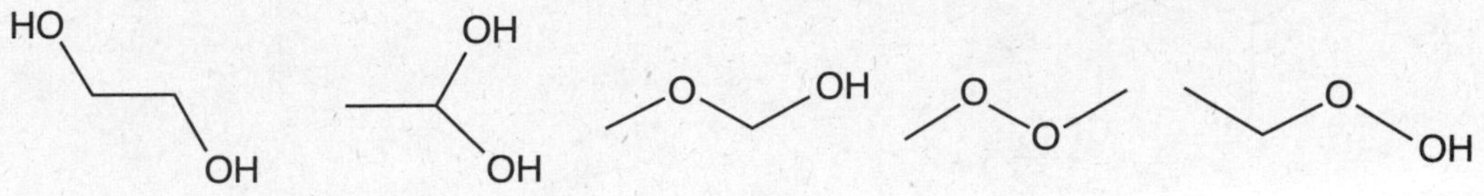

EXERCISE 5 (PAGE 216)

1.

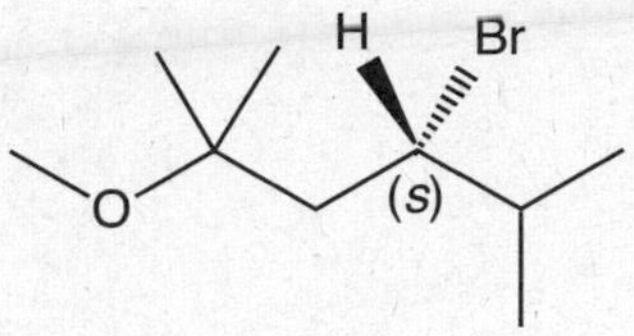

2.

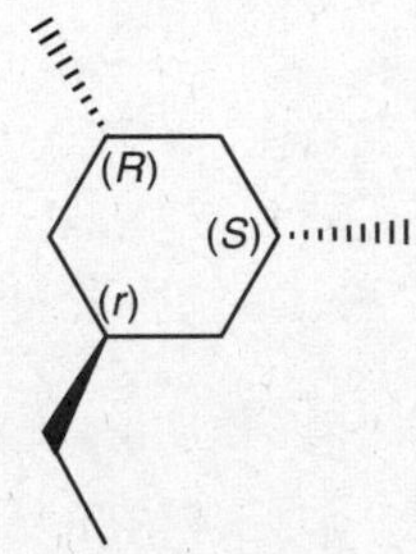

Note that this is a *meso*-compound (contains a plane of symmetry through the center of the molecule.)

3.

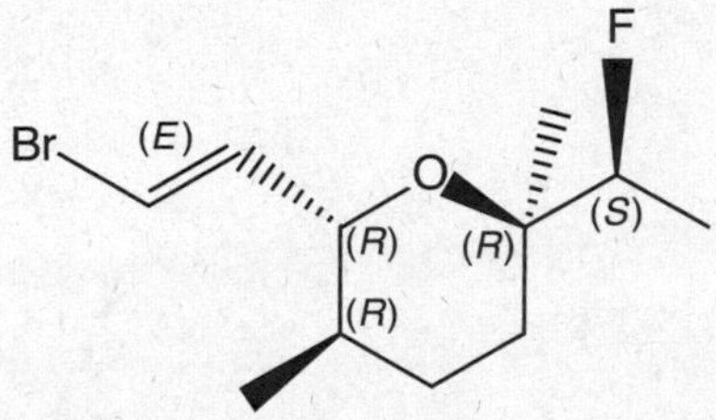

EXERCISE 6 (PAGE 220)

1.

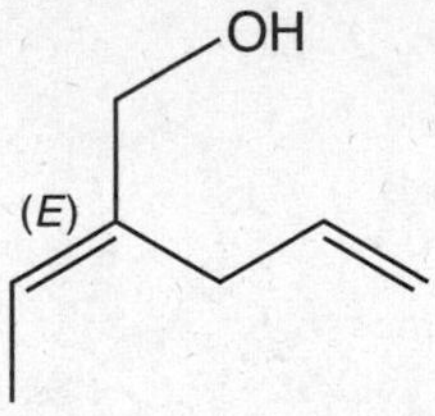

2.

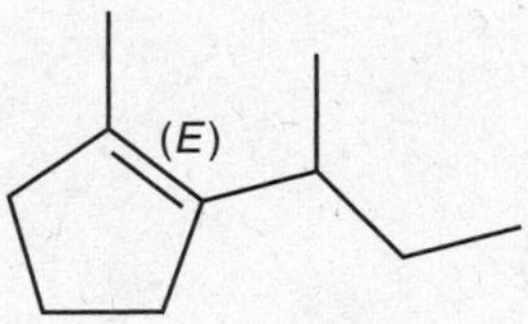

3.

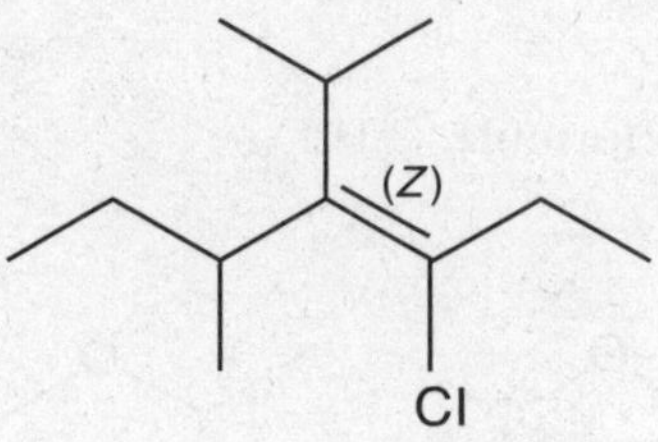

(Z)
Cl

EXERCISE 7 (PAGE 223)

1.

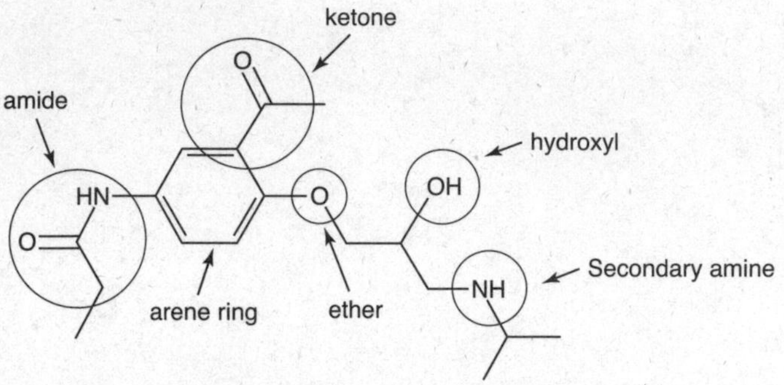

ketone

amide

hydroxyl

HN

OH

Secondary amine

O

NH

arene ring

ether

2.

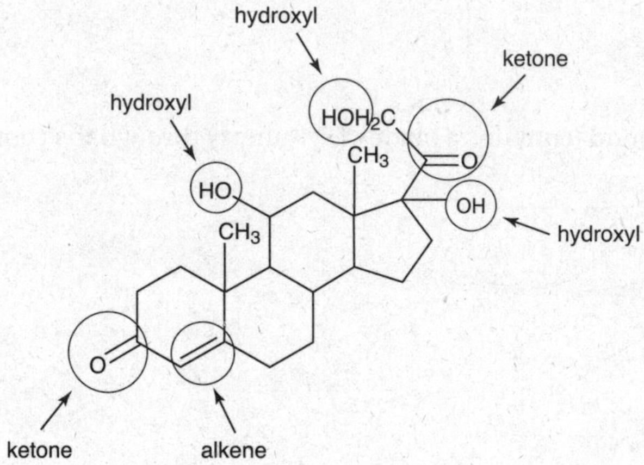

hydroxyl

hydroxyl

ketone

HOH₂C

CH₃

HO

OH

CH₃

hydroxyl

O

ketone

alkene

3.

arene
ring

sulfide

amide

hydroxyl

HO

S

O

C

N
H

N

amide

arene
ring

amide

OH

tertiary
amine

hydroxyl

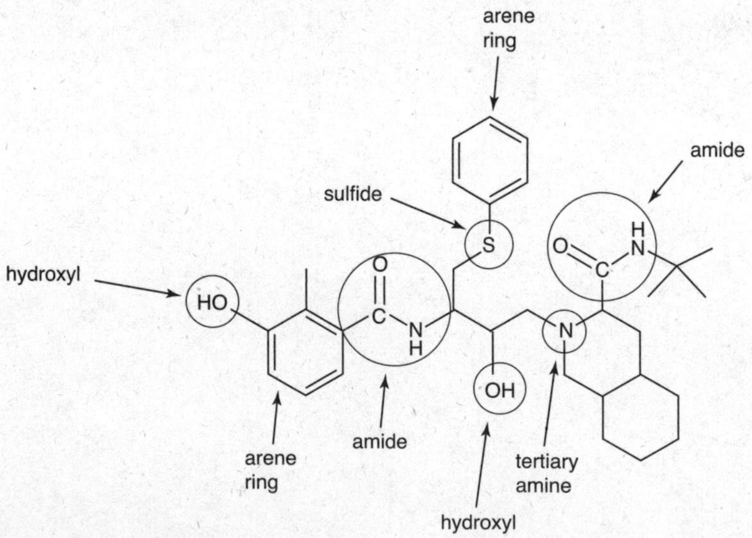

EXERCISE 8 (PAGE 228)

1.

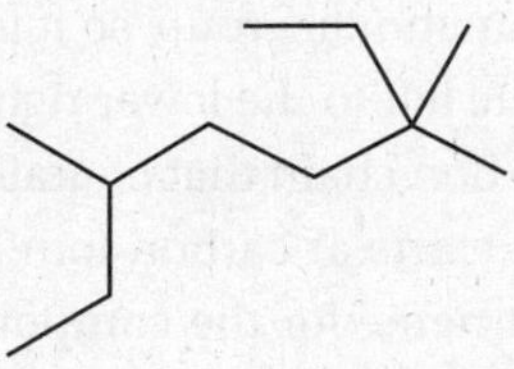

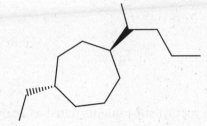

3,3,6-trimethyloctane

2.

(1*S*,4*S*)-1-ethyl-4-((*R*)-pentan-2-yl)cycloheptane

3.

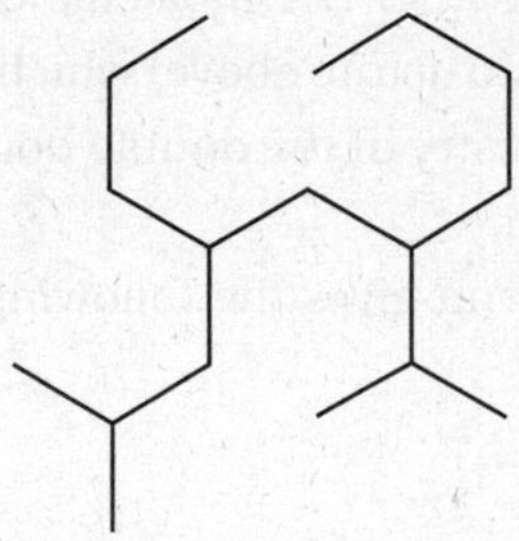

6-isopropyl-2-methyl-4-propyl decane

EXERCISE 9 (PAGE 234)

The lowest energy chair conformer for the given cyclohexane isomer is shown below (note that the *larger* ethyl group is equatorial and the *smaller* chloro group is axial).

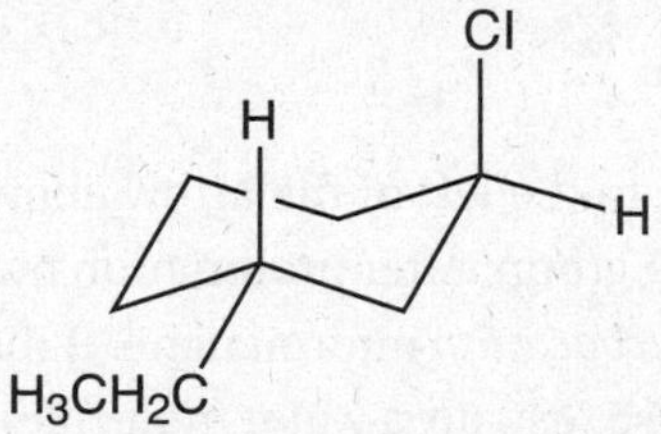

EXERCISE 10 (PAGE 239)

The compound shown contains a carbon-carbon double-bond functional group, so it is classified as an "alkene" and the -ene suffix is used. Counting from the left to the lower right side of the molecule (see structure below), the longest continuous carbon chain that contains the double bond is nine (9) carbons (non prefix). The double bond starts at carbon four (cited as "4" in the name) and terminates at carbon five. Thus the root name for the compound is "non-4-ene".

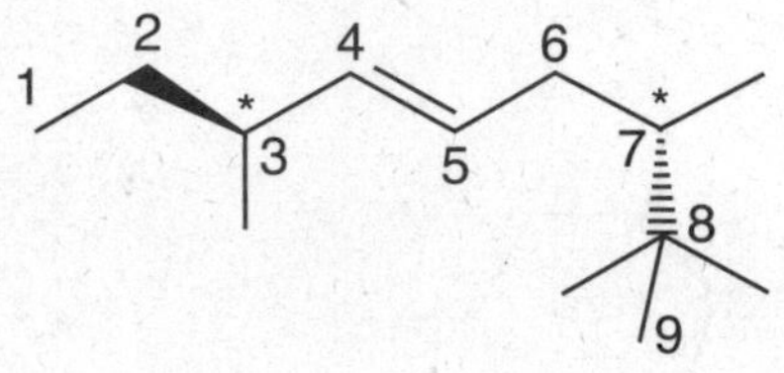

The compound's principal chain has four (4) methyl substituents (cited as *tetra*methyl), which are attached to carbons 3, 7, 8, and 8, respectively (again counting from left to right)—adding this information gives the following name: "3,7,8,8-tetramethylnon-4-ene." In addition to the cited substituents, the stereochemistry of the double bond and any chirality centers (where stereochemistry is defined) must be cited in the name. The molecule contains two chirality centers (carbons 3 and 7—the asterisks shown on structure above) which using C-I-P rules are designated *S* and *S*, respectively. The stereochemistry of the double bond (between carbons 4 and 5) is assigned as *E*, using the same approach.

Assigning the stereochemistry completes the process and gives the following full name: (3*S*,7*S*,*E*)-3,7,8,8-tetramethylnon-4-ene.

EXERCISE 11 (PAGE 241)

The conditions shown (acid and heat) will lead to alkene products (see the reaction below) via an E1 reaction process.

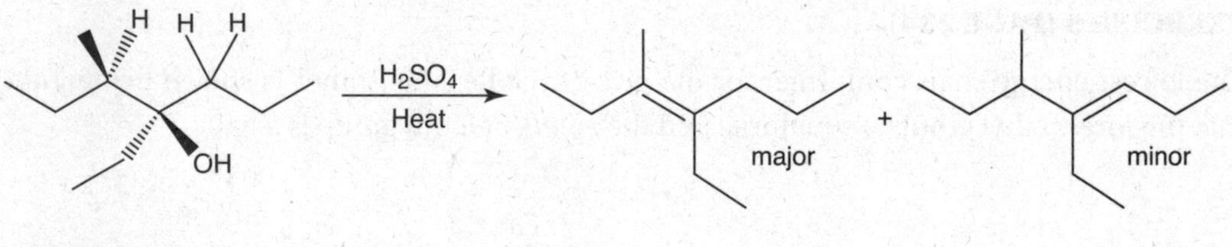

The given reactant (structure to the left of the arrow above) has reactive protons on both carbons β to the hydroxyl leaving group. After protonation by acid, the leaving group is lost as a water molecule producing a *carbocation* intermediate. If the protons on either of these carbons are abstracted by a weak base (usually a water molecule), an alkene product is produced. Loss of the proton to the *left* of the hydroxyl leaving group results in the *major* product shown above. This is the lower energy, more-substituted alkene. Losing either of the protons to the *right* of the leaving group gives the less-substituted *minor* product. Both of the products have an *E* stereochemical configuration. The reaction will also likely produce traces of the thermodynamically less stable *Z* products.

EXERCISE 12 (PAGE 244)

The best reagents to produce the products shown from the given reactant are bromine in water—see the equation below.

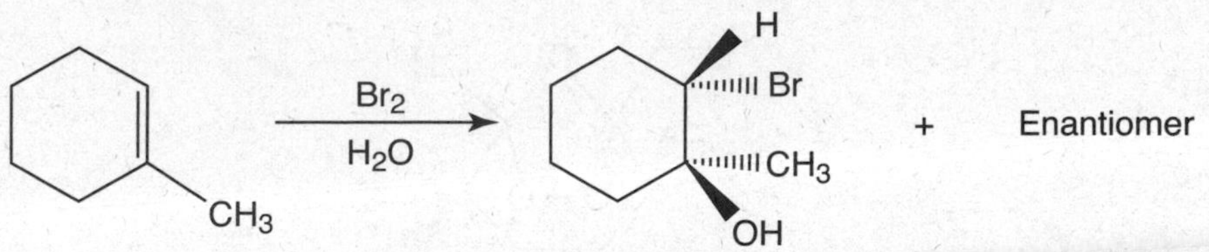

Nucleophilic attack by the alkene double bond on bromine will form a cyclic bromonium ion intermediate—see structure below.

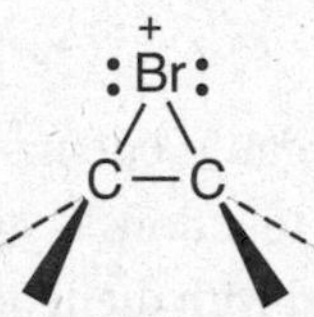

This ion will in turn undergo nucleophilic attack by water. Attack by a nucleophile can only occur from one side of the ion, because the other side is blocked by a large bromine cation. This results in a stereospecific opening of the cyclic ion and a *1,2-halohydron* product with *anti* configuration (the *bromine* atom and *hydroxyl* group will be *anti* to each other in the product). It should be noted that addition to the double bond will create two chirality centers in the product. The R and S configurations of these two centers have equal probability of forming, so the product mixture will be racemic.

EXERCISE 13 (PAGE 246)

The reaction product combined with the reagents shown in Figure 3.14 can only result from the ozonolysis of a cyclic alkene reactant—see structure below. The ozonolysis of an open-chain alkene always results in two or more (if there are additional double bonds) ketone/aldehyde fragments. There is only one product shown for this reaction, a keto-aldehyde, so the reactant must be cyclic.

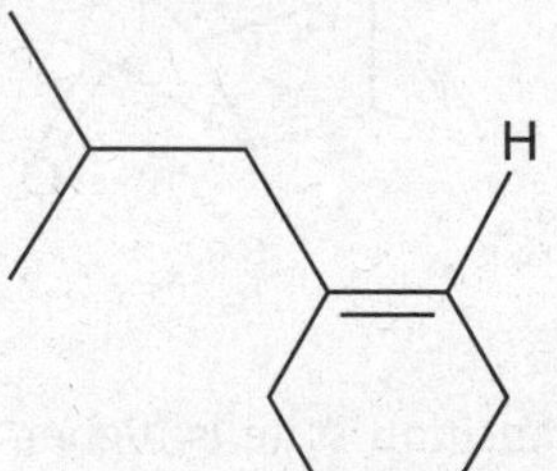

Specifically, the reactant must be a substituted cyclohexene ring because the two carbonyl groups present in the product are separated by four carbons (the two carbonyl carbons plus the four in between require a six-membered alkene ring reactant). The first step of the reaction involves ozone (O_3) reacting with the double bond shown in the reactant to form a molozonide that isomerizes to a bicyclic ozonide intermediate (see the structure below).

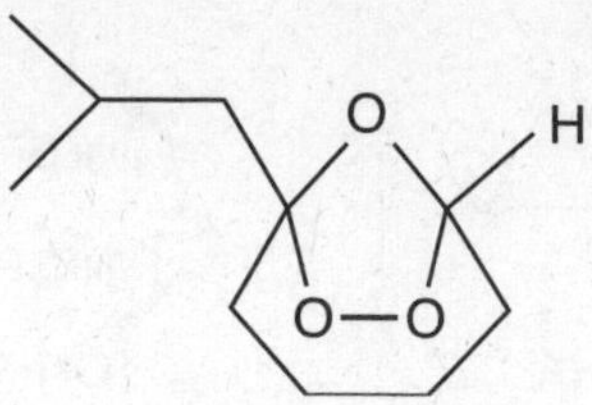

In the second step, the ozonide is reduced with acidic zinc, which results in the complete cleavage of the reactant's double bond.

EXERCISE 14 (PAGE 247)

You may recall from undergraduate organic chemistry studies that under certain circumstances, the Diels-Alder cycloaddition reaction is stereoselective. Stereochemistry is often important when *cyclic* dienes are reacted with dieneophiles to produce bridged bicyclic compounds. The predominant compound formed from the reaction shown will be bicyclic and have the stereochemistry shown in the structure below. This is termed the *endo* product.

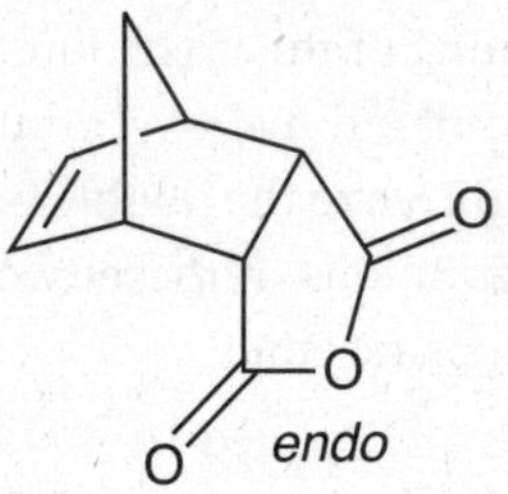

endo

In many cases, the *endo* product is formed exclusively, but sometimes it is mixed with another stereoisomer called the *exo* product (shown below).

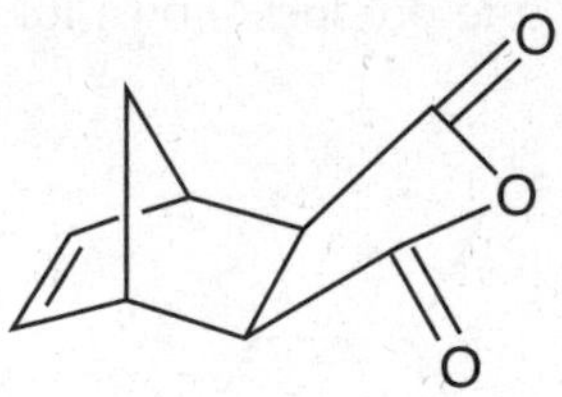

exo

The *exo* isomer's reaction transition state is higher in energy. As a result it forms more slowly than the *endo* isomer and will always be the *minor* product in such situations.

EXERCISE 15 (PAGE 248)

The compound to be named is an internal alkyne in a seven-carbon chain (heptyne) with three methyl substituents (at carbons 2, 2, and 5) and one chirality center (designated S). The alkyne's full name is shown below.

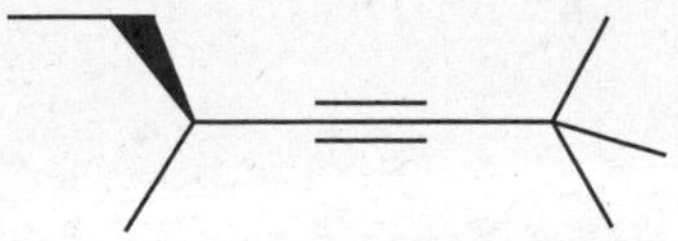

(S)-2,2,5-trimethylhept-3-yne

EXERCISE 16 (PAGE 250)

The major products that will form from the given reactant (an asymmetrical internal alkyne) and reaction conditions are shown below. The alkyne undergoes *complete* oxidative cleavage to form two different carboxylic acids.

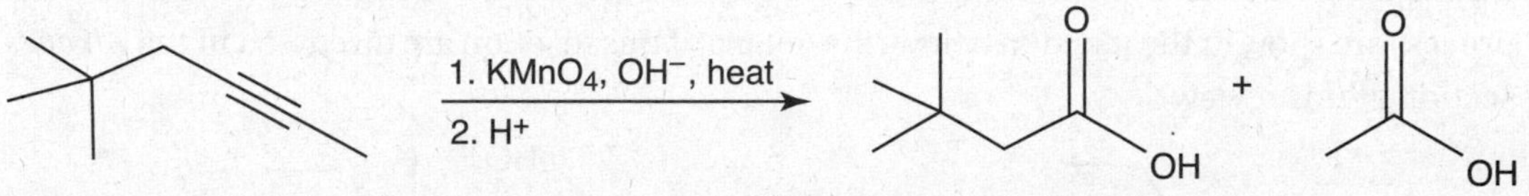

EXERCISE 17 (PAGE 253)

The compound to be named is aromatic (principal name—benzene) with two substituents (bromo and isopropyl groups listed in alphabetical order) on opposite sides of the benzene ring (*para*). The compound's full name is shown below.

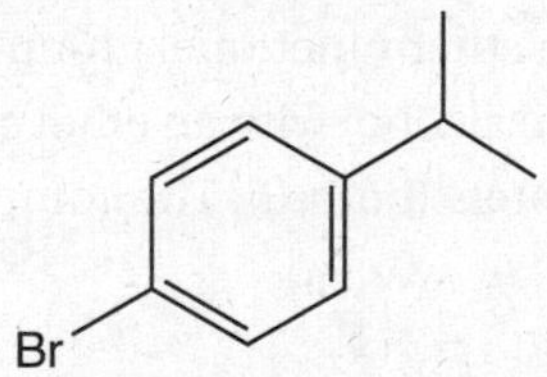

p-bromoisopropylbenzene

EXERCISE 18 (PAGE 256)

The major products that will form from the given reactant (chlorobenzene) and reaction conditions are shown below. The chloro group on the benzene ring is slightly deactivating but directs the electrophile (sulfur trioxide) to both the *ortho* and *para* positions (the *para* isomer should predominate).

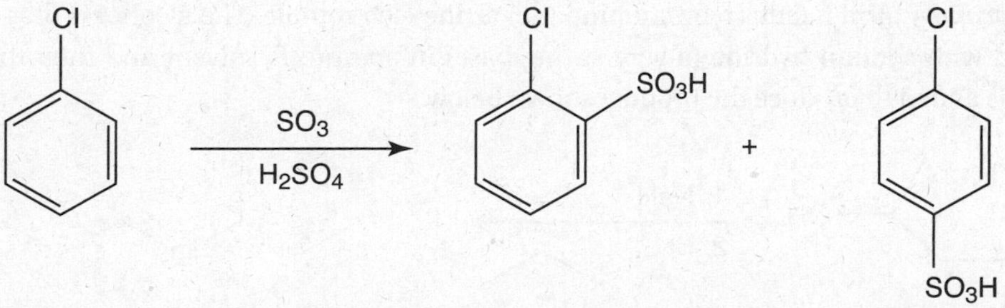

EXERCISE 19 (PAGE 259)

The compound to be named is an alcohol (hydroxyl group attached to carbon 3 of a seven-carbon principal chain—a heptanol) with three substituents (two methyl groups and an ethyl group listed in alphabetical order) and one chirality center (designated *S*). The compound's full name is shown below.

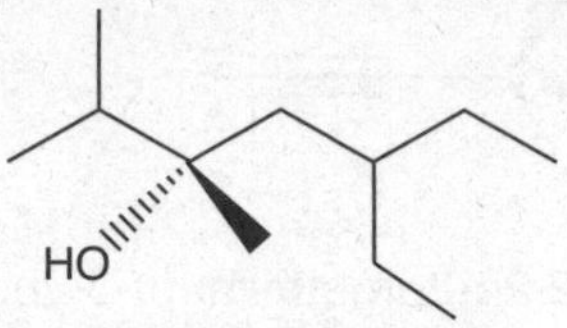

(*S*)-5-ethyl-2,3-dimethylheptan-3-ol

EXERCISE 20 (PAGE 264)

Water is being added to the alkene reactant in non-Markovnikov regiochemistry. The only way this regiochemistry can be accomplished is by hydroboration. The reagents for this two-step process are show in the reaction below (the details of this reaction are discussed in the *Alkenes* section of this review).

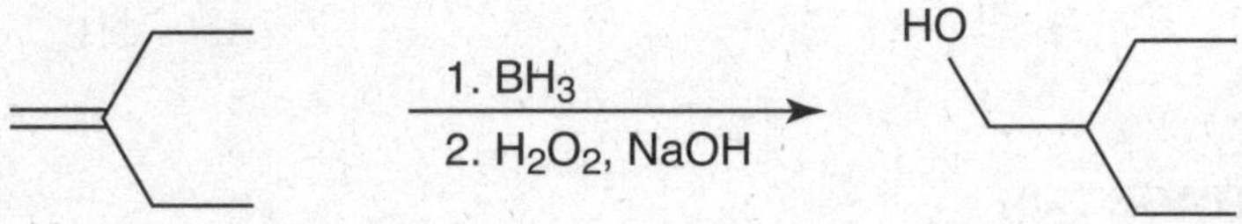

1. BH₃
2. H₂O₂, NaOH

EXERCISE 21 (PAGE 265)

The compound to be named is an *alcohol* (hydroxyl group attached to the five-carbon ring—a cyclopentanol) *ether*. Because the ether functional group is lower priority than the alcohol group, the compound is named as an alcohol with an ether substituent (2-methoxy). The molecule also contains two chirality centers (both *R*). The compound's full name is shown below.

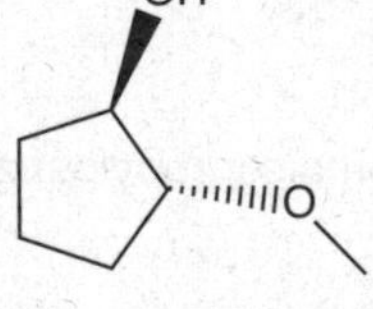

(1*R*,2*R*)-2-methoxycyclopentanol

EXERCISE 22 (PAGE 267)

The target compound is best prepared by the *Williamson ether synthesis*, an S_N2 process. For the synthesis to succeed, a branched alcohol (*sec*-butanol) should be used as the nucleophile and a *primary* alkyl halide (1-bromopropane) as the electrophile. The alcohol is first deprotonated with sodium hydride (a very strong base) in an aprotic solvent and then the alkyl halide is added to produce the product shown below.

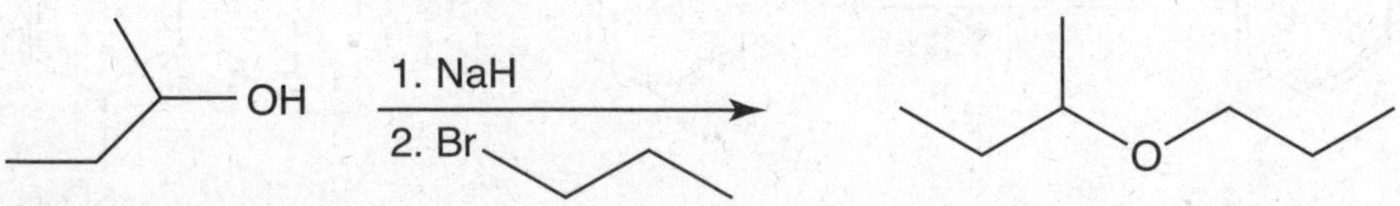

1. NaH
2. Br

EXERCISE 23 (PAGE 269)

The sodium ethoxide nucleophile will attack the epoxide ring at its least substituted carbon from both the top and bottom. Since the reactant compound already has a chirality center, this will produce two stereoisomeric products that will be *diastereomers* of each other (the S,R and S,S isomers) in *unequal* amounts. Both of these products are shown in the reaction scheme below.

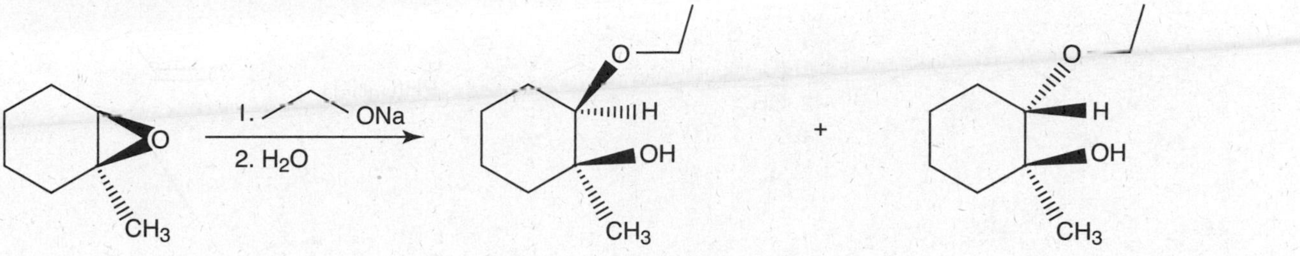

(1S,2R)-2-ethoxy-1-methylcyclohexanol   (1S,2S)-2-ethoxy-1-methylcyclohexanol

EXERCISE 24 (PAGE 271)

The compound to be named is a *ketone* (carbonyl group attached to the fourth carbon from the right in an eight-carbon principal chain—an octanone). The compound has two substituents (an ethyl and methyl group) and one chirality center (designated S). The compound's full name is shown below.

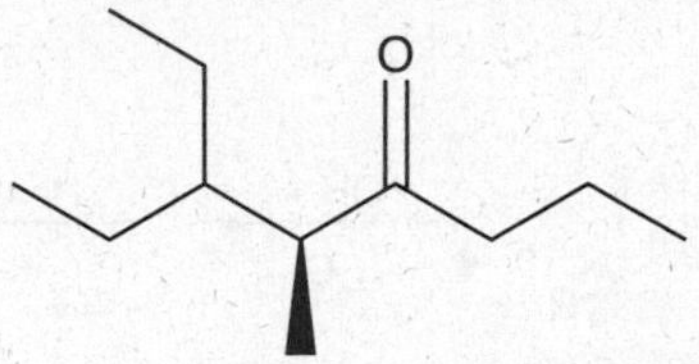

(S)-6-ethyl-5-methyloctan-4-one

EXERCISE 25 (PAGE 272)

The target compound is a methyl ketone. Starting with an alkyne (as the instructions state), a methyl ketone can be prepared by treating it with acid and a mercuric sulfate catalyst—this is a form of hydration (first an enol is formed and it isomerizes to the more stable ketone). It should be noted that the starting compound has a chirality center and will give a *racemic mixture* of the product ketone. The synthesis scheme is shown below.

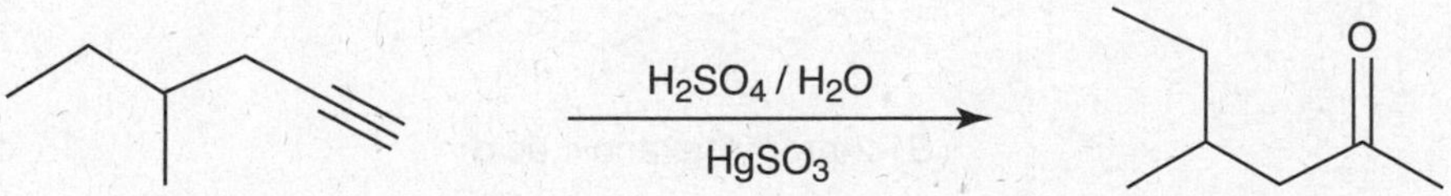

H_2SO_4 / H_2O

$HgSO_3$

EXERCISE 26 (PAGE 275)

The target alkene can be prepared from cyclopentanone and an alkyl halide (bromobutane) using the *Wittig* reaction as shown below. The process works well in this case because it starts with a primary alkyl halide to produce the required *ylide* (the ylide intermediate is formed through an S_N2 process—see the structure below after the first arrow), which is then reacted with cyclopentanone.

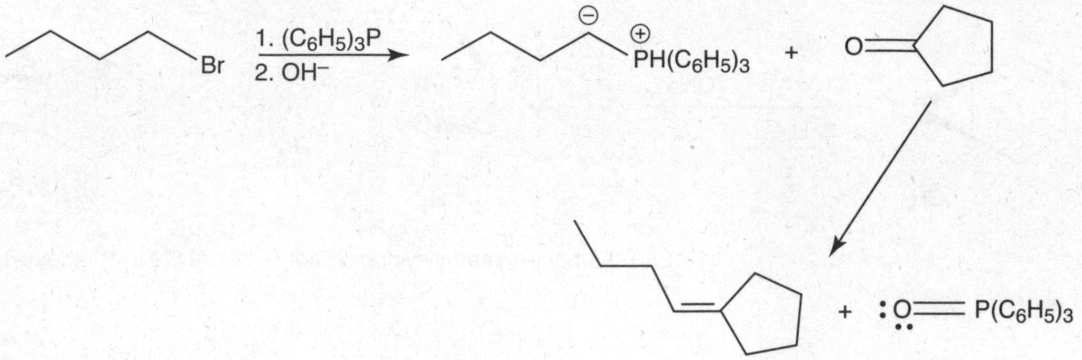

EXERCISE 27 (PAGE 278)

The given reaction sequence will produce an α, β *unsaturated aldehyde* and is formally referred to as a *Crossed Aldol* condensation. Only one product is produced (see the reaction scheme below) because the formaldehyde reactant doesn't have any α carbons.

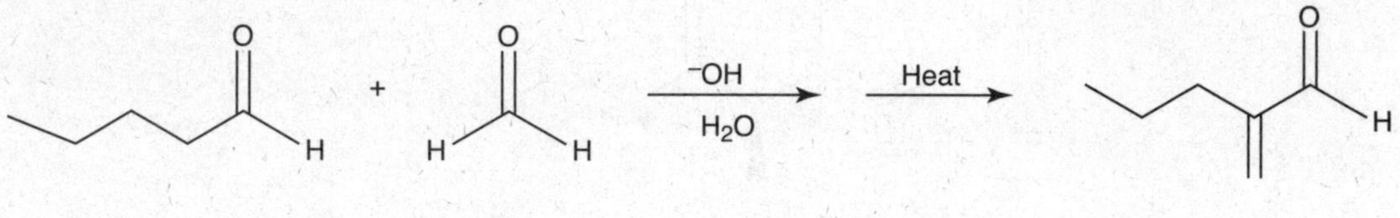

EXERCISE 28 (PAGE 280)

The compound to be named is a *carboxylic acid* (carbonyl with attached hydroxyl group terminal to a six-carbon principal chain—a hexanoic acid). The compound has one substituent (a propyl group at carbon two of the principal chain) and one chirality center (designated S). The compound's full name is shown below.

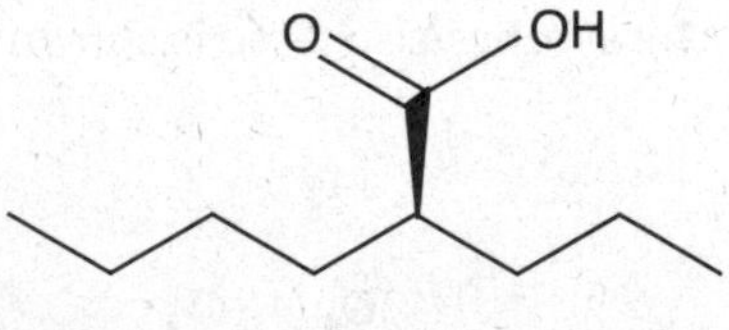

(S)-2-propylhexanoic acid

EXERCISE 29 (PAGE 282)

There are several approaches for converting an alkyl halide into a carboxylic acid. One of the most general is to produce a Grignard reagent from the reactant and then treat it with carbon dioxide and acid in succession. This approach usually produces high yields—see the synthetic scheme shown below.

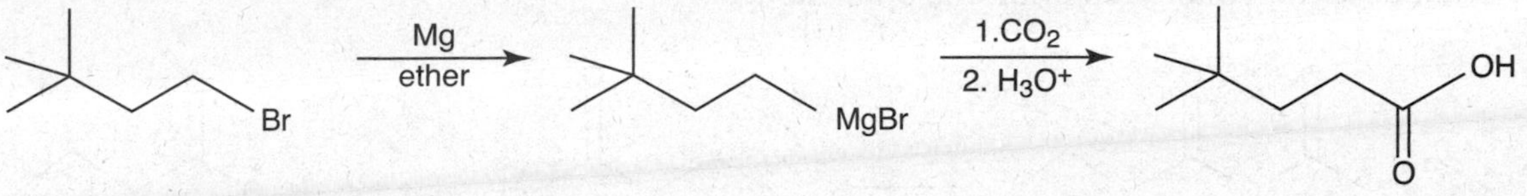

EXERCISE 30 (PAGE 284)

To synthesize the target compound (an ester), it would be best to start with benzoic acid (cheap and available), and first convert it to an acid chloride using thionyl chloride. Step one shown below—pyridine is generally used for the solvent in this process because it effectively removes the byproduct HCl from the reaction solution. Next, an alcohol is added to the acid chloride solution (step two below) to form an ester product—again, excess pyridine is used to remove HCl from the reaction mixture. There are other approaches that might work for the synthesis of the target ester, but the method described above is straightforward and should produce the compound in good yield.

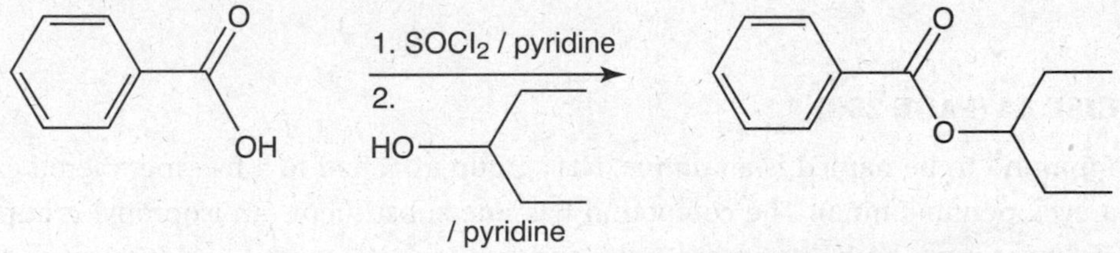

EXERCISE 31 (PAGE 294)

As the following *retrosynthetic* step shows, the target ester can be prepared from benzoic acid and *tert*-butanol. There are several ways these two reactants could be used for the synthesis, but as was shown in Exercise 30, converting the acid to an acid chloride and then reacting it with *tert*-butanol should produce a good yield of the ester product.

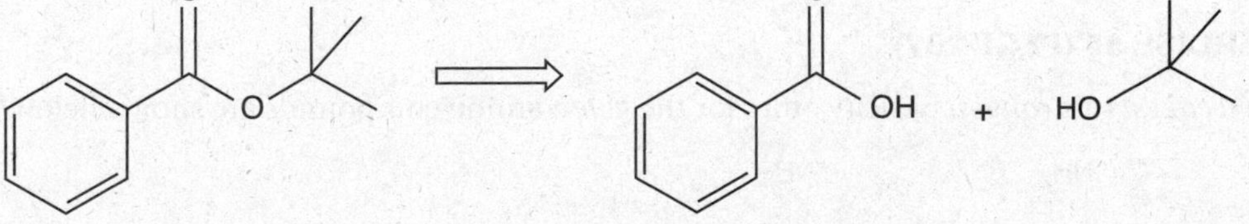

EXERCISE 32 (PAGE 294)

Similar to Exercise 31, the following retrosynthetic step provides the reactants that might be used to prepare the target anhydride. There are other approaches that might also work, but reacting an acid chloride (on the left) with a carboxylate salt (on the right) is probably the most efficient way to synthesize a mixed anhydride. The required acid chloride can be produced from thionyl chloride and butanoic acid.

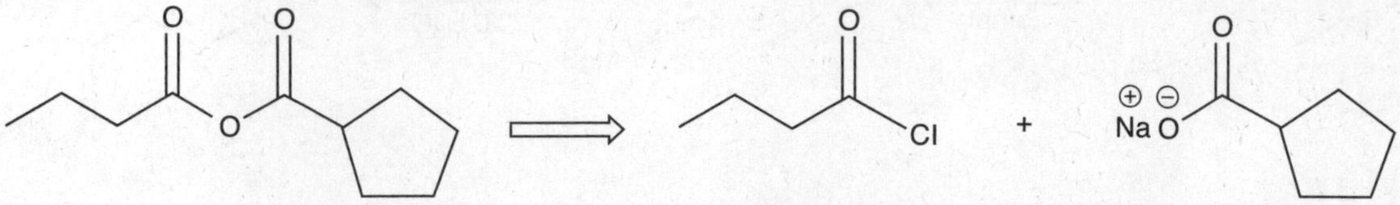

EXERCISE 33 (PAGE 294)

As shown below, under the given reaction conditions the amide reactant will be converted into a primary amine product with the loss of one carbon (originally the carbonyl carbon in the amide) as carbon dioxide. This process is referred to as the *Hofmann Rearrangement* and proceeds through an *isocyanate* intermediate.

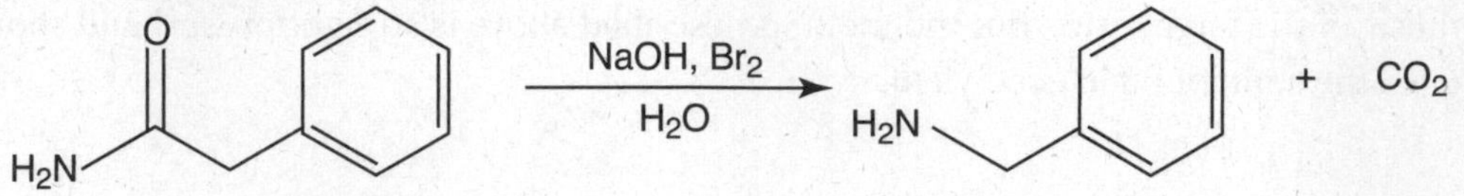

EXERCISE 34 (PAGE 296)

The compound to be named is an *amine* (NH$_2$ group attached to a five-membered carbon ring—a cyclopentanamine). The compound has one substituent (an isopropyl group) and two chirality centers (both centers are in the cyclopentane ring with S and R configurations). The compound's full name is shown below.

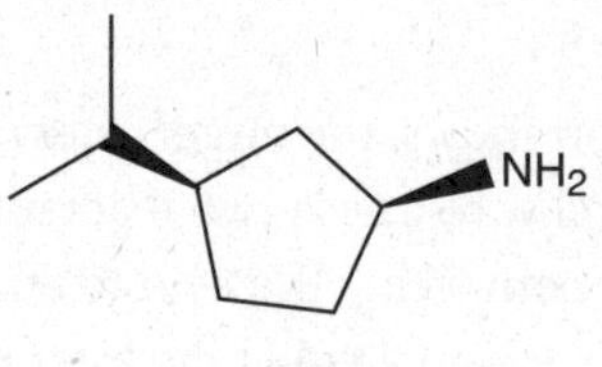

(1S,3R)-3-isopropylcyclopentanamine

EXERCISE 35 (PAGE 297)

The *weakest* to *strongest* basicity order for the given amine compounds are shown below.

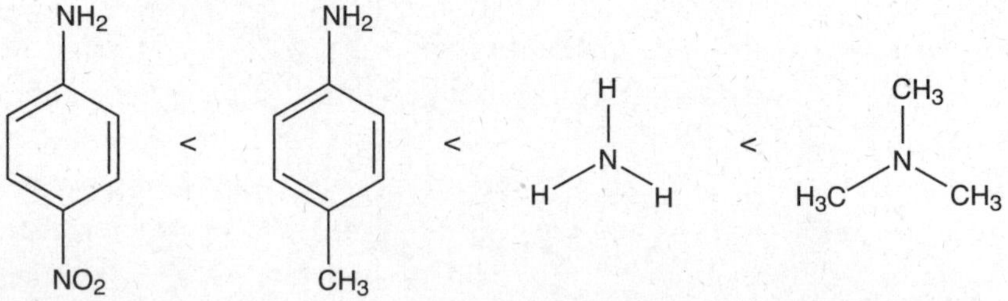

In general, due to delocalization of the amine lone pair, aromatic amines (e.g., anilines) are weaker bases than ammonia and alkyl group substituted ammonia. In this case nitro aniline is weaker than methyl aniline because the nitro group is electron withdrawing (makes the aniline lone pair less accessible due to induction) and the methyl group is electron donating. Ammonia is less basic than trimethylamine for the same reason. The methyl groups in trimethylamine donate electron density into the nitrogen center, making its lone pair electrons more nucleophilic and thus the compound more basic.

EXERCISE 36 (PAGE 301)

Starting with aniline, as required by the exercise directions, it is converted to a diazonium salt, which is then transformed to phenol, which is subsequently ethylated by *Friedel-Crafts alkylation* to form the target compound, *p*-ethylphenol. The complete synthetic scheme is shown below. It should be noted that some *o*-ethylphenol will also be produced in this process, but it should be a minor product.

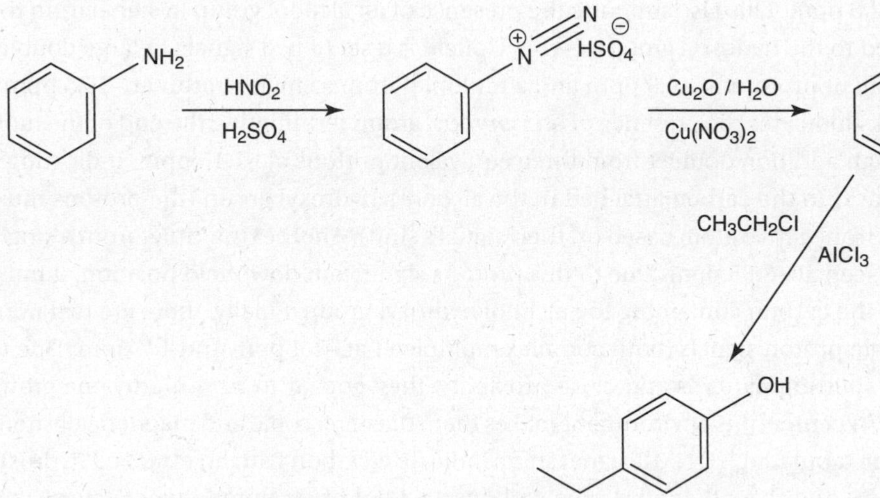

EXERCISE 37 (PAGE 310)

Using the formula on page 000, compounds C_5H_9N and $C_3H_5NO_2$ both have two degrees of unsaturation. Compound C_3H_6 has one degree and C_2Cl_6 has no degrees of unsaturation.

EXERCISE 38 (PAGE 321)

Based on the provided molecular formula ($C_5H_{10}O$), the unknown compound has one degree of unsaturation. The compound's IR spectrum shows two important bands (2,720 cm^{-1} and 1,726 cm^{-1}) in the functional group region. These bands suggest the presence of an aldehyde functional group in the compound. The ^{1}H NMR spectrum of the unknown compound contains a singlet signal at ~9.7 ppm. This also supports the presence of an aldehyde group (a signal from the proton attached to the carbonyl group: H–C=O). The other signals, all between ~2.50 ppm and .80 ppm, represent aliphatic protons attached to carbons on the other side of the aldehyde group. The splitting on these four signals is a little complex, but based on the proton numbers shown for each signal, they indicate a methyl group and three ethylene groups all connected in a chain—a total of nine protons which is consistent with the molecular formula when the aldehyde proton is included. The tabulated ^{13}C NMR signal shifts indicate a carbonyl carbon (~203 ppm) and four other alkyl type carbons—a total of five unique types (again consistent with the molecular formula).

Based on the above analysis, the structural formula that best matches the data is for the compound valeraldehyde (common name)—the structure is shown below.

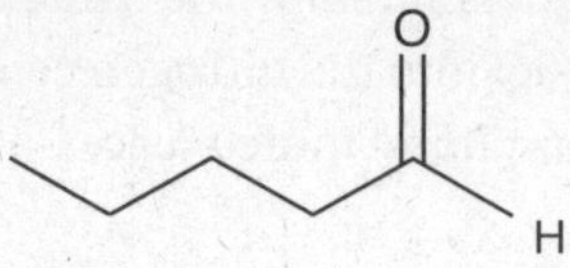

EXERCISE 39 (PAGE 322)

Based on the provided molecular formula ($C_6H_{14}O$), the unknown compound has no degrees of unsaturation. The compound's IR spectrum shows one important band (3,350 cm^{-1}) in the functional group region. This band suggests the presence of an *alcohol* (hydroxyl) functional group in the compound. The ^{1}H NMR spectrum of the unknown compound contains a singlet signal at ~2.8 ppm. This also supports the presence of an alcohol group (a signal from the proton attached to the hydroxyl group: H–O–). Upfield is a set of two signals (a large doublet from six equivalent protons at ~0.9 ppm and a multiplet from a single proton at ~1.25 ppm). This set of peaks indicates the presence of an *isopropyl* group terminating the end of the molecule. There is an addition doublet from three equivalent protons at ~1.15 ppm, indicating a methyl group next to the carbon attached to the alcohol's hydroxyl group (the protons must be near an electronegative atom based on their signal's shift). Another multiplet from a single proton can be seen at ~3.85 ppm. Due to this proton's significant downfield position, it must be attached to the carbon containing the alcohol hydroxyl group. Finally, there are two nonequivalent single proton signals (both complex multiplets) at ~1.4 ppm and 1.7 ppm. Due to their complex splitting patterns and close proximity, they appear to be a methylene group next to a *chirality* center (this environment makes them diastereotopic and magnetically nonequivalent). The tabulated ^{13}C NMR signal shifts indicate a carbon with an attached hydroxyl group (~66 ppm) and five other alkyl type carbons—a total of six unique types (consistent with the molecular formula).

Based on the above analysis, the structural formula that best matches the data is for the compound 4-methyl-2-pentanol; the structure is shown below.

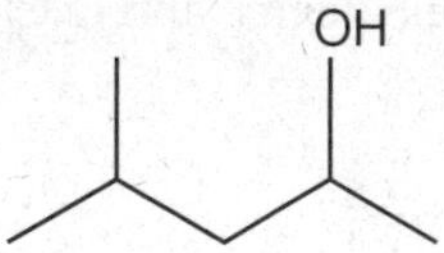

EXERCISE 40 (PAGE 323)

Based on the provided molecular formula ($C_5H_{10}O_2$), the unknown compound has one degree of unsaturation. The compound's IR spectrum shows two important bands (1,640 cm^{-1} and 1,192 cm^{-1}) in the functional group and fingerprint regions. These bands suggest the presence of an *ester* functional group in the compound. The ^{1}H NMR spectrum of the unknown compound contains an associated triplet (~1.35 ppm) from three protons and a quartet (~4.15 ppm) from two protons characteristic of an *ethyl* group attached to a very electronegative atom—in this case based on the molecular formula an oxygen atom. There is also a second similar set of signals (a triplet at ~1.15 ppm and a quartet at ~2.30 ppm) indicating another ethyl group attached to a carbonyl carbon. The two different ethyl groups contain a total of 10 protons, which is consistent with the given molecular formula. The tabulated ^{13}C NMR signal shifts indicate a carbonyl carbon (~174 ppm) and four other alkyl type carbons attached to or near oxygen atoms (based on their shift positions)—a total of five unique types (again consistent with the molecular formula).

Based on the above analysis, the structural formula that best matches the data is for the compound ethyl propionate—the structure is shown below.

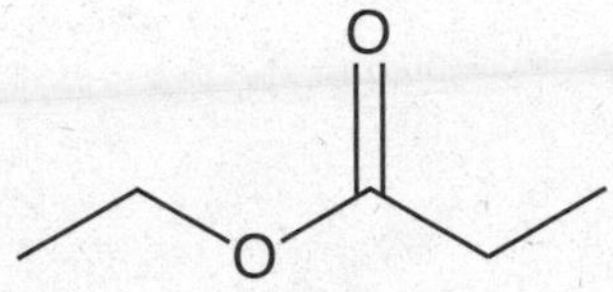

EXERCISE 41 (PAGE 338)

The most cost-effective method for the necessary separation would be *liquid-liquid* extraction. The first step would be to dissolve the mixture in a appropriate solvent such as diethyl ether (cheap and has a very low boiling point). Next, this solution would be placed in a large *separatory funnel* and shaken with a 10% by mass aqueous solution of hydrochloric acid. The diethyl ether solution and aqueous acid solution will form separate layers in the funnel under these conditions. It's generally best to conduct several small extractions with the aqueous acid (and combine the fractions) rather than one large one. As the aniline (a basic compound) is exposed to the acid solution, during extraction, it will be transformed into a hydrochloride salt and migrate into the aqueous phase. The neutral phenanthracene will be unchanged and stay in the organic phase (the diethyl either). After all the aqueous extraction fractions have been collected and combined, the solution should be cooled to ~0°C and neutralized with cold aqueous base. The solution should be checked with a pH indicator to be *sure* it is neutral or slightly basic prior to proceeding to the final step. Keeping the aqueous mixture cold will help prevent oxidation of the free amine. Finally, the free amine can be extracted from the neutral aqueous mixture with an appropriate solvent such as methylene chloride as described above, the solvent evaporated, and the aniline further dried as needed. The phenanthracene can be isolated from the diethyl ether fraction by evaporation and further dried as needed. As with most organic compound separations, chromatography could also be used for this process, but because of the large quantity of the mixture, it would be expensive and time-consuming. Recrystallization could also be tried, but this approach will likely require large quantities of organic solvents, will be messy, time-consuming, and generate a lot of waste. Also, one of the mixture components aniline is a *liquid* and won't crystallize at room temperature.

EXERCISE 42 (PAGE 338)

The answer to this question is a resounding no. The boiling point difference between benzene (~80°C) and ethyl acetate (~77°C) is only around 3°C at sea level. To effectively use simple distillation for a separation, the boiling point difference of the mixture components needs to be *at least* 30°C. Simple distillation wouldn't work for this separation.

PART FOUR

Reading Comprehension Test

Introduction

35

Reading comprehension measures your understanding of various scientific topics presented in three reading passages. Each passage contains approximately 1,500 words and is followed by 16–17 questions relating to the information, structure, or purpose of that passage. The candidate is given 60 minutes to read and answer a total of 50 multiple-choice questions related to the three passages. Having prior understanding of the science topics presented in the passages is not a prerequisite to answering any of the test questions. The reading passages require you to read, comprehend, and thoroughly analyze basic scientific information. Then you choose the best-possible response based on only information provided in the passage. The goal of this section is to test your ability to retrieve information and understand the author's intent.

This chapter presents reading comprehension strategies that you can use to master the three required reading passages and answer the questions correctly. Unfortunately, significant improvements in reading comprehension take time. They are acquired or learned skills. One goal of this section is to improve your test-taking strategies. The other goal is to help you identify cues in the questions that may help you eliminate wrong answer choices and choose one of the best remaining answers within the allotted time of 60 minutes. This section of the DAT requires no previous knowledge of dentistry, science, or scientific articles. All the information you need to answer each question is contained in the particular reading passage.

THE IMPORTANCE OF READING COMPREHENSION

Reading comprehension is a complex skill that you must develop in order to understand the depth and breadth of the dental profession. Throughout the four-year dental school experience, you are required to read, comprehend, and understand technical literature and historical knowledge from 8 specialty areas. You must first understand human biological fundamentals as they pertain to medicine and, in particular, dental medicine. The curriculum focuses on the structure and function of tissues in the head and neck. In the classroom, you are introduced to preclinical restorative dentistry with all the associated disciplines (occlusion, dental anatomy, dental materials, and behavioral science). Clinical rotations emphasize a multidisciplinary approach to solving a patient's dental health. The third and fourth years are spent visualizing the intended outcome of treatments and developing hand and eye coordination. You learn to use these skills when extracting decay from a tooth, debriding a pulp chamber of its vital components, and teaching a child to brush his or her teeth. If you do not understand the technical information that you read as a dental student, you will not succeed either in school or in a dental practice. Remember: words have no meaning without comprehension.

READING COMPREHENSION STRATEGIES

When you have no previous knowledge about the topic presented, use the following reading comprehension strategies to understand the information.

- **QUICKLY SURVEY THE PASSAGE** to determine the topic, author's writing style, and main theme. This is the time to look for important information related to the questions.

- **IDENTIFY ANY BACKGROUND KNOWLEDGE** you already have about the topic. Doing so helps in making inferences. When reading passages, you must understand the who, what, when, where, why, and how of the information. You must also associate any previous relevant knowledge you have about the topic.

- **DECODE UNFAMILIAR WORDS.** Write down key words, phrases, supporting ideas, definitions, and transitions on a separate sheet. Annotating phrases and unfamiliar words will help you pace yourself and allow you to pay close attention to the purpose of the passage.

- **PARAPHRASE THE TOPIC.** Correctly paraphrase complex details and information while reading. While reading the passage, anticipate the questions you may be asked and figure out the answers. Paraphrasing will help you recall what you read.

- **IDENTIFY KEY WORDS** to help you better understand both the passage and the questions. Before reading the passage, preview the questions. Look for key words and phrases in the questions that will help you focus when reading the passage. Pay attention to details when reading technical literature, and recognize relationships between ideas and details.

- **CHOOSE YOUR ANSWER** based on information in the passage. Read and correctly interpret the passage. Answer every question based on only information in the passage. Eliminating answer choices that are not possible will increase your chances of answering correctly.

- **PACE YOURSELF APPROPRIATELY.** Allow 10 minutes to read each passage and 10 minutes to answer the 16 or 17 questions related to the passage.

- **MAKE NOTES.** While reading each passage, highlight critical terms, dates, or numbers that may be used to answer retrieval questions.

Specific Question Types

36

The questions are always about information that is either directly stated or implied in the passage. Become familiar with each type of question. No matter the difficulty of a particular question, understanding what is being asked is the key to choosing the correct answer.

RETRIEVAL QUESTIONS

Retrieving is the process of finding something. Retrieval questions tend to be the easiest type since they simply require you to read the passage and find the answer. Look for and identify the most important word or words in the question. Then skim through the passage to identify the section or sections with the relevant information. Finally, identify the specific information being asked, such as the time, date, or numbers. Incorrect answers can be easily distinguished immediately.

➡ **Example**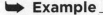

PASSAGE

Stress is exerted in a number of ways. It is tensile (stretching) if the force is acting perpendicular to and away from an object's center. The force is compressive (squeezing) if it is acting perpendicular to and toward the object's center. The force is shear (sliding) if it is acting parallel to the surface of the object. Other types of stress include residual, bending, torsional, and fatigue forces. Stress can exist inside materials when no external force is applied. Stress is inversely proportional to the cross-sectional area and directly proportional to the load.

Question

According to the information in the passage, how would you describe shear forces?

- (A) A force pulling both ends of a tube away from the center
- (B) The force of a trash compactor squeezing toward the center
- (C) The pressure of air along the front of an airplane wing
- (D) A twisting force on an iron bar
- (E) The force remaining in the material after the original forces have been removed

Reasoning

C When a question includes the phrase "according to the information in the passage," the author is directing you to a section in the passage for the answer. In this passage, the author is asking for the definition of shear force. The fourth sentence in the passage answers the question. "The force is shear (sliding) if it is acting parallel to the surface of the object." Answer choice (C) describes a force acting parallel to the surface of the object. All other responses describe different types of forces.

INFERENCE QUESTIONS

An inference is a conclusion reached on the basis of evidence and reasoning. Inference questions typically require you to make a decision, conclusion, or judgment about what the passage is saying. The answer is not easily identifiable. The reader must be able to make comparisons, find limiting words, and understand concepts and evidence to support the answer. The correct answer tends to be based on a logical sequence of words or sentences in the passage. Do not rely on answers that fail to describe or closely follow a statement in the passage. Eliminate answer choices that do not support details found in the passage.

➥ Example

PASSAGE

Water-based cements rely on an acid-base reaction. Water-based cements include glass and resin-modified glass ionomer cements, zinc polyacrylate, and zinc phosphate. The class acid-base reaction of zinc phosphate cement is the oldest and most widely used cement in dentistry. This cement requires that a combination of zinc and magnesium oxide powder be mixed together with phosphoric acid for several minutes to dissipate the heat of reaction. The mixing and placement of this cement is critical to the life of the tooth since raising the internal temperature of the tooth 6 degrees Fahrenheit or more could heat and eventually cause the pulp of the tooth to die. The powder is divided up into 6 equal amounts and placed onto one side of a "cooled" glass slab. The phosphoric acid and water mixture is dispensed in droplet form onto the opposite side. Slowly, small amounts of powder are mixed into the liquid by a stainless steel spatula and then spread over a large surface area to cool the reaction. This process continues for up to 2 minutes and stops when the cement droops 1 inch off the mixing spatula. This cement was the gold standard that all cements were measured against since the film thickness was less than 25 microns. Unfortunately, it causes hypersensitivity to the tooth due to the heat. In addition, mixing this cement properly is an extremely difficult technique. Finally, the cement has no adhesive properties other than to lock onto the tooth mechanically.

Question

What can the reader infer from the author's detailed description of mixing water-based cements?

(A)   The mixing technique has a long established history.
(B)   The proper use of mixing components is extremely important to the overall success of the tooth.
(C)   Removing heat using a cold glass slab helps distribute heat over a large surface area.
(D)   The consistency of the cement is important to insertion of the restoration.
(E)   All of the above.

Reasoning

E The information contained in the passage describes a technique for mixing water-based cements. Answer choice (E) is correct since all the other choices include correct inferences about the mixing process.

MAIN IDEA QUESTIONS

The main idea is the most important point or the theme of what is being said in the paragraph. Main idea questions ask you to point to something specific—such as a word, phrase, or sentence—to answer the question. The main idea can usually be found in the opening or closing paragraphs. The correct answer is often a paraphrase of the opening or closing paragraph.

➥ Example

PASSAGE

Casting is the process of making a metal replica using melted metal alloy that when poured into a mold, it takes the shape of the master die. Once solidified and cooled, the casting is broken out of the mold, finished and polished to improve surface appearance, ground to a specific tolerance, and/or undergoes additional heat treatment. The two basic types of molds used to cast metal fall into the expendable or nonexpendable mold patterns. Casting metal is an extremely versatile process of duplicating parts due to the wide selection of alloy types, and is the most economical way to manufacture large quantities of parts in any industry. This passage describes the fabrication methods of expendable and nonexpendable casting patterns.

Question

The main idea of the passage is to

(A) analyze expendable and nonexpendable casting methods.
(B) discuss the disadvantages to centrifugal casting.
(C) explain why the geometric properties of the master die are important to miscasting.
(D) argue about the most cost-effective method of producing a master die.
(E) discuss why investment casting is the most popular and cost-effective method of producing large quantities of parts.

Reasoning

A The main idea can be located in different places within the passage, although it is usually in the first or last paragraph. In this example, the author places the main idea in the third sentence of the passage by stating, "The two basic types of molds used to cast metal fall into the expendable or nonexpendable mold patterns." After reviewing the possible answers, only choice (A) describes the main point of the paragraph. The other choices are subsets of expendable and nonexpendable mold patterns.

SEQUENCE QUESTIONS

A sequence is the particular order in which related events follow each other. Sequence questions ask about the chronology of events. This type of question asks what happened first, second, and last. The reader usually has to identify, order, or list the events in the proper sequence.

➡ **Example** _____

PASSAGE

Mixing and placing dental amalgam involves three distinct steps.

1. Trituration is the process of mixing alloy powder with liquid mercury. Inside the pre-capsulated container, the premeasured alloy powder is separated from the mercury by a sealed membrane that, when vibrated, ruptures the membrane, releasing the mercury into the chamber and coating the metal particles. Undertriturated mixes are dull in appearance, crumble, and have poor compressive strength due to voids and other poor physical properties. Overtriturated mixes are soupy, lack strength, and display corrosion properties after setting. When properly triturated, amalgam is bright, homogenous, and dense. When correctly mixed, the physical and mechanical properties of dental amalgam determine the gamma 1 and 2 phases.

2. Condensation is packing or compressing dental amalgam into a prepared cavity or within a matrix band. Once the amalgam is exposed to air, this step must be completed rapidly since the mercury and coated alloy surfaces start transitioning from a plastic mass to a hard structure. Hand instruments are used to condense amalgam with pressure to adapt to the walls of the tooth and eliminate voids. Overpacking the restoration is required before moving on to the next step.

3. Burnishing is the procedure used to smooth the surface of a dental amalgam after the initial carving with a metal instrument. Carving helps to develop the occlusal anatomy, while burnishing seals the margins and smooths out the occlusal surface. Marginal breakdown occurs when burnishing is not performed correctly and dental amalgam around the margin of the tooth, which is the thinnest area, starts breaking away from the tooth.

Question

What is the logical sequence used to place an amalgam restoration into a large Class II cavity preparation?

(A) Condensation, burnishing, and trituration
(B) Burnishing, trituration, and condensation
(C) Trituration, burnishing, and condensation
(D) Trituration, condensation, and burnishing
(E) Condensation, trituration, and burnishing

Reasoning

D The passage describes the logical sequence of mixing and placing dental amalgam into a cavity preparation. The key is to determine what is the first step in the sequence and what is the last step in the sequence. Words such as *first, then, next,* or *finally* indicate a chronological series of events. Answer choice (D) correctly describes the logical approach to mixing and placing a dental amalgam restoration.

TONE QUESTIONS

The tone is an emotion or a feeling toward a topic or subject. Tone questions ask you to identify the attitude or style of the author. Always look for multiple descriptive adjectives or adverbs that can help you identify the author's attitude. Look for words denoting negative or positive feelings. Passages and articles about scientific principles tend to be neutral in tone.

➡ Example

PASSAGE

The conclusion made by Douglass et al. about the USPC data revealed that by the year 2020, the United States will experience a 79 percent increase in the adult population older than 55 years of age. The NHANES III report examined the percent of edentulism in the United States by estimating the need for maxillary and/or mandibular dentures as a percent of the population for each age group and an assessment of the total number of maxillary and mandibular dentures needed by the U.S. population. The report estimated the need for a maxillary denture, mandibular denture, or both. In spite of projected declining edentulism rates among adults, the report stated that the need for complete dentures would quadruple for individuals in the age range of 45 to 75+. In addition, combining edentulism rates and population projections by year and age group in thousands provided the projected estimate of the United States population in need of dentures. The conclusion is that estimates do not account for lost, broken, or worn-out dentures. Edentulous rates are higher for lower socioeconomic groups. With a slowdown in the economy and an increase in unemployment rates, there may be a rise in the edentulous rate. Finally, institutionalized elderly individuals and homebound people have a greater need for complete dentures. Data concerning the need for complete dentures in these groups tend to be underreported.

Question

The author's attitude toward recent developments in edentulous patients is best described as

(A) alarming.
(B) concerned.
(C) confused.
(D) optimistic.
(E) apathetic.

Reasoning

C The intent of the question is for you to interpret the author's tone or attitude in the passage. You can do this by examining the author's word choices. The correct answer to this question is choice (C). To answer tone questions correctly, you must understand the definition of each answer choice. The following is a list of standard definitions:

aggressive—hostile, determined, or argumentative
alarming—worrying or disturbing
ambivalent—having mixed feelings or uncertain
apathetic—showing no feelings or interest
assertive—being self-confident or strong willed
cautionary—gives warning or raises awareness
concerned—troubled, anxious, uneasy, or apprehensive
confused—unable to think clearly
defensive—justifying a certain position or being watchful
impartial—unbiased, neutral, or objective
informative—factual and educational
optimistic—hopeful and confident about the future
pensive—reflective, philosophical, or contemplative
pragmatic—realistic and sensible

EXTRAPOLATE QUESTIONS

Extrapolation means to extend a known situation to an unknown situation by assuming a similar trend will continue. Extrapolate questions are asked when graphs or tables are provided with the reading passage. To answer these questions correctly, you must identify future trends or make an estimate about known facts. Graphs and tables can be overwhelming. So be sure that you correctly identify the EXACT information being asked in the question before you try to extrapolate.

➡ Example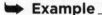

PASSAGE

After the September 2001 attacks, both the scientific and security communities believe that advances in medical technology to cure diseases such as HIV and cancer have also laid the groundwork for the potential creation of biological weapons of mass destruction. The United States is particularly vulnerable to a release of biological pathogens by rogue nations or terrorist organizations since most cities in the United States are within a 36-hour commercial flight of any area of the world. Rogue nations and terrorist organizations can replicate, mass produce, package, and deliver infectious pathogens with pinpoint accuracy to any city in the nation, resulting in high rates of morbidity and mortality. Recent terrorist attacks have prompted justified societal concerns about the hostile use of biological agents and their potential threats to health. Mortality rates associated with infectious diseases in the United States have increased by approximately 5 percent yearly since 1980. In that year, they accounted for 59 deaths per 100,000 people annually. Current research also links infectious pathogens to diseases such as diabetes, heart disease, and ulcers, which were previously thought to have been caused by environmental or lifestyle factors.

Question

Based on the 1980 infectious disease rate in the United States, how many expected deaths per 100,000 were there in the year 1990?

(A) 88.50
(B) 94.14
(C) 96.10
(D) 103.80
(E) 108.98

Reasoning

C This paragraph states the mortality rate in the United States in 1980 due to infectious diseases to be 59 deaths per 100,000. A 5 percent yearly increase would place the 1990 infectious disease rate at 96.10 deaths per 100,000. The best answer is choice (C).

DEFINITION QUESTIONS

A definition is a formal statement of the meaning or significance of a word or phrase. Definition questions are used by the author to make sure you understand a term or subject. This type of question can be identified because it includes the word "define," the phrase "is defined by," or something similar.

➡ Example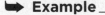

PASSAGE

The duty cycle is a number assigned to a welding machine based on the maximum current drawn at the highest amperage. The National Electrode Manufacturers sets a standard for duty cycle based on a 10-minute period. The duty cycle indicates how many minutes out of 10 that a welding machine can produce its maximum output without overheating the internal components. A welding machine rated at "50 percent duty cycle" means the welder can weld continuously for 5 minutes and then will have to let the machine rest for 5 minutes to avoid overheating the machine.

Question

How does the author define the term "duty cycle" in the passage?

(A) How many minutes of rest that a welder must stop before welding again
(B) How many minutes out of 10 that a welding machine can produce its maximum output
(C) Full capacity for 5 minutes out of every 10 minutes
(D) The force that causes current to flow in a circuit
(E) The direction the electric current is flowing

Reasoning

B This paragraph tries to throw off the reader by citing an example of duty cycle. Sentence 3 provides the definition of duty cycle. The rest of the paragraph identifies the group that sets a standard for welding machines. In this example, the only possible answer is choice (B).

CALCULATE QUESTIONS

The purpose of calculate questions is to measure your ability to use a formula or to add, subtract, or multiply numbers accurately and to choose an appropriate answer.

➡ Example _____

PASSAGE

A client is prescribed 2,000 milligrams of amoxicillin 1 hour prior to a dental root planing and scaling procedure and 500 milligrams of amoxicillin, 3 times daily, every 8 hours for the next 5 days. If the pharmacist only has 250-milligram tablets, how many should he or she dispense for the entire course of treatment?

(A) 20 tablets
(B) 25 tablets
(C) 38 tablets
(D) 40 tablets
(E) 50 tablets

Reasoning

C The answer to this question is determined by simple addition and multiplication. First understand that the initial dosage requires 2,000 milligrams (2,000 ÷ 250) = 8 tablets. The client is directed to take the prescription for an additional 5 days at a dosage of 500 milligrams 3 times a day (500 ÷ 250 × 3 × 5) = 30 tablets. Add 8 tablets plus 30 tablets to get 38 tablets, which is answer choice (C).

PART FIVE

Quantitative Reasoning Test

Introduction

37

The DAT Quantitative Section (DAT Quant) is a great opportunity for you to push up your score. It factors directly into your academic average (AA), which is one of the first things dental schools look at when evaluating you. Often, the DAT Quant is the lowest-scoring section nationally for the DAT. So don't be fooled if you think it might be "easy" due to it lacking any math beyond trigonometry. Tricky problems can easily pop up, and you might not be prepared for unusual presentations of familiar material. Another issue is time. The DAT Quant places a strong demand on your ability to manage time.

The purpose of this chapter of your *Barron's DAT* book is to bring you up to speed on the most important aspects of the DAT Quant. Emphasis has been placed on problem-solving ideas and on concepts that are generally the most stressful to students. These concepts are not easily "looked up" in textbooks. For example, we will not spend time on reducing fractions. Instead, we will focus on topics like rate problems, which sometimes require a slight twist on conventional approaches. The problems presented are a **big** portion of what makes this book unique. Some are routine. However, many encapsulate key problem-solving ideas and procedures that occur again and again in DAT Quant problems.

Another special feature of this book is the links to videos. Please take advantage of these as they extend and add to the content in this book. Everybody learns differently. A book is a great resource that is readily available and allows you to move at your own pace. Sometimes, a picture (or a video in this case) is worth a thousand words. Hopefully, the discussion of the DAT Quant here coupled with the videos will give you the best preparation possible. In psychological terms, the more modalities (senses) that are accessed, the better the learning. Some videos are clips taken from a DAT class (both small groups and regular sections containing 84 students). The background has been muted on these videos to filter out student comments and questions for the sake of brevity. Some videos have been created just for the *Barron's DAT* book. These videos appear as one-on-one problem-solving sessions.

Good Luck!

Arithmetic with Problem Solving

38

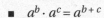

FUNDAMENTAL OPERATIONS

This book assumes that you have an understanding of fractions, exponents, roots, logarithms, absolute values, and basic operations with them. To get some practice, please consult *www.youtube.com/user/swartwoodprep*.

ONLINE TUTORIALS

- $a^b \cdot a^c = a^{b+c}$

- $\dfrac{a^b}{a^c} = a^{b-c}$

- $(a^b)^c = a^{bc}$

- $a^{-b} = \dfrac{1}{a^b}$

- $\sqrt[b]{a} = a^{\frac{1}{b}}$

- You cannot add exponents when bases are added: $a^y + a^z \neq a^{y+z}$

- $\log(ab) = \log a + \log b$

- $\log\left(\dfrac{a}{b}\right) = \log a - \log b$

- $\log a^b = b \log a$

RATES

The key formula in understanding rates is, of course, the distance formula: $d = rt$, where d is distance, r is rate, and t is time. For example, 30 miles = (10 miles per hour)(3 hours). Take the time to look at the following examples carefully as they include not only standard problems but also DAT favorites. Many of them have built into them problem-solving ideas and tips.

➡️ **Example** _____

Val travels at 30 mph for 30 minutes and then at 40 mph for 2 hours. What was his average speed for the trip?

(A) 30 mph
(B) 32 mph
(C) 35 mph
(D) 38 mph
(E) 40 mph

Solution 1

The units need to match. Convert 30 minutes into 0.5 hour so that both times are measured in hours. Use $d = rt$ twice to get the total distance.

$$d_1 = (30 \text{ mph})(0.5 \text{ hr}) = 15 \text{ miles}$$
$$d_2 = (40 \text{ mph})(2 \text{ hr}) = 80 \text{ miles}$$
$$d_{total} = 80 + 15 = 95 \text{ miles}$$
$$d_{total} = r_{average} t_{total}$$
$$95 \text{ miles} = r_{average}(2.5 \text{ hr})$$
$$r_{average} = 38 \text{ mph}$$

The answer is choice (D).

Solution 2

Test the answer choices. The average of 30 and 40 is 35. However, more time is spent at 40 mph, so the average should be closer to 40 but not 40. The only answer choice between 35 and 40 is 38. The answer is choice (D).

For another solution method, try *www.youtube.com/user/swartwoodprep*.

ONLINE TUTORIALS

➥ Example

Rila traveled from work to his house at 30 mph and returned to work at 40 mph. What was Rila's average speed for the trip?

(A) 30 mph
(B) 34.29 mph
(C) 35 mph
(D) 38.33 mph
(E) 40 mph

Solution

The issue here is that there is no given distance, but this does not stop you from creating one for your convenience. Since no distance is specified, the problem should give the answer no matter what distance is chosen. For convenience, choose a number divisible by both 30 and 40. Let's use 120. (For the remainder of the solution, units will be left out to make the solution easier to read and understand.)

$$d = rt$$
$$120 = 30t_1$$
$$t_1 = 4$$
$$120 = 40t_2$$
$$t_2 = 3$$
$$d_{total} = r_{average} t_{total}$$

The total distance there and back is $120 + 120 = 240$.

$$240 = r_{average}(t_1 + t_2)$$
$$240 = r_{average}(7)$$
$$r_{average} = 34.29$$

The answer is choice (B).

For a similar problem, see *www.youtube.com/user/swartwoodprep*.

ONLINE
TUTORIALS

WORK

Work problems are just rate problems in disguise. The distance formula can be applied in a number of settings where it is not very obvious that $d = rt$ can be employed. On occasion, the "distance" to be traveled is actually not a distance at all.

➡ Example

Peka takes 5 hours to build a car. Mickey takes 3 hours to build the same car. If they work together at their own respective rates, how long will it take them to build a car together?

(A) 8 hours

(B) 4 hours

(C) $2\frac{1}{2}$ hours

(D) $1\frac{7}{8}$ hours

(E) 1 hour

TIP

Here the trick is to set the "distance" equal to 1 car.

$$d = r_{Peka} t_{Peka}$$
$$1 = r_{Peka}(5)$$
$$r_{Peka} = \frac{1}{5}$$
$$d = r_{Mickey} t_{Mickey}$$
$$1 = r_{Mickey}(3)$$
$$r_{Mickey} = \frac{1}{3}$$
$$d = r_{combined} t_{combined}$$
$$1 = \left(\frac{1}{5} + \frac{1}{3}\right) t_{combined}$$
$$1 = \left(\frac{3}{15} + \frac{5}{15}\right) t_{combined} = \left(\frac{8}{15}\right) t_{combined}$$
$$t_{combined} = \frac{15}{8} = 1\frac{7}{8} \text{ hours}$$

ONLINE
TUTORIALS

The answer is choice (D).

For more practice, go to *www.youtube.com/user/swartwoodprep*.

PERCENTAGES

Percentages are ratios of part to whole × 100%.

You can convert from decimals to percentages by multiplying by 100%. For example:

$$\frac{1}{5} = 0.2$$

$$0.2 \times 100\% = 20\%$$

Conveniently, you can also find the decimal from the percent by dividing by 100%. For example:

$$83\% = 0.83$$

To calculate the percent increase or decrease, use the following formula:

$$\text{percent increase (or decrease)} = \frac{\text{final} - \text{initial}}{\text{initial}} \times 100\%$$

➡ **Example** _____

Gigi received a 10% raise after his first year working for a company. He then received a 20% raise on top of that the following year. What was his total percent increase from his initial salary to the end of his second year?

Solution

Assume that Gigi's initial salary was 100. After the first year, he received a 10% raise:

$$10\% \text{ of } 100 = (0.1)100 = 10$$

So Gigi's salary after the first raise was

$$10 + 100 = 110$$

After the second year, he received a 20% raise on top of his current salary at that time, 110:

$$20\% \text{ of } 110 = 0.2(110) = 22$$

Gigi's final salary was

$$22 + 110 = 132$$

Now compute the percent increase:

$$\frac{\text{final} - \text{initial}}{\text{initial}} \times 100\% = \frac{132 - 100}{100} \times 100\% = 32\%$$

The usefulness of picking 100 for Gigi's initial salary is that the computations are very quick.

Try out this one: *www.youtube.com/user/swartwoodprep*.

TIP

When working with percentages, always use 100 or a similar number—such as 10—when choosing test numbers.

ONLINE TUTORIALS

RATIOS

A key component when attacking problems involving ratios is to make sure that corresponding parts match. In the following example, notice how the number of boys at the beginning is matched to the number of boys at the end and how the number of girls at the beginning is matched to the number of girls at the end.

➡ Example _____

The ratio of boys to girls at a club event is three to four. There are originally 210 people present at the event. If the number of girls is doubled, how many total people are now present at the event?

(A) 9
(B) 120
(C) 180
(D) 240
(E) 330

Solution

This problem is trickier than it looks but will give us good practice using ratios. Here is one way of solving the problem. The number of girls originally at the event is $\frac{\text{girls}}{\text{boys}}$ (total originally). Note that $\frac{4}{3}(210) = 280$ is *not* the answer as the ratio $\frac{4}{3}$ matches the number of girls to the number of boys. Instead, we need the ratio of the number of girls to the total number of people initially at the event. Use the ratio $\frac{4}{3+4}$ because it matches the number of girls to the total number of people. So the number of girls originally present is $\frac{4}{3+4}(210) = 120$. Naturally, the number of boys originally present is $210 - 120 = 90$. Since the number of girls was then doubled to 240, the total number of people at the event is now $240 + 90 = 330$. The answer is choice (E).

Algebra

LINEAR EQUATIONS AND SYSTEMS OF LINEAR EQUATIONS

Make sure you are comfortable setting up and solving simple linear equations. These are popular on the DAT. Here are some classics to give you a bit of practice.

➥ Example

Val is twice Paola's age now. In ten years from now, Paola's age at that time will be three-fourths Val's age at that time. How old is Paola now?

(A) 5
(B) 10
(C) 15
(D) 20
(E) 25

Solution

Val (V) is now twice Paola's age (P):

$$V = 2P$$

In ten years from now, Paola will be $\frac{3}{4}$ of Val's age at that time:

$$P + 10 = \frac{3}{4}(V + 10)$$

You now have 2 equations with 2 unknowns. Solve for P:

$$\frac{3}{4}(2P + 10) = P + 10$$
$$1.5P + 7.5 = P + 10$$
$$0.5P = 2.5$$
$$P = 5$$

The answer is choice (A).

If two sandwiches and three colas cost 8 dollars and if three sandwiches and four colas cost 11 dollars, then how much does a sandwich and a cola cost?

(A) $1
(B) $2
(C) $3
(D) $4
(E) $5

Solution

There is a very fast way to do this problem. Please consult _www.youtube.com/user/swartwoodprep_ for a quick method. However, since the point of this problem is to practice general techniques, let's solve this using a system of linear equations (which sounds much worse than it really is). Let S represent the price of one sandwich. Let C represent the price of one cola. Then the problem can be written as:

$$2S + 3C = 8$$
$$3S + 4C = 11$$
$$S + C = ?$$

ONLINE TUTORIALS

Can you see the shortcut? If not, look at _www.youtube.com/user/swartwoodprep_ after reading through this solution.

The long solution: We can solve for either S or C in one equation, substitute that answer into the other equation, and solve for $S + C$. Instead, we will multiply the first equation by –4 and the second by 3:

$$-8S + (-12C) = -32$$
$$9S + 12C = 33$$

Now add the two new equations together to eliminate C:

$$S = 1$$

Solve for C by plugging $S = 1$ back into either of the original two equations. For this problem, let's use the first equation. Then solve for the price of one sandwich and one cola:

$$2S + 3C = 8$$
$$2(1) + 3C = 8$$
$$3C = 6$$
$$C = 2$$
$$S + C = 3$$

The answer is choice (C).

LINEAR INEQUALITIES

Linear inequalities can be solved just as you do for linear equations but with the following caveat. You must remember that multiplication or division by a negative number switches the direction of the inequality sign.

➡ Example _____

If $-2y + 16 \leq 32$, then what is true of y?

(A) $y \leq -8$

(B) $y \leq 8$

(C) $y \geq -8$

(D) $y \geq 8$

(E) $y = 8$

Solution

Solving this problem gives you practice with manipulating inequalities. Believe it or not, you could actually see a problem like this on the DAT. First subtract 16 from both sides:

$$-2y + 16 \leq 32$$
$$-2y \leq 16$$

Now divide both sides by -2. **This changes the direction of the inequality sign:**

$$y \geq -8$$

The correct answer is choice (C).

A WORD ABOUT NOTHING

Zero is a key player in multiplication and division. The DAT knows that fact. Anytime multiplying numbers results in zero, one of the numbers being multiplied must be zero. Division by zero is not possible.

> **TIP**
>
> Adding or subtracting by a negative number does not change the direction of the inequality sign.

➡ Example _____

$(a \cdot b^2 \cdot c^{-2} \cdot d \cdot \pi) = 0$. Which of the following must be true?

(A) a, b, c, and d must all be zero.

(B) a, b, c, and d cannot be zero.

(C) c^{-2} can be zero.

(D) b^2 can be zero, but b cannot.

(E) a, b, or d must be zero.

Solution

One of the multiplied numbers must be zero, but they do not all have to be. So both choices (A) and (B) are incorrect. Choice (C) is incorrect because c^{-2} cannot be zero.

$$c^{-2} = 0 \rightarrow \frac{1}{c^2} = 0 \rightarrow 1 = 0, \text{ if } c^2 \neq 0$$

If $c^2 = 0$, then $\frac{1}{c^2} = \frac{1}{0}$ makes no sense. There is no reason why both b and b^2 cannot be zero. So choice (D) is incorrect. Since zero is the product and c cannot be zero, a, b, or d must be zero. The correct answer is choice (E).

QUADRATICS AND FACTORING

It is useful to know the following three identities:

$$(a+b)^2 = a^2 + 2ab + b^2$$
$$(a-b)^2 = a^2 - 2ab + b^2$$
$$(a+b)(a-b) = a^2 - b^2$$

You should also be familiar with FOIL and reverse FOIL (a form of *factoring*). Examples of each are found in Figures 39.1 and 39.2.

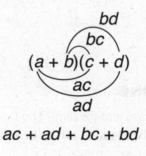

Figure 39.1. FOIL

$$\underbrace{x^2 + (a+b)x + ab}$$
$$(x+a)(x+b)$$

Figure 39.2. Reverse FOIL (factoring)

➡ Example

What are the x-intercepts of the parabola $y = x^2 + 5x + 6$?

(A) (0, 3), (0, –3)
(B) (3, 0), (–3, 0)
(C) (2, 0), (0, –2)
(D) (2, 0), (–3, 0)
(E) (–2, 0), (–3, 0)

Solution

The x-intercepts of a graph are the points where the graph crosses the x-axis. These must always have y-coordinates of zero. So only answer choices (B), (D), and (E) are viable. You can use reverse FOIL (factoring) since the y-coordinate must be zero:

$$0 = x^2 + 5x + 6$$
$$0 = (x + 2)(x + 3)$$

Since $(x + 2)$ and $(x + 3)$ multiply to give you zero, one of them must equal zero for the equation to work. Set each one equal to zero to find solutions for x:

$$(x + 2) = 0 \qquad (x + 3) = 0$$
$$x = -2 \qquad\quad x = -3$$

The only options for the x-intercepts are (–2, 0) and (–3, 0). The answer is choice (E).

If using reverse FOIL does not work to solve a problem, you could always use the quadratic formula. See *www.youtube.com/user/swartwoodprep* for an application. For a quadratic equation in the form $ax^2 + bx + c = 0$:

$$x = \frac{-b \pm \sqrt{b^2 - 4ac}}{2a}$$

ONLINE TUTORIALS

Geometry

40

PARALLEL LINES AND VERTICAL ANGLES

Vertical angles are formed when straight lines cross. Two sets of vertical angles are shown in Figure 40.1. Angles *a* and *b* are vertical; they are equal in measure. Angles *b* and *c* are vertical; they are equal in measure.

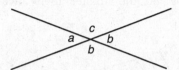

Figure 40.1. Vertical angles

Matching angles (corresponding angles) are formed when parallel lines are intersected by another line (transversal). In Figure 40.2, two sets of matching angles are created.

In the diagram below, *a–h* represent the measures of the respective engles.

a = *b*, *c* = *d*, *e* = *f*, and *g* = *h*

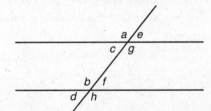

After adding information about vertical angles being equal in measure, we obtain:

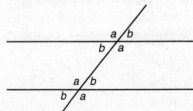

Figure 40.2. Matching angles (corresponding angles)

TRIANGLES I

Triangles are very important in geometry. The following are some important facts about triangles that might come in handy on the DAT. Learn them.

Triangle Fact 1

The sum of the measures of the interior angles in any triangle always adds up to 180°. See Figure 40.3.

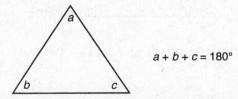

$a + b + c = 180°$

Figure 40.3. The sum of the interior angles in a triangle always equals 180°.

Triangle Fact 2

The sum of the lengths of any two sides of a triangle is always greater than the length of the third side. Likewise, the difference between the lengths of any two sides of a triangle is always less than the length of the third side. See Figure 40.4.

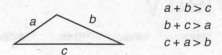

$$a + b > c$$
$$b + c > a$$
$$c + a > b$$

Figure 40.4. The relationship among side lengths in any triangle

Triangle Fact 3

Given any two angles in a triangle, the smaller angle always faces the smaller side. See Figure 40.5.

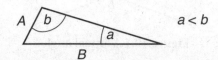

$$a < b$$

Figure 40.5. Angle *a* is smaller than angle *b*. Side *A* is shorter than side *B*.

➥ Example

Achilles decides to walk 3 miles in one direction and then 5 miles in another direction. If the two directions are not the same and are not opposite, which of the following could be the distance between his starting and ending locations?

(A) 1 mile
(B) 2 miles
(C) 3 miles
(D) 8 miles
(E) 9 miles

Solution

Think of the 3 miles and 5 miles that Achilles walked as being the sides of a triangle. You are now trying to figure out something about the third side. Draw a triangle, and label the known sides.

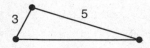

By Triangle Fact 2, the third side must be bigger than $5 - 3 = 2$ but smaller than $5 + 3 = 8$. Only answer choice (C) works.

TRIANGLES II (PYTHAGOREAN THEOREM)

Based on their angles, triangles can be classified in one of three ways:

1. **Acute:** the angles are all less than $90°$
2. **Obtuse:** one angle is greater than $90°$
3. **Right:** one angle is exactly $90°$

Based on their sides, triangles can also be classified in one of three ways:

1. **Scalene:** all three sides have different lengths
2. **Isosceles:** two sides have the same length
3. **Equilateral:** all three sides have the same length

Make sure you know the following facts about triangles.

Triangle Fact 4

In an isosceles triangle, the angles facing sides of equal length are of equal measure.

Triangle Fact 5

All three angles in an equilateral triangle are of equal length.

Triangle Fact 6

In a right triangle, the Pythagorean theorem lets us know that $a^2 + b^2 = c^2$ when side c is opposite the right angle. The side opposite the right angle is called the *hypotenuse*. See Figure 40.6.

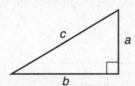

Figure 40.6. The Pythagorean theorem
applies to right triangles: $a^2 + b^2 = c^2$.

The Pythagorean theorem actually gives us a sense of distance in the plane and in space. Make sure you know these two fundamental Pythagorean triples as the DAT loves them. The first is

$$3^2 + 4^2 = 5^2$$

Triangles having these lengths, or a multiple of them, are often referred to as 3-4-5 triangles. The second Pythagorean triple is

$$5^2 + 12^2 = 13^2$$

Triangles having these lengths, or a multiple of them, are often referred to as 5-12-13 triangles.

Note that any multiples of these two special triplets work as well. For example, 6, 8, 10 are the lengths of the sides of a right triangle since $6 = 2 \times 3$, $8 = 2 \times 4$, and $10 = 2 \times 5$. We will look at some examples after covering perimeter and area.

The Pythagorean Theorem applies only to right triangles. If the longest side (hypotenuse) is side c, then $a^2 + b^2 = c^2$.

TRIANGLES III (SPECIAL TRIANGLES)

You should know there are two special right triangles. The first is the 45°-45°-90° right triangle. Its angles are 45°, 45°, and 90°. The ratios of the lengths of the respective sides are $a:a:a\sqrt{2}$, as you can see in Figure 40.7.

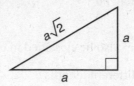

Figure 40.7. A 45°-45°-90° right triangle
with side lengths a, a, and $a\sqrt{2}$

The second special right triangle is the 30°-60°-90° right triangle. Its angles are 30°, 60°, and 90°. The ratios of the lengths of the respective sides are $a:a\sqrt{3}:2a$. See Figure 40.8.

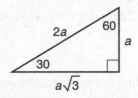

Figure 40.8. A 30°-60°-90° right triangle
with side lengths of a, $a\sqrt{3}$, and $2a$

The properties of 45°-45°-90° and 30°-60°-90° right triangles can be proven with the Pythagorean theorem. You should be very comfortable using these triangles when taking the DAT.

➠ **Example** _____

What is the length of side b in the figure shown below?

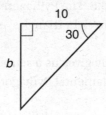

(A) $\dfrac{10\sqrt{3}}{3}$

(B) $\dfrac{\sqrt{3}}{10}$

(C) $10\sqrt{3}$

(D) $3\sqrt{10}$

(E) 20

Solution

In the diagram, you are given two angles: 30° and 90° (shown by the box symbol). Based on Triangle Fact 1, the missing angle must equal 60° since 30° + 60° + 90° = 180°. So this is a 30°-60°-90° right triangle. Use the known relationships among the sides of a 30°-60°-90° right triangle to find the length of side b. The side with length b is opposite the 30° angle. The side with length 10 is opposite the 60° angle. Therefore, 10 must equal $b\sqrt{3}$. Solve for b:

$$b\sqrt{3} = 10$$

$$b = \frac{10}{\sqrt{3}}$$

You must rationalize the denominator, which means getting rid of the radical sign. Just multiply the fraction by $\frac{\sqrt{3}}{\sqrt{3}}$, which equals 1, and, therefore, does not change the value of the fraction:

$$\frac{10}{\sqrt{3}} \cdot \frac{\sqrt{3}}{\sqrt{3}} = \frac{10\sqrt{3}}{3}$$

The answer is choice (A).

PERIMETER AND AREA

Figure 40.9 shows a quick summary of the perimeter (the length "around" the figure) and the area of several plane figures. These formulas are often employed on the DAT.

Shape	Perimeter	Area
Square 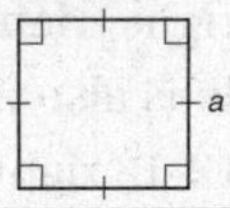	$4a$	a^2
Rectangle 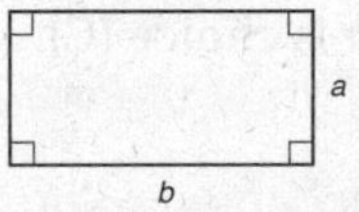	$2a + 2b$	ab
Parallelogram 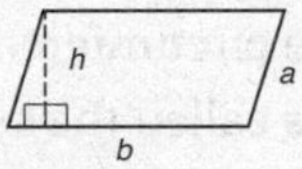	$2a + 2b$	bh
Triangle 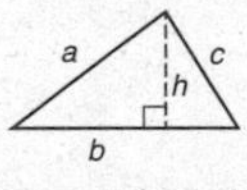	$a + b + c$	$\frac{1}{2}bh$
Trapezoid 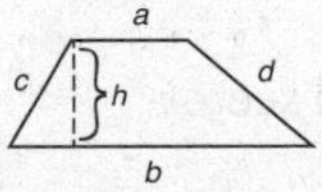	$a + b + c + d$	$\left(\frac{a+b}{2}\right)h$
Circle 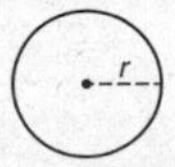	$2\pi r$	πr^2

Figure 40.9. The perimeter and area of plane figures

What is the area of rectangle A in the diagram?

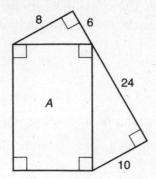

(A)   120 square units
(B)   130 square units
(C)   260 square units
(D)   320 square units
(E)   520 square units

Solution

While you can use the Pythagorean theorem to solve for the missing lengths, try using this shortcut. You are told (by the box symbol) that the upper triangle is a right triangle. Since $6 = 2 \times \underline{3}$ and $8 = 2 \times \underline{4}$, the upper triangle must be a 3-4-5 right triangle. The hypotenuse must therefore be $2 \times \underline{5} = 10$. Likewise, the triangle on the side is also a right triangle. Since $24 = 2 \times \underline{12}$ and $10 = 2 \times \underline{5}$, the triangle on the side must be a 5-12-13 right triangle. The hypotenuse must therefore be $2 \times \underline{13} = 26$. The length of the rectangle is 10, and the width is 26. So the area of the rectangle is $10 \times 26 = 260$. The correct answer is choice (C).

CIRCLES

Circles deserve special attention. The section of the circumference shown in Figure 40.10 is the arc subtended by angle A. The length of the section of the circumference is called the arc length. The area of the part of the circle enclosed by angle A is called the sector.

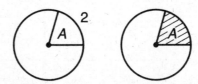

Figure 40.10. Arc, arc length, and sector

The key to solving arc length and sector area problems is to use proportions.

➡ Example

If the arc length of a portion of a circle subtended by angle θ is 5π, what is the area of the sector enclosed by angle θ? The radius of the circle is 10. (It is assumed that units are consistent.)

(A) 5π

(B) 20π

(C) 25π

(D) 100π

(E) 200π

Solution

In case you are rusty with the jargon, *subtended* means "enclosed." The key is to set up a proportion. Remember that a proportion is when two ratios are set equal to each other. The circumference of the circle is $2\pi r = (2)(\pi)(10) = 20\pi$. The total area of the circle is $\pi r^2 = (\pi)(10)^2 = 100\pi$. Remember to match part to whole:

$$\frac{\text{part}}{\text{whole}} = \frac{\text{part}}{\text{whole}}$$

$$\frac{\text{part}}{\text{whole}} = \frac{\text{arc}}{\text{circumference}} = \frac{5\pi}{20\pi}$$

$$\frac{\text{part}}{\text{whole}} = \frac{\text{sector angle}}{\text{total angle}} = \frac{\theta}{360°}$$

$$\frac{5\pi}{20\pi} = \frac{\theta}{360°}$$

$$\theta = 90°$$

Now use the angle of the sector to set up the proportion for the areas:

$$\frac{\text{part}}{\text{whole}} = \frac{\text{sector area}}{\text{total area}} = \frac{90°}{360°}$$

$$\frac{\text{sector area}}{100\pi} = \frac{90°}{360°}$$

$$\text{sector area} = 25\pi$$

The answer is choice (C).

3D FIGURES

Figure 40.11 shows a summary of the surface area and volume formulas for common solid figures.

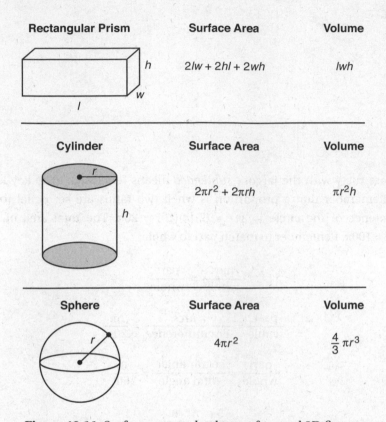

Rectangular Prism	Surface Area	Volume
	$2lw + 2hl + 2wh$	lwh

Cylinder	Surface Area	Volume
	$2\pi r^2 + 2\pi rh$	$\pi r^2 h$

Sphere	Surface Area	Volume
	$4\pi r^2$	$\frac{4}{3}\pi r^3$

Figure 40.11. Surface area and volume of several 3D figures

➡ **Example** _____

A room in the shape of a rectangular prism has dimensions of 9 feet by 12 feet by 36 feet. What is the distance from one corner of the room to the opposite corner?

(A) 13 feet
(B) 26 feet
(C) 39 feet
(D) 108 feet
(E) 130 feet

Solution

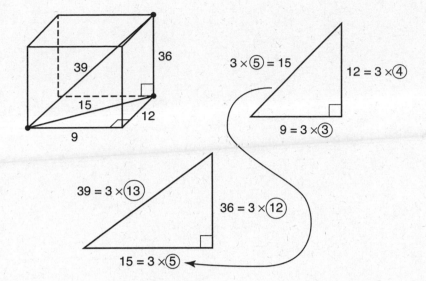

The diagram shows that we can reduce this problem to two right triangles. As is usually the case on the DAT, the right triangles involved are "special." Instead of computing, we can notice that $9 = 3 \times \underline{3}$ and that $12 = 3 \times \underline{4}$. This gives us a 3-4-5 right triangle. So the hypotenuse (which is the length across the floor in the diagram) is $3 \times 5 = 15$. For the second triangle, we again use a cheap trick. $15 = 3 \times \underline{5}$, and $36 = 3 \times \underline{12}$. So, there is a 5-12-13 right triangle. Get used to this sort of thinking; the DAT loves it. The missing hypotenuse must be $3 \times \underline{13} = 39$. The correct answer is choice (C). Shortcuts are key to time management.

See *www.youtube.com/user/swartwoodprep.*

Analytic Geometry

41

LINES

You should understand both the point-slope form and the slope-intercept form of the equation of a line. For a brief description of these equations as well as a discussion of slope itself, please go to *www.youtube.com/user/swartwoodprep*.

ONLINE TUTORIALS

> **SLOPE-INTERCEPT FORM**
> $y = mx + b$

In the slope-intercept form, $y = mx + b$, m represents the slope $= \dfrac{\text{rise}}{\text{run}} = \dfrac{\Delta \text{ vertical}}{\Delta \text{ horizontal}}$ and b represents where the line intercepts the y-axis.

➡ Example

What is the equation of the line that passes through $(3, 9)$ with a slope of 10?

(A) $y = 9x + 3$
(B) $y = 3x + 9$
(C) $y = 10x + 9$
(D) $y = 10x + 3$
(E) $y = 10x - 21$

Solution

One strategy is to plug in 3 for x and plug in 9 for y into each answer choice and see which equation works. Note that the slope is 10, so choices (C), (D), and (E) are the only viable answers. Now, plug in to solve for b:

$$9 = 10(3) + b$$
$$9 = 30 + b$$
$$-21 = b$$
$$y = 10x - 21$$

The correct answer is choice (E).

> **POINT-SLOPE FORM**
> $y - y_1 = m(x - x_1)$

In point-slope form, $y - y_1 = m(x - x_1)$, the variables x_1 and y_1 represent the x- and y-coordinates, respectively, of a point on the line. The variable m represents the slope.

Example

What is the equation of the line passing through (3, 9) with a slope of 10?

(A) $y - 10 = 3(x - 9)$
(B) $y - 10 = 9(x - 3)$
(C) $y - 3 = 9(x - 10)$
(D) $y - 3 = 10(x - 9)$
(E) $y - 9 = 10(x - 3)$

Solution

Again, we can use the fact that the slope is 10 to narrow the options to choices (D) and (E). Since 9 must be subtracted from y and 3 must be subtracted from x, the answer is choice (E).

PARALLEL AND PERPENDICULAR LINES

Two lines are parallel if their slopes are the same. Two lines are perpendicular if their slopes are negative reciprocals of one another. In symbol form, $\ell_1 \parallel \ell_2 \Leftrightarrow m_1 = m_2$ and $\ell_1 \perp \ell_2 \Leftrightarrow m_1 = -\dfrac{1}{m_2}$.

To illustrate, the lines $y = 3x + 12$ and $y = 3x - 75$ are parallel because they both have the same slope, 3. In contrast, the lines $y = 3x + 12$ and $y = -\dfrac{1}{3}x - 75$ are perpendicular because their slopes are the negative reciprocals of each other, 3 and $-\dfrac{1}{3}$.

See *www.youtube.com/user/swartwoodprep* for an example.

CIRCLES

A circle is a collection of points a fixed distance r from the *center* of the circle. The defining equation for a circle with its center at the origin can be found using the Pythagorean theorem.

> **FORMULA FOR A CIRCLE CENTERED AT THE ORIGIN**
>
> $x^2 + y^2 = r^2$

Not all circles have their center at the origin. Another formula can be used for all circles, no matter the location of their center.

> **FORMULA FOR A CIRCLE CENTERED AT (h, k)**
>
> $(x - h)^2 + (y - k)^2 = r^2$

Example

What is the equation of a circle centered at (3, 4) with a radius of 2?

(A) $(x-3)^2 + (y-2)^2 = 4$
(B) $(x-4)^2 + (y-3)^2 = 2$
(C) $(x-3)^2 + (y-4)^2 = 2$
(D) $(x-2)^2 + (y-4)^2 = 4$
(E) $(x-3)^2 + (y-4)^2 = 4$

Solution

We just plug and chug. Since the circle is centered at (3, 4), only choices (C) and (E) are options. Since the radius is 2, the right-hand side of the equation must be $2^2 = 4$. The correct answer is choice (E).

ELLIPSES

Ellipses are basically stretched circles. Start by thinking of a circle centered at (0, 0) with a radius of 1. Its equation is $x^2 + y^2 = 1$. Now stretch the circle by a units in the x-direction and by b units in the y-direction to find the equation of an ellipse.

> **EQUATION OF AN ELLIPSE CENTERED AT (0, 0)**
>
> $$\frac{x^2}{a^2} + \frac{y^2}{b^2} = 1$$

> **EQUATION OF AN ELLIPSE CENTERED AT (h, k)**
>
> $$\frac{(x-h)^2}{a^2} + \frac{(y-k)^2}{b^2} = 1$$

Make sure you understand Figure 41.1 and the terminology.

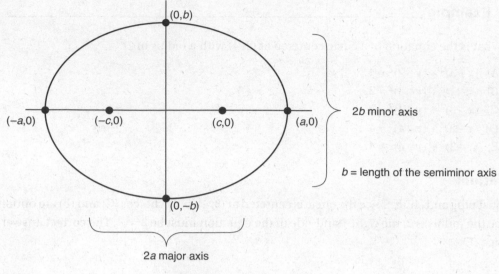

(0,*b*)

(−*a*,0)   (−*c*,0)   (*c*,0)   (*a*,0)

2*b* minor axis

b = length of the semiminor axis

(0,−*b*)

2*a* major axis

a = length of the semimajor axis

Figure 41.1. An ellipse

There is something more to be said of ellipses. Just as circles are created using a compass placed at the center of a circle, ellipses are created using two pins placed at locations called the *foci* (singular *focus*). A piece of string is tied from one focus to the other focus and stretched as far as it can reach. Then a pencil is placed at the most outstretched point and dragged around the foci. The figure traced out is an ellipse. So what is the upshot of this for the DAT?

Since the length of the string is fixed, **the distance from one focus to the ellipse to the other focus is always the same**. In fact, that length is 2*a*. That length is called the **major axis**, assuming that the ellipse is wider than it is tall. (If the ellipse is taller than it is wide, the length of the major axis is 2*b*.) **The length *a* is called the length of the semimajor axis.** See *www.youtube.com/user/swartwoodprep* for a more complete description.

➡ Example

What is the distance traversed by a light ray as it leaves one focus, arrives at the point

(0, 3), and returns to the other focus to form an ellipse with the equation $\frac{x^2}{5^2} + \frac{y^2}{3^2} = 1$?

(A) 3
(B) 5
(C) 9
(D) 10
(E) 25

Solution

The distance traversed is the length of the major axis, which is 2*a* = 2(5) = 10. The correct answer is choice (D).

Trigonometry

42

TRIGONOMETRY FUNCTIONS (SOHCAHTOA)

You are likely familiar with the fundamental trigonometry functions: sine, cosine, tangent, cosecant, secant, and cotangent. The acronym SOHCAHTOA stands for **S**ine = **O**pposite over **H**ypotenuse, **C**osine = **A**djacent over **H**ypotenuse, and **T**angent = **O**pposite over **A**djacent. Figure 42.1 shows the opposite side (y), adjacent side (x), and hypotenuse (r) in a right triangle.

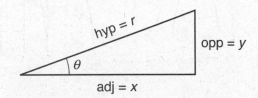

Figure 42.1. Opposite, adjacent, and hypotenuse
in a right triangle based on angle

> ### BASIC TRIGONOMETRY FUNCTIONS
>
> $$\sin \theta = \frac{\text{opp}}{\text{hyp}} = \frac{y}{r} \qquad\qquad \csc \theta = \frac{\text{hyp}}{\text{opp}} = \frac{r}{y}$$
>
> $$\cos \theta = \frac{\text{adj}}{\text{hyp}} = \frac{x}{r} \qquad\qquad \sec \theta = \frac{\text{hyp}}{\text{adj}} = \frac{r}{x}$$
>
> $$\tan \theta = \frac{\text{opp}}{\text{adj}} = \frac{y}{x} \qquad\qquad \cot \theta = \frac{\text{adj}}{\text{opp}} = \frac{x}{y}$$

Notice that in a given row in the box showing the basic trigonometry functions, the functions in the right column are reciprocals of the functions in the left column. For example,

$$\csc \theta = \frac{1}{\sin \theta}$$

Figure 42.2 shows the graph of the basic trigonometry functions. Note that the angles shown in the graphs are in radians.

> ### RELATING RADIANS AND DEGREES
> π radians = 180°

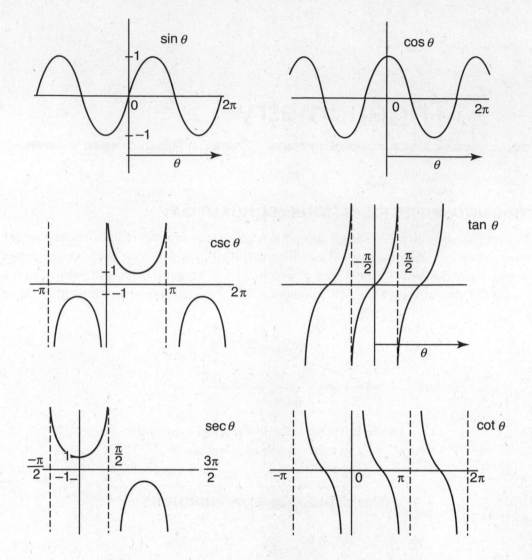

Figure 42.2. Graphs of the basic trigonometry functions

The next problem is probably one of the DAT's all-time favorites.

➡ Example _____

If $\sin \theta = \dfrac{3}{5}$, then what is $\cos \theta$?

(A) $\dfrac{3}{4}$

(B) $\dfrac{4}{5}$

(C) $\dfrac{3}{7}$

(D) $\dfrac{4}{7}$

(E) $\dfrac{5}{7}$

Solution

We can use any triangle that has $\sin\theta = \frac{3}{5}$. So use one that has sides 3, b, and 5. Draw 3 as the length of the side opposite to θ, b as the length adjacent to θ, and 5 as the hypotenuse. By using the Pythagorean theorem, we determine that b is 4. So $\cos\theta = \frac{4}{5}$. The correct answer is choice (B).

See *www.youtube.com/user/swartwoodprep* for a discussion of the unit circle.

You should memorize the sine, cosine, and tangent for the angles in 30°-60°-90° and 45°-45°-90° triangles. These values are shown in Figure 42.3.

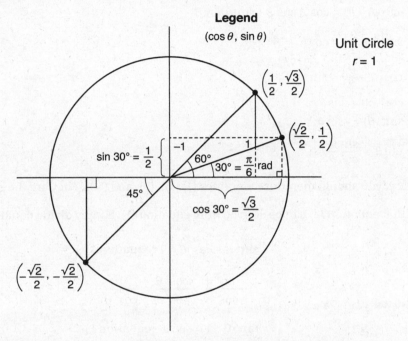

	0°	30°	45°	60°	90°
$\sin\theta$	0	$\frac{1}{2}$	$\frac{\sqrt{2}}{2}$	$\frac{\sqrt{3}}{2}$	1
$\cos\theta$	1	$\frac{\sqrt{3}}{2}$	$\frac{\sqrt{2}}{2}$	$\frac{1}{2}$	0
$\tan\theta$	0	$\frac{\sqrt{3}}{3}$	1	$\sqrt{3}$	und.

Figure 42.3. Trigonometric functions in special triangles

TRIGONOMETRIC IDENTITIES

Here are a few trigonometric identities that are useful to know for the DAT.

1. $\sin^2\theta + \cos^2\theta = 1$

2. $\tan^2\theta + 1 = \sec^2\theta$

3. $\cos\left(\dfrac{\pi}{2} - \theta\right) = \sin\theta$

   $\sin\left(\dfrac{\pi}{2} - \theta\right) = \cos\theta$

4. $\sin(A \pm B) = \sin A \cos B \pm \cos A \sin B$

5. $\cos(A + B) = \cos A \cos B - \sin A \sin B$

   $\cos(A - B) = \cos A \cos B + \sin A \sin B$

6. $\sin\left(\theta + \dfrac{\theta}{2}\right) = \cos\theta$

7. $\cos\left(\theta - \dfrac{\theta}{2}\right) = \sin\theta$

8. $\cos(-\theta) = \cos\theta$

9. $\sin(-\theta) = -\sin\theta$

10. $\tan\theta = \dfrac{\sin\theta}{\cos\theta}$

Of these, you should memorize identities (1), (8), (9), and (10). They are the most important.

Note that equation (2) can be derived from equation (1). Simply divide equation (1) by $\cos^2\theta$:

$$\sin^2\theta + \cos^2\theta = 1 \text{ (equation 1)}$$

$$\frac{\sin^2\theta}{\cos^2\theta} + \frac{\cos^2\theta}{\cos^2\theta} = \frac{1}{\cos^2\theta}$$

$$\tan^2\theta + 1 = \sec^2\theta \text{ (equation 2)}$$

➡ Example

$$3\sin^2\left(\frac{\theta}{2} + \theta\right) + 3\cos^2\left(\frac{\theta}{2} + \theta\right) = ?$$

(A) 1

(B) 1.5

(C) 3

(D) 3.5

(E) 5

Solution

Use $\sin^2\theta + \cos^2\theta = 1$. We use $\propto$ instead of θ to avoid confusion.

Let $\propto = \left(\dfrac{\theta}{2} + \theta\right)$. Then $3\sin^2\propto + 3\cos^2\propto = 3(\sin^2\propto + \cos^2\propto) = 3(1) = 3$.

Probability

43

THE COUNTING PRINCIPLE

Counting is one of the main reasons that students tend to hate probability questions on the DAT. The principles are not that bad. If you are the type who loves algorithms, most likely you will be among those who find this section to be one of your least favorites. Students often complain, "I don't know where to start. If I did, it would be a piece of cake." Hopefully, this lesson will help rectify this.

Most of the effort you exert will be invested in learning when and how to apply probability principles. The key to solving probability questions on the DAT is learning the approaches to problem solving.

It might seem easy, but even the counting principle can lead to challenging problems on the DAT. Informally, the counting principle states that whenever you run multiple experiments (or actions), such as choosing a shirt color (RED, BLUE, GREEN) and choosing another garment to wear (BLUE JEANS, SLACKS, SKIRT) to make an outfit, you need to multiply the number of outcomes in each experiment to get the total number of outcomes. Here, the 3 outcomes of shirt color and 3 outcomes for lower garment type give us $3 \times 3 = 9$ total outcomes.

To convince yourself that this works, imagine making a table with RED, BLUE, and GREEN shirts for the row labels and BLUE JEANS, SLACKS, and SKIRT for the column labels, as seen in Table 43.1. You can see that each square is an outcome, such as RED SHIRT and SKIRT. To get the number of squares, you really do multiply.

TIP

You have to learn only a few basic probability principles.

Table 43.1. Outcomes

	BLUE JEANS	SLACKS	SKIRT
RED SHIRT	RED SHIRT, BLUE JEANS	RED SHIRT, SLACKS	RED SHIRT, SKIRT
BLUE SHIRT	BLUE SHIRT, BLUE JEANS	BLUE SHIRT, SLACKS	BLUE SHIRT, SKIRT
GREEN SHIRT	GREEN SHIRT, BLUE JEANS	GREEN SHIRT, SLACKS	GREEN SHIRT, SKIRT

We won't go into this much detail on every topic, but the counting principle is the start of it all.

See *www.youtube.com/user/swartwoodprep* for another version.

ONLINE TUTORIALS

➡ Example _____

A pizza must be ordered for an event. There are three types of crust, five vegetable options, and ten meat toppings. If the pizza ordered has one type of crust, one choice of vegetables, and one meat topping, how many different pizzas can be delivered to the event?

(A) 27
(B) 50
(C) 125
(D) 150
(E) 1,000

Solution

You have 3 possibilities for the type of crust, 5 for the vegetable option, and 10 for the meat topping. So there are $3 \times 5 \times 10 = 150$ different total pizzas. The correct answer is choice (D).

➡ Example _____

There are three different treatment options for patients with a particular disease: drug 1, drug 2, or both. If a treatment plan for 5 specific patients is to be made, how many different ways can this be done? Note that every patient receives a treatment option.

(A) 15
(B) 60
(C) 125
(D) 243
(E) 3,125

Solution

It might be helpful to look at how these answer choices came about.

Choice (A) is $3 \times 5 = 15$.
Choice (B) is $5 \times 4 \times 3 = 60$.
Choice (C) is $5 \times 5 \times 5 = 125$.
Choice (D) is $3 \times 3 \times 3 \times 3 \times 3 = 243$.
Choice (E) is $5 \times 5 \times 5 \times 5 \times 5 = 3,125$.

Some students pick choice (A) because they think that there are 3 choices for the treatments and 5 for the patients, but this would compute the number of ways for one patient to be treated.

For the moment, let's compute the actual answer. (We will talk about some of the other answer choices later.) "A treatment plan for 5 specific patients" means that each patient must be assigned drug 1, drug 2, or both. For convenience, let's label the patients as P1, P2, P3, P4, and P5. P1 has 3 choices of treatment. P2 has 3 choices. P3 has 3 choices, and so on. Thus, we have $3 \times 3 \times 3 \times 3 \times 3 = 243$ outcomes. If you understand this, then you have a head start on what's coming up. If not, do not let this discourage you. Stick with it, and you will be fine. The correct answer is choice (D).

k-PERMUTATIONS

A k-permutation ("permutation" for us) is best explained with an example.

➡ **Example** _____

There are 10 candidates for three positions: president, vice president, and treasurer. Any person can occupy only one position at a time. How many ways can the president, vice president, and treasurer be chosen?

(A) 27
(B) 30
(C) 720
(D) 1,000
(E) 1,320

Solution

Imagine picking the president. There are 10 different possibilities. After you pick the president, there are only 9 people left to pick the vice president from, and after that, 8 for the treasurer. Since there are 10 outcomes for the first experiment or action, 9 for the second action, and 8 for the third action, the counting principle says that there are $10 \times 9 \times 8 = 720$ total outcomes. The correct answer is choice (C).

Now that we have seen a permutation in action, let's identify some conditions where they are used before we talk about a formula.

1. **ORDER MATTERS.** When you are counting and the order matters, you are likely dealing with a permutation of some sort.

    Notice in the previous problem that nothing about order was mentioned, but it was implied by the labels: president, vice president, and treasurer. In other words, it matters whether Bill, Ted, and Fred are the president, vice president, and treasurer, respectively, or whether Ted, Bill, and Fred are the president, vice president, and treasurer, respectively.

2. **THERE IS NO REPLACEMENT.** Whenever a choice is made (for example, Bill for president), that entity chosen (Bill) cannot be chosen again.

TIP

Don't forget that order can masquerade as labels.

Before we derive the formula for permutation, we need some notation. The notation $n!$ indicates the product of the numbers $n(n-1)(n-2)\ldots(1)$. The notation $n!$ is called "n factorial." Look at these examples of factorials.

$$4! = 4 \times 3 \times 2 \times 1 = 24$$
$$3! = 3 \times 2 \times 1 = 6$$
$$10! = 10 \times 9 \times 8 \times 7 \times 6 \times 5 \times 4 \times 3 \times 2 \times 1 = 3,628,800$$

In the previous example, we let n equal the number of people we choose from and k equal the number of positions we are filling (president, vice president, treasurer). We can find the answer using the following equation:

$$\frac{n!}{(n-k)!}$$

In our example, $\dfrac{10!}{(10-3)!}$. You can think of n as the number of entities to choose from and k as the number of ordered choices you will make. You may just want to skip the formula and think "$10 \times 9 \times 8$" as we did in the example.

Extra: (You can skip this section if you are happy with using the formula. Looking at this section, though, may help you get a "feel" for problems of this sort.)

Let's take a brief moment to explain the permutation equation in the context of our previous example. To arrive at a general formula, we would like to use "!" (factorial) notation. Let $n = 10$ (number of things to choose from) and $k = 3$ (number of ordered choices to make). 10! is not the answer. You already know the answer is $10 \times 9 \times 8$. So what does 10! count? It counts making 10 ordered choices (choosing people for 10 different jobs or positions). To find the correct answer to the question on page 409, though, we need to divide out the unnecessary factors from $10 \times 9 \times 8 \times (7 \times 6 \times 5 \times 4 \times 3 \times 2 \times 1)$. Note that the "bad" factors are in parentheses. They multiply to 7! You might want to think of it this way. We need to fill only 3 positions (president, vice president, treasurer). So the rest (7 "bad" positions = 10 total positions – 3 "good" positions) must be discarded. This gives us the $(10-3)!$ or $(n-k)!$ that must be divided out. Once we do this, we have what we need: $\dfrac{10!}{(10-3)!} = \dfrac{10!}{7!} = 10 \times 9 \times 8 = 720$.

➡ Example _____

Three people must be seated at a table from left to right. If there are 5 people to choose from, how many seating arrangements are possible?

(A) 6
(B) 27
(C) 30
(D) 60
(E) 125

Solution

Important!

1. Order matters since you are placing people from left to right.
2. There is no replacement since a person cannot sit in two seats at the same time.

This is a permutation.

There are 5 choices for the seat on the left, 4 remaining choices for the middle seat, and 3 choices for the seat on the right. Hence, there are $5 \times 4 \times 3 = 60$ arrangements. You can also use the formula:

$$\frac{n!}{(n-k)!} = \frac{5!}{(5-3)!} = \frac{5 \times 4 \times 3 \times 2 \times 1}{2 \times 1} = 5 \times 4 \times 3 = 60$$

The correct choice is answer (D).

COMBINATIONS

We've dealt with permutations, where order matters. Now it is time to handle problems where the order does not matter, but there is still no replacement. When looking at a DAT combination problem be aware of the following.

1. Order does NOT matter.
2. There is no replacement.

➡ Example

There are 5 people at a party. How many ways can 3 of them be chosen to pick up food?

(A) 10
(B) 30
(C) 60
(D) 75
(E) 125

Solution

This problem looks suspiciously like the previous one. However, the problem itself is fundamentally different. In the previous example, order mattered since we were seating people from left to right. In this example, though, order does *not* matter since we do not care who is picked first, second, and third. All we care about is who is going to get the food. The group of Bob, Ted, and Fred is the same group as Fred, Bob, and Ted.

Let's do some strategic thinking before we figure out the solution. We already know how to compute the answer if order mattered. That answer would be 60. Since order does not matter, the number of outcomes must be reduced (remember: Bob, Ted, Fred = Fred, Bob, Ted). So the actual answer must be less than 60. The possible answers are narrowed down to choices (A) or (B). If you had to guess, 50:50 odds are much better than 1:4 odds.

The problem is that 60, choice (C), assumes that order matters. To make things concrete, imagine that the 3 people we have picked are X, Y, and Z. Our count of 60 (where order matters) differentiates X, Y, Z from Y, Z, X. However, these are both the same group of people. For every set of three people, such as X, Y, Z, we have overcounted.

Imagine counting the number of oven mittens a group of cooks is using (assuming each cook has a pair). If you ended up with 20 oven mittens, that does not mean that you have 20 people since for each person, you have overcounted twice. To fix the count, you must divide 20 by 2.

Likewise, for our group of three people—X, Y, Z—we have overcounted 6 times (XYZ, XZY, YXZ, YZX, ZXY, ZYX). Actually, we do this for every group of 3 we pick. To fix the count, we must divide by 6. The answer is $\frac{60}{6} = 10$. The correct answer is choice (A).

The explanation to the previous problem is fine. However, we should have a more systematic way of solving combination problems since they come up often on the DAT. With three people (X, Y, Z), the number of ways to arrange them in order is $3 \times 2 \times 1 = 6$. So, the formula for a combination must divide out the overcounting. The formula to solve a combination problem is shown below, where n is the number of people or items we choose from and k is the number of people or items in each group:

$$\frac{n!}{(n-k)!k!}$$

So if there are 5 people and 3 of them are chosen, you can calculate the number of possible groups using $\frac{5!}{(5-3)!3!}$. In other words, this combination is actually a permutation dividing out the overcount of $k!$. In the last problem, $\frac{5!}{(5-3)!3!} = 10$.

> ### A SPECIAL SYMBOL
> Combinations are such a common form of counting that a special symbol is given to them:
>
> $$\binom{n}{k}$$
>
> This reads as "n choose k."

➥ Example

Ten different books lie on a shelf. How many different pairs of books can we pick?

(A) 2

(B) 20

(C) 45

(D) 90

(E) 100

Solution

Since we are picking 2 books and do not care about their order, this is a combination. Remember that n = number of things to choose from, which is 10 books. Also, remember that k = the number of choices to make, which is 2 books.

$$\frac{n!}{(n-k)!k!}$$

$$\frac{10!}{(10-2)!2!}$$

$$\frac{10 \times 9 \times 8!}{8!2!}$$

$$\frac{10 \times 9}{2 \times 1} = 45$$

ONLINE TUTORIALS

The correct answer is choice (C).

See a video version at *www.youtube.com/user/swartwoodprep*.

MULTINOMIAL

Forget the name *multinomial*. What matters is how to handle the problem type. This topic is somewhat rare but can occur on the DAT.

As before, let's start with an example.

➡ Example

How many 11-letter "words" can the letters in MISSISSIPPI be rearranged to spell? (Here the "words" are just collections of letters written from left to right; they do not actually have to be words in a language. For example, SSSSPPIIIIM is fine.)

(A) $11!$

(B) $\dfrac{11!}{4!(11-4)!}$

(C) $\dfrac{11!}{2!2!4!}$

(D) $\dfrac{11!}{2!4!4!}$

(E) $\dfrac{11!}{4!4!4!}$

Solution

Let's start with what we know. We know that arranging all 11 letters from left to right is a permutation of 11 items. So, there are $11!$ ways to do this. However, we have overcounted since $11!$ assumes that every letter is different. Here, for example, the letter P appears 2 times.

Let's take SSSSPPIIIIM as an example. If we incorrectly answered $11!$, we would have treated each P as being different: SSSS*PP*IIIIM and SSSS*PP*IIIIM. The two versions given are only different if you can tell each P apart. Since we can't, we have overcounted twice. To fix this, we need to divide by $2! = 2$. How about each S? There are 4. So in $11!$ the S has been overcounted $4!$ times. (Imagine lining up the 4 S's and pretending they are different. How many ways can this be done? $4!$) To fix the S overcount as well as the I count, we have to divide by $4!$ (for the S) and by another $4!$ (for the I).

The correct answer is $\dfrac{11!}{2!4!4!}$, which is answer choice (D).

The previous example gives us a general formula:

$$\frac{n!}{a!b!c!}$$

In the formula, n is the number of items we are arranging and a, b, and c represent the number of repeats. We don't have to end at c. We can keep adding more "repeats" to divide out as necessary. In other words, if 5 different items are repeated, the formula would have a denominator of $a!b!c!d!e!$

NAIVE PROBABILITY

In DAT problems, you should think of probability as "the number of desirable outcomes" divided by "the total number of possible outcomes." That's really all there is to it. Everything else is what we did before, counting. For example: what is the probability of rolling a "1" on a 6-sided die? There is one way to roll a "1" and 6 possible outcomes, so the probability is $\frac{1}{6}$.

> **PROBABILITY FORMULA**
>
> $$\text{probability} = \frac{\text{number of desirable outcomes}}{\text{total number of possible outcomes}}$$

The set of all outcomes is called the sample space. A subset of the sample space (for example, getting a "1") is an event. We will not need much of that terminology here, but it is always good to state the "official terms" just in case.

➡ Example

A bag has 2 red balls, 2 orange balls, and 2 black balls in it. If Miranda picks two balls without replacement, what is the probability they are both red?

(A) $\frac{2}{15}$

(B) $\frac{1}{15}$

(C) $\frac{1}{3}$

(D) $\frac{8}{15}$

(E) $\frac{14}{15}$

> **DENOTING PROBABILITY**
> For future reference, we will denote the probability of event A occurring as $P(A)$.

Solution

In this problem, it does not matter which red ball Miranda picks first. She is simply picking 2 red balls without replacing them. So this is a combination. Miranda has $\binom{2}{2} = 1$ ways of getting 2 red balls from the 2 red balls available. She also has $\binom{6}{2} = 15$ ways for the total number of possibilities since she can pick any 2 of the 6. That is, there is only one way to have both balls be red. To find the final answer, calculate the following:

$$\text{probability} = \frac{\text{number of desirable outcomes}}{\text{total number of possible outcomes}}$$

$$\frac{\binom{2}{2}}{\binom{6}{2}} = \frac{1}{15}$$

The correct answer is choice (B).

THE COMPLEMENT OF AN EVENT

If there is a 30% chance it will rain, then there is a 70% chance it will not rain. The complement of event A is what is left over in the sample space when you remove event A. So the probability of obtaining the complement is (1 – the probability of event A). For example, the probability of rolling anything but a "1" on a 6-sided die is (1 – the probability of rolling a "1") = $1 - \frac{1}{6} = \frac{5}{6}$.

We will denote the complement of event A as A^c.

THE COMPLEMENT
OF EVENT A

$P(A^c) = 1 - P(A)$

THE PROBABILITY OF A UNION OF EVENTS

The probability of rolling a "1" on a 6-sided die is $\frac{1}{6}$, and the probability of rolling a "2" is $\frac{1}{6}$. It stands to reason that the probability of rolling either a "1" or a "2" is $\frac{1}{6} + \frac{1}{6} = \frac{2}{6}$. There is one catch. If the events we are taking together have some outcomes in common, then we overcount by simply adding the probabilities. For example, the probability of rolling a "1" or an "odd number" is not $\frac{1}{6} + \frac{1}{2} = \frac{2}{3}$ since the number "1" is both "1" and "an odd number." To fix the overcount, we need to subtract the probability of obtaining the outcomes in common. Hence, $\frac{1}{6} + \frac{1}{2} - \frac{1}{6} = \frac{1}{2}$ is correct. We call the joining of two events the *union* of the events. We call the set containing the outcomes that overlap for two events the *intersection* of the events.

UNIONS AND INTERSECTIONS OF EVENTS

The union of events is symbolized by ∪.
The intersection of events is symbolized by ∩.
The union of events is often indicated by the word "OR" in problems.
The intersection of events is often indicated by the word "AND" in problems.

Let's use symbols to look again at the probability of rolling a "1" or an "odd number" using a 6-sided die. We'll let $P(A)$ be the probability of rolling a "1" and $P(B)$ be the probability of rolling an "odd number." In symbols, this can be displayed as the following:

$$P(A \cup B) = P(A) + P(B) - P(A \cap B)$$

You do not need to memorize the symbols. You just need to understand the idea.

For example, Miranda picks 1 ball from a bag containing 2 red, 3 blue, and 5 green balls. What is the probability that she picks either a red ball OR a green ball? Here, you can compute this directly as 7 desirable outcomes out of 10 possible outcomes. However, you can also think of this as $\frac{2}{10}$ for the probability of picking a red ball and $\frac{5}{10}$ for the probability of picking a green ball. So the probability of the union is $\frac{2}{10} + \frac{5}{10} = \frac{7}{10}$. Note that the probability of the intersection is 0 since there are no balls that are simultaneously red and green. This might seem like overkill for a simple problem, but understanding the logic will help us later.

CONDITIONAL PROBABILITY

Conditional probability is at the heart of probability. In effect, conditional probability is a readjustment of probability based on known information. For example, what is the probability of "1" being the number you rolled on a 6-sided die if you know that the number rolled was even? The answer is 0 since "1" is an odd number. Conditional probability, which is denoted as $P(A|B)$, can be defined formally as:

$$P(A|B) = \frac{P(A \cap B)}{P(B)}$$

This formula deserves some explanation. $P(A|B)$ is read, "The probability of event A occurring given that event B has occurred." Event B is the event that has already occurred and, hence, gives us additional knowledge. Although we will not be formal about showing why this definition works, you should note that the equation follows the form of "desirable divided by possible." If event B has occurred, the only possibilities include event B. If what is desired is event A, the only way to obtain event A while stuck in event B is $(A \cap B)$. Clearly, this is only an analogy as we are speaking of events and the definition of conditional probability entails probabilities.

The question now is how we should approach problems on the DAT. Although you can use the formula, this following shortcut—demonstrated in a problem—will likely prove to be easier to implement in practice.

Let's redo a previous problem by using conditional probability.

➡ Example _____

A bag has 2 red balls, 2 orange balls, and 2 black balls in it. If Miranda picks two balls without replacement, what is the probability they are both red?

(A) $\frac{2}{15}$

(B) $\frac{1}{15}$

(C) $\frac{1}{3}$

(D) $\frac{8}{15}$

(E) $\frac{14}{15}$

Solution

We want the probability that both are red. Let B = the event that the first ball is red and A = the event that the second ball is red. Then $P(A|B) = \frac{P(A \cap B)}{P(B)}$ tells us that $P(A \cap B) = P(A|B)P(B)$ by rearranging the equation. $P(B) = \frac{2}{6}$ because there are 2 red balls out of 6 total balls. To compute $P(A|B)$, first assume that event B has happened. Then compute event A using the information available since event B occurred. If the first ball chosen is red (B), then there are 5 balls left. Thus, $P(A|B) = \frac{1}{5}$. The final answer is $\left(\frac{2}{6}\right)\left(\frac{1}{5}\right) = \frac{2}{30} = \frac{1}{15}$. The correct answer is choice (B).

INDEPENDENCE OF EVENTS

Two events are independent if information that either event has occurred does not affect the likelihood of the other event occurring. In other words, $P(A|B) = P(A)$. Thus, knowing that event B has occurred has no effect on the probability that event A will occur. The formula to use when events A and B are independent is the following:

$$P(A \cap B) = P(A)P(B)$$

➡ Example _____

(not DAT multiple choice) A set of cards contains 20 cards. Half are red, and half are black. Half of the red cards are numbered 1–5, and the other half are lettered A–E. The same is true of the black cards. A random card is selected. Are the events A = "the card is a number" and B = "the card is red" independent?

Solution

Yes, the events are independent. $P(A) = \dfrac{10}{20}$ since half of the total number of cards are numbered. $P(B) = \dfrac{10}{20}$ since half of the cards are red. $P(A \cap B) = \dfrac{5}{20}$ since 5 of the cards are both red and numbered. If $P(A)P(B) = P(A \cap B)$, the events are independent.

$$P(A)P(B) = \left(\frac{10}{20}\right)\left(\frac{10}{20}\right) = \frac{100}{400} = \frac{5}{20} = P(A \cap B)$$

$$P(A)P(B) = P(A \cap B)$$

The events are independent.

See *www.youtube.com/user/swartwoodprep* for a slightly more complicated example.

BABY BINOMIAL

A common problem type encountered on the DAT involves binomial distributions. Spending a lot of time on binomial distributions may well be overkill on the DAT. So, instead we will cover this sort of problem using the techniques we have already developed without turning to the official formula. In class, I often refer to this as "baby binomial." The conditions for baby binomial are as follows.

1. You have only two options: success or failure.
2. Each trial is independent.
3. Each trial is identical with respect to its probability of success.

➥ Example_____

A fair coin is flipped 3 times. What is the probability that exactly 2 heads result?

(A) $\dfrac{2}{3}$

(B) $\dfrac{1}{2}$

(C) $\dfrac{3}{8}$

(D) $\dfrac{1}{4}$

(E) $\dfrac{1}{8}$

Solution

There are only two options: heads (success) and tails (failure). Each flip does not affect the probability of getting a heads on the next flip (independent trials). The probability of getting a heads on each flip is the same. So we are dealing with a baby binomial. The probability of getting HHT is $\left(\dfrac{1}{2}\right)\left(\dfrac{1}{2}\right)\left(\dfrac{1}{2}\right) = \dfrac{1}{8}$ since each flip is independent of one another. Likewise, the probability of HTH occurring is $\dfrac{1}{8}$. There are three different ways of getting 2 heads and 1 tail: HHT, HTH, THH. You can see this by noticing that the position of the "T" determines the rest of the setup and there are only three places at which the "T" can be. Since the three events (HHT, HTH, and THH) are mutually exclusive, their intersections have zero probability.

We can use $P(A \cup B) = P(A) + P(B) - P(A \cup B)$ with $P(A \cap B) = 0$. That simplifies to $P(A \cup B) = P(A) + P(B)$. Technically, we have three events in this problem:

$$P(A \cup B \cup C) = P((A \cup B) \cup C) = P(A \cup B) + P(C) = P(A) + P(B) + P(C)$$

$$P(\text{HHT, HTH, THH}) = \dfrac{1}{8} + \dfrac{1}{8} + \dfrac{1}{8} = \dfrac{3}{8}$$

The correct answer is choice (C).

Statistics

44

MEASURES OF CENTRAL TENDENCY

There are three measures of central tendency (average representative number) that you should be familiar with on the DAT:

1. **Mode:** the number that occurs the most often in a group of numbers
2. **Median:** the middle number when a group of numbers is arranged from lowest to highest
3. **Mean:** the traditional average obtained by adding up the numbers and dividing by the quantity of numbers

➡ Example

For the set of numbers {1, 1, 1, 1, 2, 2, 2, 2, 2, 3, 3, 3, 3}, what are the mode, median, and mean, respectively?

(A) 1, 1, 1
(B) 2, 2, 2
(C) 3, 3, 3
(D) 2.5, 2, 2
(E) 2, 2.5, 2

Solution

The most often seen score is 2. The numbers in the set are organized from lowest to highest. So the median, which is the middle number, is 2. You can see this by crossing off the highest and lowest numbers and then repeating the procedure for the remaining numbers until one is left. If two numbers are left, you take the mean of the two. The mean is

$$1 + 1 + 1 + 1 + 2 + 2 + 2 + 2 + 2 + 3 + 3 + 3 + 3$$

divided by 13. This is also 2. The correct answer is choice (B).

The symbolic way of computing the mean is $\dfrac{\sum\limits_{i=1}^{n} x_i}{N}$, where x_i represents the ith number and N represents the total quantity of numbers.

MEASURES OF DISPERSION

There are three measures of dispersion with which you should be comfortable:

1. **Range:** the difference of the highest and lowest numbers
2. **Variance:** a value that indicates how far from the mean the numbers are *on average*
3. **Standard deviation:** the square root of the variance

Example

For the set of numbers {1, 1, 1, 1, 2, 2, 2, 2, 2, 3, 3, 3, 3}, what is the range?

(A) 0

(B) 1

(C) 2

(D) 3

(E) 4

Solution

The range is $3 - 1 = 2$. The correct answer is choice (C).

The variance deserves some special attention. It is a measure of how far from the mean the numbers are *on average*. The formula to calculate variance is $\dfrac{\sum\limits_{i=1}^{n}(x_i - \text{mean})^2}{N}$, where x_i represents the ith number and N represents the total quantity of numbers.

1. Find the mean of the numbers.
2. Find the difference between each number and the mean ($x_i - \text{mean}$).
3. Square each difference found in step (2): $(x_i - \text{mean})^2$.
4. Add the squares found in step (3) to get the numerator of the variance formula: $\sum\limits_{i=1}^{n}(x_i - \text{mean})^2$.
5. Find the average of the result of step (4) by dividing that value by the number of scores to complete the variance formula: $\dfrac{\sum\limits_{i=1}^{n}(x_i - \text{mean})^2}{N}$.

To find the standard deviation of a set of numbers, take the square root of the variance.

Example

For the set of numbers {1, 1, 1, 1, 2, 2, 2, 2, 2, 3, 3, 3, 3}, what is the variance and the standard deviation, respectively?

(A) $\dfrac{60}{13}, \sqrt{\dfrac{60}{13}}$

(B) 2, 2

(C) 1, 1

(D) $\dfrac{8}{13}, \sqrt{\dfrac{8}{13}}$

(E) 0, 0

Solution

Calculate the variance. First find the mean:

$$\frac{1 + 1 + 1 + 1 + 2 + 2 + 2 + 2 + 2 + 3 + 3 + 3 + 3}{13} = \frac{26}{13} = 2$$

Find the difference between each number and the mean. Square each difference. Then find the average of those numbers. This is shown in one step:

$$\frac{(1-2)^2+(1-2)^2+(1-2)^2+(1-2)^2+(2-2)^2+(2-2)^2+(2-2)^2+(2-2)^2+(2-2)^2+(3-2)^2+(3-2)^2+(3-2)^2+(3-2)^2}{13}=\frac{8}{13}$$

The variance is $\frac{8}{13}$. Since the standard deviation is the square root of the variance, the standard deviation is $\sqrt{\frac{8}{13}}$. The answer is choice (D).

PROPERTIES OF MEAN AND VARIANCE

With respect to properties under addition and multiplication, the mean is nice while the variance is not.

1. If two sets of numbers, $\{x_1,..., x_n\}$ and $\{y_1,..., y_n\}$, have their corresponding numbers added together to form a new set, $\{x_1+y_1, x_1+y_2,..., x_n+y_n\}$, the mean of the new set of numbers is the **sum of the means of each of the original sets**.
2. If a set of numbers has each value multiplied by a fixed number a, the mean of the new set is the **mean of the original set multiplied by a**.
3. If a set of numbers has each value added to a fixed number a, the mean of the new set is the **mean of the original set plus a**.
4. If a set of numbers has each value multiplied by a fixed number a, the variance of the multiplied numbers is the **variance of the original set multiplied by a^2**.
5. If a set of numbers has each value added to a fixed number a, the variance of the summed numbers is the **variance of the original set**.

These rules are best illustrated with examples.

➡ **Example** _____

The mean and variance of $\{1, 1, 1, 1, 2, 2, 2, 2, 2, 3, 3, 3, 3\}$ are 2 and $\frac{8}{13}$, respectively.

What are the mean and variance of $\{2, 2, 2, 2, 4, 4, 4, 4, 4, 6, 6, 6, 6\}$?

(A) $3, \frac{21}{13}$

(B) $3, \frac{32}{13}$

(C) $4, \frac{21}{13}$

(D) $4, \frac{24}{13}$

(E) $4, \frac{32}{13}$

Solution

The numbers in the second set are twice the numbers in the first set. To find the mean of the second set, multiply the mean of the first set by 2:

$$2 \times 2 = 4$$

To find the variance of the second set, multiply the variance of the first set by the square of 2:

$$\frac{8}{13} \times 2^2 = \frac{8}{13} \times 4 = \frac{32}{13}$$

The answer is choice (E).

➡ **Example** _____

The mean and variance of {1, 1, 1, 1, 2, 2, 2, 2, 2, 3, 3, 3, 3} are 2 and $\frac{8}{13}$, respectively.

What are the mean and variance of {2, 2, 2, 2, 3, 3, 3, 3, 3, 4, 4, 4, 4}?

(A) 3, $\frac{8}{13}$

(B) 2, $\frac{8}{13}$

(C) 3, $\frac{21}{13}$

(D) 3, $\frac{24}{13}$

(E) 3, $\frac{32}{13}$

Solution

The numbers in the second set are the numbers in the first set plus 1. The mean of the second set is the mean of the first set plus 1:

$$2 + 1 = 3$$

The variance of the second set is the same as the variance of the first set, $\frac{8}{13}$. The answer is choice (A).

Special Question Types

45

The DAT incorporates two special question types you may not be used to answering:

1. Quantitative comparison questions
2. Data sufficiency questions

QUANTITATIVE COMPARISON

Quantitative comparison questions do not necessarily ask you to compute an answer. In fact, in many cases, doing so would be a detriment. Instead, the task is to look at two columns (A and B) and decide based on the information presented whether:

(A) Column A is greater.
(B) Column B is greater.
(C) Columns A and B are equal.
(D) Cannot be determined.

Choice (D), "Cannot be determined," is correct when one of the three previous answers cannot be confirmed based on the information presented in the columns. For ease of notation, we will write "A," "B," "=," or "cannot be determined" for the answer choices when explaining the solutions to the following problems.

A number of useful strategies can be applied when answering quantitative comparison questions. Feel free to visit *www.youtube.com/user/swartwoodprep* for examples and strategies.

ONLINE TUTORIALS

Theme: Don't Do Unnecessary Computations!

➡ **Example** _____

$$3x + 4y = 5$$
$$4x + 5y = 7$$

Column A	Column B
$x + y$	2

(A) Column A is greater.
(B) Column B is greater.
(C) Columns A and B are equal.
(D) Cannot be determined.

Solution

Although this problem can be solved by substitution or elimination, the point is to avoid doing unnecessary computations. Instead of solving for x and solving for y, solve for $x + y$ since that is what you are actually comparing to 2. Subtract the top equation from the bottom equation:

$$\begin{array}{r} 4x + 5y = 7 \\ -\ (3x + 4y = 5) \\ \hline x + y = 2 \end{array}$$

Columns A and B are equal. The answer is choice (C).

ONLINE TUTORIALS

See *www.youtube.com/user/swartwoodprep* for another example.

Theme: Make the Columns Look Similar

➡ **Example** _____

Column A	Column B
$15^{30} + 15^{31}$	15^{32}

(A) Column A is greater.
(B) Column B is greater.
(C) Columns A and B are equal.
(D) Cannot be determined.

Solution

Column B is larger. The one answer you should NOT pick is "Cannot be determined" as these are fixed numbers. The DAT writers probably do not expect you to punch 15×15 into your calculator over and over again. Instead, try to make the columns look as similar as possible. It is tempting just to combine the exponents in column A. However, doing so is a trap as the bases are not being multiplied. Remember that $15^{30} + 15^{31} \neq 15^{61}$. The best we can do is factor out 15^{30} from both columns:

Column A	Column B
$15^{30}(1 + 15^1)$	$15^{30}(15^2)$

ONLINE TUTORIALS

It is now easy to see that $1 + 15^1 = 16$ is less than 15^2. The solution is choice (B).
See *www.youtube.com/user/swartwoodprep* for another example.

Theme: Try Out Numbers

➥ **Example** _____

$$x > 0, \, y > 0$$

Column A	Column B
$x^2 + y^2$	$2xy$

(A) Column A is greater.

(B) Column B is greater.

(C) Columns A and B are equal.

(D) Cannot be determined.

Solution

Method 1:

For many problems of this type, picking numbers is key. Good numbers to pick are zero, positives, negatives, and fractions. Here, we cannot choose zero. Simpler is always better. Let's pick $x = 1 = y$. This is a lucky choice.

Column A	Column B
$x^2 + y^2 = (1)^2 + (1)^2 = 2$	$2xy = 2(1)(1) = 2$

Since we picked numbers, we cannot be certain the answer is choice (C) "=." We have to try at least one other set of numbers since "Cannot be determined" may still be an answer. Let's pick $x = 1$ and $y = 2$.

Column A	Column B
$x^2 + y^2 = (1)^2 + (2)^2 = 5$	$2xy = 2(1)(2) = 4$

In this case, column A is greater. So the answer must be "Cannot be determined" because column A is not always equal to column B and because column A is not always greater. The correct answer is choice (D).

Method 2:

Although using method 1 is recommended, you can also approach the problem more algebraically. The expressions $x^2 + y^2$ and $2xy$ are special in that they are related by $(x - y)^2 = x^2 - 2xy + y^2$.

This gives us a hint to look at $(x - y)^2$. Since $(x - y)^2$ is a square, it is ≥ 0.

$$(x - y)^2 \geq 0$$
$$x^2 - 2xy + y^2 \geq 0$$
$$x^2 + y^2 \geq 2xy$$

Since column A could be either larger than or equal to column B, the correct answer is choice (D).

Note: If the initial conditions had included $x \neq y$, the answer would have been choice (A). For more examples, see *www.youtube.com/user/swartwoodprep*.

ONLINE TUTORIALS

DATA SUFFICIENCY

Data sufficiency questions may be new to you. Like quantitative comparison questions, you are often rewarded for not computing the answer directly. Generally, in data sufficiency questions, two statements are presented along with information and a question. Your task is to determine which of the following answer choices is correct.

    (A) Statement (1) alone is sufficient, but statement (2) alone is not sufficient.
    (B) Statement (2) alone is sufficient, but statement (1) alone is not sufficient.
    (C) Both statements together are sufficient, but neither statement alone is sufficient.
    (D) Each statement alone is sufficient.
    (E) Statements (1) and (2) together are not sufficient.

What do these answer choices mean? Choice (A) means that statement (1) provides enough information by itself to solve the problem. However, statement (2) does not. Choice (B) means that statement (2) provides enough information by itself to solve the problem. However, statement (1) does not. Choice (C) means that you need both statements combined to solve the problem. Choice (D) means that statement (1) is sufficient and so is statement 2. Finally, choice (E) means that even when statements (1) and (2) are combined, you do not have enough information to solve the problem.

> ## REMEMBER
>
> **You do not actually have to solve the problem. Just figure out if the statements provide enough information to solve the problem.**

Theme: Try Each Statement One at a Time

➡ Example

How much money does Dino make in a week?

(1) Dino works 25.5 hours per week.
(2) Dino makes $35.50/hr.

    (A) Statement (1) alone is sufficient, but statement (2) alone is not sufficient.
    (B) Statement (2) alone is sufficient, but statement (1) alone is not sufficient.
    (C) Both statements together are sufficient, but neither statement alone is sufficient.
    (D) Each statement alone is sufficient.
    (E) Statements (1) and (2) together are not sufficient.

Solution

Try each statement one at a time. Knowing the number of hours (1) Dino works is not enough information since you do not know his pay rate. Knowing just his rate per hour (2) is not sufficient since you do not know how many hours Dino works. Knowing both allows you to answer the question since 25.5×35.50 equals the answer. (Remember—you do not need to calculate the actual amount of money Dino earns each week.) The answer is choice (C).

➡ Example _____

What is the area of the square in the figure below?

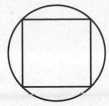

(1) The length of the diameter of the circumscribed circle is 10.
(2) The length of a diagonal of the square is 10.

(A) Statement (1) alone is sufficient, but statement (2) alone is not sufficient.
(B) Statement (2) alone is sufficient, but statement (1) alone is not sufficient.
(C) Both statements together are sufficient, but neither statement alone is sufficient.
(D) Each statement alone is sufficient.
(E) Statements (1) and (2) together are not sufficient.

Solution

If we know the length of the diameter of the circle, we also know the length of the diagonal of the square since they are the same. Once the length of the diagonal of the square is known, we can use the fact that the diagonal and two adjacent sides of the square form a 45°-45°-90° right triangle. This gives us a way to find the length of the legs of the right triangle. This length is also the side of the square. We can then use the length of the side of the square to compute the area as the length squared. The point is not to compute but to know that the computation could be done if you knew the length of the diameter. So statement (1) is sufficient. Since statement (2) gives the diagonal of the square, the same procedure guarantees that statement (2) is sufficient. Note that for this problem, knowing statement (1) is equivalent to knowing statment (2) and vice versa. So only choices (D) and (E) are options. The answer is choice (D).

Conversions

46

METRIC

Believe it or not, the DAT tests you on your knowledge of units. The metric system is key. Everything in the metric system is based on units of 10. Table 46.1 shows the most common prefixes used with the metric system.

Table 46.1. Common Metric Prefixes

Abbreviation	Unit	Meaning
Mega-	M	10^6
Kilo-	k	10^3
Deci-	d	10^{-1}
Centi-	c	10^{-2}
Milli-	m	10^{-3}
Micro-	μ	10^{-6}
Nano-	n	10^{-9}

When working with the metric system, remember the following.

1. For length, the metric system uses the unit meters (m).
2. For time, the metric system uses the unit seconds (s).
3. For volume, the metric system uses the unit cubic meters (m^3) and and also the unit liters (L). Note that $1 \text{ cm}^3 = 1 \text{ mL}$ and that $1{,}000 \text{ L} = 1 \text{ m}^3$.
4. For mass, the metric system uses the unit kilograms (kg).
5. For weight, the metric system uses the unit newtons (N).

U.S. CUSTOMARY UNITS

Table 46.2 shows the units, abbreviations, and conversions used in the U.S. customary system.

Table 46.2.
The U.S. Customary System of Measurements

Length
1 foot (ft or ') = 12 inches (in. or ")
1 yard (yd) = 3 ft
1 mile (mi) = 5,280 ft = 1,760 yd
Fluid Volume
1 fluid ounce (fl oz)
1 cup (c) = 8 fl oz
1 pint (pt) = 2 c
1 quart (qt) = 2 pt
1 gallon (gal) = 4 qt
Weight
1 ounce (oz)
1 pound (lb) = 16 oz
1 ton (1 short ton) = 2,000 lb

➡ Example

How many ounces are in 2 pounds?

(A) 2 oz
(B) 16 oz
(C) 32 oz
(D) 40 oz
(E) 64 oz

Solution

Use unit conversions to find the answer:

$$2 \text{ lb} \times \frac{16 \text{ oz}}{\text{lb}} = 32 \text{ oz}$$

The correct answer is choice (C).

CELSIUS AND FAHRENHEIT

In modern chemistry, temperature is typically measured in kelvin, as discussed in the chemistry section of *Barron's DAT* book. However, Celsius and Fahrenheit still both thrive as units for measuring temperature. As a result, we must be able to convert between the different systems. Table 46.3 shows how to do this.

Table 46.3. Converting Temperatures

Celsius to Kelvin
($°C$ + 273.15) = K
Celsius to Fahrenheit
$\frac{9}{5}°C + 32 = °F$
Fahrenheit to Celsius
$\frac{5}{9}(°F - 32) = °C$

➡ **Example** _____

59°F is what temperature in the Celsius scale?

(A) 50°C
(B) 29°C
(C) –15°C
(D) –3°C
(E) –27°C

Solution

Choose the correct formula to do the conversion:

$$\frac{5}{9}(°F - 32°) = °C$$

$$\frac{5}{9}(5° - 32°) = °C$$

$$\frac{5}{9}(-27°) = °C$$

$$-15°C$$

The correct answer is choice (C).

PART SIX

Perceptual Ability Test

Introduction

47

WHAT IS THE PERCEPTUAL ABILITY TEST?

The Perceptual Ability Test (PAT) is perhaps the most unusual component of the DAT. It is a measure of your ability to perceive and consider two- and three-dimensional forms and is probably unlike any other type of test you have taken. The test is composed of six parts that appear in the following order: aperture passing, orthographic projection, angle discrimination, paper folding, cubes, and form development.

DETAILS OF THE TEST

The PAT is administered second, directly following the Survey of the Natural Sciences. There is a total of 90 items on the PAT, divided evenly among the six parts (15 questions each). Although there are 90 questions, only 75 of them are scored. The remaining 15 are experimental questions that are scattered randomly throughout the PAT sections. You will *not* be able to identify these experimental questions. You are given 60 minutes to complete the 90 questions.

The six parts of the PAT are arranged in sections of 15 questions. However, even though the sections are discrete, they are administered as a unit with no time breaks between them. This means that you have the freedom to skip ahead to a particular section first, if you wish, and later return to address the skipped sections. Within the 60-minute time frame, you may address the PAT as you wish.

TAKING THE TEST

Considering the allotted time and the number of test items, you have an average of 40 seconds to complete each question and an average of 10 minutes to complete each section. As you will come to discover through practice, some questions are quite time consuming, while others have answers that seem readily apparent.

There is no right number of seconds or minutes to spend on each question and section. Perhaps the best rule to follow is that you should progress through the test to completion at a productive pace. If you find yourself spending too much time on a difficult item and thus failing to maintain your established pace, you should leave that question and later, time permitting, return to it. As you take the practice tests in this book, you should time yourself on at least one of the two tests. It might be useful to complete one test at a comfortable pace, but record precisely how long you spent on each perceptual ability section. This will give you an index of the relative time it took you to complete each group of questions.

PERCEPTUAL ABILITY? I JUST WANT TO BECOME A DENTIST

In examining the utility of the PAT, the American Dental Association ran a study to assess the correlation between performance on this test and preclinical performance in laboratory settings that require a high degree of manual dexterity. The result is not surprising—performance on the PAT and preclinical performance in laboratory settings are indeed significantly correlated. The study and the practice of dentistry demand the ability to conceive of objects spatially. A strong performance on the PAT reflects the sort of mental agility useful in the profession.

Additionally, it should be mentioned that, in light of the correlation between PAT scores and performance in dental school, Admissions Committees hold the PAT score in high regard. These committees examine with particular care two scores that reflect performance on the DAT: (1) total academic and (2) perceptual ability. Arguably, since several individual scores are figured into the total academic score, the perceptual ability score is the single most important score on the DAT.

HOW CAN I IMPROVE MY PERCEPTUAL ABILITY?

You will quickly come to learn that perceptual ability (as it is measured by the PAT) is not something that you either *have* or *don't have*. It is a quality that can be nurtured, developed, and enhanced through training. The following review is a comprehensive preparation guide that addresses the details of what to expect on the test and provides explanatory figures and practice exercises.

The components that you need to perfect are: visual perception and visualization and mental imagery. Even if you have perfect vision, you will find that discipline and practice are needed in order to perceive minuscule details. (If you suspect that you don't have very good vision, now is a good time to invest in a pair of glasses.)

The ability to make use of visualization and mental imagery also improves with practice. As you are preparing for the PAT, continue to challenge yourself with mental imagery tasks even after you close this book. Imagine, for example, how the room you are sitting in would be oriented if the entire unit (the room and all its contents) were rotated and flipped. Try to identify the new positionings of various objects in the room. Exercises like this one will help keep your *mind's eye* active throughout the day.

There are also several creative activities, such as origami, that rely on the same skills you will be refining for the PAT. Origami, the Japanese art of paper folding, is a discipline that requires a lot of structure and precision. The intricate origami folds transform a flat piece of paper into a multidimensional form. Involvement in origami will expand your ability to recognize how flat paper can take on a multitude of forms. This activity is most applicable to the part of the PAT called "form development" but will also contribute to your preparation for the paper-folding questions.

Be creative in choosing supplementary activities for your additional practice. By stacking sugar cubes or children's building blocks, you can create cube formations like those illustrated in this book or you can create your own. This offers further practice for the painted-surface-counting questions in the cube section of the PAT. Additionally, by using dice, you can practice imagining the location of the surface dots after repositioning each die. This will contribute to enhanced performance on aperture passing and form development questions.

Preparing for the PAT can actually be quite enjoyable. The following preparation review offers clear, easy to understand approaches to each part of the PAT. In each section of the review are highly useful descriptions of the nature of the test questions and appropriate practice exercises. While the additional activities suggested above will help you to generally improve your perceptual abilities, the exercises in each review section are designed to "target train" your perception, visualization and mental imagery, and logical reasoning skills as they apply specifically to the questions on the DAT.

Aperture Passing

48

INTRODUCTION

The first section of the PAT is aperture passing. Here you will be presented with an image of a three-dimensional object and the outlines of five different apertures. Your task is to identify the aperture (or opening) that could accommodate the insertion of the solid object.

An aperture is much like a keyhole. It is an opening through which an object can pass. An aperture-passing item as it appears on the DAT is governed by a number of rules, which are outlined below.

- Although the object is presented in a particular position, it may be turned in any direction prior to insertion.
- Once the object has been started through the opening, it may not be rotated, turned, or twisted in any way.
- Both the aperture and the object are drawn to the same scale.
- There are no irregular or surprising shapes in any portion of the object that are not in clear view as is presented in the three-dimensional rendering.
- The correct aperture is always the exact shape of the object's silhouette.
- In each group of apertures, there is only one aperture that can be used to pass the solid object.

A thorough understanding of these parameters will further enhance your ability to make use of strategy. Perhaps more so than on any other section of the PAT, the questions on aperture passing exploit your understanding of the rules.

Each rule stated above has a number of consequences that can help you locate the correct answer quickly. Also, when in doubt, application of the rules will help you to eliminate one or more incorrect answer choices, thus improving your chances of selecting the correct response.

THE RULES, THEIR CONSEQUENCES, AND YOUR STRATEGY

Although the object is presented in a particular position, it may be turned in any direction prior to insertion. Usually the three-dimensional form will need to be turned or oriented in a position different from the initial presentation. The aperture-passing questions are largely a test of your ability to mentally maneuver obscure forms and to identify appropriate corresponding silhouettes. For this reason, you should assume that most times a degree of maneuvering is required. You may need to imagine either turning the object to align a particular side, or rotating the object horizontally or vertically in order to accommodate the orientation of the aperture.

Each object has six distinct sides: top, bottom, left, right, front, and rear. This first rule implies that the object may be inserted into the aperture top first, bottom first, or any of the sides first. You need not consider any angular insertions that deviate from a distinct side or top entry. Below is an example of an aperture-passing question. The object is pictured at the left.

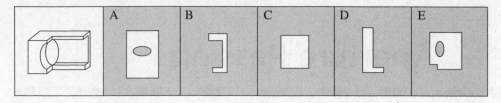

Before examining the possible apertures, choices A–E, it is important that you identify the significance of each line in the three-dimensional drawing. The subtleties of the lines are often overlooked. Also, the aperture shapes can bias your viewing, causing you to overlook the intricate detail of the object. You set yourself up for failure if you examine the apertures before thoroughly understanding the drawing.

The subtleties that you should look for in the drawing are reflected in the following questions:

- Are the outermost surfaces of the object (front, rear, top, bottom, and left and right sides) flat, or are there slopes or protrusions?
- From which direction are protrusions noticeable and unnoticeable?
- Are there any holes or recesses in the form? Where are they?
- Are there any stairlike edges? Are the stairs of equal height?

The second rule states that, *once the object has been started through the opening, it may not be rotated, turned, or twisted in any way.* Although there are six sides to choose from as the entry side, in actuality you need to consider only three sides. Remember that, not only must a side be able to enter the aperture, but also the entire form must be able to follow through. Thus, you need consider only three possibilities: a top/bottom entry and the two different side entries (see figures below).

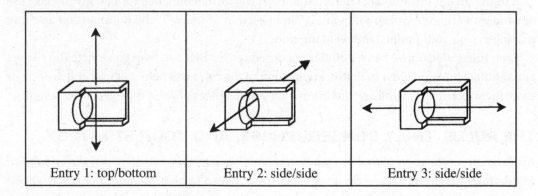

| Entry 1: top/bottom | Entry 2: side/side | Entry 3: side/side |

After you are familiar with the form of the object, you should begin to identify what each of the three silhouettes looks like. A silhouette is an outline of a form that contours the outermost edge. Keep in mind that a silhouette is a contour on a single plane that does not reveal any information about the object's depth. Although the depth of the object is not indicated on a silhouette, all of the points of the object (including the ones that recede into space) will take part in the formation of the silhouette if they extend beyond the image created from the surface being considered. In the following illustration, each of the three silhouettes corresponds to one of the images presented above:

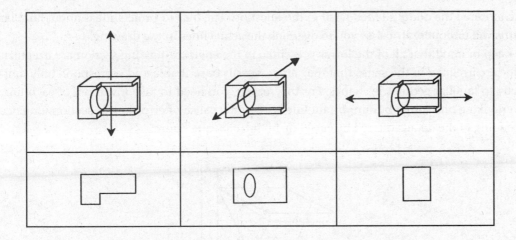

Since, as the third rule states, *both the aperture and the object are drawn to the same scale*, you need to rely heavily on precise comparison between the projected silhouette and the aperture opening. The aperture must accommodate the size of the silhouette. A perfect but smaller silhouette would not allow the three-dimensional shape to be inserted. Hence, it is possible for the aperture to be the same shape but too small for the object. According to the publishers of the DAT, the differences in size are "large enough to be judged by [the precise] eye." You are cautioned, however, to take great care in looking for small differences in size.

Although you are presented with a drawing in which three sides are exposed, there are portions of the object that are not visible in the view that is displayed. The fourth rule states that *there are no irregular or surprising shapes in any portion of the object that are not in clear view as is presented in the three-dimensional rendering*. If, however, the object has symmetric indentations, the hidden portion will be symmetric with the part shown. As a rule, enough information will be presented to allow you to make an informed decision concerning the appropriate opening.

According to the last two rules, *the correct aperture is always the exact shape of the object's silhouette* and *in each group of apertures, there is only one aperture that can be used to pass the solid object*. These rules are clearly to your advantage. Unlike questions that challenge you to select the *best* answer, your task here is to select the *only* answer. Regarding the last rule, if you find that two openings appear to accommodate the object, you are probably overlooking a detail of form or have failed to recognize that one opening is too small. Consider, if you are stumped by multiple answer choices, that you are committing one of the above errors.

With all six of these rules in mind, the appropriate answer to the aperture-passing question on page 440 is easily located. Careful consideration of the silhouette helps to eliminate choices (B), (D), and (E). Choice (A) closely approximates "Entry 3: side/side," but the darkened oval shape is slightly misplaced. Choice (C) shows the correct aperture through which the object under consideration could pass (see "Entry 3: side/side," on page 440).

LINES AS "BUILDERS OF THE FORM"

You need to practice the discipline of attending to lines as "builders of the form." There is a human tendency to approach an oddly shaped, irregular drawing with a mental stereotype of a familiar (household or geometric) form. A desire to deal with the familiar often overshadows the reality of what is presented. If you approach this section of the PAT by attending to lines as "followers of the form," you will unfortunately overlook quite a bit. Most likely you have never encountered the oddly shaped form in the question. The bias to project ideas about familiar forms will undoubtedly cause you to overlook the actual lines in the drawing.

Keep in mind that all of the forms presented in the aperture-passing section are irregular. They are irregular in the sense that they are not easily describable and correspond only indirectly to familiar geometric shapes. For this reason, you need to take inventory of each line. Overlooking one subtle but important line is often the cause of error in this section. Practice attending to the details offered by each line in the following figure:

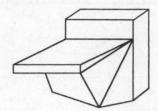

This is a highly complex figure. What makes it so difficult to deal with is the heavy reliance on the lines that is required in order to determine the many spatial planes.

Below is the same figure reproduced with visual cues and spatial guidelines.

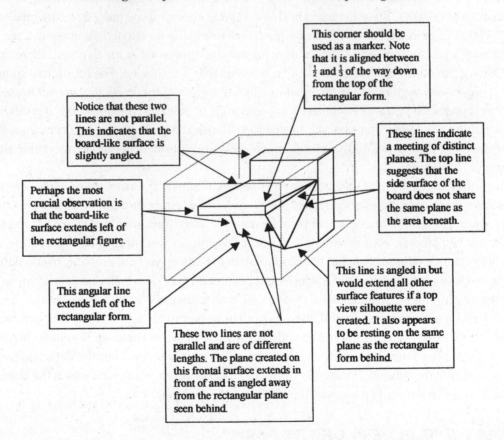

Now consider the various silhouettes that would be produced from both side/side angles and from the top/bottom angle.

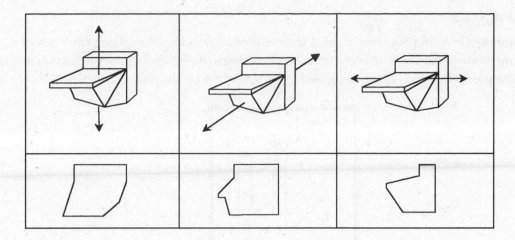

As you work through this section of the PAT, try to maintain a productive, steady pace. Do not let any one question drain you of too much time. If you find that you are stumped on a question, it is to your advantage to move on and return later if time permits. Often, a second consideration of a complex three-dimensional form will bring a fresh perspective if you allow yourself to concentrate on other forms in the meantime.

REVIEW

- Although the object is presented in a particular position, it may be turned in any direction prior to insertion. The three-dimensional form will most often need to be turned or oriented in a position different from the initial presentation.

- You may need to imagine either turning the object to align a particular side, or rotating the object horizontally or vertically in order to accommodate the orientation of the aperture.

- The object may be inserted into the aperture top first, bottom first, or any side first. You need not consider any angular insertions that deviate from a distinct side or top entry.

- Always examine the intricate lines of the object prior to reviewing the aperture choices. The aperture shapes can bias your viewing, causing you to overlook subtle details of the object.

- After you are familiar with the form, you should identify what each of the three silhouettes looks like—side/side, side/side, and top/bottom. Recall that the aperture and the object are drawn to the same scale. Hence, the aperture must be no smaller than the silhouette.

- Only one of the possible five apertures will allow the object to be inserted. If you find that two openings appear to accommodate the object, you are probably overlooking a feature detail or have failed to recognize that an opening is too small.

- Carefully attend to each line. Remember that the forms in aperture passing are highly irregular. Consider the lines to be "builders of the form" rather than "followers of the form."

- Parts of the object that are out of view will not contain any surprising shapes. However, if the object has symmetric indentations, the hidden portion will be symmetric with the part shown.

- Keep to a productive, steady pace. If you find that you are stumped on a question, move on and return later if time permits.

EXERCISE 1

Examine the form presented in each framed box. After carefully studying the lines of the form, create a silhouette for every direction of viewing in the boxes below. Practice visualizing and representing each silhouette scaled to the size of the small image with arrows.

1.

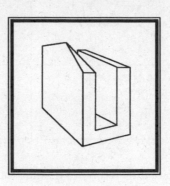

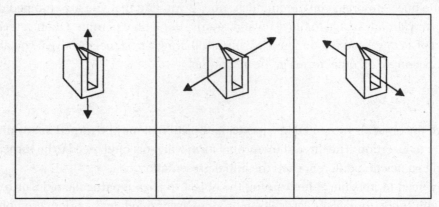

2.

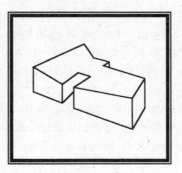

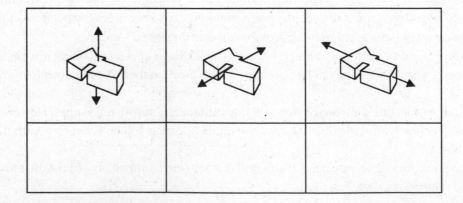

3.

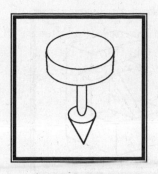

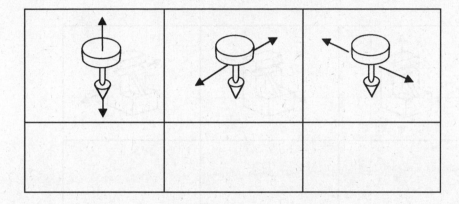

4.

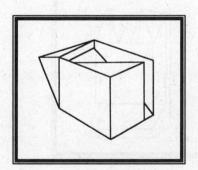

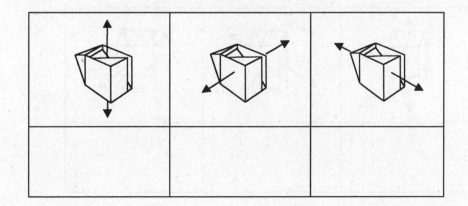

5.

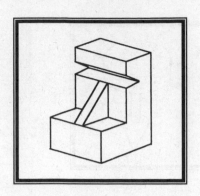

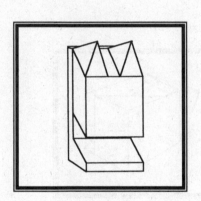

6.

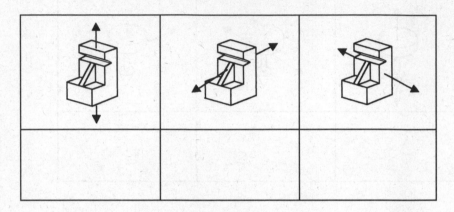

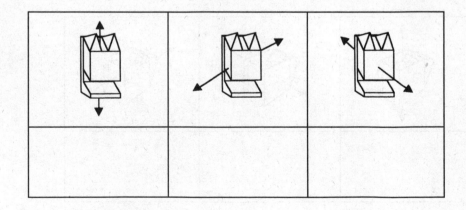

7.

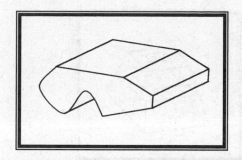

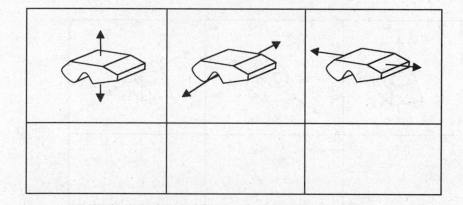

8.

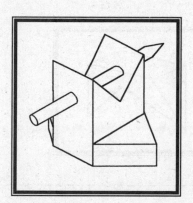

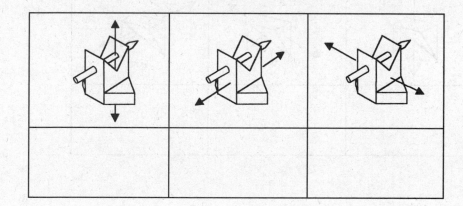

9.

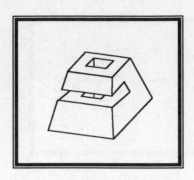

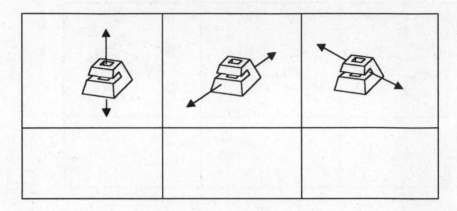

10.

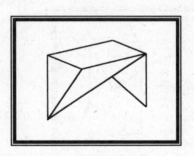

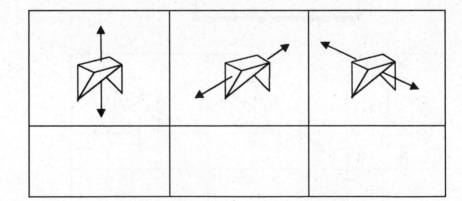

EXERCISE 2

This exercise follows the same format and directions that apply to the aperture-passing questions on the PAT. Examine the figure shown to the far left. Then choose the aperture that would allow the object to completely pass through the opening if the proper side was inserted first.

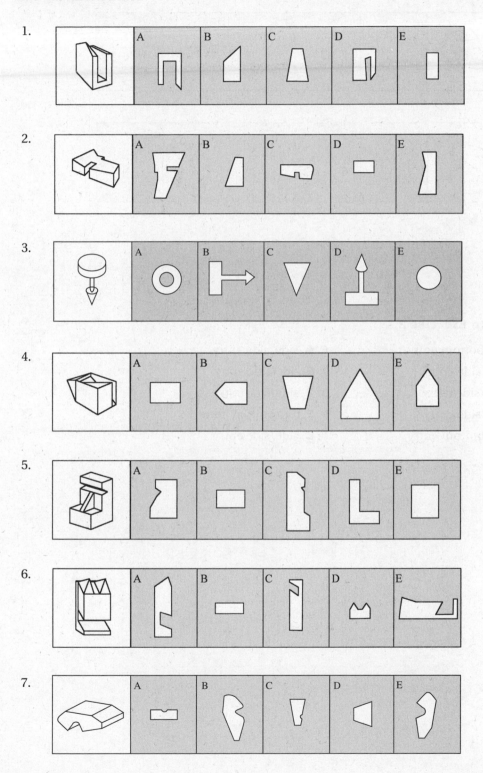

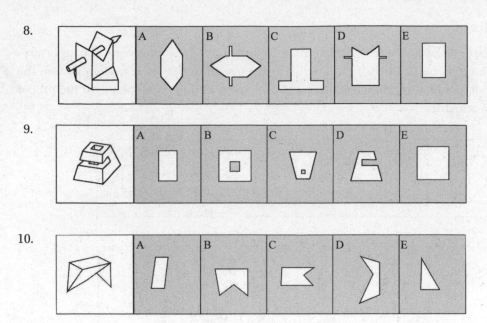

Answers to Exercise 2

1. **C**, top/bottom entry
2. **E**, side/side entry
3. **D**, side/side entry
4. **E**, side/side entry
5. **E**, top/bottom entry
6. **A**, side/side entry
7. **E**, side/side entry
8. **C**, side/side entry
9. **E**, top/bottom entry
10. **C**, side/side entry

Orthographic Projections

49

INTRODUCTION

The second section of the PAT is orthographic projections. Here you will be shown two views of an object. Given the information presented by the two views, your task is to select the third view that correctly describes the object.

WHAT IS AN ORTHOGRAPHIC PROJECTION?

Engineers and architects heavily rely on orthographic projections when they draft plans for construction. Orthographic projections are sets of descriptive drawings that serve to portray and clarify the complexity and uniqueness of the objects being considered.

An orthographic projection is a series of two-dimensional views of an object. Below is an example of how an orthographic projection series is laid out.

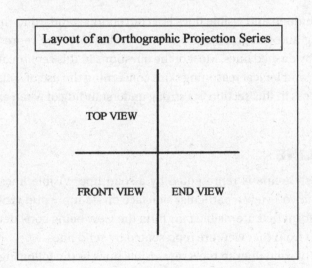

The orthographic projections on the DAT are composed of three views: the top view, front view, and end view. Each of the views is rendered *without perspective*. In other words, each view is drawn as it would appear head on with its planes parallel to the viewer.

In the example of a brick below, examine both the labeled brick shown at the left and its corresponding orthographic projection at the right.

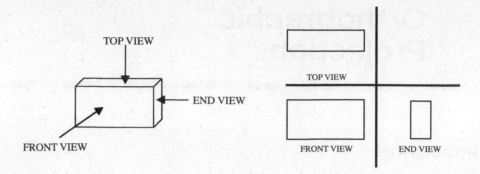

Notice the orientation of each projected image. It is as though the viewer examined each side in turn, walking around the object so that a perfect head-on view could be seen of each face (top, front, and end). Consider each display box (created by the crossed lines) to be a frame for the projection as seen from that particular viewing direction.

On the DAT, the projection layout is identical to that in the example above. The projection looking down at the object is displayed in the upper left-hand corner of the projection layout and is labeled "TOP VIEW." The projection looking at the object from the front is displayed in the lower left-hand corner and is labeled "FRONT VIEW." Lastly, the projection looking at the object from the end (or side) is displayed in the lower right-hand corner and is labeled "END VIEW."

The use of both hidden and visible lines is a convention standard to the practice of creating and interpreting an orthographic projection. Visible lines are represented by the solid lines; hidden lines, by dashed lines. Most of the questions in this section of the PAT challenge your understanding and logical reasoning skills concerning the use of solid and dashed lines. Crucial to your success in this section is a strong understanding of when each of the two lines is used.

THE VISIBLE LINE

As mentioned, a visible line is represented by a solid line. Visible lines are lines that are exposed to you when you view a particular side face on—simply put, visible lines are *visible* to you. Changes in form that are visible *only* from the view being considered and the outline of the object as seen from that view are represented by solid lines.

Examine the use of solid lines to represent visible lines in the following two examples:

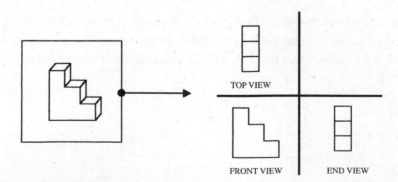

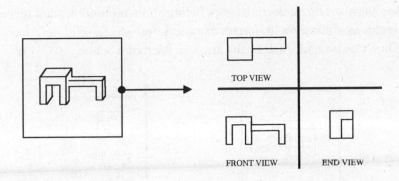

Study the figures carefully, and be sure that you are able to identify the correspondence between each projection line and the object. For clarification, refer to the following:

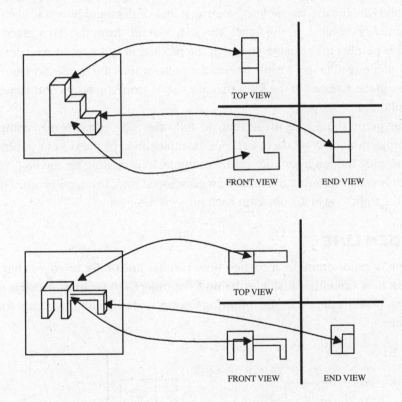

Now notice the slight modification of the second object that has occurred. Instead of a benchlike extension, this object now has a slide that extends from the central unit.

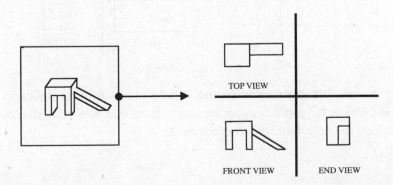

Comparison between the projection series before and after modification reveals that only the front view changes. It is most important to understand why the end view does not change. Examine the line that is highlighted by the arrow in the figure below.

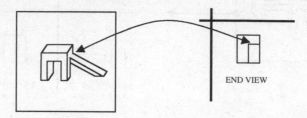

It may not be initially obvious why the end view does not change. To fully understand the use of the solid line (or the *visible line*), you must first understand how it is used in the end view of the modified object. In the figure, the slide extends from the flat surface that is just above it and is parallel to the plane on which the projection is rendered. Any deviation from this parallel plane results in a visible line at the point where the transition from parallel to angular takes place. Creases in the form that are visible from the projection view will always result in a solid line.

Lastly, the point should be made that, to fully describe some highly complex forms, additional projections may be necessary. For example, none of the views examined thus far addresses the wide hidden leg of the second example. In preparing for the PAT, you need be concerned only with mastering the three views discussed (top, front, and end). The end view will refer to the right side of the object in each projection series.

THE HIDDEN LINE

A hidden line is represented by a dashed line. Hidden lines refer to edges that cannot be seen because they are either inside or behind the object. These lines provide meaningful cues about an object's depth. In the following examples dashed lines indicate the presence of hidden lines.

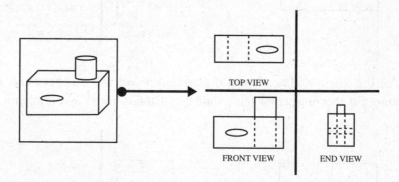

In the first example, the drawing at left shows only a brick with an object on top and an oval on the side. The orthographic projection views reveal that these oval shapes are tubular and travel through the height and width of the brick.

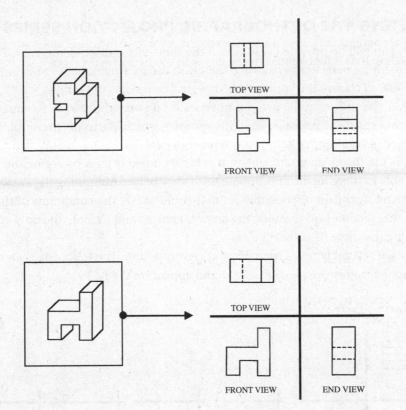

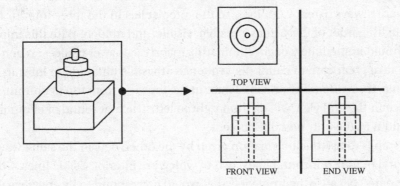

In the second and third examples, notice that the width of the object can be identified by the vertical lines; solid and dashed, in the top view. The lengths of these lines match the width in the end view.

Now examine the following series:

Here, the front and end views are identical. Also notice that these views provide the information that the narrowest cylinder is the only form that extends through the entire height of the object. The widest cylinder rests on top of the square base with the middle cylinder passing through it. The middle cylinder also rests on the base.

Note: When a hidden line is exactly behind a visible line, the part of the dashed line that coincides with the solid (visible) line remains solid. When two hidden lines overlap, the resulting line remains dashed.

COMPLETING THE ORTHOGRAPHIC PROJECTION SERIES

On the PAT, you will be provided with two of the three views discussed earlier. You will *not* be presented with a perspective drawing; but given the information contained in the views, you will be able to choose the appropriate view that completes the series.

On the PAT the orthographic projection series is laid out with two views and a question mark in place of the third, missing view. This section is much like trying to complete a puzzle. In the absence of a guiding image, you will need to examine each possibility in order to see what logically fits the given arrangement. It is highly unlikely that, by seeing the two views, you will be able to imagine the appropriate third view before examining the answer choices. There will be many third-view possibilities that could satisfy the conditions of the first two. Your job in this section is to examine the answer choices and identify the only correct view by eliminating the three incorrect choices.

Expect to see several types of each missing view question. The following is an example of an orthographic projection question as it would appear on the PAT:

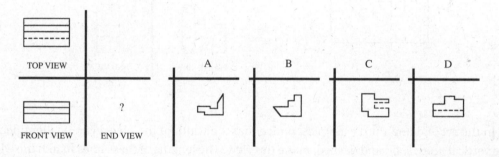

Choose the correct END VIEW.

TOP VIEW / FRONT VIEW / END VIEW / A / B / C / D

Your first strategy should be to identify the number of visible lines and hidden lines in one of the two views given. In this example, the top view has five horizontal lines. The top and bottom line are always exterior outlines, so the interest lies in the three interior lines. From top to bottom, the order of these lines is visible, visible, and hidden. With this information in mind, you should immediately begin eliminating incorrect answer choices. When examining the choices, take great care to count the sequence of visible and hidden lines in the proper order. As a rule, if you identify horizontal lines in the top view from top to bottom, their order of appearance in the end view will be from right to left. The first round of elimination leaves answers A and B as the only possible choices.

The next step is to use the information given by the other view in the same way. The front view has a total of four horizontal lines, two of which are interior visible lines. Choice A can now be eliminated because the front view that would correspond to its end view would have the following lines from bottom to top: visible, hidden, visible, and visible (not including the outlines). Choice B is the correct answer.

If after counting the number and pattern of visible and horizontal lines you have a match between two or more answer choices, verify for each choice that the lines are in the proper locations relative to each other and to the perimeter of the side being considered. For each group of projections, there will be only one answer that satisfies the conditions set forth by the two given views.

This strategy of identifying the number, order, and placement of appropriate lines can be highly effective and time saving. It will be necessary, however, to fully understand the logic of projected lines so that you can easily make transitions among different views.

If you find that you have difficulty with transitions among different types of absent views, it is suggested that you identify the projection series that you can most easily solve. Then, to remain clearly focused throughout this section, first solve the sets that you are most comfortable with; for example, solve all the problems that have a top and front view. Then return to all of one of the remaining types, for example, the front and end view problems. Lastly, address the questions of the third type (absent front view). This approach will help you keep track of each perspective and will serve to "warm you up" for questions of greater challenge.

REVIEW

- The orthographic projections on the PAT are composed of three views: the top view, front view, and end view. Each of the views is rendered without perspective.
- The end view refers to the right side of the object in each projection series.
- Visible lines are represented by solid lines, while hidden lines are represented by dashed lines.
- Changes in form that are visible only from the view being considered and from the outline of the object as seen from that view are represented by solid lines.
- Any deviation from the parallel viewing plane results in a visible line at the point where the transition from parallel to angular takes place. Creases in the form that are visible from the projection view always result in solid lines.
- Hidden lines, shown as dashed lines, refer to edges that cannot be seen because they are either inside or behind the object.
- When a hidden line is exactly behind a visible line, the part of the dashed line that coincides with the solid (visible) line remains solid. When two hidden lines overlap, the resulting line remains dashed.
- Your job in this section is to examine the answer choices and identify the only possible view by eliminating the three incorrect choices.
- When examining answer choices, take great care to count the sequence of visible and hidden lines in the proper order.
- The strategy of identifying the number, order, and placement of appropriate lines is highly effective and time saving.

EXERCISE 1

In each case, examine the three-dimensional image presented in the box. Then, to the right of each image, draw in the appropriate views. Use of a straightedge is suggested for this exercise.

1.

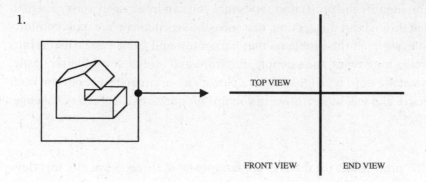

TOP VIEW

FRONT VIEW   END VIEW

2.

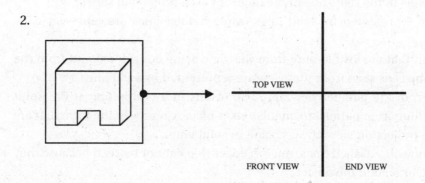

TOP VIEW

FRONT VIEW   END VIEW

3.

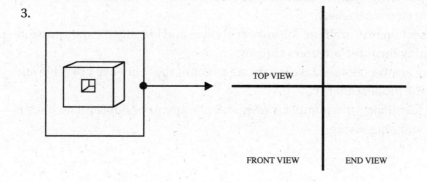

TOP VIEW

FRONT VIEW   END VIEW

Answers to Exercise 1

1.

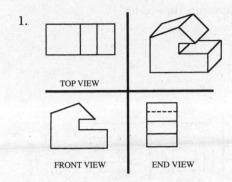

TOP VIEW

FRONT VIEW   END VIEW

2.

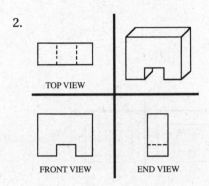

TOP VIEW

FRONT VIEW   END VIEW

3.

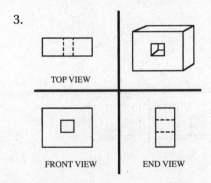

TOP VIEW

FRONT VIEW   END VIEW

EXERCISE 2

Choose the correct view to complete each orthographic projection series.

1. Choose the correct END VIEW.

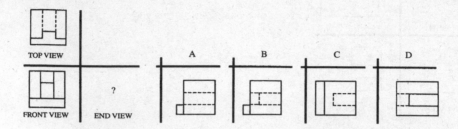

2. Choose the correct TOP VIEW.

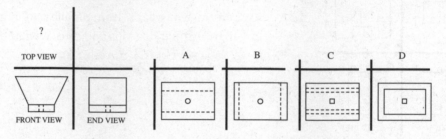

3. Choose the correct FRONT VIEW.

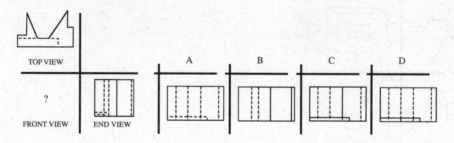

4.

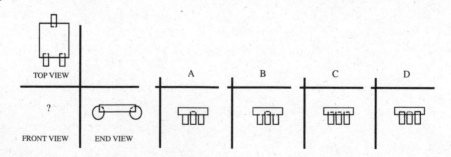

Answers to Exercise 2

1. **B**   2. **B**   3. **D**   4. **D**

Angle Discrimination

50

INTRODUCTION

The third section of the PAT is angle discrimination. This is the only portion of the PAT that involves flat renderings representing two-dimensional space that you need not mentally rotate.

Angle discrimination questions ask you to rank angles by size, from smallest to largest. With practice, you will be able to sharpen your angle-estimation skills and thus avoid pitfalls that are meant to complicate the task of discriminating between similar angles.

ANGLE RANKING

As a warmup to this section, spend some time reviewing the illustrations below. Begin by ranking the four angles in each of the following examples from smallest to largest.

➦ **Example 1** _____

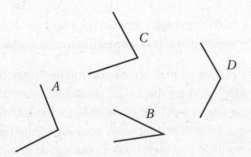

The correct ranking is *B, C, A, D*. Most likely, you were able to quickly choose angle *B* as the smallest angle and angle *D* as the largest. Angles *A* and *C*, however, are relatively close in size. The first rule to follow in this section is to always begin by identifying the smallest and largest angles, which will generally be apparent upon initial inspection. Even if just the largest angle is obvious, your odds of answering correctly have been increased (more on this later).

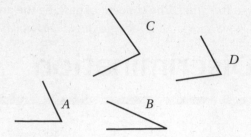

The correct ranking is *B, A, D, C.*

The angles in the following example are closer in size.

➡ **Example 3**

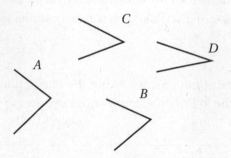

The correct ranking is *D, C, B, A.* In this example, the two angles closest in measurement are *B* and *A.* Angle *D* clearly appears smallest, but it is somewhat unclear which angle is largest.

In determining the rankings of two similar-appearing angles, refer to Exercise 1. One strategy that is often useful is called "parking the angle." When you have two angles of varying degrees, one angle (the larger angle) will always be able to "house" the other angle. In other words, the smaller angle can be inserted into the opening of the larger angle. Hence, the notion of *parking the angle* can help you identify the rankings of angles. To illustrate the application of this method, angle *C* from Example 1 above may be "parked" within angle *A* as follows:

Employment of the parking method depends largely on mental imagery. Asking the question, "Could angle *X* fit within angle *Y* or vice-versa?" often helps illuminate an intuitive hunch that one angle is smaller than the other. The concept of parking the angle applies also to angles with varying leg lengths. Basically stated, *a larger angle will always accommodate a smaller angle regardless of the length of the angles' legs.* From Example 3, angle *B* is parked within angle *A* as shown below.

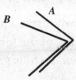

EXERCISE 1

In each of the following 10 sets of angles, determine which angle is larger.

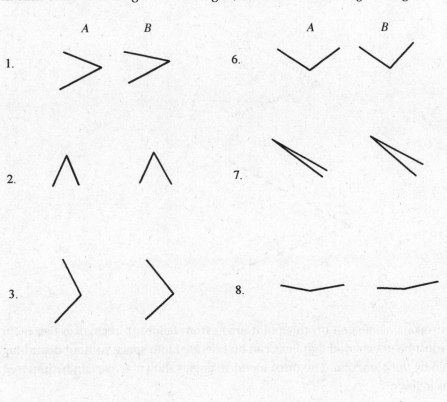

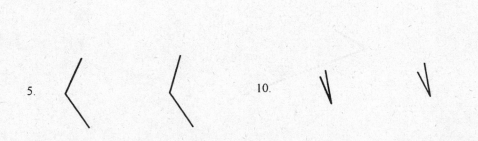

Answers to Exercise 1

1. **A** 2. **B** 3. **A** 4. **A** 5. **B** 6. **A** 7. **B** 8. **B** 9. **A** 10. **B**

If you have identified several of the larger angles incorrectly, return to the angle sets repeatedly until you are able to perceive the subtle differences. It is often helpful to review these angle sets several times before moving on to further examples and explanations.

An angle is created by the joining of two distinct legs. Crucial to your success on the angle discrimination section is an understanding of the following rule: *The length of an angle's legs is independent of its angular measurement.* To fully grasp this rule, examine the angles below, which share the same angular measurement.

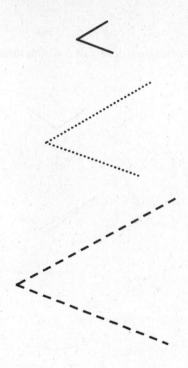

For most test-takers, confusion on this point arises from failure to recognize two main points. First, it must be understood that lines can be extended into space without disturbing the angle created by their junction. The three identical angles shown above can be imposed on each other as follows:

TIP

The length of an angle's legs is independent of its angular measurement.

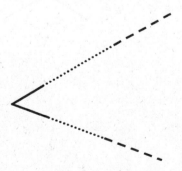

The three sets of legs (or rays) are extensions of the same angle.

The second crucial point is concerned with how an angle is measured. On the DAT you will not be permitted to make use of any measuring device (including your fingers and test-taking materials). You must rely on visual acuity to "eyeball" relative sizes. One method of eyeing an angle is to examine the mouth at a set distance from the joining point of the legs. This technique can be helpful as long as you use great caution. To implement the procedure correctly, *you must compare all the angles at the same distance from the joining point.* The following figure illustrates this point.

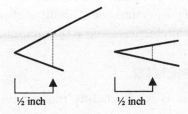

It can be inferred that the angle on the left is the larger angle. *When comparing angles, a greater measured distance between two legs will imply a larger angle if and only if the measurement is taken at the same distance from each angle's vertex.*

To practice your understanding of this rule, examine the two angles below.

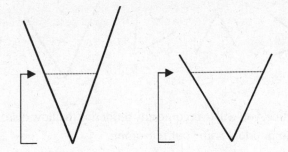

When the horizontal dotted lines at the same distance from each angle's vertex are compared, it is readily apparent that the angle on the right is larger. Keep in mind that you will not be permitted to use any measurement devices on the DAT. The horizontal lines shown in the figures above are there to illustrate the viewing path that you may take when comparing angles.

WHERE TO LOOK

Another useful method of angle comparison relies heavily on viewing only a discrete area of the angle, namely, the niche. The niche of the angle is the tightest part of the corner created by the two joining legs. This method also takes practice. Since your eye wants to traverse the extended lines away from the vertex, you must practice the restraint necessary to make angle comparisons at the niche. In the following examples, which highlight the viewing of an angle's niche, the angles are ordered from small to large:

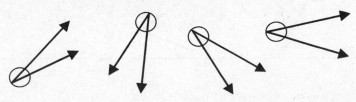

Paramount to your success on the angle discrimination questions is a solid understanding of the basic laws and methods of angle comparison:

- Always begin by establishing a largest or smallest angle, or both if possible.
- Regardless of leg size, a smaller angle can always be inserted within the opening of a larger angle. Hence, the method of "parking an angle" can be useful in conceptualizing the task at hand.
- The length of an angle's legs is independent of its angular measurement.
- When comparing angles, a greater measured distance between two legs will imply a larger angle if and only if the measurement is taken at the same distance from each angle's vertex.

COMPLEX ARRANGEMENTS

The task of comparing angles is made slightly more complex by oblique positioning. Certainly it will not be possible to rotate the computer screen in order to view the angles at similar positions. For this reason, as you practice the comparison of angles, refrain from angling the book to accommodate your view of particular angles.

The following arrangement is made with identical angles. Notice how the oblique positioning of angles coupled with varying leg lengths affects your visual sensibility.

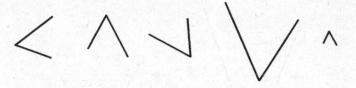

With repeated practice, you will overcome any tendency to allow distortions of angle orientation and leg length to interfere with your reasoning.

EXERCISE 2

The following exercise will help you overcome distortion interference. In each set of three angles, two angles are identical and one angle is different. Select the angle that is different from the other two angles; then determine whether it is smaller or larger.

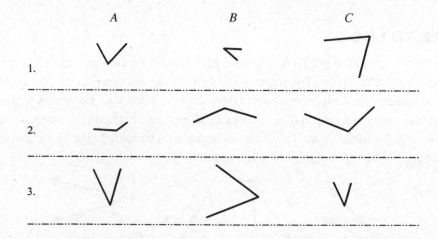

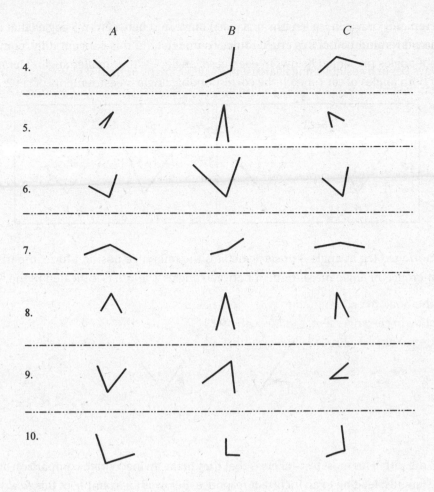

	A	B	C
4.			
5.			
6.			
7.			
8.			
9.			
10.			

Answers to Exercise 2

1. **B** (smaller)   4. **A** (smaller)   7. **A** (smaller)   10. **C** (larger)

2. **C** (smaller)   5. **C** (larger)   8. **A** (larger)

3. **B** (larger)   6. **A** (larger)   9. **C** (smaller)

You are not expected to score perfectly on this exercise. With continued exposure to these and other angle discrimination problems, however, you will develop the agility necessary to move from angle to angle with a keen eye.

VARIED LEG LENGTHS IN AN ANGLE

You have now been exposed to a variety of angles positioned uniquely and having different leg lengths. Another form of perceptual interference is due to a mixed set of leg lengths in a given angle. If, however, you are careful to employ the techniques discussed thus far, you will find that angles with mixed leg lengths are actually helpful. Since your eye tends naturally to rush to the end of the line to make the angular comparison, the presence of a shorter leg helps you to avoid making an inaccurate comparison at the end of the line. Recall that, when comparing angles, a greater measured distance between two legs implies a larger angle *if and only if the measurement is taken at the same distance from each angle's vertex.*

A discrepancy between leg lengths in a given angle and between two angles that are compared should remind you of this crucial rule. To understand this concept fully, compare the two sets of angles presented below. In each case, angle *A* is the smaller angle. The measurements of both angles of set 1 match the corresponding angle measurements of set 2.

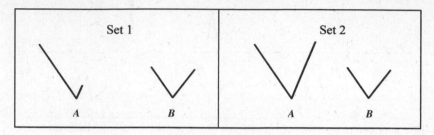

The shortened leg in angle *A* of set 1 dictates the reference position for comparison. The subtle difference in angle measurement between angles *A* and *B* is indicated in the following diagram.

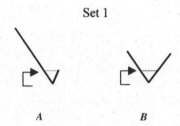

Again, the pitfall for most test-takers is that they make an inaccurate comparison at the end of the leg lengths, leading to an incorrect response. Below is an example of this *faulty* reasoning taken from set 2.

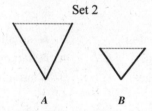

GENERAL STRATEGY

Without becoming unduly suspicious, be aware that both the angles and answer choices on the PAT may tempt faulty reasoning. Rely heavily on the methods discussed, and rehearse the implementation of visual reasoning skills on angles you encounter.

Questions on the PAT show sets of four angles. You are asked to select, from four choices, the correct ranking of the angles from small to large. With a bit of test-taking logic and your heightened awareness of discriminating between like angles, you will be able to greatly improve your odds of scoring highly on these questions.

As already mentioned, you first should identify the smallest or largest angle, or both if possible. Then, before proceeding, examine the answer choices. Many times you will be able to eliminate one or two choices before examining the remaining angles. If the angle you selected as smallest is represented in two choices as the smallest angle, you can begin eliminating the other choices. Next examine whether the angle you think is largest is also listed as largest in one of the two choices you are considering. At this point, you may be able to select the correct answer.

Maintaining a fast pace throughout this section will allow you to concentrate longer on other items of the Perceptual Ability Test that require additional time. In order to stay organized while working quickly, it is recommended that you keep track of your angle discrimination decisions on the erasable board provided. For example, upon your initial inspection for the largest and smallest angles, write down any decisions you can make before looking at the answer choices.

To keep track of choices that you have eliminated and answers you are still considering, you should jot down the answer choices on your erasable board, and cross numbers off as you delete the corresponding choices. Simply writing "1," "2," "3," and "4" will enable you to stay organized, and it should take you only a few seconds to make these notes. Under test-taking circumstances, you can easily become confused in your decision making without these and similar brief notations. Most students who are skilled test-takers make use of minimal notes such as the ones suggested here.

Because of the computer format of the DAT, you will not be able to mark decision-making notations directly on the test. Hence, part of your preparation for the DAT should include practice in using scratch paper effectively. Below is an example of a typical PAT angle discrimination question and the use of the erasable board.

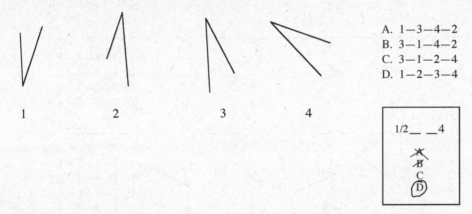

A. 1—3—4—2
B. 3—1—4—2
C. 3—1—2—4
D. 1—2—3—4

REVIEW

- The length of an angle's legs is independent of its angular measurement.
- You must compare all the angles at the same distance from the joining point of the legs. When comparing angles, a greater measured distance between two legs will imply a larger angle if and only if the measurement is taken at the same distance from each angle's vertex.
- A useful method of angle comparison relies heavily on viewing only a discrete area of the angle, namely, the niche. The niche of the angle is the tightest part of the corner created by the two joining legs.
- When ranking angles, you first should identify the smallest or largest angle, or both if possible. Then begin eliminating answer choices.

EXERCISE 3

The following sets of angles are provided for your additional practice. They are structured in the same manner as angle discrimination problems from previous versions of the DAT. In each case, select the ranking that appropriately orders the angles from small to large.

1.

1 2 3 4

A. 1–3–2–4
B. 3–4–1–2
C. 2–1–4–3
D. 1–2–3–4

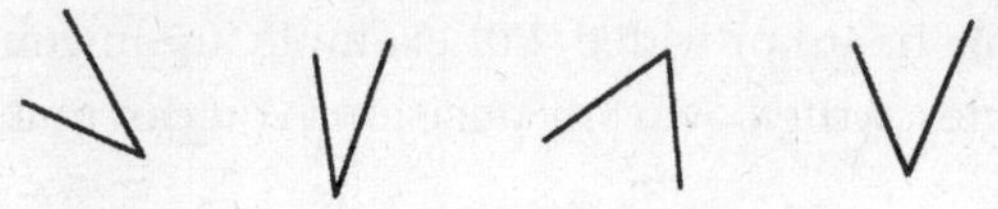

2.

1 2 3 4

A. 4–2–3–1
B. 2–4–3–1
C. 2–4–1–3
D. 4–3–2–1

3.

1 2 3 4

A. 4–1–2–3
B. 4–1–3–2
C. 1–4–2–3
D. 1–4–3–2

4.

1 2 3 4

A. 3–1–4–2
B. 1–3–4–2
C. 3–2–1–4
D. 1–3–2–4

5.

1 2 3 4

A. 3–1–2–4
B. 1–3–4–2
C. 3–2–1–4
D. 1–3–2–4

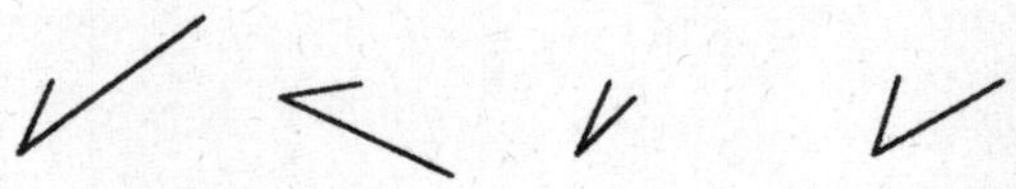

6.

1 2 3 4

A. 2–1–3–4
B. 2–3–1–4
C. 2–1–4–3
D. 2–3–4–1

7.

1 2 3 4

A. 4–3–2–1
B. 2–4–1–3
C. 4–2–3–1
D. 2–4–3–1

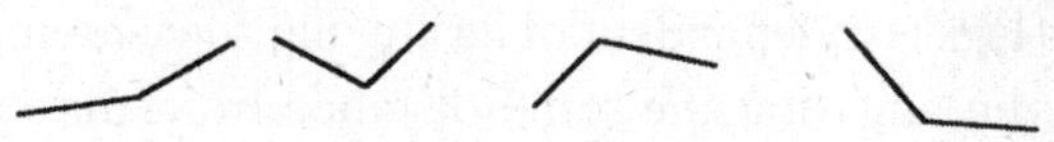

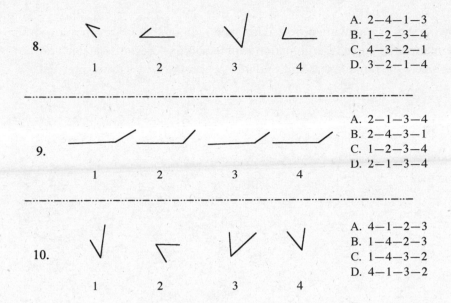

8.

1   2   3   4

A. 2—4—1—3
B. 1—2—3—4
C. 4—3—2—1
D. 3—2—1—4

9.

1   2   3   4

A. 2—1—3—4
B. 2—4—3—1
C. 1—2—3—4
D. 2—1—3—4

10.

1   2   3   4

A. 4—1—2—3
B. 1—4—2—3
C. 1—4—3—2
D. 4—1—3—2

Answers to Exercise 3

1. **C**, 2—1—4—3
2. **B**, 2—4—3—1
3. **D**, 1—4—3—2
4. **D**, 1—3—2—4
5. **A**, 3—1—2—4
6. **D**, 2—3—4—1
7. **D**, 2—4—3—1
8. **B**, 1—2—3—4
9. **B**, 2—4—3—1
10. **C**, 1—4—3—2

Paper Folding

INTRODUCTION

The fourth section of the PAT is paper folding. Beginning with a square, you are presented with a series of progressive folds that the initial square undergoes. After the folds have been completed, a hole is punched somewhere in the final form. The task of this section is to mentally unfold the paper and determine the precise positioning of the one or more holes resulting from the punch.

RULES

The parameters of paper folding are straightforward:

- The initial paper will always be square.
- The paper will never be twisted.
- The orientation of the paper will remain the same.
- All folds will result in forms that are contained within the imaginary perimeter of the initial square.
- Dashed lines indicate the absence of paper due to a fold.
- Solid lines indicate either a crease or the paper's edge.
- Only after all folds have been completed will a hole be punched.
- One or more holes may be punched.
- The hole may penetrate one layer or multiple layers of the paper.

Success on the paper-folding section relies heavily on the understanding of a few basic principles. With practice, you should be able to answer the paper-folding questions in a short time and with little error.

FORMAT OF THE FOLDING SEQUENCE

The paper-folding sequence is presented as a series of two to four images arranged side by side. The series is laid out progressively, beginning with the first fold, then the second, and so on. Although not shown, the starting form is always assumed to be a square. The final image of the sequence is identical to the next to last image but shows the placement of the hole punch.

Below is an example of a typical paper-fold sequence.

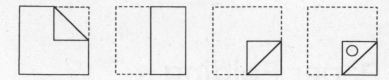

The dashed lines indicate absence of the paper (due to folding) from the original square. A solid line marks either a crease in the paper (seen only from frontal viewing) or the paper's edge. In the last image, the circle marks the location of the hole punch.

The following illustration includes guide arrows for clarification.

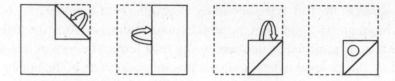

In this sequence, there are three folds. Prior DATs indicate that you can expect to see mostly two- and three-fold sequences.

THE PUNCH GRID

Presented with the folding sequence are five possible answers as to where the punched holes are located on the paper. These choices are presented in the form of punch grids. The blackened circles on the grid indicate the locations of punched holes. Below are five possible answer choices for the sequence presented above.

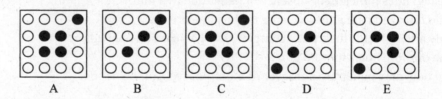

The punch grid is a standard configuration that is used in all types of folding sequences. Examination of the general punch grid offers important information concerning the nature of the types of folds that can be used in folding series.

The punch grid is composed of 16 possible holes, evenly arranged in rows and columns. A folding pattern will never result in hole punches that stray from the possibilities offered in the punch grid. With this fact in mind, it is evident that the folds must maintain the integrity of the four ordered rows and columns.

EXERCISE 1

The following exercise will help you better understand the relationship between folding patterns and punched-hole outcomes. Remove the exercise punch grids found in pages 00–00. Using these punch grids and a hand-held hole puncher, complete each of the following folding patterns and punch a hole in the place as indicated. Blacken the appropriate holes of the answer punch grid for each sequence *after* unfolding the hole-punched exercise punch grid.

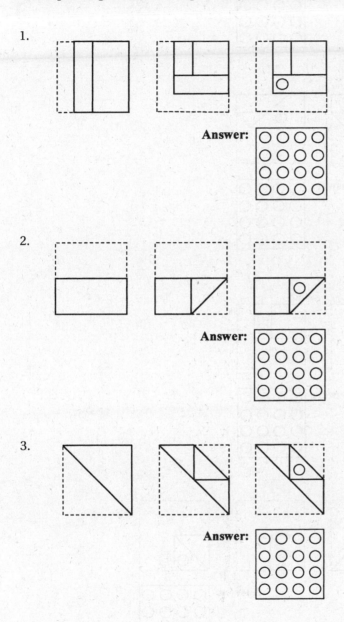

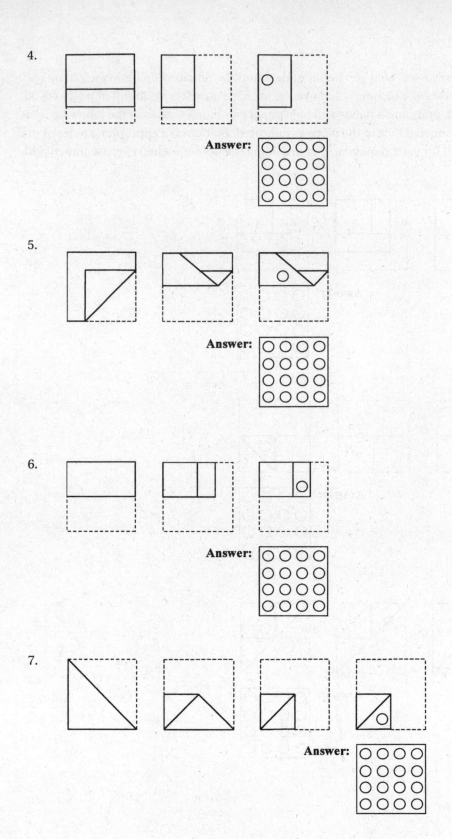

4.

Answer:

5.

Answer:

6.

Answer:

7.

Answer:

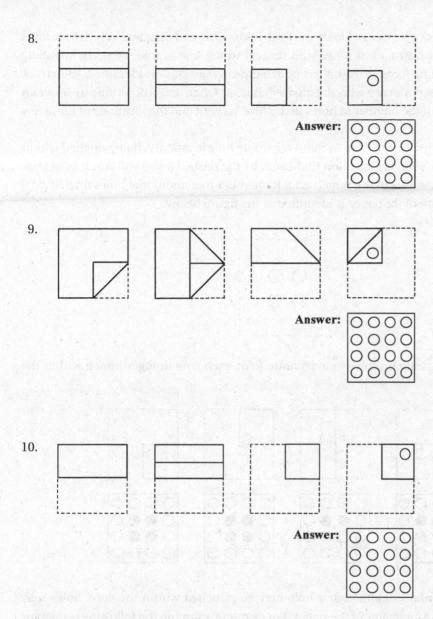

8.

Answer:

9.

Answer:

10.

Answer:

THE LOGIC OF FOLDS AND HOLES

With an understanding of the basic logic that underlies this section, you will be able to quickly identify the correct answer from the array of choices presented. Having completed Exercise 1, you have probably made the basic observation that *the number of resulting holes is equivalent to the number of paper layers through which the hole is punched.* You will often find that several answer choices can be disregarded as having too few or too many holes. In some cases, you may be left with only one choice, thus allowing you to select the correct answer without even considering the location of the holes. For this reason, your initial step should be to determine the number of paper layers *at the location of the punched hole.* Then quickly scan the answer choices to identify the punch grids that have the same number of blackened holes as the number of paper layers you identified.

The next step in arriving at the correct answer efficiently is to pinpoint the locations of holes. If you have narrowed the answer choices to just a few candidates, it may not be necessary to identify the locations of all the holes.

You will encounter three types of folds: vertical, horizontal, and diagonal. All of these folds will reveal holes that mirror each other with respect to the line of fold. Begin by mentally unfolding the paper and locating the holes one at a time. As each hole is identified, keep track of the pattern's correspondence with the answer choices. Often you will be able to select an answer on the basis of the number of holes in the final pattern and the locations of just a few holes.

There are a few principles to keep in mind regarding hole location. A hole punched within the core of the paper's original position (indicated by the dashed lines) will result in at least one hole located in the core of the punch grid. Remember that additional holes may lie outside the core. The core of the paper is identified in the figure below.

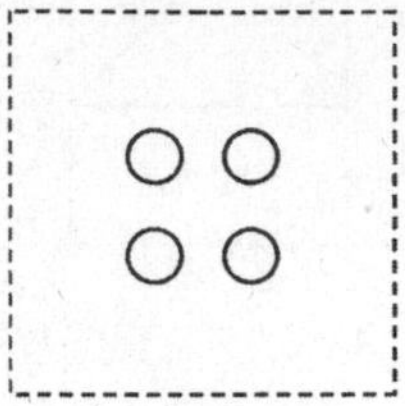

The following illustration shows four separate folds each containing a punch within the core.

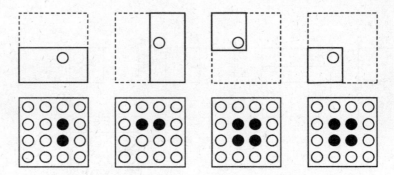

As previously mentioned, although a hole may be punched within the core, holes may also occur around the perimeter of the paper. For example, examine the following sequence:

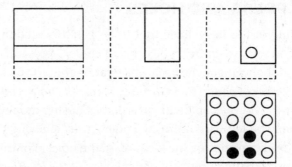

As a general rule, if the final form has a hole punched within the core of the form created by the original square (indicated by the dashed lines), the resulting punch grid will have at least one core hole. This general rule may be used to eliminate improbable answer choices.

Holes punched around the perimeter of the original square will result in forms that have at least one perimeter hole. Perimeter hole punches may be located in any of the positions indicated below.

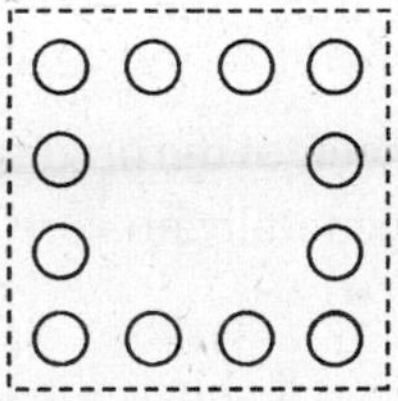

The restraint that the paper must stay within the confines of the original square makes it difficult to obtain an interior core hole from a perimeter punch. With this restriction, the only way to obtain interior core holes from a perimeter punch is to have a folding segment that quarters the length or width of the paper to the edge of the original square. Examples of the resulting forms are seen in the figure below.

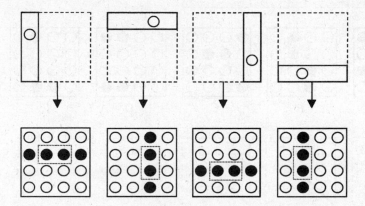

Most of the folds necessary to create an interior core hole from a punch around the perimeter would resemble those in the following sequence:

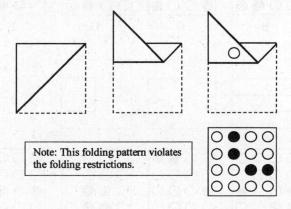

Note: This folding pattern violates the folding restrictions.

REVIEW

- First establish how many paper layers were penetrated by the hole punch. Eliminate answer choices that have too few or too many holes.
- Identify the locations of the punched holes. Remember that each fold will produce mirrored holes with respect to the line of fold.
- If the final form has a hole punched within the core of the form created by the original square (indicated by the dashed lines), the resulting punch card will have at least one core hole.
- Holes punched around the perimeter of the original square will result in forms that have at least one perimeter hole and generally no core hole (see the illustration on page 479 for exceptional folds).

EXERCISE 2

The following folding sequence questions are provided for additional practice.

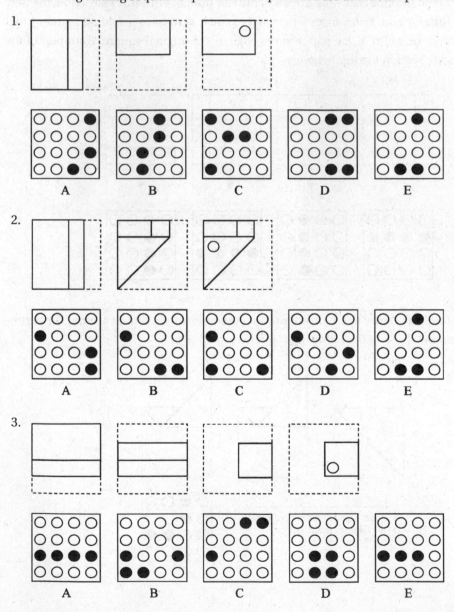

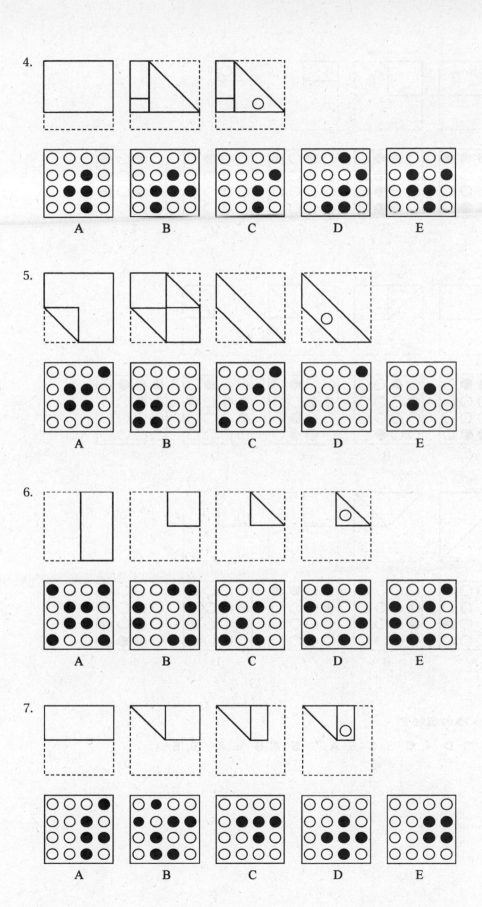

8.

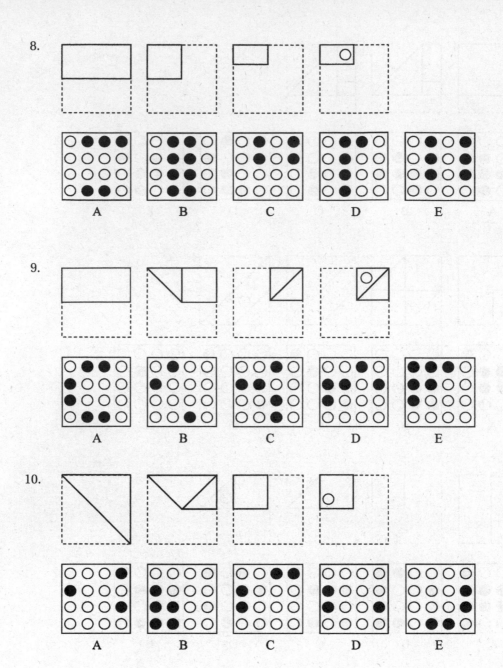

9.

10.

Answers to Exercise 2

1. **D**   2. **B**   3. **D**   4. **C**   5. **C**   6. **A**   7. **E**   8. **B**   9. **A**   10. **E**

The following punch grids are provided for use in the folding exercises. Using scissors, cut along the perimeter of each grid.

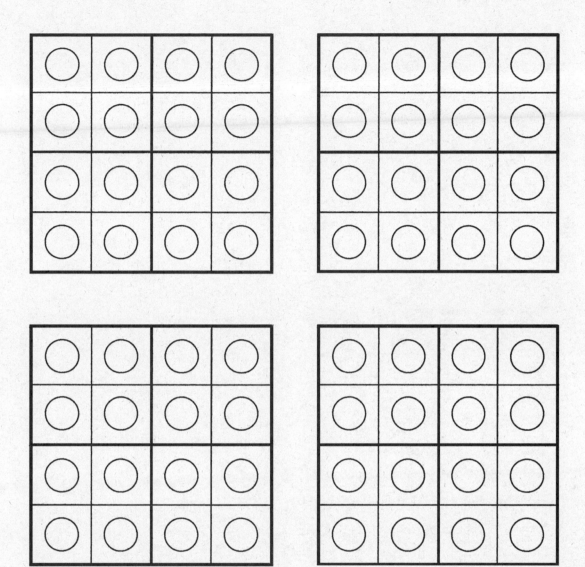

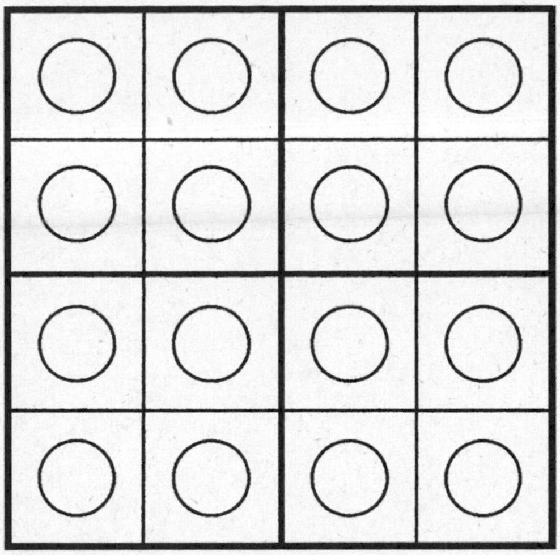
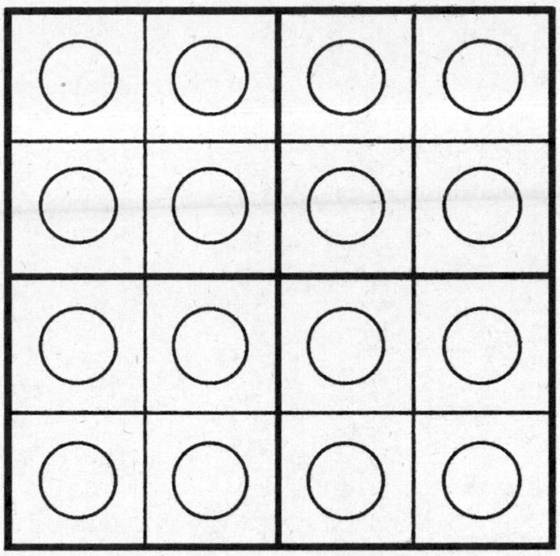
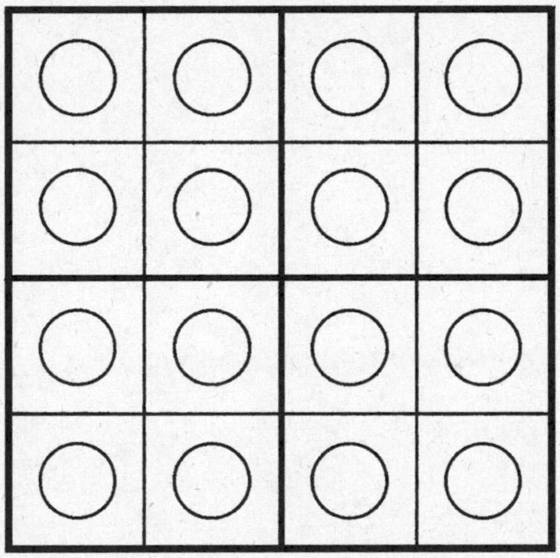
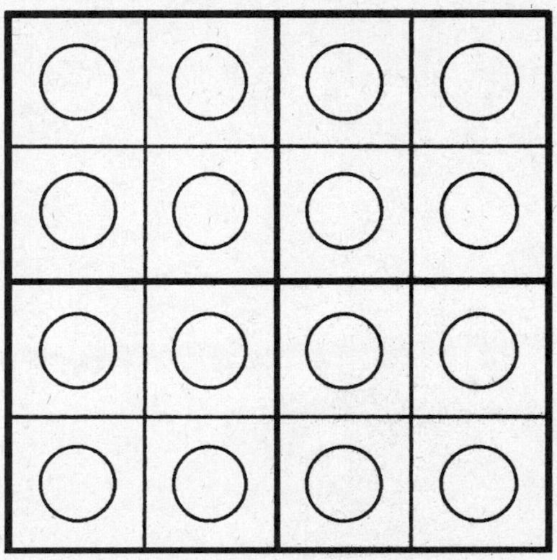

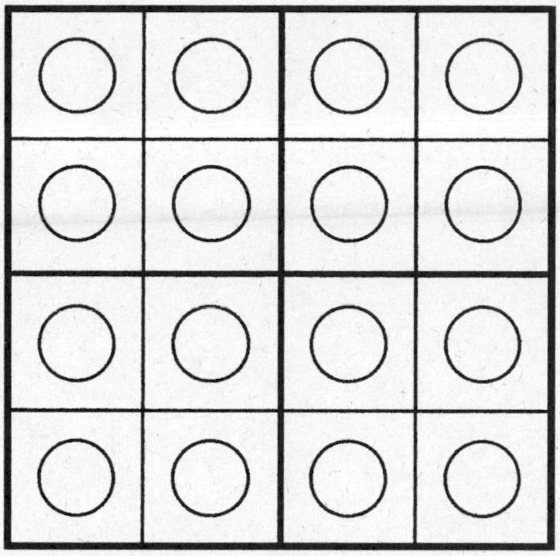
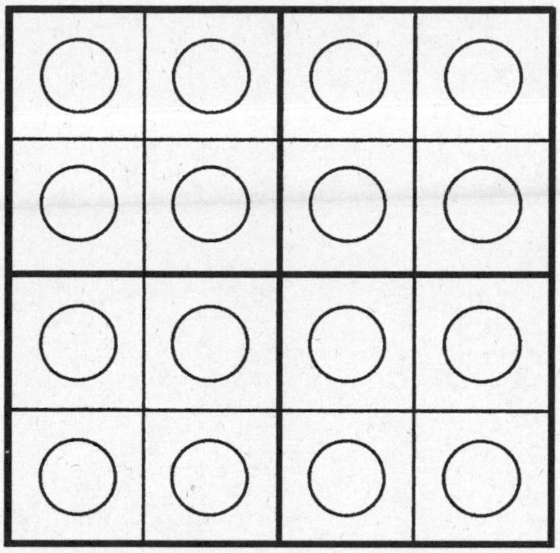
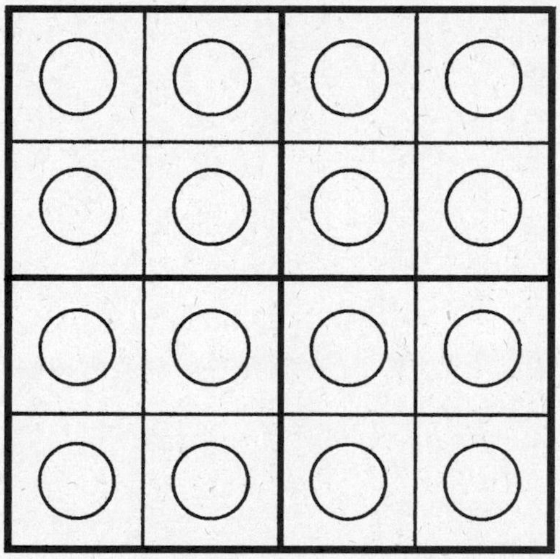
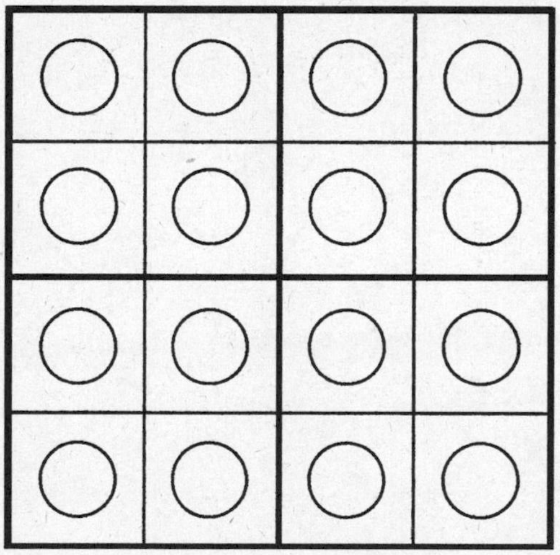

Cubes

52

INTRODUCTION

The fifth section of the PAT involves counting the painted surfaces of cubes. In this section, you will be presented with formations of stacked cubes. Groups of questions will correspond to the cube formations. The questions will ask you to determine how many cubes have a particular number of painted surfaces.

What distinguishes this section is the ease with which an answer can be quickly generated. For most test-takers, this section presents the fewest difficulties. In fact, with careful preparation and strategy, you can expect to answer these questions both efficiently and accurately. Because of the relative ease of this section in comparison to the other perceptual ability sections, you are cautioned to *not overlook* the use of strategy and preparative measures necessary for exceptional scoring. A high score on this group of questions will play an important role in achieving an overall high score on the PAT. Remember as you review for the cube questions that you are aiming for a nearly perfect score on these questions, which count no less than other, seemingly more difficult questions in the perceptual ability section of the DAT.

CUBE COUNTING

Below is an example of a basic cube formation. This example is used to illustrate the basic assumptions that should underlie your reasoning throughout the cube section. The cube formations on the actual test will not be labeled and will be more complex than the simple example that follows. Further testlike examples will be offered after the introductory explanations.

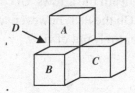

Notice that there appear to be three cubes in the above formation. In this section, you must pay careful attention to any hidden or obscured cubes. Realizing that cube *A* is above cubes *B* and *C*, you should infer that there exists cube *D*, which is out of view. Hence, there are four cubes in this simple formation. The assumption of *necessary support,* that is, that any cube above the first level must be supported by underlying cubes, is the first crucial assumption that you should make throughout this section.

To review your understanding of this basic assumption, practice counting the number of cubes in the following formation.

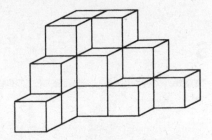

If you counted 18 cubes, you have answered correctly. If you failed to identify all 18 cubes, chances are that you either lacked organization as you counted or you did not attend to the assumption of necessary support. An organized count might begin at the top and work downward. (Additionally, for more complex arrangements, the direction of count would move from left to right for each level.) In this fashion, you would first identify the top 3 cubes. Then, following the assumption of necessary support, you would identify the 3 hidden cubes plus the additional 3 visible cubes on the second level. Thus, the second level has a total of 6 cubes. The bottom level has 6 hidden and 3 visible cubes, totaling 9 cubes. The grand total is 3 + 6 + 9 = 18.

Again, practice arriving at a total cube count by using the following formation.

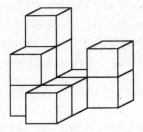

The correct answer is 10 cubes (1 + 3 + 6 = 10).

The second assumption that you should make in dealing with the cube section is that an *empty "ceiling" implies that there are no hidden cubes beneath*. For example, in the following formation examine the columns beneath the arrows. Of course, in real life a cube *could* exist on the first level that is out of view. On the PAT, however, an empty ceiling (top level) implies an empty column if the column is entirely out of view.

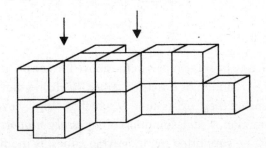

In the figure shown above, there are 6 cubes on the top level and 9 cubes on the bottom level. Here, the arrows draw your attention to empty columns. On the PAT, however, there will not be arrows to indicate empty columns. You will need to rely on your knowledge of the two assumptions discussed on page 489 in order to make appropriate judgments concerning the absence or presence of cubes out of view.

Now, try a more complex arrangement.

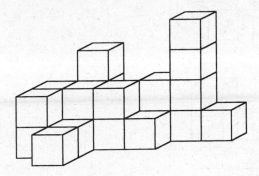

The correct answer is 21 cubes.

The initial counting of cubes is an important step that should precede any reasoning concerning the painted surface questions. Although no questions will ask you to simply identify the total number of cubes, an initial cube count takes little time and helps you avoid the trap of failing to identify hidden cubes. Additionally, the cube count will serve as a self-check in figuring your answers.

EXERCISE 1

The following cube formations are provided to help you achieve greater speed and accuracy in counting cubes.

How many cubes are there in each formation?

1.

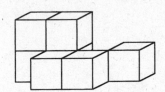

2.

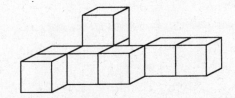

3.

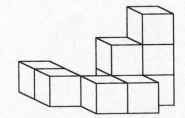

4.

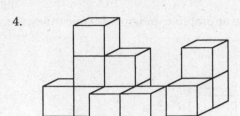

5.

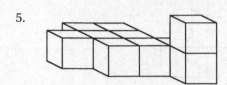

6.

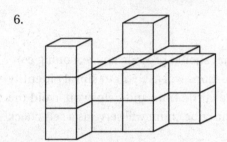

7.

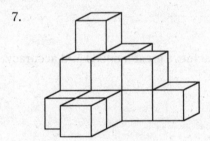

8.

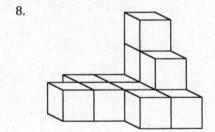

9.

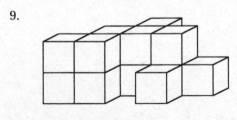

10.

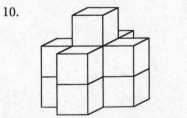

Compare your cube count totals with the answers provided below:

Answers to Exercise 1

1. **8** 2. **7** 3. **9** 4. **11** 5. **10** 6. **20** 7. **15** 8. **12** 9. **14** 10. **11**

Counting Painted Surfaces

The task in the cube section of the PAT is to count painted surfaces. Imagine that the formation below has been painted with white paint on all exposed sides. The exposed sides are the sides that would reflect light if light were projected from the front, the back, and the left and right sides of the formation.

What is the total number of painted surfaces (or cube sides) in the formation shown below?

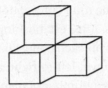

The total number of painted surfaces (or cube sides) of this formation is 15. In counting, it is a common mistake to overlook the exposed sides of blocks that are not visible to the respondent.

Below is a block separation of the basic figure considered above. Notice that the blackened areas are the surfaces that either sit on the imaginary floor or are shared between two blocks. These blackened areas are never to be counted as painted surfaces.

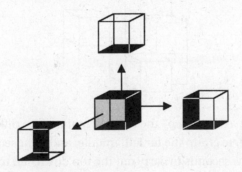

Actual painted surface questions that have appeared on previous DAT exams had this form:

In figure X, how many cubes have

    A. one of their exposed sides painted?

    B. two of their exposed sides painted?

    C. four of their exposed sides painted?

On the test approximately three painted surface questions refer to each formation. For this reason, it is crucial to follow a consistent methodology when counting painted surfaces. Failure to accurately identify all the cubes in a particular formation could result in incorrect responses to several questions.

Note that no cube should ever have six painted surfaces. Although there are six surfaces to a cube, the cube will always be resting against the imaginary floor or another cube. Also note that there will be instances in which a given cube will have no painted surface. This will occur when there are neighboring cubes on all sides and another cube rests above the cube in question. In general, your success in counting painted surfaces will depend on your ability to mentally meander around the far corners of the arrangement that are out of view. As is true for all sections of the DAT, with practice you will notice improvement.

Since the DAT will be administered on the computer, you will need to make good use of available scratch board. The painted cube questions, perhaps more than any other type, will reflect your ability to remain organized under test-taking circumstances.

STRATEGY

As stated previously, you should count the total number of cubes before addressing the issue of painted surfaces. (Remember to use an organized count—top down, left to right, and back in space.) This preliminary count will serve two purposes. First, it will help you identify all the obscured or hidden cubes. Second, the total cube count will serve as a self-check when you tally the numbers of painted surfaces. After establishing a total count, begin identifying (by cube) the number of painted surfaces on each cube. Follow the same pathway that you used to count the number of cubes (top down, left to right, and back in space). On your scratch paper create a vertical list that assigns a number of painted surfaces to each cube.

After counting the cube surfaces in the top level, draw a horizontal line to indicate the counting of cubes in a new level. Insert a horizontal line after each level. Finally, before answering the questions, check that the number of cubes you have tallied matches the total cube count that you identified initially.

To review the suggested counting methodology, consider the following example:

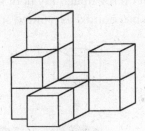

Although it is tempting to "break up" the cube formation into different sections for counting purposes (for example, to group the far left, middle, and right sections), this is *not* recommended. It takes only a few seconds to carry out the top down, left to right, and back in space procedure, and a consistent direction of count helps you remain accurate from formation to formation despite the differences between formations. The use of an organized procedure such as the one recommended above and illustrated below helps ensure that you will properly identify all hidden cubes.

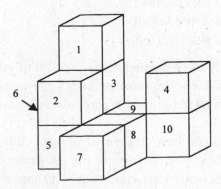

On your erasable board, note the total cube count before proceeding. Next, begin your vertical list of numbers that correspond to painted surfaces. For the above example, the list would be written as follows:

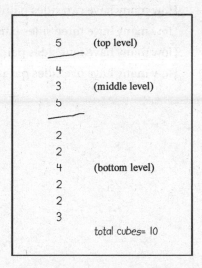

As mentioned previously, the cube count serves as a means of self-checking. Before responding to questions, verify that the number of cube surfaces you have identified matches the total number of cubes. If you find that you have made a mistake at some point, recheck your scratch work level by level (as separated by the horizontal lines in your list) to find where the skipped item was omitted.

At this point, you are ready to efficiently answer questions regarding the number of painted surfaces. Consider the following questions:

In the figure above, how many cubes have two of their exposed sides painted?
How many cubes have three of their exposed sides painted?
How many cubes have four of their exposed sides painted?
How many cubes have five of their exposed sides painted?

A helpful method for combing your list is to employ a circle, the letter X, and a squiggle to identify like numbers. A basic method of this sort helps avoid the fatal flaw of overlooking a crucial number. Failure to identify how many cubes share a certain number of painted sides can lead to incorrect choices on the test. Using an active rather than a passive method at each stage of developing your final answer will enable you to avoid mistakes.

Below is an example of the circle, X, and squiggle method for establishing the final answers to the questions given above. You can develop additional forms of notation that catch your eye at a glance.

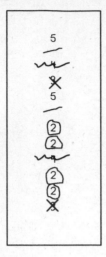

How many have two sides painted? 4

How many have three sides painted? 2

How many have four sides painted? 2

How many have five sides painted? 2

REVIEW

- According to the assumption of necessary support, any cube above the first level must be supported by underlying cubes.
- An empty ceiling (top level) implies an empty column if the column is entirely out of view.
- The initial counting of cubes is an important step that should precede any reasoning concerning painted surface questions.

EXERCISE 2

Practice is necessary to develop speed and accuracy in the employment of the various methods discussed above. Turn to pages 481–482, and answer the following questions for each of the 10 formations:

  a. How many cubes have one exposed side painted?

  b. How many cubes have two exposed sides painted?

  c. How many cubes have three exposed sides painted?

  d. How many cubes have four exposed sides painted?

  e. How many cubes have five exposed sides painted?

Answers to Exercise 2

  1. 0, 1, 2, 4, 1
  2. 0, 1, 2, 3, 1
  3. 0, 1, 3, 4, 1
  4. 0, 2, 3, 4, 2
  5. 1, 2, 5, 1, 1
  6. 3, 7, 6, 1, 2 (Note: One cube has no painted surface.)
  7. 1, 6, 3, 3, 1
  8. 2, 3, 4, 2, 1
  9. 2, 3, 4, 5, 0
  10. 0, 0, 4, 4, 1 (Note: Two cubes have no painted surface.)

Form Development

53

INTRODUCTION

The last section of the PAT is form development. In this section, you are presented with a flat pattern that is to be folded into a three-dimensional form. Your task is to select the appropriate three-dimensional rendering of the flattened image from four possible choices.

This section has the power to consume a tremendous amount of valuable test time. One of your many goals for this section is to be able to recognize when it is prudent to skip questions too difficult to be solved at first try. Although form development is a challenge for most test-takers, it offers the opportunity to integrate the skills mastered for other sections of the PAT. This section need not be construed as formidable; careful use of strategy will enhance your ability to recognize the appropriate answer without delay.

THE FLATTENED IMAGE

The flattened image is a rendering of what you would have if a three-dimensional object was opened at its edges with each surface "unwrapped" and the whole form flattened on one plane. The following is an example of a flattened image.

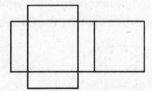

Notice that the flattened image is one complete unit. Although sides have been cut at the edges, each panel has at least one edge joined with another surface. On some flattened images, shaded regions or designs mark the surfaces. Keep in mind that each line that is part of the flattened image indicates one of the following: (1) a bend, (2) an edge, or (3) the outline of a shaded region.

CONSTRUCTION OF THE THREE-DIMENSIONAL IMAGE

Your task in the form development section is to select the correct or appropriate three-dimensional image constructed from the flattened figure. The three-dimensional figures will be rendered as isometric drawings. An isometric drawing is a representational drawing in which all faces of the image are shown with equal inclination and all the lines are drawn to their true lengths. Below is an example of a three-dimensional construction of the flattened image shown above.

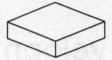

The orientation of the three-dimensional image will vary from question to question. After the form is constructed, it may be turned on its side or upside down. The following two examples illustrate how the same flattened image may be represented three dimensionally in two different ways.

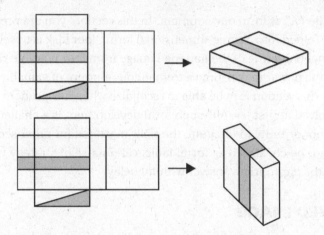

Likewise, there is no standard orientation of the flattened image that relates to the direction of fold used to construct the three-dimensional image. In the following example, the flattened pattern is oriented in four different positions. What is later perceived as the figure's top may seem to be a likely bottom when viewing the flattened image.

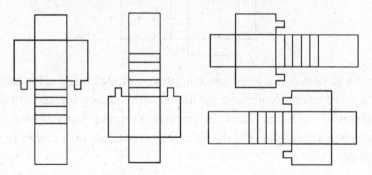

Any of the flattened images above could be used to describe *all* of the following three-dimensional forms:

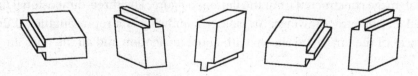

Often, the orientation of the flattened image biases your thinking in regard to where the folding begins and how you conceive of the folding direction. Such a bias may interfere with the ability to regard certain answer choices as possible accurate renderings. For this reason, it is important to develop a strategy that leads you to the correct answer regardless of the orientation or positioning of the flattened form or of the three-dimensional answer choices.

ATTENTION TO DETAIL

Perhaps the quickest way to identify an appropriate three-dimensional rendering of the flattened form is to utilize details of each drawing (flattened figures and three-dimensional answer choices). Consider the following flattened form and corresponding answer choices:

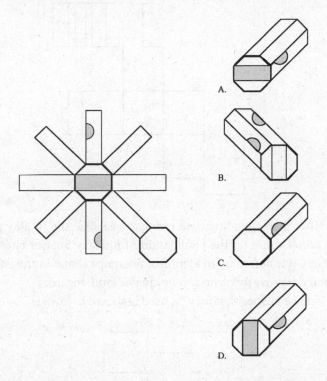

In this example, the details that stand out are the shaded half-circles and the shaded rectangle. *Whenever shading is used, first examine the answer choices to eliminate any that have an inappropriate positioning of the shaded region or design.* Take note of the precise positioning of a shaded region. It is not necessary to initially check each design for the positioning of each shaded region. Often you can eliminate several choices by checking the positioning of just one shaded region. As you narrow the choices, you can expand the degree of detail on which you will base your final judgment. In the example above, the first detail check might be to scan for the distance between the half-circle and the rectangular figure. Noticing that both half-circles are positioned closer to the blank hexagon than to the hexagon with the rectangle, you can eliminate choices A, B, and D. With little effort, you realize that the correct answer is C. This answer was arrived at without considering the angle of view or the spacing between marked sides. By keeping to a simplistic plan such as detail scanning, you save a tremendous amount of time and energy.

Although detail scanning is extremely helpful in questions that contain shaded regions or designs, in other questions you will be confronted with complex flattened images that contain no distinct feature markings.

COMPLEX FORMS

Some flattened forms will be difficult to visualize in three dimensions. The shape may be unusual, or the number of folds necessary to arrive at the final form may be unusually high. The form below would be considered complex in both regards.

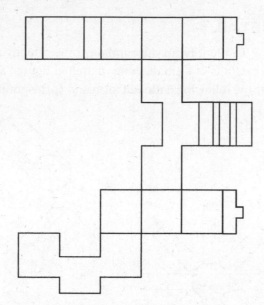

In such cases, rather than spending time trying to visualize the totality of the final three-dimensional form, concentrate on the elimination of unlikely answer choices. To begin the process of elimination, it is necessary to identify a reference shape in the flattened form. This reference shape should be easy to locate and unique in some regard.

One of many reference shapes that may be used is shown below:

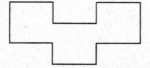

This particular form happens to be the largest unfolded portion of the flattened figure. It also appears twice in the flattened image. Often, a pair of identical large regions serves the three-dimensional image as the sides or the top and bottom.

Once you have identified the reference shape you wish to use, examine the answer choices. Check each choice to see whether the shape is reproduced correctly, the neighboring sides make logical sense given the joining shapes in the flattened form, and the shape is repeated the correct number of times.

Now, considering the form given above, try these strategies on the answer choices below.

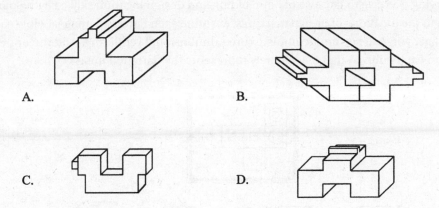

A.

B.

C.

D.

The correct answer is D.

REVIEW

- The orientation of the three-dimensional image will vary from question to question. After the form is constructed, it may be turned on its side or upside down. Likewise, there is no standard orientation of the flattened image in relation to the direction of fold used to construct the three-dimensional image.
- Each line that is part of the flattened image indicates one of the following: (1) a bend, (2) an edge, or (3) the outline of a shaded region.
- Whenever shading is used, first search your answer choices to eliminate any that have an inappropriate positioning of a shaded region or design. Remember that it is not necessary to initially check each design for the positioning of every shaded region. You are often able to eliminate several choices by checking the positioning of just one shaded region.
- When confronted with a complex form, concentrate on the elimination of unlikely answer choices. To begin the process of elimination, identify a reference shape in the flattened form. Check each answer choice to see whether the shape is reproduced correctly, the neighboring sides make logical sense given the joining shapes in the flattened form, and the shape is repeated the correct number of times.
- Use your time carefully. Do not allow yourself to dwell on any one question. Skip a question if you cannot effectively eliminate answer choices at the first try.

EXERCISE 1

The following exercise makes use of both folding and design location skills. Paying particular attention to the locations of design markings, examine each flattened image. Below each flattened image, you will see an incomplete three-dimensional rendering. Add the appropriate marking to each cube so that it accurately represents the flattened image.

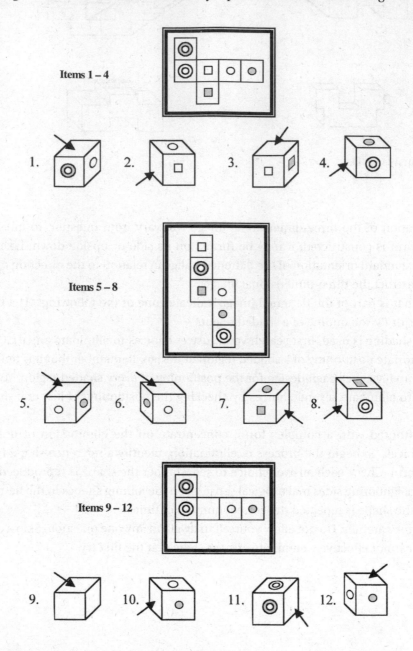

Answers to Exercise 1

1. Shaded circle
2. Shaded ring
3. White circle
4. Shaded square

5. White square
6. Shaded square
7. White ring
8. Shaded ring

9. White circle or white ring
10. (Blank)
11. Shaded circle
12. Shaded ring

EXERCISE 2

This exercise is formatted identically to the way in which form development questions appear on the DAT. In each case, choose the correct three-dimensional representation of the flattened image shown at left.

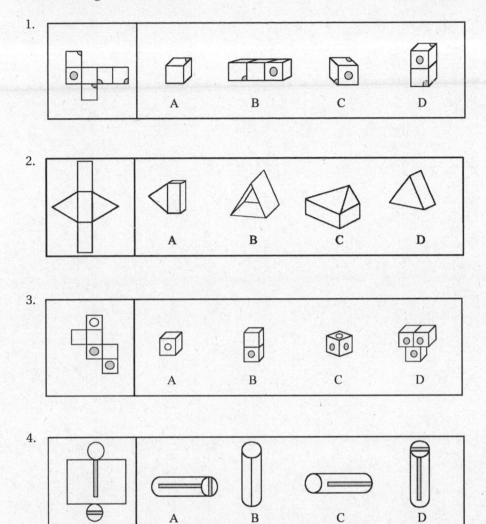

Answers to Exercise 2

(It is suggested that you complete Exercise 3 before checking your answers to Exercise 2.)

1. **C**   2. **D**   3. **A**   4. **B**   5. **D**

EXERCISE 3

On the following pages you will find reproductions of all the flattened forms discussed in the form development section. Carefully cut out each form and create three-dimensional forms by folding the cutouts. Then use the three-dimensional figures to review the strategic discussions and Exercises 1 and 2.

Carefully remove each flattened figure by cutting around its perimeter. Then construct a three-dimensional form by folding. Clear tape may be used to fasten the sides.

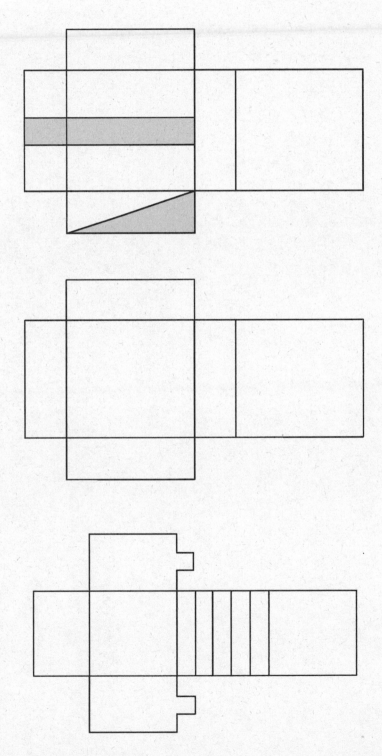

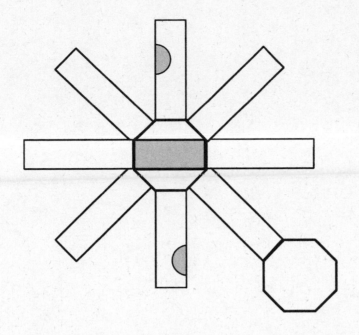

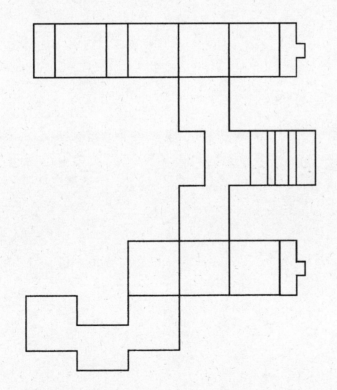

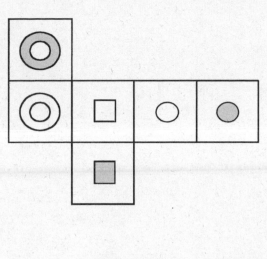

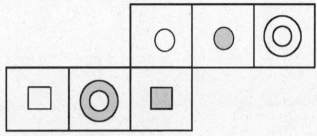

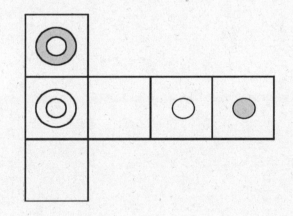

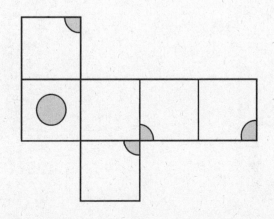

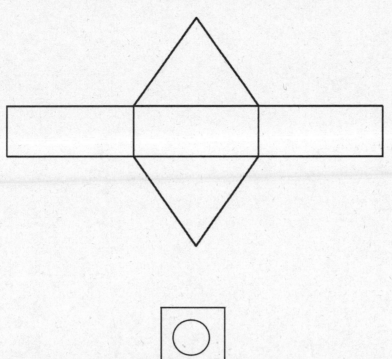

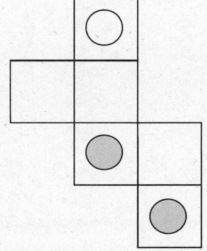

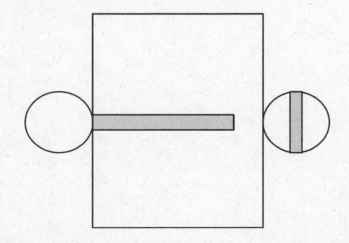

ANSWER SHEET
Practice Test 1

Survey of the Natural Sciences Test

1. Ⓐ Ⓑ Ⓒ Ⓓ Ⓔ	26. Ⓐ Ⓑ Ⓒ Ⓓ Ⓔ	51. Ⓐ Ⓑ Ⓒ Ⓓ Ⓔ	76. Ⓐ Ⓑ Ⓒ Ⓓ Ⓔ
2. Ⓐ Ⓑ Ⓒ Ⓓ Ⓔ	27. Ⓐ Ⓑ Ⓒ Ⓓ Ⓔ	52. Ⓐ Ⓑ Ⓒ Ⓓ Ⓔ	77. Ⓐ Ⓑ Ⓒ Ⓓ Ⓔ
3. Ⓐ Ⓑ Ⓒ Ⓓ Ⓔ	28. Ⓐ Ⓑ Ⓒ Ⓓ Ⓔ	53. Ⓐ Ⓑ Ⓒ Ⓓ Ⓔ	78. Ⓐ Ⓑ Ⓒ Ⓓ Ⓔ
4. Ⓐ Ⓑ Ⓒ Ⓓ Ⓔ	29. Ⓐ Ⓑ Ⓒ Ⓓ Ⓔ	54. Ⓐ Ⓑ Ⓒ Ⓓ Ⓔ	79. Ⓐ Ⓑ Ⓒ Ⓓ Ⓔ
5. Ⓐ Ⓑ Ⓒ Ⓓ Ⓔ	30. Ⓐ Ⓑ Ⓒ Ⓓ Ⓔ	55. Ⓐ Ⓑ Ⓒ Ⓓ Ⓔ	80. Ⓐ Ⓑ Ⓒ Ⓓ Ⓔ
6. Ⓐ Ⓑ Ⓒ Ⓓ Ⓔ	31. Ⓐ Ⓑ Ⓒ Ⓓ Ⓔ	56. Ⓐ Ⓑ Ⓒ Ⓓ Ⓔ	81. Ⓐ Ⓑ Ⓒ Ⓓ Ⓔ
7. Ⓐ Ⓑ Ⓒ Ⓓ Ⓔ	32. Ⓐ Ⓑ Ⓒ Ⓓ Ⓔ	57. Ⓐ Ⓑ Ⓒ Ⓓ Ⓔ	82. Ⓐ Ⓑ Ⓒ Ⓓ Ⓔ
8. Ⓐ Ⓑ Ⓒ Ⓓ Ⓔ	33. Ⓐ Ⓑ Ⓒ Ⓓ Ⓔ	58. Ⓐ Ⓑ Ⓒ Ⓓ Ⓔ	83. Ⓐ Ⓑ Ⓒ Ⓓ Ⓔ
9. Ⓐ Ⓑ Ⓒ Ⓓ Ⓔ	34. Ⓐ Ⓑ Ⓒ Ⓓ Ⓔ	59. Ⓐ Ⓑ Ⓒ Ⓓ Ⓔ	84. Ⓐ Ⓑ Ⓒ Ⓓ Ⓔ
10. Ⓐ Ⓑ Ⓒ Ⓓ Ⓔ	35. Ⓐ Ⓑ Ⓒ Ⓓ Ⓔ	60. Ⓐ Ⓑ Ⓒ Ⓓ Ⓔ	85. Ⓐ Ⓑ Ⓒ Ⓓ Ⓔ
11. Ⓐ Ⓑ Ⓒ Ⓓ Ⓔ	36. Ⓐ Ⓑ Ⓒ Ⓓ Ⓔ	61. Ⓐ Ⓑ Ⓒ Ⓓ Ⓔ	86. Ⓐ Ⓑ Ⓒ Ⓓ Ⓔ
12. Ⓐ Ⓑ Ⓒ Ⓓ Ⓔ	37. Ⓐ Ⓑ Ⓒ Ⓓ Ⓔ	62. Ⓐ Ⓑ Ⓒ Ⓓ Ⓔ	87. Ⓐ Ⓑ Ⓒ Ⓓ Ⓔ
13. Ⓐ Ⓑ Ⓒ Ⓓ Ⓔ	38. Ⓐ Ⓑ Ⓒ Ⓓ Ⓔ	63. Ⓐ Ⓑ Ⓒ Ⓓ Ⓔ	88. Ⓐ Ⓑ Ⓒ Ⓓ Ⓔ
14. Ⓐ Ⓑ Ⓒ Ⓓ Ⓔ	39. Ⓐ Ⓑ Ⓒ Ⓓ Ⓔ	64. Ⓐ Ⓑ Ⓒ Ⓓ Ⓔ	89. Ⓐ Ⓑ Ⓒ Ⓓ Ⓔ
15. Ⓐ Ⓑ Ⓒ Ⓓ Ⓔ	40. Ⓐ Ⓑ Ⓒ Ⓓ Ⓔ	65. Ⓐ Ⓑ Ⓒ Ⓓ Ⓔ	90. Ⓐ Ⓑ Ⓒ Ⓓ Ⓔ
16. Ⓐ Ⓑ Ⓒ Ⓓ Ⓔ	41. Ⓐ Ⓑ Ⓒ Ⓓ Ⓔ	66. Ⓐ Ⓑ Ⓒ Ⓓ Ⓔ	91. Ⓐ Ⓑ Ⓒ Ⓓ Ⓔ
17. Ⓐ Ⓑ Ⓒ Ⓓ Ⓔ	42. Ⓐ Ⓑ Ⓒ Ⓓ Ⓔ	67. Ⓐ Ⓑ Ⓒ Ⓓ Ⓔ	92. Ⓐ Ⓑ Ⓒ Ⓓ Ⓔ
18. Ⓐ Ⓑ Ⓒ Ⓓ Ⓔ	43. Ⓐ Ⓑ Ⓒ Ⓓ Ⓔ	68. Ⓐ Ⓑ Ⓒ Ⓓ Ⓔ	93. Ⓐ Ⓑ Ⓒ Ⓓ Ⓔ
19. Ⓐ Ⓑ Ⓒ Ⓓ Ⓔ	44. Ⓐ Ⓑ Ⓒ Ⓓ Ⓔ	69. Ⓐ Ⓑ Ⓒ Ⓓ Ⓔ	94. Ⓐ Ⓑ Ⓒ Ⓓ Ⓔ
20. Ⓐ Ⓑ Ⓒ Ⓓ Ⓔ	45. Ⓐ Ⓑ Ⓒ Ⓓ Ⓔ	70. Ⓐ Ⓑ Ⓒ Ⓓ Ⓔ	95. Ⓐ Ⓑ Ⓒ Ⓓ Ⓔ
21. Ⓐ Ⓑ Ⓒ Ⓓ Ⓔ	46. Ⓐ Ⓑ Ⓒ Ⓓ Ⓔ	71. Ⓐ Ⓑ Ⓒ Ⓓ Ⓔ	96. Ⓐ Ⓑ Ⓒ Ⓓ Ⓔ
22. Ⓐ Ⓑ Ⓒ Ⓓ Ⓔ	47. Ⓐ Ⓑ Ⓒ Ⓓ Ⓔ	72. Ⓐ Ⓑ Ⓒ Ⓓ Ⓔ	97. Ⓐ Ⓑ Ⓒ Ⓓ Ⓔ
23. Ⓐ Ⓑ Ⓒ Ⓓ Ⓔ	48. Ⓐ Ⓑ Ⓒ Ⓓ Ⓔ	73. Ⓐ Ⓑ Ⓒ Ⓓ Ⓔ	98. Ⓐ Ⓑ Ⓒ Ⓓ Ⓔ
24. Ⓐ Ⓑ Ⓒ Ⓓ Ⓔ	49. Ⓐ Ⓑ Ⓒ Ⓓ Ⓔ	74. Ⓐ Ⓑ Ⓒ Ⓓ Ⓔ	99. Ⓐ Ⓑ Ⓒ Ⓓ Ⓔ
25. Ⓐ Ⓑ Ⓒ Ⓓ Ⓔ	50. Ⓐ Ⓑ Ⓒ Ⓓ Ⓔ	75. Ⓐ Ⓑ Ⓒ Ⓓ Ⓔ	100. Ⓐ Ⓑ Ⓒ Ⓓ Ⓔ

ANSWER SHEET
Practice Test 1

Perceptual Ability Test

Part 1: Aperture Passing

1. Ⓐ Ⓑ Ⓒ Ⓓ Ⓔ   5. Ⓐ Ⓑ Ⓒ Ⓓ Ⓔ   9. Ⓐ Ⓑ Ⓒ Ⓓ Ⓔ   13. Ⓐ Ⓑ Ⓒ Ⓓ Ⓔ
2. Ⓐ Ⓑ Ⓒ Ⓓ Ⓔ   6. Ⓐ Ⓑ Ⓒ Ⓓ Ⓔ   10. Ⓐ Ⓑ Ⓒ Ⓓ Ⓔ   14. Ⓐ Ⓑ Ⓒ Ⓓ Ⓔ
3. Ⓐ Ⓑ Ⓒ Ⓓ Ⓔ   7. Ⓐ Ⓑ Ⓒ Ⓓ Ⓔ   11. Ⓐ Ⓑ Ⓒ Ⓓ Ⓔ   15. Ⓐ Ⓑ Ⓒ Ⓓ Ⓔ
4. Ⓐ Ⓑ Ⓒ Ⓓ Ⓔ   8. Ⓐ Ⓑ Ⓒ Ⓓ Ⓔ   12. Ⓐ Ⓑ Ⓒ Ⓓ Ⓔ

Part 2: Orthographic Projections

16. Ⓐ Ⓑ Ⓒ Ⓓ   20. Ⓐ Ⓑ Ⓒ Ⓓ   24. Ⓐ Ⓑ Ⓒ Ⓓ   28. Ⓐ Ⓑ Ⓒ Ⓓ
17. Ⓐ Ⓑ Ⓒ Ⓓ   21. Ⓐ Ⓑ Ⓒ Ⓓ   25. Ⓐ Ⓑ Ⓒ Ⓓ   29. Ⓐ Ⓑ Ⓒ Ⓓ
18. Ⓐ Ⓑ Ⓒ Ⓓ   22. Ⓐ Ⓑ Ⓒ Ⓓ   26. Ⓐ Ⓑ Ⓒ Ⓓ   30. Ⓐ Ⓑ Ⓒ Ⓓ
19. Ⓐ Ⓑ Ⓒ Ⓓ   23. Ⓐ Ⓑ Ⓒ Ⓓ   27. Ⓐ Ⓑ Ⓒ Ⓓ

Part 3: Angle Discrimination

31. Ⓐ Ⓑ Ⓒ Ⓓ   35. Ⓐ Ⓑ Ⓒ Ⓓ   39. Ⓐ Ⓑ Ⓒ Ⓓ   43. Ⓐ Ⓑ Ⓒ Ⓓ
32. Ⓐ Ⓑ Ⓒ Ⓓ   36. Ⓐ Ⓑ Ⓒ Ⓓ   40. Ⓐ Ⓑ Ⓒ Ⓓ   44. Ⓐ Ⓑ Ⓒ Ⓓ
33. Ⓐ Ⓑ Ⓒ Ⓓ   37. Ⓐ Ⓑ Ⓒ Ⓓ   41. Ⓐ Ⓑ Ⓒ Ⓓ   45. Ⓐ Ⓑ Ⓒ Ⓓ
34. Ⓐ Ⓑ Ⓒ Ⓓ   38. Ⓐ Ⓑ Ⓒ Ⓓ   42. Ⓐ Ⓑ Ⓒ Ⓓ

Part 4: Paper Folding

46. Ⓐ Ⓑ Ⓒ Ⓓ Ⓔ   50. Ⓐ Ⓑ Ⓒ Ⓓ Ⓔ   54. Ⓐ Ⓑ Ⓒ Ⓓ Ⓔ   58. Ⓐ Ⓑ Ⓒ Ⓓ Ⓔ
47. Ⓐ Ⓑ Ⓒ Ⓓ Ⓔ   51. Ⓐ Ⓑ Ⓒ Ⓓ Ⓔ   55. Ⓐ Ⓑ Ⓒ Ⓓ Ⓔ   59. Ⓐ Ⓑ Ⓒ Ⓓ Ⓔ
48. Ⓐ Ⓑ Ⓒ Ⓓ Ⓔ   52. Ⓐ Ⓑ Ⓒ Ⓓ Ⓔ   56. Ⓐ Ⓑ Ⓒ Ⓓ Ⓔ   60. Ⓐ Ⓑ Ⓒ Ⓓ Ⓔ
49. Ⓐ Ⓑ Ⓒ Ⓓ Ⓔ   53. Ⓐ Ⓑ Ⓒ Ⓓ Ⓔ   57. Ⓐ Ⓑ Ⓒ Ⓓ Ⓔ

Part 5: Cubes

61. Ⓐ Ⓑ Ⓒ Ⓓ Ⓔ   65. Ⓐ Ⓑ Ⓒ Ⓓ Ⓔ   69. Ⓐ Ⓑ Ⓒ Ⓓ Ⓔ   73. Ⓐ Ⓑ Ⓒ Ⓓ Ⓔ
62. Ⓐ Ⓑ Ⓒ Ⓓ Ⓔ   66. Ⓐ Ⓑ Ⓒ Ⓓ Ⓔ   70. Ⓐ Ⓑ Ⓒ Ⓓ Ⓔ   74. Ⓐ Ⓑ Ⓒ Ⓓ Ⓔ
63. Ⓐ Ⓑ Ⓒ Ⓓ Ⓔ   67. Ⓐ Ⓑ Ⓒ Ⓓ Ⓔ   71. Ⓐ Ⓑ Ⓒ Ⓓ Ⓔ   75. Ⓐ Ⓑ Ⓒ Ⓓ Ⓔ
64. Ⓐ Ⓑ Ⓒ Ⓓ Ⓔ   68. Ⓐ Ⓑ Ⓒ Ⓓ Ⓔ   72. Ⓐ Ⓑ Ⓒ Ⓓ Ⓔ

Part 6: Form Development

76. Ⓐ Ⓑ Ⓒ Ⓓ   80. Ⓐ Ⓑ Ⓒ Ⓓ   84. Ⓐ Ⓑ Ⓒ Ⓓ   88. Ⓐ Ⓑ Ⓒ Ⓓ
77. Ⓐ Ⓑ Ⓒ Ⓓ   81. Ⓐ Ⓑ Ⓒ Ⓓ   85. Ⓐ Ⓑ Ⓒ Ⓓ   89. Ⓐ Ⓑ Ⓒ Ⓓ
78. Ⓐ Ⓑ Ⓒ Ⓓ   82. Ⓐ Ⓑ Ⓒ Ⓓ   86. Ⓐ Ⓑ Ⓒ Ⓓ   90. Ⓐ Ⓑ Ⓒ Ⓓ
79. Ⓐ Ⓑ Ⓒ Ⓓ   83. Ⓐ Ⓑ Ⓒ Ⓓ   87. Ⓐ Ⓑ Ⓒ Ⓓ

Reading Comprehension Test

1. Ⓐ Ⓑ Ⓒ Ⓓ Ⓔ   14. Ⓐ Ⓑ Ⓒ Ⓓ Ⓔ   27. Ⓐ Ⓑ Ⓒ Ⓓ Ⓔ   40. Ⓐ Ⓑ Ⓒ Ⓓ Ⓔ
2. Ⓐ Ⓑ Ⓒ Ⓓ Ⓔ   15. Ⓐ Ⓑ Ⓒ Ⓓ Ⓔ   28. Ⓐ Ⓑ Ⓒ Ⓓ Ⓔ   41. Ⓐ Ⓑ Ⓒ Ⓓ Ⓔ
3. Ⓐ Ⓑ Ⓒ Ⓓ Ⓔ   16. Ⓐ Ⓑ Ⓒ Ⓓ Ⓔ   29. Ⓐ Ⓑ Ⓒ Ⓓ Ⓔ   42. Ⓐ Ⓑ Ⓒ Ⓓ Ⓔ
4. Ⓐ Ⓑ Ⓒ Ⓓ Ⓔ   17. Ⓐ Ⓑ Ⓒ Ⓓ Ⓔ   30. Ⓐ Ⓑ Ⓒ Ⓓ Ⓔ   43. Ⓐ Ⓑ Ⓒ Ⓓ Ⓔ
5. Ⓐ Ⓑ Ⓒ Ⓓ Ⓔ   18. Ⓐ Ⓑ Ⓒ Ⓓ Ⓔ   31. Ⓐ Ⓑ Ⓒ Ⓓ Ⓔ   44. Ⓐ Ⓑ Ⓒ Ⓓ Ⓔ
6. Ⓐ Ⓑ Ⓒ Ⓓ Ⓔ   19. Ⓐ Ⓑ Ⓒ Ⓓ Ⓔ   32. Ⓐ Ⓑ Ⓒ Ⓓ Ⓔ   45. Ⓐ Ⓑ Ⓒ Ⓓ Ⓔ
7. Ⓐ Ⓑ Ⓒ Ⓓ Ⓔ   20. Ⓐ Ⓑ Ⓒ Ⓓ Ⓔ   33. Ⓐ Ⓑ Ⓒ Ⓓ Ⓔ   46. Ⓐ Ⓑ Ⓒ Ⓓ Ⓔ
8. Ⓐ Ⓑ Ⓒ Ⓓ Ⓔ   21. Ⓐ Ⓑ Ⓒ Ⓓ Ⓔ   34. Ⓐ Ⓑ Ⓒ Ⓓ Ⓔ   47. Ⓐ Ⓑ Ⓒ Ⓓ Ⓔ
9. Ⓐ Ⓑ Ⓒ Ⓓ Ⓔ   22. Ⓐ Ⓑ Ⓒ Ⓓ Ⓔ   35. Ⓐ Ⓑ Ⓒ Ⓓ Ⓔ   48. Ⓐ Ⓑ Ⓒ Ⓓ Ⓔ
10. Ⓐ Ⓑ Ⓒ Ⓓ Ⓔ   23. Ⓐ Ⓑ Ⓒ Ⓓ Ⓔ   36. Ⓐ Ⓑ Ⓒ Ⓓ Ⓔ   49. Ⓐ Ⓑ Ⓒ Ⓓ Ⓔ
11. Ⓐ Ⓑ Ⓒ Ⓓ Ⓔ   24. Ⓐ Ⓑ Ⓒ Ⓓ Ⓔ   37. Ⓐ Ⓑ Ⓒ Ⓓ Ⓔ   50. Ⓐ Ⓑ Ⓒ Ⓓ Ⓔ
12. Ⓐ Ⓑ Ⓒ Ⓓ Ⓔ   25. Ⓐ Ⓑ Ⓒ Ⓓ Ⓔ   38. Ⓐ Ⓑ Ⓒ Ⓓ Ⓔ
13. Ⓐ Ⓑ Ⓒ Ⓓ Ⓔ   26. Ⓐ Ⓑ Ⓒ Ⓓ Ⓔ   39. Ⓐ Ⓑ Ⓒ Ⓓ Ⓔ

Quantitative Reasoning Test

1. Ⓐ Ⓑ Ⓒ Ⓓ Ⓔ   11. Ⓐ Ⓑ Ⓒ Ⓓ Ⓔ   21. Ⓐ Ⓑ Ⓒ Ⓓ Ⓔ   31. Ⓐ Ⓑ Ⓒ Ⓓ Ⓔ
2. Ⓐ Ⓑ Ⓒ Ⓓ Ⓔ   12. Ⓐ Ⓑ Ⓒ Ⓓ Ⓔ   22. Ⓐ Ⓑ Ⓒ Ⓓ Ⓔ   32. Ⓐ Ⓑ Ⓒ Ⓓ Ⓔ
3. Ⓐ Ⓑ Ⓒ Ⓓ Ⓔ   13. Ⓐ Ⓑ Ⓒ Ⓓ Ⓔ   23. Ⓐ Ⓑ Ⓒ Ⓓ Ⓔ   33. Ⓐ Ⓑ Ⓒ Ⓓ Ⓔ
4. Ⓐ Ⓑ Ⓒ Ⓓ   14. Ⓐ Ⓑ Ⓒ Ⓓ   24. Ⓐ Ⓑ Ⓒ Ⓓ Ⓔ   34. Ⓐ Ⓑ Ⓒ Ⓓ Ⓔ
5. Ⓐ Ⓑ Ⓒ Ⓓ Ⓔ   15. Ⓐ Ⓑ Ⓒ Ⓓ Ⓔ   25. Ⓐ Ⓑ Ⓒ Ⓓ   35. Ⓐ Ⓑ Ⓒ Ⓓ Ⓔ
6. Ⓐ Ⓑ Ⓒ Ⓓ Ⓔ   16. Ⓐ Ⓑ Ⓒ Ⓓ Ⓔ   26. Ⓐ Ⓑ Ⓒ Ⓓ Ⓔ   36. Ⓐ Ⓑ Ⓒ Ⓓ Ⓔ
7. Ⓐ Ⓑ Ⓒ Ⓓ Ⓔ   17. Ⓐ Ⓑ Ⓒ Ⓓ Ⓔ   27. Ⓐ Ⓑ Ⓒ Ⓓ Ⓔ   37. Ⓐ Ⓑ Ⓒ Ⓓ Ⓔ
8. Ⓐ Ⓑ Ⓒ Ⓓ Ⓔ   18. Ⓐ Ⓑ Ⓒ Ⓓ Ⓔ   28. Ⓐ Ⓑ Ⓒ Ⓓ Ⓔ   38. Ⓐ Ⓑ Ⓒ Ⓓ Ⓔ
9. Ⓐ Ⓑ Ⓒ Ⓓ Ⓔ   19. Ⓐ Ⓑ Ⓒ Ⓓ Ⓔ   29. Ⓐ Ⓑ Ⓒ Ⓓ Ⓔ   39. Ⓐ Ⓑ Ⓒ Ⓓ Ⓔ
10. Ⓐ Ⓑ Ⓒ Ⓓ Ⓔ   20. Ⓐ Ⓑ Ⓒ Ⓓ Ⓔ   30. Ⓐ Ⓑ Ⓒ Ⓓ Ⓔ   40. Ⓐ Ⓑ Ⓒ Ⓓ Ⓔ

Practice Test 1

SURVEY OF THE NATURAL SCIENCES TEST

TIME LIMIT: 90 MINUTES

> **Directions:** The following items are questions or incomplete statements. Read each item carefully, and then choose the best answer. Blacken the corresponding space on the answer sheet.

1. Each one of the following is an element in the periodic table. All EXCEPT one are members of the nonmetal group essential for the growth of cells. Which one is the EXCEPTION?

   (A) H
   (B) O
   (C) C
   (D) As
   (E) N

2. Allostearic enzymes

   (A) function by phosphorylating the substrate.
   (B) have binding sites for coenzymes.
   (C) are required for regulation of metabolic pathways.
   (D) are key components of the electron transport chain.
   (E) convert glycogen to glucose.

3. The biological membrane that surrounds all cells is

   (A) a hydrophilic protein bilayer.
   (B) a hydrophobic lipid barrier.
   (C) devoid of proteins.
   (D) used for photosynthesis by plant cells.
   (E) a complex of proteins covalently cross-linked to phospholipids.

4. Which one of the following statements best describes the effect of osmosis on cells?

   (A) Cells plasmolyze when the concentration of solutes is highest inside the cell.
   (B) Water rapidly enters when the concentration of solutes is highest outside the cell.
   (C) Water rapidly exits when the concentration of solutes is highest inside the cell.
   (D) Osmotic pressure is greater from the outside when cells are in an isotonic solution.
   (E) Solute concentration equilibrates inside and outside through a semipermeable membrane.

5. Prokaryotic cells contain each of the following structures or organelles EXCEPT one. Which one is the EXCEPTION?

   (A) Nuclear membrane
   (B) Chromosome
   (C) Ribosomes
   (D) Cytoplasmic membrane
   (E) Cell Wall

6. A virus that infects a prokaryotic cell is known as a

(A) plasmid.
(B) transposon.
(C) chloroplast.
(D) lysosome.
(E) bacteriophage.

7. Each of the following organelles contains membranes EXCEPT one. Which one is the EXCEPTION?

(A) Chloroplast
(B) Mitochondrion
(C) Ribosome
(D) Golgi Complex
(E) Endoplasmic Reticulum

8. The organelle responsible for ATP synthesis in a eukaryotic cell is the

(A) cell membrane.
(B) endoplasmic reticulum.
(C) peroxisome.
(D) mitochondrion.
(E) Golgi complex.

9. The conversion of one mole of glucose to pyruvic acid during glycolysis typically yields

(A) four moles of NADH.
(B) four moles of NAD.
(C) two moles of ATP.
(D) four moles of ATP.
(E) four moles of ADP.

10. In a typical fermentation reaction

(A) ATP is made in the Krebs cycle.
(B) ATP is made in the Calvin cycle.
(C) oxygen is an electron acceptor.
(D) pyruvic acid is the final end product.
(E) a six-carbon sugar is converted to smaller carbon end products.

11. Which statement concerning aerobic respiration is true?

(A) Alcohol is produced from pyruvic acid.
(B) ATP yield per mole of glucose in respiration is greater than that in fermentation.
(C) Kreb cycle intermediates are used by the cell to make nucleic acids.
(D) A cytochrome usually serves as a terminal electron acceptor.
(E) Glucose is made from carbon dioxide.

12. The chemiosmotic theory explains how

(A) ATP synthesis is coupled to the electron transport chain.
(B) nutrients enter the cell by active transport.
(C) nucleic acids are made.
(D) the archaea differ from prokaryotic cells.
(E) plants obtain energy from carbon dioxide.

13. Which statement concerning photosynthesis is true?

(A) In the light reaction, chlorophylls capture energy from light.
(B) The light and dark reactions take place in mitochondria.
(C) Only heterotrophs can make glucose from carbon dioxide.
(D) ATP is made by substrate level phosphorylation reactions.
(E) Only the dark reaction takes place in chloroplasts.

14. Each of the following phases is part of the cell cycle EXCEPT one. Which one is the EXCEPTION?

(A) G_1 (gap 1)
(B) G_2 (gap 2)
(C) M (mitosis)
(D) S (DNA synthesis)
(E) D (division)

15. Each of the following is a phase in mitosis EXCEPT one. Which one is the EXCEPTION?

    (A) Nucleophase
    (B) Prophase
    (C) Metaphase
    (D) Anaphase
    (E) Telophase

16. The endosymbiotic theory explains the

    (A) evolution of eukaryotes from prokaryotes.
    (B) evolution of mitochondria.
    (C) discovery of the archaea.
    (D) ability of fungi and algae to form lichens.
    (E) development of an oxygen atmosphere on early earth.

17. Members of which one of the following kingdoms reproduce by alteration of generations?

    (A) Bacteria (Monera)
    (B) Protozoa (Protista)
    (C) Chromista
    (D) Fungi
    (E) Animalia

18. Primates belong to which one of the following phyla?

    (A) Arthropoda
    (B) Chordata
    (C) Mollusca
    (D) Nematoda
    (E) Porifera

19. Which one of the following mathematical formulas can be used to determine if evolution has occurred between generations in a population?

    (A) Principles of inheritance
    (B) Allele frequency
    (C) Alteration of generations
    (D) Hardy-Weinberg principle
    (E) Malthusian growth model

20. Which one of the following is a consequence of evolution?

    (A) Extinction
    (B) Genetic drift
    (C) Genetic recombination
    (D) Heredity
    (E) Natural selection

21. If a genetic cross is set up in a Punnett square so that a male heterozygous for brown eyes (Bb) is mated with a female having blue eyes (bb), what would be the predicted outcome of the offspring?

    (A) 25% brown eyes and 75% blue eyes
    (B) 75% brown eyes and 25% blue eyes
    (C) 50% brown eyes and 50% blue eyes
    (D) 100% brown eyes
    (E) 100% blue eyes

22. Since there is a difference between the sex chromosomes in human males (XY) and females (XX), there are consequences related to X-linked and Y-linked inheritance. Which one of the following statements about sex-linked inheritance is true?

    (A) Recessive X-linked traits typically affect the phenotype of male offspring.
    (B) X-linked traits can be inherited by male offspring from the father.
    (C) Males can be carriers for recessive X-linked traits
    (D) Y-linked traits can be inherited from the mother.
    (E) There are no known Y-linked traits.

23. During embryogenesis in animals, development of the zygote into a gastrula requires

    (A) invagination.
    (B) formation of a notochord.
    (C) formation of mesoderm.
    (D) organogenesis.
    (E) formation of a blastula.

24. Each of the following is a function of the human integumentary system EXCEPT one. Which one is the EXCEPTION?

    (A) It acts as a protective barrier against invading microorganisms.
    (B) It removes excess lymph from the body.
    (C) It aids in the elimination of waste products.
    (D) It protects other organs.
    (E) It acts as a sensory interface with the environment.

25. Skeletal muscle contraction and relaxation is dependent on the interaction between two proteins in the myofibrils of muscle cells. These two proteins are

    (A) melatonin and myosin.
    (B) pepsin and actin.
    (C) myosin and actin.
    (D) myelin and actin.
    (E) hemoglobin and lysozyme.

26. Each of the following is a type of white blood cell present in the buffy coat of separated human blood EXCEPT one. Which one is the EXCEPTION?

    (A) Erythrocyte
    (B) Lymphocyte
    (C) Neutrophil
    (D) Eosinophil
    (E) Basophil

27. Oxygen is transported to the tissues and cells of the body by the most abundant type of cell in blood. The oxygen binding site of this cell is a cofactor containing which one of the following ions?

    (A) Mn^{2+}
    (B) Mg^{2+}
    (C) Ca^{2+}
    (D) Fe^{2+}
    (E) K^+

28. The primary action of bile in the duodenum is to

    (A) increase the pH to denature proteins in the chime.
    (B) act as a surfactant to emulsify fats in the chime.
    (C) deliver bilirubin that breaks down mucus in the small intestine.
    (D) deliver amylase to break down complex carbohydrates in the chime.
    (E) maintain the balance of salts in the small intestine.

29. Features common to the structures of all the immunoglobulin isotypes are

    (A) two light chains and multiple heavy chains.
    (B) a single Fc region that binds to complement.
    (C) two antigen binding sites.
    (D) synthesis by T cells.
    (E) recognition of a single specific antigen.

30. The autonomic nervous system is divided into the sympathetic and parasympathetic systems. The function of the parasympathetic nervous system is to control

    (A) resting activities of the body, such as salivation, digestion, and urination.
    (B) voluntary actions performed by skeletal muscles.
    (C) signals originating only from the spinal cord.
    (D) physiological reactions in response to stress stimuli.
    (E) signals originating only from the brain.

31. Axons transmit electrochemical signals in the form of a wave known as an action potential. Action potentials are

    (A) created when the membrane potential increases from a resting potential of –70 mV to a maximum potential of –55 mV.
    (B) dependent on the movement of sodium and potassium ions across the axon membrane.
    (C) passed only to motor neurons by neural transmitters.
    (D) stronger in glial cells than in neurons.
    (E) are not required for the transmission of electrochemical signals in the parasympathetic nervous system.

32. Which one of the following hormones is made in the pituitary gland?

    (A) Insulin
    (B) Estrogen
    (C) Melatonin
    (D) Calcitonin
    (E) Luteinizing hormone

33. During oogenesis, polar bodies are formed when the secondary oocyte develops from the primary oocyte in meiosis I and when the secondary oocyte develops into the ovum during meiosis II. The main purpose of the polar bodies is to

    (A) eliminate the extra haploid set of chromosomes formed during meiosis.
    (B) bind excess sperm to ensure that the ovum is fertilized by a single sperm.
    (C) produce follicle-stimulating hormone (FSH).
    (D) induce a new menstruation cycle.
    (E) help release the zygote from the ovary.

34. Certain types of microorganisms are essential for the maintenance of the nitrogen cycle because

    (A) plants cannot obtain nitrogen compounds from the soil.
    (B) animals release large amounts of gaseous nitrogen (N_2) as waste.
    (C) bacteria cannot convert ammonia (NH_4^+) and nitrate (NO_3^+) to gaseous nitrogen (N_2).
    (D) plants cannot use the gaseous form of nitrogen (N_2).
    (E) herbivores fix large amounts of gaseous nitrogen (N_2) denitrification.

35. The primary energy producers in a food cycle in an ecosystem are

    (A) omnivores.
    (B) autotrophs.
    (C) detritivores.
    (D) heterotrophs.
    (E) predators.

36. An important function of the Loop of Henle in the nephron of the kidney is to

    (A) filter the blood that enters and leaves the Bowman's capsule.
    (B) remove the red blood cells that enter the glomerulus.
    (C) return dissolved oxygen to the renal corpuscle.
    (D) increase the calcium concentration in the urine.
    (E) create a salt gradient in the medulla to concentrate the urine.

37. During what stage of the ovarian cycle do levels of luteinizing hormone and estradiol increase dramatically?

(A) Just prior to follicle release (day 0)
(B) During follicle release (days 0–14)
(C) Just prior to ovulation (days 14–16)
(D) During formation of the corpus luteum (days 20–24)
(E) Luteinizing hormone and estradiol levels do not significantly increase during the menstruation cycle.

38. The result of spermatogenesis is the production of spermatids that are haploid. This outcome is important because

(A) primary spermatocytes are formed from spermatogonia during meiosis.
(B) a diploid zygote must be produced when a sperm cell fertilizes an ovum.
(C) primary spermatocytes are haploid.
(D) all alleles on the Y chromosome must be represented in the sperm.
(E) every sperm cell produced during spermatogenesis must be identical.

39. When the interaction between two species in a community of organisms is beneficial to both species, it is known as

(A) competitive.
(B) predatory.
(C) parasitism.
(D) commensalism.
(E) mutualism.

40. Which one of the following statements is false about kin selection?

(A) The individual exhibiting the behavior experiences a fitness loss.
(B) The individual receiving the effects of the behavior experiences a fitness gain.
(C) It is an instinctive behavior based on a "releasing" stimulus.
(D) The behavior enhances the reproductive success of the receiving individual.
(E) Among insects, such as ants and bees, the behavior is known as group selection.

41. How many moles of oxygen (O) are in 2 moles of $Ca(NO_3)_2$?

(A) 1
(B) 2
(C) 3
(D) 6
(E) 12

42. Hexafluorosilicic acid, $(H_3O)_2SiF_6$, is commonly used to fluorinate water. At neutral pH, hexafluorosilicic acid hydrolyzes by the following unbalanced equation:

$$\_NaOH + \_H_2SO_4 \rightarrow \_Na_2SO_4 + \_H_2O$$

What is the correct order for the coefficients?

(A) 4, 2, 2, 4
(B) 1, 2, 2, 1
(C) 2, 1, 1, 2
(D) 1, ½, ½, 1
(E) It is already balanced.

43. What is the percent composition of oxygen in sulfuric acid (H_2SO_4)?

(A) 2.055%
(B) 65.24%
(C) 32.69%
(D) 16.31%
(E) 34.76%

44. Which of the following statements about the kinetic molecular theory of gases is false?

(A) Gas molecules do not interact with each other.
(B) The average kinetic energy of a gas molecule depends only on the temperature.
(C) The space that a gas occupies is negligible.
(D) Gas molecules are not elastic.
(E) The pressure of gas is due to the molecules colliding with the container.

45. A flexible container holds 18.9 L of propane, C_3H_8, at 760 mm Hg and 25°C. What is the volume of the propane at 42°C?

   (A) 31.8 L
   (B) 17.9 L
   (C) 0.0263 L
   (D) 20.0 L
   (E) 22.4 L

46. Which statement about the ideal gas law is true?

   (A) The ideal gas law combines Boyle's law and Charles's law, but not Avogadro's law.
   (B) At standard temperature and pressure, the volume of 1 mole of a liquid is 22.4 L.
   (C) The standard temperature is 298K.
   (D) The ideal gas law assumes that gases behave ideally and that the molecules have no interactions.
   (E) Both (C) and (D) are correct.

47. How many atoms are inside the unit cell shown?

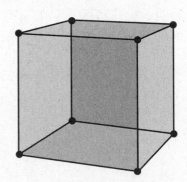

   (A) 1
   (B) 2
   (C) 3
   (D) 4
   (E) 5

48. Which statement about vapor pressure is true?

   (A) The higher the boiling point, the higher the vapor pressure.
   (B) The vapor pressure equals the external pressure at the boiling point.
   (C) The higher the temperature, the lower the vapor pressure.
   (D) The lower the temperature, the higher the vapor pressure.
   (E) The stronger the intermolecular forces, the higher the vapor pressure.

49. Which intermolecular force is the principle force in solvating ions in aqueous solutions?

   (A) Dipole-dipole
   (B) Induced-dipole
   (C) Hydrogen bonding
   (D) Ion-dipole
   (E) Covalent

50. What is the molality of a solution prepared by dissolving 40.0 grams of sodium hydroxide (40.0 g/mol) into 500 mL of ethanol (D = 0.789 g/mL)?

   (A) 0.08 m
   (B) 0.002 m
   (C) 2.00 m
   (D) 2.30 m
   (E) 2.53 m

51. 50.00 mL of perchloric acid ($HClO_4$) are titrated to the phenolphthalein end point using 43.91 mL of 0.08775 M potassium hydroxide (KOH) solution. What is the concentration of the original perchloric acid solution?

   (A) 0.09992 M
   (B) 0.07706 M
   (C) 0.01926 M
   (D) 0.02502 M
   (E) 0.05172 M

52. What is the correct setup for the K_{eq} of $3A \rightleftharpoons 2B + C$ based on the K_{eq} of the following reactions?

$$A \rightleftharpoons 2d \qquad K_1 = 1.2$$
$$4B + 2C \rightleftharpoons 4d \qquad K_2 = 4.4$$

(A) $(1.2)^3 \cdot \left(\dfrac{1}{4.4}\right)^{\frac{1}{2}}$

(B) $(1.2)^3 \cdot (4.4)^{\frac{1}{2}}$

(C) $(1.2)^3 \cdot (4.4)^2$

(D) $(1.2)^3 + (4.4)^2$

(E) $(1.2 \cdot 3) + \left(\dfrac{4.4}{2}\right)$

53. What is the pK_a of the following reaction at 25°C?

$$NH_4^+(aq) + H_2O(l) \rightleftharpoons NH_3(aq) + H_3O^+(aq)$$

$$K_a = 5.8 \times 10^{-10}$$

(A) $pK_a = 5.8$
(B) $pK_a = 0.58$
(C) $pK_a = 7.0$
(D) $pK_a = 9.2$
(E) $pK_a = -5.8$

54. Adding EDTA to the below reaction will result in which if the following?

$$Fe^{3+}(aq) + 2H_2O(l) \rightleftharpoons Fe(OH)^{2+}(aq) + H_3O^+(aq)$$

(A) A decrease in $[Fe^{3+}]$, resulting in a shift toward reactants
(B) A decrease in $[Fe^{3+}]$, resulting in a shift toward products
(C) An increase in $[Fe^{3+}]$, resulting in a shift toward reactants
(D) An increase in $[Fe^{3+}]$, resulting in a shift toward products
(E) Adding EDTA doesn't affect the equilibrium

55. Determine the enthalpy of

$$2Fe(s) + 3Cl_2(g) \rightarrow 2FeCl_3(g)$$

based on the enthalpies given:

$$FeCl_2(s) \rightarrow Fe(s) + Cl_2(g) \qquad \Delta H_1 = 25.6 \text{ kJ}$$
$$2FeCl_2(s) + Cl_2(g) \rightarrow 2FeCl_3(s) \quad \Delta H_2 = -35.8 \text{ kJ}$$

(A) +80.7 kJ
(B) −10.2 kJ
(C) −61.4 kJ
(D) −48.6 kJ
(E) −87.0 kJ

56. Which of the following is an example of a decrease in entropy?

(A) Melting
(B) Condensation
(C) Mixing two solutions together
(D) Sublimation
(E) $2H_2O(g) \rightarrow 2H_2(g) + O_2(g)$

57. What is the activation energy for the *reverse* reaction?

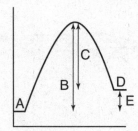

(A) A
(B) B
(C) C
(D) D
(E) E

58. How many half-lives has C-14 undergone if the initial mass is 24 g and the final mass is 0.75 g?

(A) 2
(B) 3
(C) 4
(D) 5
(E) 6

59. Which statement is NOT correct for the following reaction?

$$MnO_2(s) + 4H^+(aq) + 2Cl^-(aq) \rightarrow$$
$$Mn^{2+}(aq) + 2H_2O(l) + Cl_2(g)$$

(A) MnO_2 is the reducing agent.
(B) The presence of H^+ means this occurred under acidic conditions.
(C) Cl^- was oxidized.
(D) Mn^{2+} has an oxidation state of 2+.
(E) All of the above are correct.

60. What is E°_{cell} for the following reaction?

$$3Ag^+ + Fe(s) \rightarrow 3Ag(s) + Fe^{3+}(aq) \quad E^\circ_{cell}$$

Half reactions with cell potentials:

$$Ag^+(aq) + e^- \rightarrow Ag(s) \qquad E^\circ = +0.80$$
$$Fe^{3+}(aq) + 3e^- \rightarrow Fe(s) \qquad E^\circ = -0.04$$

(A) −2.44
(B) +0.76
(C) +0.84
(D) +2.44
(E) −1.36

61. How many neutrons does carbon-13 have?

(A) 13
(B) 12
(C) 7
(D) 5
(E) 1

62. Which statement is true about the Pauli-exclusion principle?

(A) Protons cannot occupy the same orbital with the same spin type.
(B) Neutrons cannot occupy the same orbital as an electron.
(C) Neutrons cannot occupy the same orbital as a proton.
(D) Electrons cannot occupy the same orbital with the same spin type.
(E) Electrons with the same spin can occupy the same orbital.

63. Which is the correct Lewis electron dot structure for $BFCl_2$ (lone pairs are excluded)?

(A)
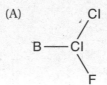

(B)
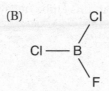

(C)
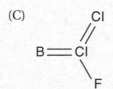

(D) B —— F —— Cl_2

(E) F —— B —— Cl_2

64. Based on the periodic table, electronegativity tends to increase

(A) down a column.
(B) across a row from left to right.
(C) toward the middle.
(D) up a group.
(E) Both (B) and (D)

65. Which statement is false about the Group I elements?

(A) They are called the alkali metals.
(B) They are the elements lithium, sodium, potassium, rubidium, cesium, and francium.
(C) They are all soft, silver metals.
(D) They have relatively low first ionization energies.
(E) They are not very reactive.

66. Which of the following is a covalent compound?

    (A) Magnesium sulfide
    (B) Manganese (IV) oxide
    (C) Carbonate
    (D) Carbon trioxide
    (E) Ammonium carbonate

67. What element is missing in this alpha decay:

$$^{210}_{84}Po \rightarrow {}^{4}_{Z}X + \alpha$$

    (A) $^{210}_{84}Po$

    (B) $^{4}_{2}He$

    (C) $^{214}_{86}RN$

    (D) $^{210}_{83}Bi$

    (E) $^{206}_{82}Pb$

68. Which of the following statements about errors is false?

    (A) Systematic errors tend to shift all measurements in a systematic way.
    (B) Small systematic errors will nearly always be present in an experiment.
    (C) Random errors fluctuate.
    (D) Random errors are avoidable.
    (E) Random errors distribute about a mean value.

69. Which of the following is not basic PPE?

    (A) Goggles/glasses
    (B) Gloves
    (C) Lab coats
    (D) Closed-toed shoes
    (E) Radiation suit

70. If your working concentration of a solution is 100 mM, what would be a reasonable stock solution concentration?

    (A) 5 M
    (B) 0.05 M
    (C) 500 M
    (D) 0.001 M
    (E) 0.025 M

71. What reagents would best accomplish the following substitution reaction?

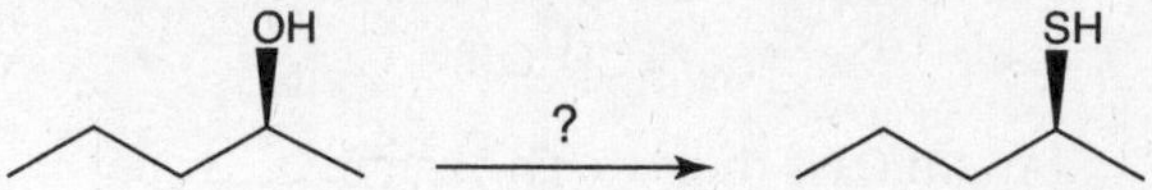

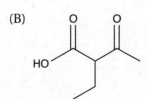

    (A) NaSH, DMSO
    (B) 1. TsCl, pyridine; 2. NaSH, DMSO
    (C) 1. TsCl, pyridine; 2. NaI, DMSO; 3. NaSH, DMSO
    (D) 1. NaI, DMSO; 2. NaSH, DMSO
    (E) 1. H_3O^+; 2. NaSH, DMSO

72. Consider the keto ester shown below.

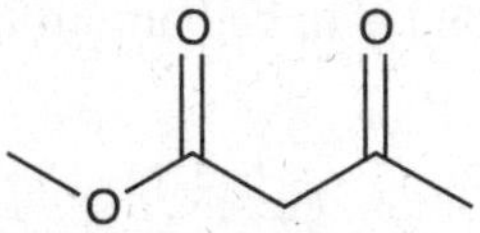

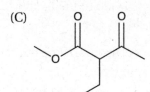

What is the major product if this compound is treated (in sequence) with the following reagents? 1. $CH_3O^- Na^+$, 2. CH_3CH_2I; followed by 1. H_3O^+, 2. heat

    (A)

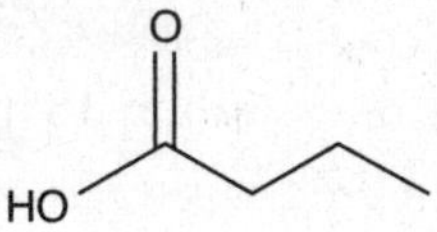

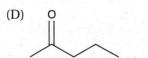

    (B)

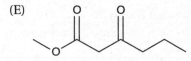

    (C)

    (D)

    (E)

73. Which of the following is the *strongest* Brönsted-Lowry acid?

(A)

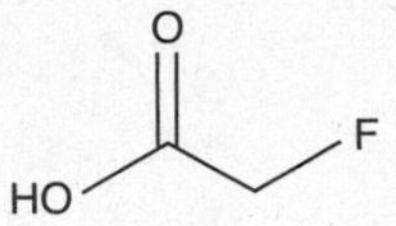

(B)

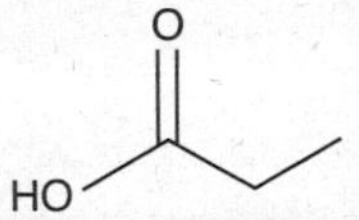

(C)

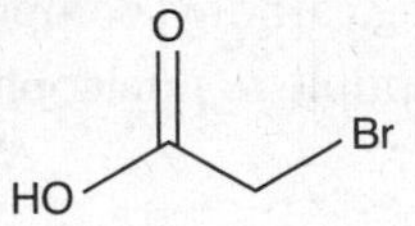

(D)

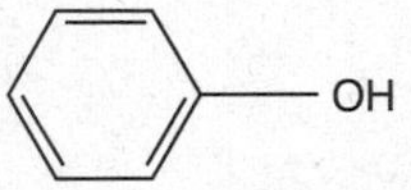

(E)

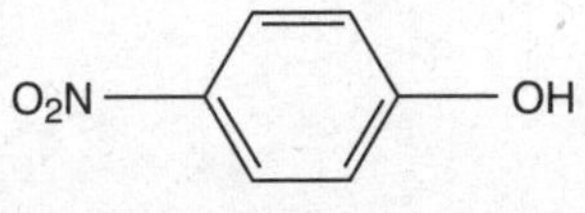

74. The dynamic equilibrium between the keto and enol forms of a compound is *best* termed

(A) reduction.
(B) isomerization.
(C) oxidation.
(D) tautomerization.
(E) racemization.

75. Which of the following statements is false?

(A) *Trans* alkene isomers tend to be more stable (lower in energy) than *cis* isomers.
(B) An *anti*-periplaner bond geometry between a hydrogen being abstracted by a base and an adjacent leaving group is necessary for an E2 reaction to proceed at a reasonable rate.
(C) *cis* alkene isomers are usually more polar than *trans* isomers.
(D) Alkenes are less reactive and less polarizable than their alkane counterparts.
(E) Alkenes of low molar mass are important precursors in the production of many commodity-based polymers (plastics).

76. The reaction below can be classified as which of the following?

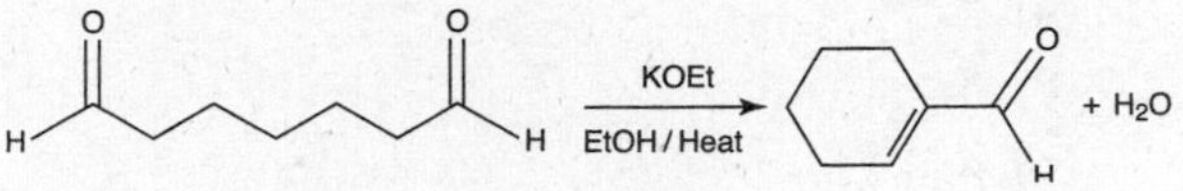

(A) A Robinson annulation
(B) An intermolecular Claisen condensation
(C) A mixed aldol condensation
(D) A Michael addition
(E) An intermolecular aldol condensation

77. The most likely product(s) of the following sequence of reactions is (are)?

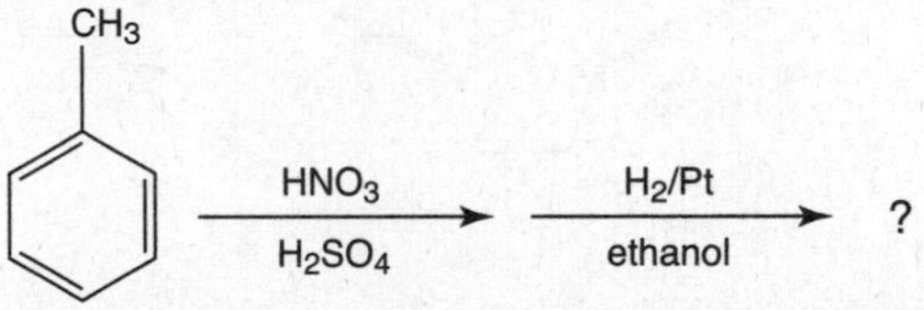

(A)

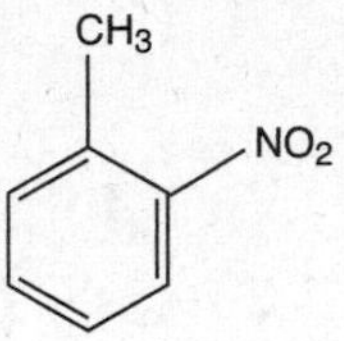

(B)

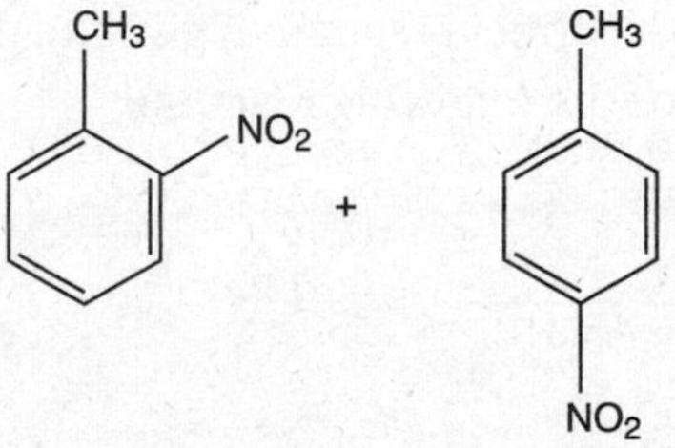

(C)

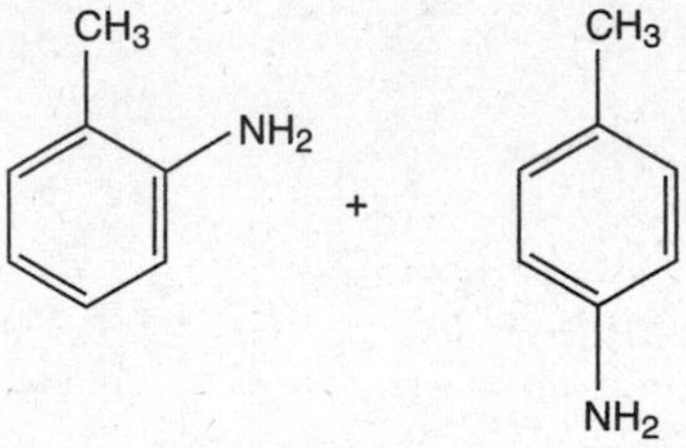

(D)

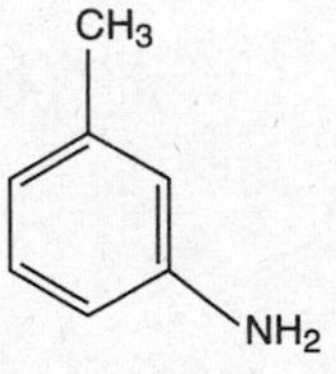

(E)

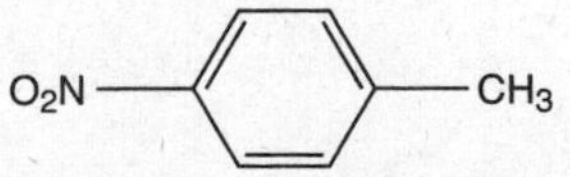

78. How many isomers are possible for the molecular formula C_4H_8?

(A) 2
(B) 3
(C) 4
(D) 5
(E) 6

79. Select the answer with the correct absolute stereochemical assignments for the chirality centers, proceeding clockwise around the ring from center 1 to center 3, shown in the following molecule.

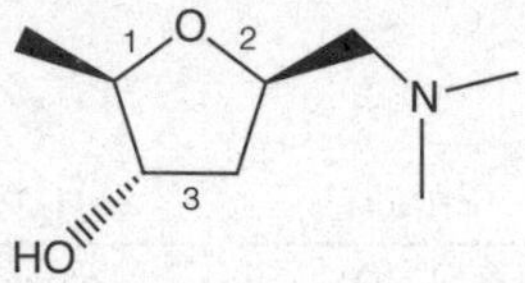

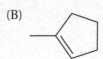

(A) *R, R, R*
(B) *S, S, S*
(C) *R, R, S*
(D) *S, S, R*
(E) *S, R, S*

80. Select the correct reactant to give the product shown for the following reaction.

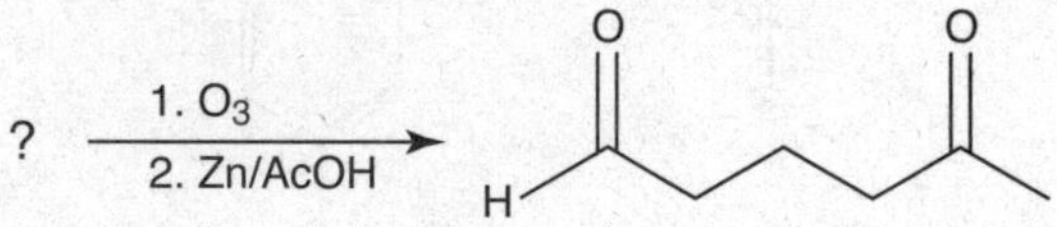

(A)

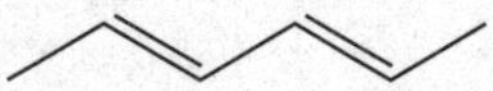

(B)

(C)

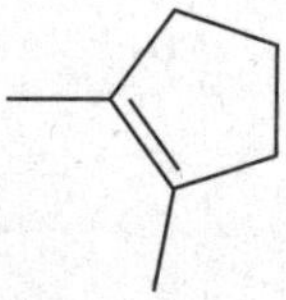

(D) 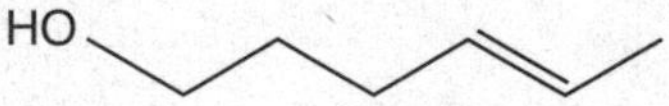 HO

(E)

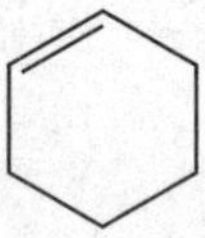

81. The conversion of cyclohexanone to cyclohexanol using H_2/Pt is best classified as what type of reaction?

(A) Substitution
(B) Reduction
(C) Rearrangement
(D) Oxidation
(E) Elimination

82. Which of the following carbonyl compounds would be most susceptible to nucleophilic attack?

(A)

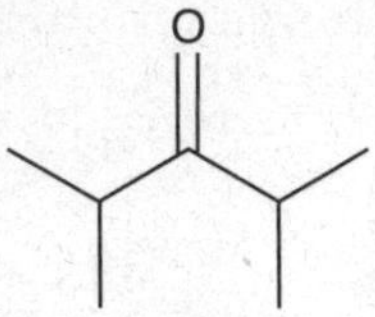

(B)

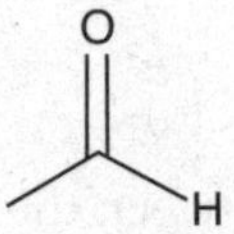

(C)

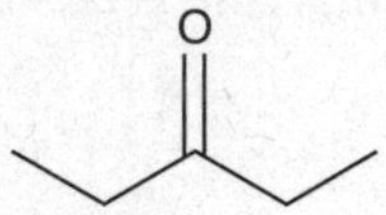

(D)

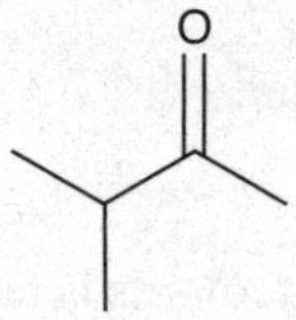

(E)

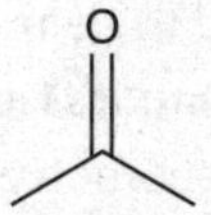

83. Which of the following nitrogen-containing compounds is the least basic?

(A) 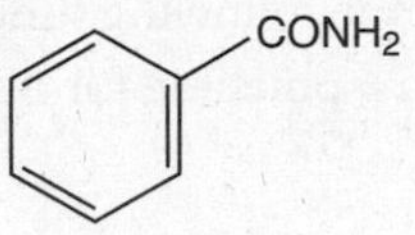 [benzamide structure with CONH₂ group]

(B) 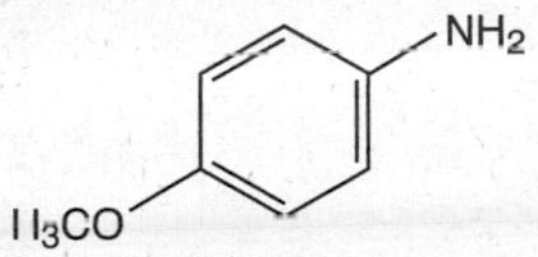 [aniline structure with NH₂ and H₃CO groups]

(C) 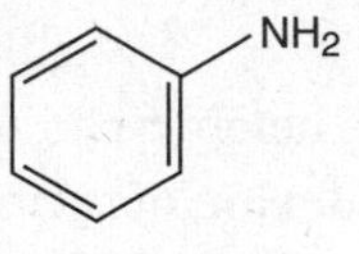 [aniline structure with NH₂ group]

(D) 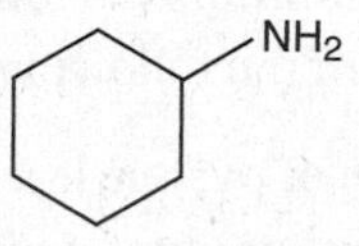 [cyclohexylamine structure with NH₂ group]

(E) 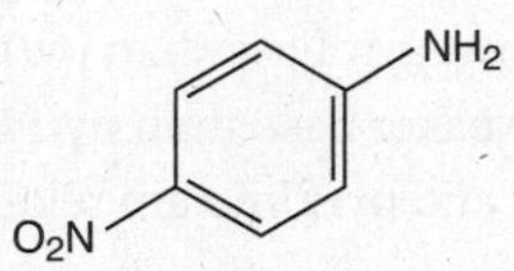 [aniline structure with NH₂ and O₂N groups]

84. Alcohols are slightly acidic and can usually be deprotonated with

(A) sodium hydroxide.
(B) sodium hydride.
(C) potassium ethoxide.
(D) potassium carbonate.
(E) None of the above

85. Comparing the two species shown below, the following can be concluded:

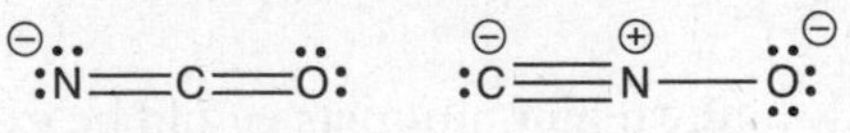

[Lewis structures: :N=C=Ö: and :C≡N—Ö:]

(A) They are resonance forms.
(B) They are structural isomers.
(C) They are neither resonance forms nor structural isomers.
(D) They are both resonance forms and structural isomers.
(E) They are stereoisomers.

86. For the structure shown below, what is the ^{1}H NMR splitting pattern for the hydrogens indicated with the arrow?

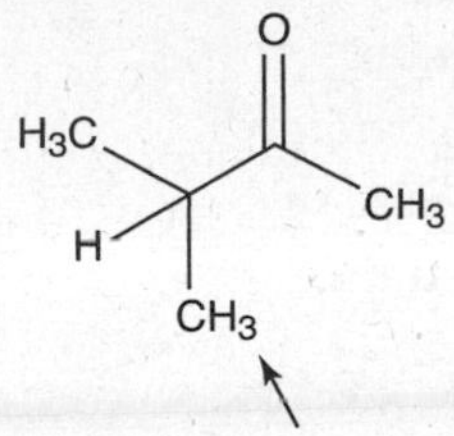

[structure showing 3-methyl-2-butanone type compound with H₃C, O, CH₃, H, CH₃ groups and arrow pointing to CH₃]

(A) Singlet
(B) Doublet
(C) Triplet
(D) Quartet
(E) Septet

87. Which reagent shown below would best complete the following reaction?

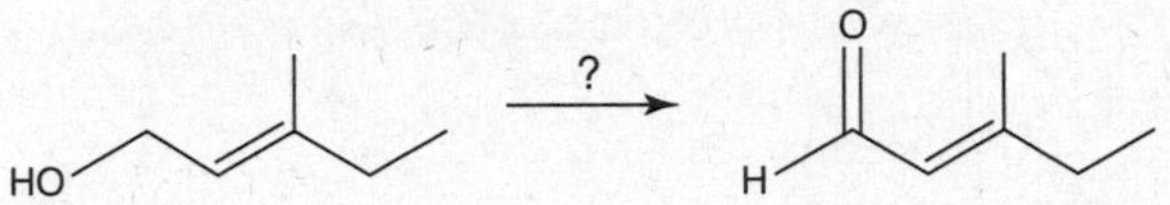

[reaction: HO-containing alkene → aldehyde with structure]

(A) PCC
(B) $KMnO_4$
(C) OsO_4
(D) 1. O_3; followed by 2. $(CH_3)_2S$
(E) $Na_2Cr_2O_7$, H_2SO_4

88. Select the correct name for the following compound structure.

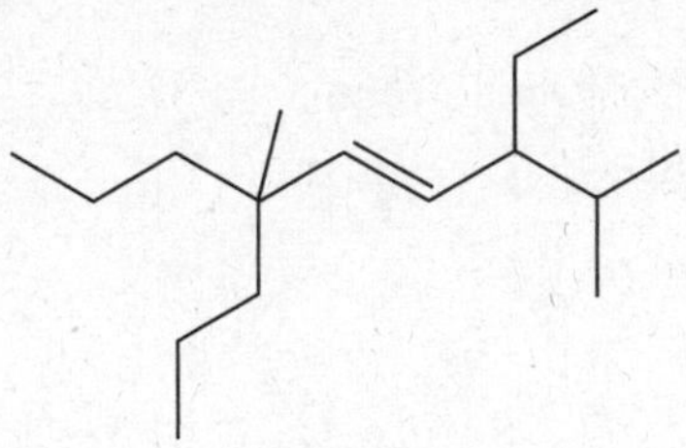

[branched alkene structure]

(A) (Z)-3-ethyl-2,6-dimethyl-6-propylnon-4-ene
(B) (E)-3-ethyl-2,6-dimethyl-6-propylnon-4-ene
(C) (Z)-7-ethyl-4,8-dimethyl-4-propylnon-5-ene
(D) (E)-7-ethyl-4,8-dimethyl-4-propylnon-5-ene
(E) cis-3-ethyl-2,6-dimethyl-6-propylnon-4-ene

89. The relatively high energy associated with the gauche conformation of butane is primarily due to

    (A) angle strain.
    (B) torsional strain.
    (C) steric strain.
    (D) orbital strain.
    (E) ring strain.

90. In what positions (axial/equatorial) would the substituents of the lowest energy conformation of the following compound be found?

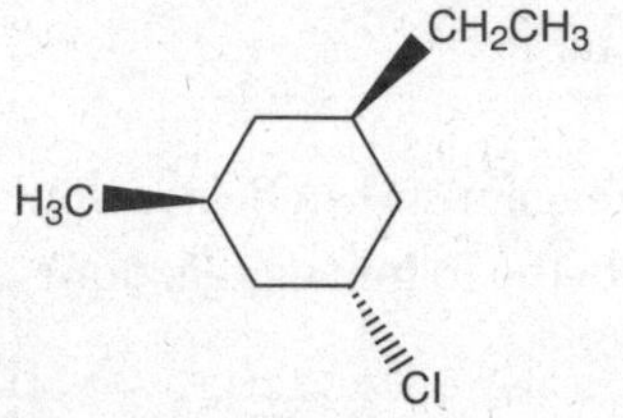

    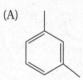

    (A) All axial
    (B) All equatorial
    (C) Methyl and chlorine axial, ethyl equatorial
    (D) Methyl and ethyl equatorial, chlorine axial
    (E) Methyl and ethyl axial, chlorine equatorial

91. Which of the following compounds is aromatic?

    (A)
    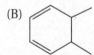

    (B)
    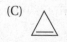

    (C)
    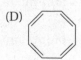

    (D)
    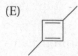

    (E)

92. IR spectroscopic analysis of an unknown sample gives a very strong absorption band at 1,730 cm^{-1}. Which of the following functional groups is most likely responsible for this absorption band?

    (A) Hydroxyl
    (B) Amine
    (C) Alkyne
    (D) Alkene
    (E) Aldehyde or ketone

93. Pyrrole and pyridine are heterocyclic amines. The pK_a of the ammonium ion of pyrrole is ~0.40. The pK_a of the ammonium ion of pyridine is ~5.3. Which of the following is true?

    (A) The ammonium ion of pyrrole is a weaker acid than the ammonium ion of pyridine.
    (B) Pyrrole is a stronger base than pyridine.
    (C) Pyrrole is a weaker base than pyridine.
    (D) Both pyrrole and pyridine are relatively strong acids.
    (E) The ammonium ions of pyrrole and pyridine are weak bases.

94. Which of the following compounds cannot be oxidized by a mixture of sodium dichromate and sulfuric acid?

    (A) 2-methyl-2-propanol
    (B) 2-methyl-1-propanol
    (C) 2-butanol
    (D) 1-propanol
    (E) 2-propanol

95. How many major products would be expected from the reaction of 1,5-heptadiyne with excess HBr?

    (A) 1
    (B) 2
    (C) 3
    (D) 4
    (E) 5

96. Which of the protons (1, 2, 3, and 4) specified on the following compound is the most acidic?

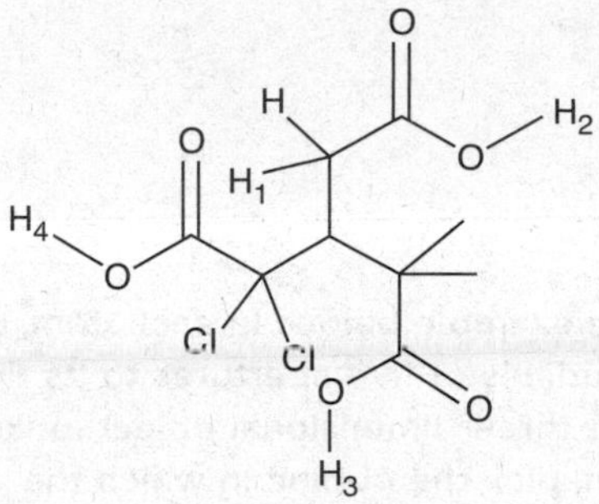

(A) H-1
(B) H-2
(C) H-3
(D) H-4
(E) They are all approximately the same.

97. A Grignard reagent is prepared by mixing which of the following reagents in a dry argon atmosphere?

(A) Pentane and $MgBr_2$ in diethyl ether
(B) Pentane and $MgBr_2$ in ethanol
(C) 1-bromopentane and $Mg_{(s)}$ in ethanol
(D) 1-bromopentane and $Mg_{(s)}$ in diethyl ether
(E) Pentane, $Mg_{(s)}$, and $Br_{2(l)}$ in diethyl ether

98. An alkyl carbocation may be formed when an alcohol is heated with a strong acid (i.e., sulfuric acid). The first step of this process is

(A) the loss of a proton by the alcohol.
(B) the elimination of water from the alcohol.
(C) the loss of the hydroxyl group from the alcohol.
(D) the protonation of the hydroxyl group of the alcohol.
(E) a nucleophilic attack of the alcohol by the acid.

99. Esters can be synthesized by combining an alcohol with an anhydride under the appropriate conditions. Which of the following compounds (again, under the appropriate conditions) could *best* replace an anhydride for the synthesis of an ester?

(A) A ketone
(B) An amide
(C) A carboxylic acid
(D) An aldehyde
(E) An acid chloride

100. The most likely product of the following reaction sequence is?

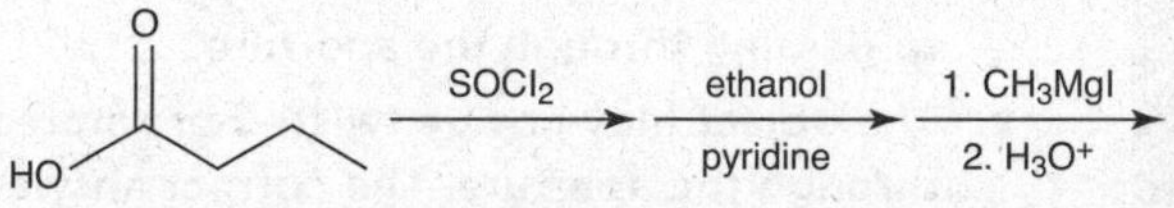

(A)

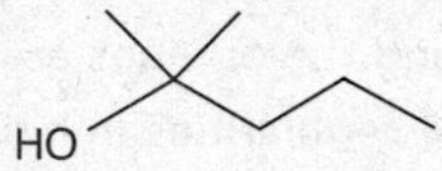

(B)

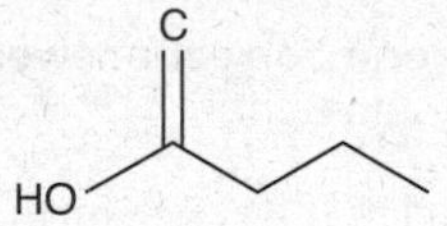

(C)

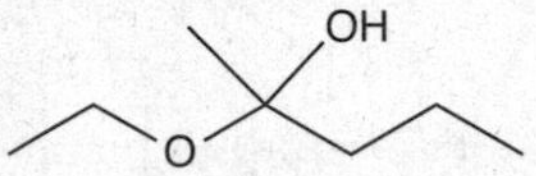

(D)

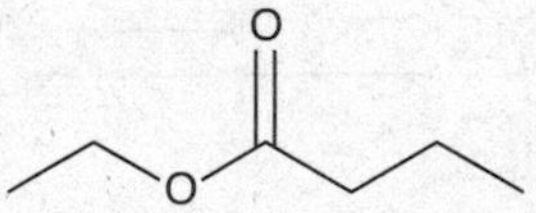

(E)

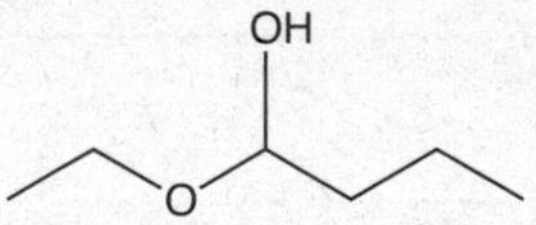

PRACTICE TEST 1

TIME LIMIT: 60 MINUTES

Part 1: Aperture Passing

Directions: For questions 1 through 15:

This section of the exam consists of 15 items similar to the example below. In each item, a three-dimensional object is shown on the left, followed by outlines of five apertures to its right.

The task is the same for each item. Conceptualize how the three-dimensional object looks from each possible side (in addition to the side shown). Then, pick the outline in which the three-dimensional object could pass if the proper side were inserted. Choose the letter corresponding to the correct aperture.

Here are rules for Part 1, the aperture section:

1. The irregular solid three-dimensional object on the left can be rotated in any direction prior to passing through the aperture.

2. The object may not be twisted or rotated in any way once it has started to be passed through the aperture. The correct answer is the exact representation of the external outline of the object viewed from the appropriate side.

3. The objects and the outlines are drawn to the same scale.

4. There are no irregularities in hidden portions of the objects. If the figure has symmetric indentations, it is assumed that the hidden portion is symmetric with the portion shown.

5. There is only one correct answer.

EXAMPLE

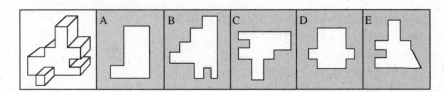

The correct answer is C.

1.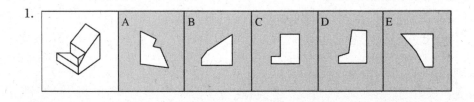

2.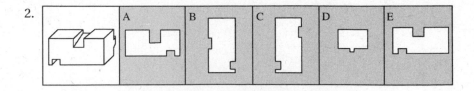

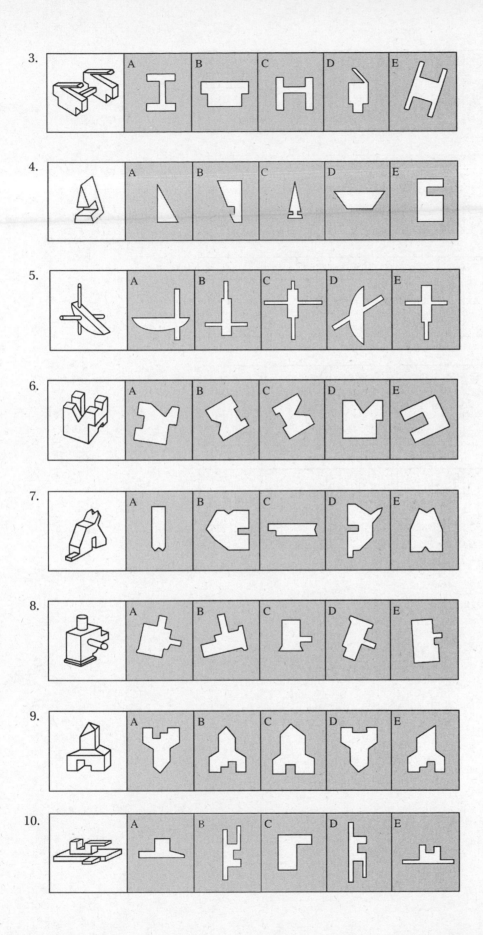

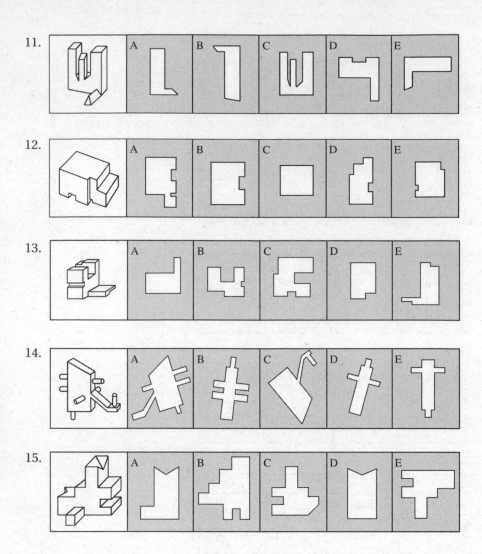

Part 2: Orthographic Projections

Directions: For questions 16 through 30:

The pictures that follow are representations of solid objects from three different views: top, front, and end views. The pictures are views drawn without perspective: the surface viewed is along parallel lines of vision. The projection that is labeled TOP VIEW is shown looking DOWN on its top surface and is pictured in the upper-left corner. The projection labeled FRONT VIEW is shown looking at the object from the FRONT and is pictured in the lower-left corner. The projection labeled END VIEW is shown looking at the object from the END (or side) and is pictured in the lower-right corner. These three views are always in their respective corners and labeled accordingly.

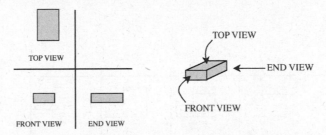

If there were a hole in the figure, it would be represented like this:

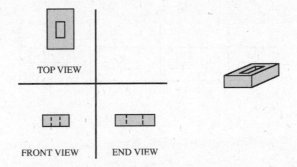

DOTTED lines indicate lines that exist but cannot be seen in the perspective shown.

In the following problems, TWO of the previous three views discussed will be shown with four alternatives to the right. Choose the correct letter that represents the correct view that completes the set.

EXAMPLE

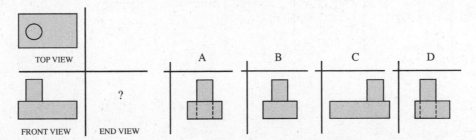

The FRONT VIEW shows that there is a smaller block on top of a larger block and there is no hole. The TOP VIEW shows that the top block is round and is centered on a rectangular block. From this information gathered in the two views given, the correct answer must be B.

In the following problems, one of the three views will be omitted; it is not always the END VIEW as shown in the example.

16. Choose the correct FRONT VIEW.

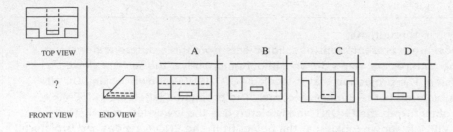

TOP VIEW

?　FRONT VIEW　END VIEW　A　B　C　D

17. Choose the correct FRONT VIEW.

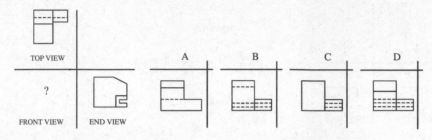

TOP VIEW

?　FRONT VIEW　END VIEW　A　B　C　D

18. Choose the correct TOP VIEW.

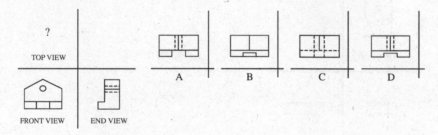

?　TOP VIEW

FRONT VIEW　END VIEW　A　B　C　D

19. Choose the correct END VIEW.

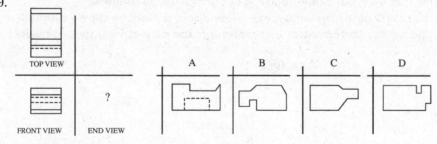

TOP VIEW

FRONT VIEW　?　END VIEW　A　B　C　D

20. Choose the correct FRONT VIEW.

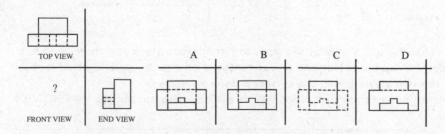

TOP VIEW

?　FRONT VIEW　END VIEW　A　B　C　D

21. Choose the correct END VIEW.

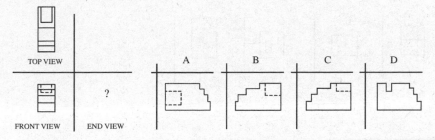

22. Choose the correct TOP VIEW.

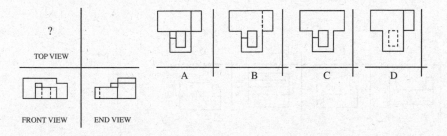

23. Choose the correct END VIEW.

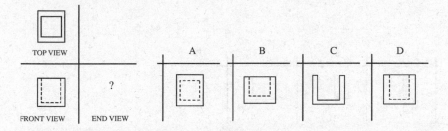

24. Choose the correct FRONT VIEW.

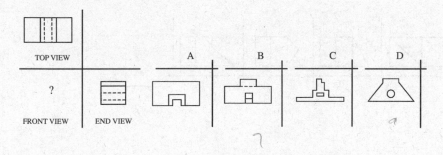

25. Choose the correct FRONT VIEW.

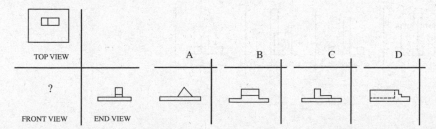

26. Choose the correct TOP VIEW.

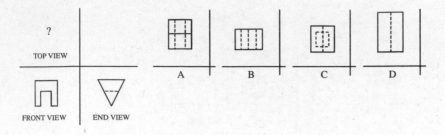

27. Choose the correct END VIEW.

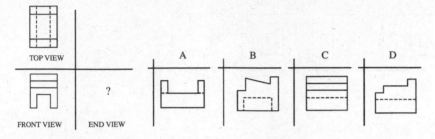

28. Choose the correct END VIEW.

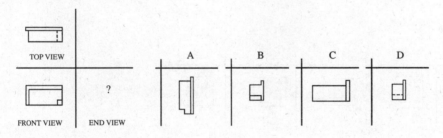

29. Choose the correct TOP VIEW.

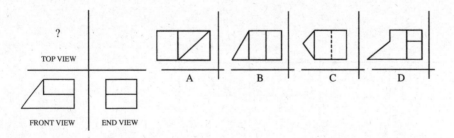

30. Choose the correct TOP VIEW.

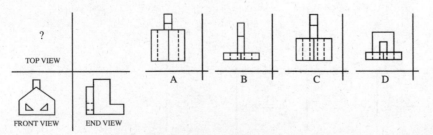

Part 3: Angle Discrimination

Directions: For questions 31 through 45:

Examine the INTERNAL ANGLES and rank them in terms of degrees from SMALL to LARGE. Select the alternative that represents the correct ranking.

EXAMPLE

1   2   3   4

A. 1 - 2 - 4 - 3
B. 2 - 1 - 4 - 3
C. 3 - 4 - 2 - 1
D. 3 - 4 - 1 - 2

The correct ranking is 2 – 1 – 4 – 3. Therefore, the correct answer is B.

31.

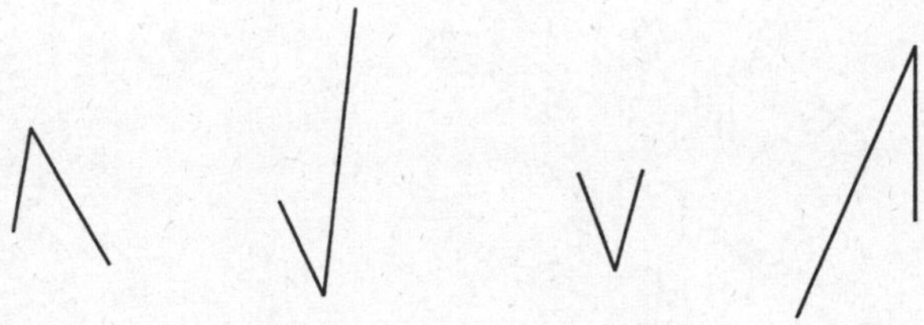

1   2   3   4

A. 2 – 4 – 3 – 1
B. 4 – 2 – 3 – 1
C. 4 – 2 – 1 – 3
D. 2 – 3 – 4 – 1

32.

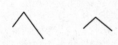

1   2   3   4

A. 3 – 4 – 1 – 2
B. 1 – 3 – 2 – 4
C. 3 – 1 – 4 – 2
D. 1 – 3 – 4 – 2

33.

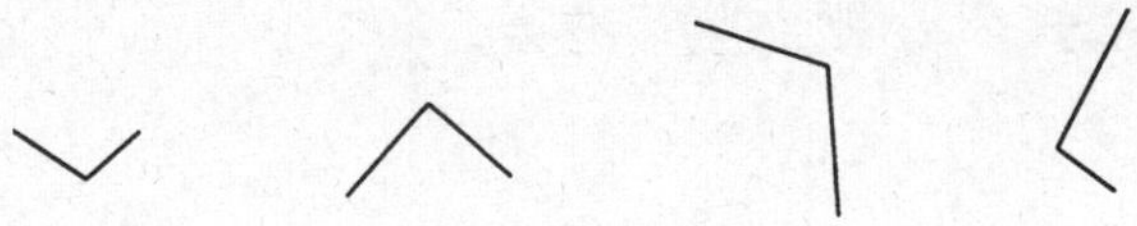

1   2   3   4

A. 1 – 2 – 4 – 3
B. 2 – 4 – 1 – 3
C. 4 – 1 – 2 – 3
D. 1 – 4 – 2 – 3

34.

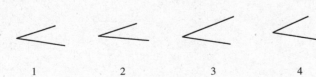

1   2   3   4

A. 2 – 1 – 3 – 4
B. 2 – 1 – 4 – 3
C. 2 – 4 – 1 – 3
D. 2 – 4 – 3 – 1

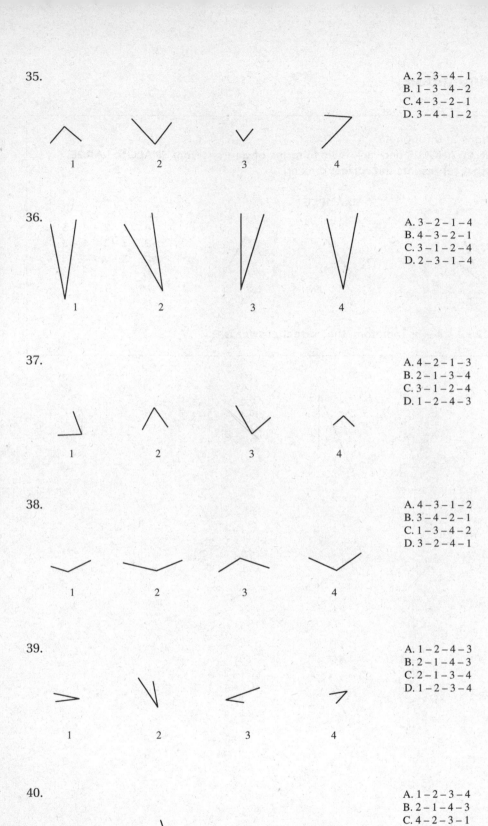

35.
A. 2 – 3 – 4 – 1
B. 1 – 3 – 4 – 2
C. 4 – 3 – 2 – 1
D. 3 – 4 – 1 – 2

1   2   3   4

36.
A. 3 – 2 – 1 – 4
B. 4 – 3 – 2 – 1
C. 3 – 1 – 2 – 4
D. 2 – 3 – 1 – 4

1   2   3   4

37.
A. 4 – 2 – 1 – 3
B. 2 – 1 – 3 – 4
C. 3 – 1 – 2 – 4
D. 1 – 2 – 4 – 3

1   2   3   4

38.
A. 4 – 3 – 1 – 2
B. 3 – 4 – 2 – 1
C. 1 – 3 – 4 – 2
D. 3 – 2 – 4 – 1

1   2   3   4

39.
A. 1 – 2 – 4 – 3
B. 2 – 1 – 4 – 3
C. 2 – 1 – 3 – 4
D. 1 – 2 – 3 – 4

1   2   3   4

40.
A. 1 – 2 – 3 – 4
B. 2 – 1 – 4 – 3
C. 4 – 2 – 3 – 1
D. 2 – 4 – 1 – 3

1   2   3   4

41.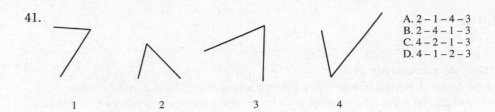

A. 2 – 1 – 4 – 3
B. 2 – 4 – 1 – 3
C. 4 – 2 – 1 – 3
D. 4 – 1 – 2 – 3

42.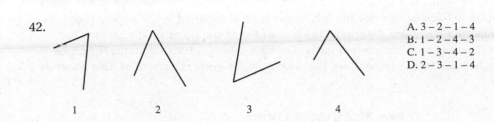

A. 3 – 2 – 1 – 4
B. 1 – 2 – 4 – 3
C. 1 – 3 – 4 – 2
D. 2 – 3 – 1 – 4

43.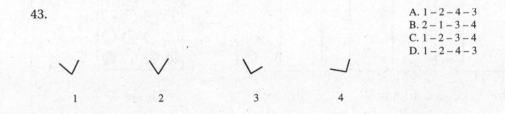

A. 1 – 2 – 4 – 3
B. 2 – 1 – 3 – 4
C. 1 – 2 – 3 – 4
D. 1 – 2 – 4 – 3

44.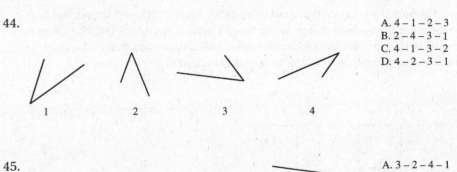

A. 4 – 1 – 2 – 3
B. 2 – 4 – 3 – 1
C. 4 – 1 – 3 – 2
D. 4 – 2 – 3 – 1

45.

A. 3 – 2 – 4 – 1
B. 4 – 3 – 2 – 1
C. 4 – 3 – 1 – 2
D. 3 – 4 – 2 – 1

Part 4: Paper Folding

Directions: For questions 46 through 60:

A flat, square piece of paper is folded one or more times starting from the left, proceeding stepwise to the illustrations to the right. The original position of the paper is represented by broken lines. The solid line indicates edges of the folded paper. The piece of paper is never twisted or turned and always remains within the outline of the original square. There may be ONE FOLD, TWO FOLDS, or THREE FOLDS in each item. After the last fold, a hole is punched in the paper. Your task is to unfold the paper in your mind and determine the placement of the holes on the original flat, square piece of paper. There is only one correct pattern of hole punches for each item. The black circles indicate hole punches. Choose the pattern that indicates the correct pattern of hole punches in the unfolded paper.

PRACTICE ILLUSTRATIONS:

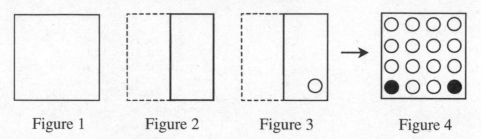

Figure 1   Figure 2   Figure 3   Figure 4

In this example, Figure 1 shows the original flat, square piece of paper. Figure 2 shows the first fold. Figure 3 shows the location of the hole punch in the folded paper. The black circles in Figure 4 show the pattern of the hole punches on the unfolded paper. The answer has two holes since the paper was two layers thick in the position where the hole was punched.

EXAMPLE

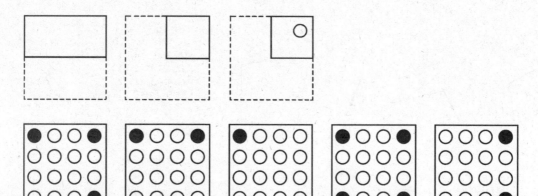

A   B   C   D   E

The correct answer is D. The paper was four thicknesses and, therefore, has four hole punches. The punch was made in the corner, so the four hole punches in the four corners are shown in black in the correct pattern.

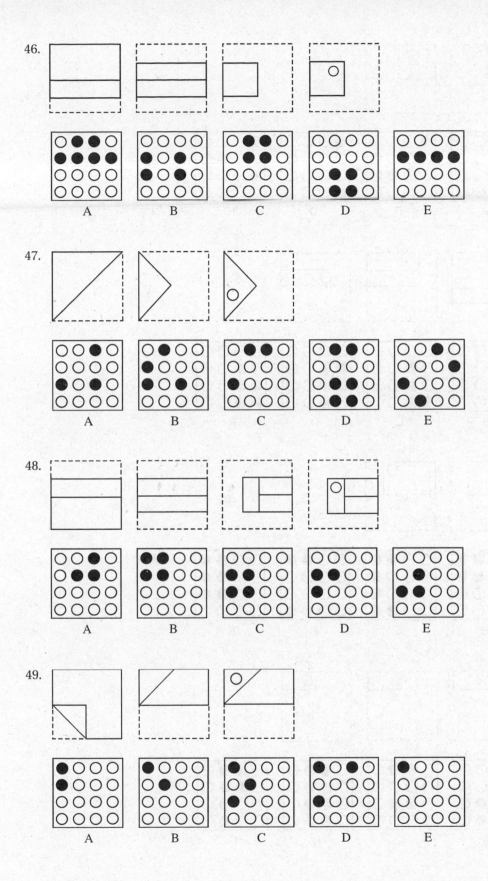

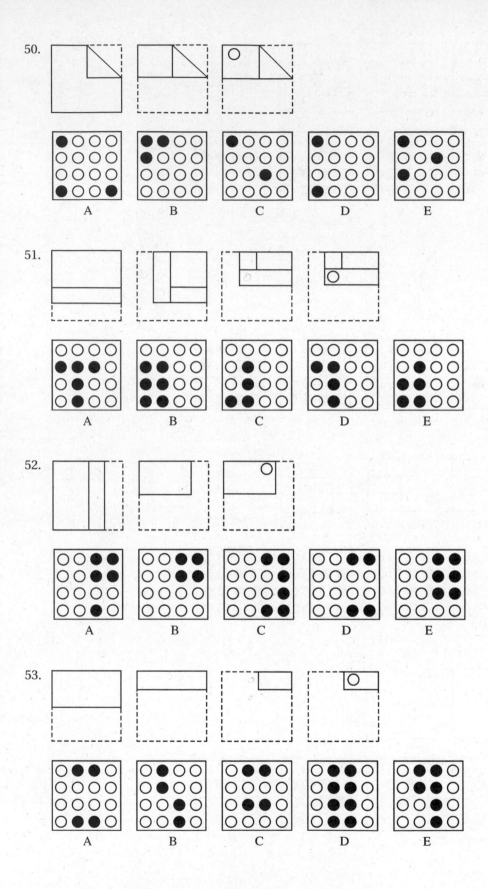

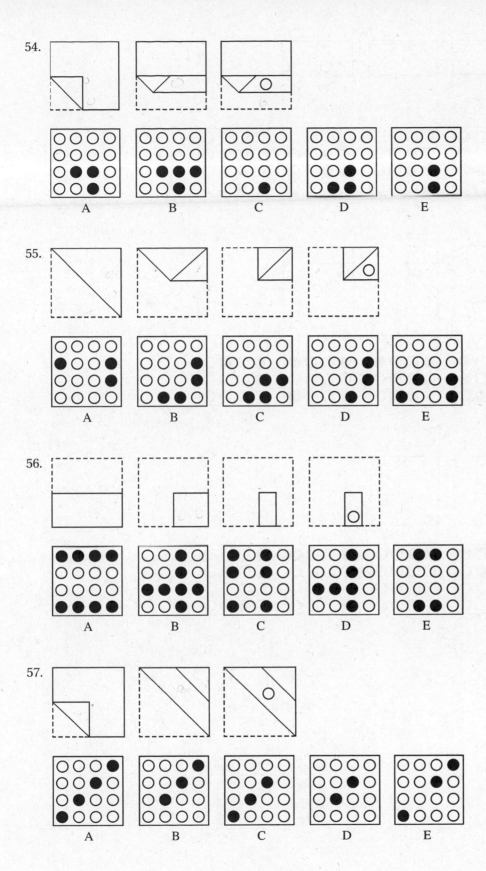

58.

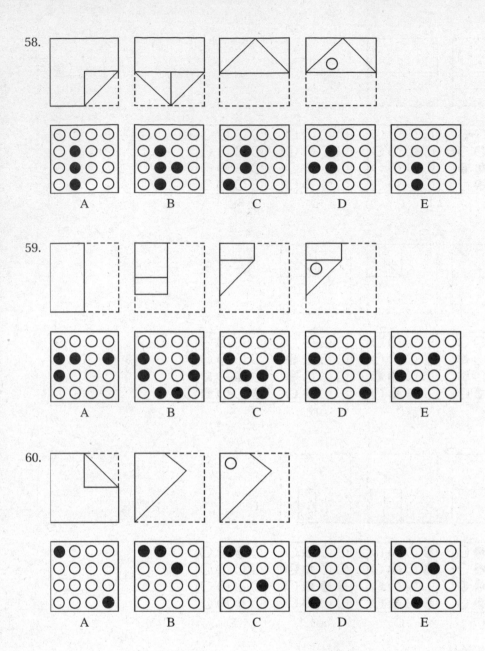

Part 5: Cubes

Directions: For questions 61 through 75:

Each of the figures in this section is representative of cubes of the same size that have been cemented together. After the cubes were cemented, the group of cubes was painted on each of the exposed sides WITH EXCEPTION TO THE BOTTOM SIDE ON WHICH THE FIGURE IS RESTING. Some illustrations contain hidden cubes. The only hidden cubes are cubes that are necessary to support other cubes.

In each item you are to determine how many cubes have

- ONE side painted,
- TWO sides painted,
- THREE sides painted,
- FOUR sides painted, or
- FIVE sides painted.

There are no problems that will ask for the number of cubes that have none (zero) of their sides painted.

EXAMPLE

In Figure A, how many cubes have two of their sides painted?

(A) 1 cube
(B) 2 cubes
(C) 3 cubes
(D) 4 cubes
(E) 5 cubes

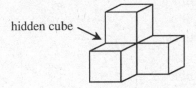

FIGURE A

There are four cubes in Figure A (one is hidden supporting the top cube). The top cube has five sides painted. The hidden cube supporting it has two sides painted. The two cubes in the foreground each have four sides painted. Therefore, there is only one cube that has just two sides painted and the correct answer is A.

Choose the letter that corresponds to the correct number of cubes with the given number of sides painted. Remember that THE BOTTOM OF THE CUBE IS NOT PAINTED.

61. In Figure A, how many cubes have two of their exposed sides painted?

(A) 1 cube
(B) 2 cubes
(C) 3 cubes
(D) 4 cubes
(E) 5 cubes

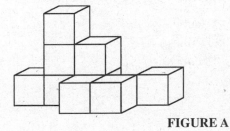

FIGURE A

62. In Figure A, how many cubes have three of their exposed sides painted?

(A) 1 cube
(B) 2 cubes
(C) 3 cubes
(D) 4 cubes
(E) 5 cubes

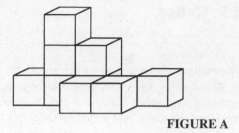

FIGURE A

63. In Figure A, how many cubes have four of their exposed sides painted?

(A) 1 cube
(B) 2 cubes
(C) 3 cubes
(D) 4 cubes
(E) 5 cubes

64. In Figure A, how many cubes have five of their exposed sides painted?

(A) 1 cube
(B) 2 cubes
(C) 3 cubes
(D) 4 cubes
(E) 5 cubes

65. In Figure B, how many cubes have two of their exposed sides painted?

(A) 1 cube
(B) 2 cubes
(C) 3 cubes
(D) 4 cubes
(E) 5 cubes

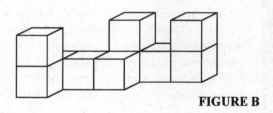

FIGURE B

66. In Figure B, how many cubes have five of their exposed sides painted?

(A) 1 cube
(B) 2 cubes
(C) 3 cubes
(D) 4 cubes
(E) 5 cubes

67. In Figure C, how many cubes have
    two of their exposed sides painted?

    (A) 1 cube
    (B) 2 cubes
    (C) 3 cubes
    (D) 4 cubes
    (E) 5 cubes

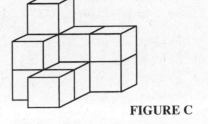

FIGURE C

68. In Figure C, how many cubes have three
    of their exposed sides painted?

    (A) 1 cube
    (B) 2 cubes
    (C) 3 cubes
    (D) 4 cubes
    (E) 5 cubes

69. In Figure C, how many cubes have five
    of their exposed sides painted?

    (A) 1 cube
    (B) 2 cubes
    (C) 3 cubes
    (D) 4 cubes
    (E) 5 cubes

70. In Figure D, how many cubes have
    two of their exposed sides painted?

    (A) 1 cube
    (B) 2 cubes
    (C) 3 cubes
    (D) 4 cubes
    (E) 5 cubes

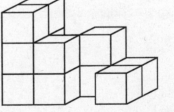

FIGURE D

71. In Figure D, how many cubes have three
    of their exposed sides painted?

    (A) 1 cube
    (B) 2 cubes
    (C) 3 cubes
    (D) 4 cubes
    (E) 5 cubes

72. In Figure D, how many cubes have four
of their exposed sides painted?

(A) 1 cube
(B) 2 cubes
(C) 3 cubes
(D) 4 cubes
(E) 5 cubes

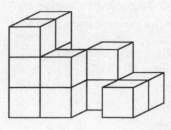

FIGURE D

73. In Figure E, how many cubes have
one of their exposed sides painted?

(A) 1 cube
(B) 2 cubes
(C) 3 cubes
(D) 4 cubes
(E) 5 cubes

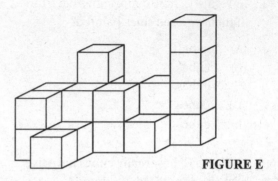

FIGURE E

74. In Figure E, how many cubes have two
of their exposed sides painted?

(A) 2 cubes
(B) 3 cubes
(C) 4 cubes
(D) 5 cubes
(E) 6 cubes

75. In Figure E, how many cubes have four of
their exposed sides painted?

(A) 1 cube
(B) 2 cubes
(C) 3 cubes
(D) 4 cubes
(E) 5 cubes

Part 6: Form Development

Directions: For questions 76 through 90:

A flat pattern will be presented in the box to the left. Your task is to mentally fold this pattern into a three-dimensional figure and choose the correct representation from the choices to the right. There is only one correct choice for each item.

EXAMPLE

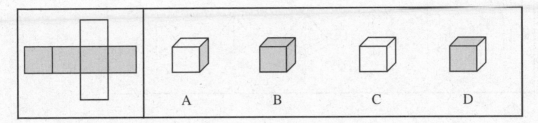

Folding the pattern in the left-most box can form only one of the figures to the right. The only figure that accurately represents the shaded areas once the pattern is folded is D.

Choose the letter that represents the three-dimensional object that correctly represents the folded pattern.

76.

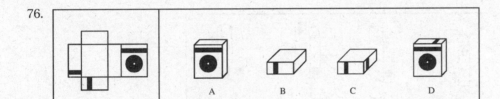

77.

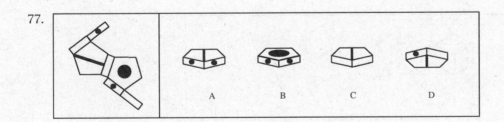

78.

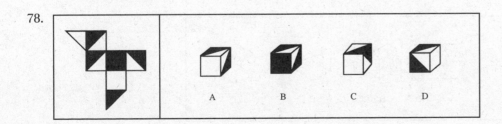

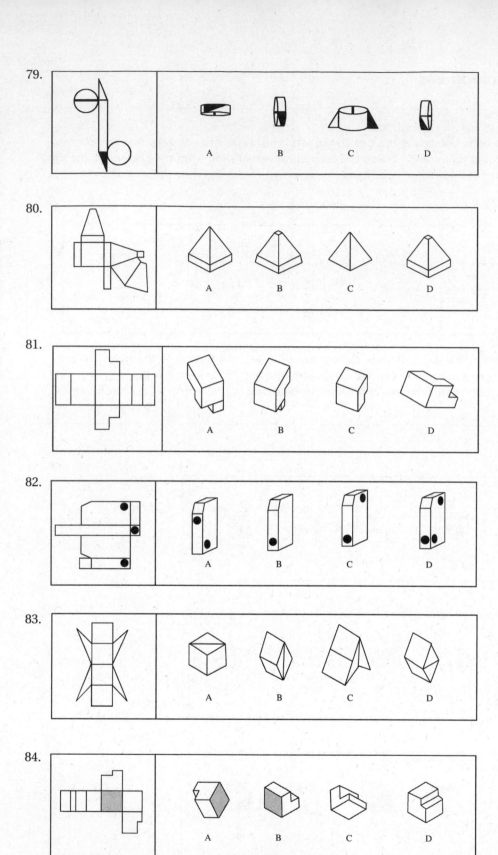

79.

A   B   C   D

80.

A   B   C   D

81.

A   B   C   D

82.

A   B   C   D

83.

A   B   C   D

84.

A   B   C   D

85.

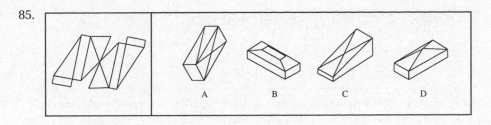

86.

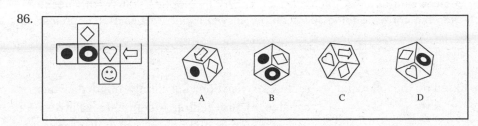

87.

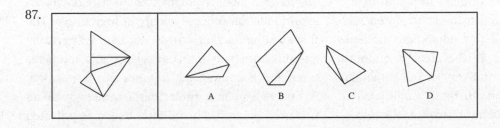

88.

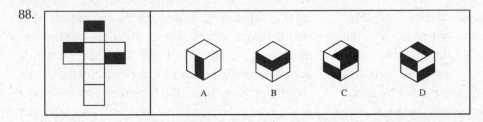

89.

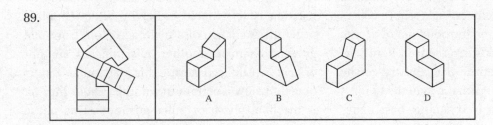

90.

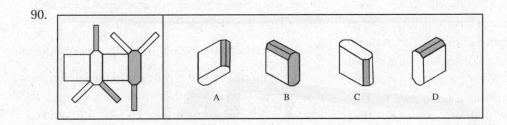

PRACTICE TEST 1

TIME LIMIT: 60 MINUTES

> **Directions:** This section consists of three passages, with questions and/or incomplete statements following each passage. Read each passage; then read the questions and/or incomplete statements and answer choices carefully. For each question and/or incomplete statement, choose the best answer and blacken the corresponding space on the answer sheet. This section contains 50 items.

Questions 1 through 17 are based on the following passage.

1. There are a limited number of dental materials used in rendering prosthetic treatment for the partially and completely edentulous patient. The two materials used in the greatest quantity are metal alloys and dental acrylic. Dental acrylic comprises the bulk of the prosthesis and is used to replace resorbed soft and hard tissues in the maxillary or mandibular dental arch. It is manufactured using a liquid-powder resin system. The liquid component is unpolymerized methyl methacrylate with small amounts of hydroquinone acting as an inhibitor, while the powder component consists of prepolymerized spheres of poly(methyl methacrylate) and a small amount of benzoyl peroxide as the initiator. Spurred on by Dr. Wright's 1937 clinical evaluations of methyl methacrylate resin (a plastic denture-base material), the introduction of acrylic resin was a significant advancement in dentistry. With the growth of synthetic resin chemistry, acrylic resins represent the first synthetic material to meet requirements for an improved denture-base material used to replace vulcanite. Throughout the first 65 years of their existence, acrylic resins have been used for inlays, onlays, crowns, and fixed partial restorations. Acrylic polymers have also been made to simulate the color and consistency of gingival tissue and natural teeth. The function of the acrylic polymer is to support artificial teeth and replace missing osseous tissue that was resorbed after natural tooth extraction.

2. Polymers consist of large molecules and a molecular structure limited in configurations. The process of polymerization is a repetitive inter-molecular reaction, covalently bonded, which is capable of proceeding indefinitely, allowing for various numbers of monomers of molecular weight 100 to form a linear polymer chain. The polymerization reaction process occurs in four stages. The first stage, *induction*, consists of benzoyl peroxide splitting into two free radicals at low temperatures and becoming the initiator of the reaction. A free radical is a molecular fragment with an unpaired electron. The initiator becomes activated with ultraviolet light, visible light, heat, or energy from another compound to form free radicals that interact with the monomer molecules. The second stage, *propagation*, is the free radical reacting with the double bonds of the methyl methacrylate monomer molecules. The reaction proceeds very quickly until most of the monomer is converted to a polymer. The third stage is *termination*. The reaction is terminated either by direct coupling or by the exchange of a hydrogen atom from one growing chain to another. A significant amount of heat is produced during this reaction and must be held below a certain maximum. *Chain transfer* is the final phase of polymerization. This phase occurs when an activated radical is transferred to an inactive molecule and a new nucleus is created. The polymerization reaction is as shown:

Methyl Methacrylate → Poly(methyl methacrylate)

3. Polymerization is rarely completed fully. As a result, residual monomer molecules can leach from the polymeric materials. The organic matrix that makes up the dental acrylic includes a variety of dimethyl acrylates and compounds depending on whether the polymerization is chemical, light, or heat activated. The components include

initiators: benzoyl peroxide or camphoquinones; accelerators: toluidines, anilines, or amino benzoic acid; and inhibitors: hydroquinonmonomethylene. Polymerization often fails to complete itself for four main reasons. First, several reactive groups may not participate in the process. Second, the surface layer exposed to oxygen/air is polymerized incompletely. Third, the dental acrylic lacks adequate chemical and physical properties, and last, many operators fail to follow the recommended manufacturer's instructions. The thickness of the oxygen-inhibited layer that is unpolymerized determines the percentage of residual monomer. According to the McCabe and Baker studies of residual monomer content in dentures, the residual monomer content levels can range as high as 1.85 percent in chemical-activated acrylic resin and between 0.045 and 0.103 percent in heat-activated resins, a difference of 18 to 40 fold, depending on the technique.

4. Until recently, almost all national and international dental standards and testing programs focused entirely on physical and chemical properties. Published clinical studies and clinical utilization of materials help set forth specifications for these materials, which are then codified by standards organizations. The American Dental Association (ADA), for example, mandates that ideal dental materials should be harmless to all oral tissues—gingival, mucosa, pulp, and bone. Materials should not be toxic, leachable, or diffusible into the circulatory system where they could cause systemic toxic responses that could elicit sensitization or an allergic response in a sensitized patient.

5. Since 1976, the United States Medical Service Amendments has emphasized the need for biological testing of dental materials. In 1984, the Federal Drug Administration (FDA) established a system for individuals to report side effects of dental restorative materials. Unfortunately, there is a growing body of evidence to suggest that residual methyl methacrylate provokes allergic responses in the oral cavity. The following definitions should help clarify some of the fundamental principles that describe immune responses of the human body.

A. **Absolute irritants:** substances that are intrinsically damaging to the skin, are often corrosive, and rapidly injure the skin.

B. **Allergic contact stomatitis:** a reaction of the oral mucosa to a dental material that results in burning, mild and visible erythematous, or white hyperkeratosis lesion.

C. **Positive patch test:** consists of erythema, mild edema, and small, closely set vesicles.

D. **Sensitivity:** the minimum amount of contaminates that can repeatedly be detected by an instrument.

E. **Sensitization:** the process of rendering an individual sensitive to the action of a chemical. Once sensitized, an individual's immune system will react in a damaging manner if exposed to the antigen again.

F. **Sensitizer:** a material that can cause an allergic reaction of the skin or respiratory system.

6. The National Health Interview Survey (NHIS) is responsible for reporting estimated national rates of edentulism in the United States. The edentulous rates in the United States in 1957 and 1971 were 13 and 11.2 percent, respectively, for all ages. In 2002, Douglas, Shih, and Ostry evaluated edentulism based on a shift in the American population's size and age. The research was based on two nationally funded studies: the 1996 United States Population Census (USPC) and the 1989–1991 National Health and Nutrition Examination Survey (NHANES III). After analyzing the USPC census projections for 2000, 2010, and 2020 (seen below on Table 1), Douglas, Shih, and Ostry extrapolated the following data points:

- The total adult population will increase from 187 million to more than 245.1 million people by 2020.
- The number of senior citizens over the age of 75 will increase by 61 percent from 13.5 million to 21.9 million people.
- The adult population from the age 55 through 74 will increase from 39.2 million to 73.1 million people.

Table 1. Population Projection by Year and Age Group

Age Group	1991	2000	2010	2020
18–24	26,351,000	26,258,000*	30,138,000	29,919,000
25–34	42,889,000	37,233,000	30,138,000	29,919,000
35–44	39,268,000	44,659,000	38,521,000	39,612,000
45–54	25,743,000	37,030,000	43,564,000	37,740,000
55–64	21,006,000	23,962,000	35,283,000	41,714,000
65–74	18,274,000	18,136,000	21,057,000	31,385,000
75–84	10,311,000	12,315,000	12,680,000	15,375,000
85+	3,178,000	4,259,000	5,671,000	6,460,000
Total	187,020,000	203,852,000	225,206,000	245,139,000

*Middle estimates of population size.

7. By the year 2020, the United States will experience a 79 percent increase in the adult population older than 55 years of age. The NHANES III report examined the percent of edentulism in the United States by estimating the need for maxillary and/or mandibular dentures as a percent of the population for each age group and an assessment of the total number of maxillary and mandibular dentures needed by the U.S. population. This was the first report to estimate the need for both maxillary dentures and mandibular dentures. The report discovered that in spite of projected declining edentulism rates among adults, the need for complete dentures will quadruple for individuals in the age range of 45 to 75+.

8. Combining edentulism rates and population projections by year and age group in thousands, Table 2 provides the projected estimate of the United States population in need of dentures. Below are some points to keep in mind while examining the data.

- The estimates do not account for lost, broken, or worn-out dentures.
- Edentulous rates are higher for lower socioeconomic groups. With a slowdown in the economy and increase in unemployment rates, there may be a rise in the edentulous rate.
- Institutionalized elderly and homebound people have greater needs for complete dentures and tend to be underreported in the national data.
- Members of the Armed Forces are underreported in the national data.

9. Prosthetic dentistry is responsible for the majority of acrylics used throughout dentistry, principally to support artificial teeth in a complete

Table 2. Number of U.S. Adults Who Need One or Two Dentures

Age Group	1991	2000	2010	2020
25–34	858,000	670,000	613,000	601,000
35–44	3,770,000	3,841,000	2,928,000	2,614,000
45–54	5,612,000	7,332,000	7,711,000	5,850,000
55–64	7,667,000	7,836,000	10,232,000	10,595,000
65–74	7,675,000	6,837,000	7,054,000	9,164,000
75–84	6,166,000	6,613,000	5,934,000	6,381,000
85+	1,900,000	2,287,000	2,654,000	2,681,000
Total # of adults	33,648,000	35,416,000	37,126,000	37,886,000
Demand at 90% utilization	30,283,000	31,874,000	33,413,000	34,097,000
Total # of edentulous	53,839,000	56,493,000	59,265,000	61,043,000

or partial denture. To avoid the potential negative effects of liquid monomers, researchers have been looking at new materials to fabricate dental prostheses. Several companies offer thermoplastic injectable resin for use in creating complete dentures, flexible partial dentures, and combinations of metal with flexible components. The advantage is a monomer-free material with superior flexibility, transparency for optimal esthetics, and biocompatibility. The increasing population of edentulous adults in America should be a major concern for all dental practitioners.

1. In the data provided in Table 1, what trend can be extrapolated for the 18–34 age group between the years 2000 and 2020?

   (A) 0.35% increase in population
   (B) 0.7% decline in population
   (C) 6.1% decline in population
   (D) 12.1% decline in population
   (E) 15.2% increase in population

2. Which of the following would not be a reason a polymerization reaction fails to go to completion?

   (A) The thickness of the oxygen-inhibited layer that is unpolymerized determines the percentage of residual monomer.
   (B) The dental acrylic lacks adequate chemical and physical properties.
   (C) Reactive groups may not participate in polymerization.
   (D) The surface layer exposed to oxygen/air is polymerized incompletely.
   (E) The operator fails to follow the manufacturer's recommended instructions.

3. Based on the information in the passage, the Federal Drug Administration

   (A) determined the safe dosage of residual monomer content in dentures.
   (B) described a method for testing dental materials.
   (C) reported on the best technique to cure methyl methacrylate.
   (D) established a system to report side effects of dental restorative materials.
   (E) None of the above

4. What is the term for when an "activated radical is transferred to an inactive molecule, and a new nucleus is created"?

   (A) Termination
   (B) Propagation
   (C) Induction
   (D) Chain transfer
   (E) None of the above

5. Based on the American Dental Association Specification #41, you could infer that dental acrylic would cause which of the following immune responses?

   (A) Intrinsic damage and corrosive and rapid injury to the skin
   (B) An allergic reaction of the skin or respiratory system
   (C) Renders an individual sensitive to the action of a chemical
   (D) An erythema, mild edema, and small, closely set vesicles
   (E) None of the above

6. Which is the most appropriate title for this passage?

   (A) History of Methyl Methacrylate
   (B) Reasons for the Projected Increases in the Edentulous Population
   (C) Higher Edentulous Rates for the Lower Socioeconomic Population
   (D) The Use of Methyl Methacrylate in the Edentulous Population
   (E) Reasons That Justify a 79 Percent Increase in the Adult Population

7. According to the passage, what study was responsible for reporting an 11.2% edentulism rate in the United States?

(A) National Health and Nutrition Examination Study, 1991
(B) United States Population Census, 1996
(C) National Health Interview Survey, 1971
(D) National Health and Nutrition Examination Study, 1989
(E) American Dental Association, Specification #41

8. The main benefit of a complete denture is to

(A) simulate the color and consistency of lost gingival tissue.
(B) replace missing osseous tissue.
(C) support artificial teeth.
(D) allow a patient to masticate food.
(E) All of the above

9. What was a conclusion that was reported in the National Health and Nutrition Examination Study III in the United States?

(A) This study was the first to report the percent of edentulism by age and year for maxillary and mandibular dentures.
(B) The adult population greater than 55 years old will experience a 79% increase in edentulism.
(C) The need for complete dentures will quadruple for individuals in the age range 45 through 75+.
(D) None of the above
(E) All of the above

10. According to Table 1, which age group will experience the highest percentage of growth when comparing 2000 and 2020 population projections?

(A) 25–34
(B) 35–44
(C) 55–64
(D) 75–84
(E) 85+

11. The author's attitude toward recent developments in edentulous patients is best described as

(A) alarming.
(B) concerned.
(C) confused.
(D) optimistic.
(E) apathetic.

12. Which of the following assumptions can be made about the future number of adults needing dentures in the year 2020?

(A) There will be a lesser demand for complete dentures for lower socioeconomic groups.
(B) Members of the Armed Forces have a higher demand for complete dentures.
(C) The high number of adults requiring single or complete dentures will be the 65–74 age group.
(D) Lost or broken denture rates are higher than average.
(E) Homebound elderly people have a lesser need for complete dentures.

13. According to this passage, which of the following can you infer would most likely be true with a slowdown in the economy and increase in unemployment rates?

(A) The need for dentures will decrease.
(B) The need for dentures should stay the same.
(C) The need for dentures will increase.
(D) None of the above
(E) All of the above

14. The author's purpose of writing this passage is to

    I. identify and address future health problems by estimating the increasing numbers of adverse reactions on future edentulism rates.

    II. review the history of flexible dentures and describe how methyl methacrylate affects population groups by ethnicity.

    III. review the science behind methyl methacrylate and understanding of the polymerization process.

(A) I only
(B) II only
(C) III only
(D) I and II only
(E) I and III only

15. The process of polymerization consists of

(A) large molecules ionically bonded.
(B) small molecules bonded covalently to form branched chains.
(C) molecules repetitively covalently bonded to form a linear chain.
(D) CH_3 groups attached by van der Waals forces to a definite length.
(E) None of the above

16. Initiation of the polymerization process involves

(A) toluidines, anilines, or amino benzoic acid.
(B) reactive groups exposed to oxygen or air.
(C) heat, chemical, or light activators.
(D) benzoyl peroxides or camphoquinones.
(E) hydroquinonmonomethylene.

17. Based on the McCabe and Baker studies, one could reasonably conclude that residual monomer remaining in heat-activated acrylic resin has a

    I. higher content due to a more effective polymerization.

    II. lower content due to a more effective polymerization.

    III. higher content due to a thicker oxygen-inhibited layer.

    IV. lower content due to a thinner oxygen-inhibited layer.

(A) I only
(B) II only
(C) III only
(D) I and III only
(E) II and IV only

Question 18 through 34 are based on the following passage.

1. A mere six diseases account for 90 percent of all deaths from infectious diseases throughout the world—54 million per year or one-third of all mortality. There is a growing body of scientific literature tracing the rise of newly emerging infectious and biologic diseases and evaluating their effects on our nation's health, economics, and national security. Well-known illnesses thought to be under control are being reported to county and state public health officials at an increasing rate of 5 percent per year. The reason for this alarming increase in the United States is due to four factors: (1) 57 million U.S. citizens undertake international travel for tourism or business purposes yearly; (2) increasing immigration of more than 1.5 million people, both legally and illegally per year; (3) returning military forces from all regions of the world infected indirectly by coalition forces or indigenous population; and (4) globalization of food imports into the United States to feed a diverse population.

2. These diseases threaten U.S. vital interests, endanger citizens at home and abroad, and threaten U.S. armed forces deployed overseas. Well-known illnesses thought to be under control

are reemerging and pose a serious global health threat, affecting political stability of developed and developing countries and posing significant security concerns for all nations. Infectious disease is the leading cause of death globally, accounting for a quarter to one-third of the estimated deaths in 1998. The Center for Disease Control and Prevention (CDC) defines infectious diseases as "diseases of infectious origin whose incidence in humans has increased within the past two decades or threatens to increase in the near future."

3. After the events leading to the September 11, 2001 attacks, both the scientific and security communities believe that advances in medical technology to cure diseases, such as HIV and cancer, has also laid the groundwork for the potential creation of biological weapons of mass destruction. The United States is particularly vulnerable to a release of biological pathogens by rogue nations or terrorist organizations since most cities in the United States are within a 36-hour commercial flight of any area of the world. Rogue nations and terrorist organizations can replicate, mass-produce, package, and deliver biologic, infectious pathogens with pinpoint accuracy to any city in the nation, resulting in high rates of morbidity and mortality. Recent terrorist attacks have prompted justified societal concerns about the hostile use of biological agents and their potential threats to health. Mortality rates associated with infectious diseases in the United States have increased by approximately 5 percent yearly, since 1980, to account for 59 deaths per 100,000 people annually. Current research also links infectious pathogens to diseases, such as diabetes, heart disease, and ulcers, previously thought to have been caused by environmental or lifestyle factors.

4. Infectious disease rates are increasing and appear to be virulent in the United States due to the following environmental and lifestyle changes:

- **International travel.** More than 57 million U.S. citizens traveled outside the United States for recreational and business purposes in 1998. In addition, tens of millions of foreign-born travelers enter the United States every year. Travelers on commercial flights can reach most U.S. cities before the incubation period of many infectious diseases.

- **Immigration.** In 1998, one million immigrants and refugees entered the United States legally, often from countries with a high prevalence of infectious diseases. For every one million people that enter legally, it is estimated that several hundred thousand enter illegally. At every port of entry, immigration officials have the authority to isolate or provisionally release people that show the symptoms of disease in category A or B.

- **Returning U.S. Military Forces.** United States military forces are currently stationed within every country of every continent in the world. Soldiers are immunized against many infectious diseases and are sensitized to detecting any symptoms before or after their return. Unfortunately, Reserve and National Guard soldiers must rely on the civilian health care system to diagnosis and treat postdeployment infections and illnesses.

- **Globalization of Food Supplies.** As the numbers of food imports have doubled over the past 5 years, food-borne illnesses have become a common problem. Depending upon the season, more than 75 percent of the fruits and vegetables available for consumption are imported, potentially infected with pathogenic microorganisms.

5. The United States Public Health System classifies biological and infectious agents based on rates of morbidity and mortality. In addition, infectious diseases can be classified based on the speed and geographical area they affect.

Category A
Anthrax (Bacillus anthraces)
Botulism (Clostridium botulinum toxin)
Plaque (Yersinia pestis)
Smallpox (variola major)
Tularemia (Francisella tularenis)
Viral hemorrhagic fever (Ebola) and areanaviruses (Lassa)

Category B
Brucellosis (Brucella species)
Epsilon toxin of Clostridium perfingens
Food safety threats (Salmonella species, E. coli)
Glanders (Burkholderia mallei)
Meliodosis (Burkholderia pseudomallei)
Psittacosis (Chlamydia burnetii)
Q fever (Coxiella burnetii)

Ricin toxin from Ricinus communes

Staphylococcal entertoxin B

Typhus fever (Rickettsia prowazekii)

Viral enchalitis (encephalitis)

Water safety threats (vibo cholerae)

Category C

Emerging infectious disease threats, such as Nipah virus and hantavirus

6. Endemic refers to the presence of a disease or infectious agent within a geographical area. An example would be the incidence of malaria around equatorial nations due to temperature and environmental conditions. An epidemic is the outbreak of disease or illness in excess of what may be expected on the basis of past experience for a given population. For instance, the emergence of the swine flu in the United States several years ago led to an epidemic. A pandemic is a worldwide epidemic affecting an exceptionally high proportion of the global population. An example is HIV/AIDS. Pandemics are becoming increasingly common due to the ease of travel, flow of imports/exports, and large numbers of continuously moving refugees and displaced persons throughout the world. The Center for Disease Control identifies threats based on the following categories:

Category A is high-priority pathogens that pose a major threat to national security. These include diseases that can be easily disseminated or transmitted from person to person, resulting in the highest mortality rates and has potential for major public health impact, public panic, and social disruption.

Category B includes pathogens that pose a more moderate risk to national security. These diseases are relatively easy to disseminate, result in moderate morbidity rates and low mortality rates, and require specific enhancements of CDC's diagnostic disease surveillance.

Category C agents are emerging pathogens that could be engineered for mass dissemination in the future due to the availability and ease of production and dissemination and potential for high morbidity and mortality rates.

There are 3 major groups of disease pathogens: viruses, bacteria, and protozoa.

7. Within each group are numerous species, which differ in shape, size, and structure. These pathogens are affected by a multitude of changes in human behavior, as well as social, economic, and technological changes.

- **Environment Changes.** Short term changes, such as the change of seasons, the amount of rainfall, or periods of drought, are often considered dangerous, but minor threats. When the balance of species is changed between microbe, human, and animal, infectious diseases multiply rapidly and increase the risk of exposing humans that share the same environment. Long-term changes permanently alter the interactions of species living in an affected area.

- **Human Behavior.** Frequent and sudden population movements of people due to ethnic conflict, civil war, and famine continue to spread diseases rapidly in affected areas. It was estimated that more than 120 million people lived outside the country in which they were born in 1998, causing migration of nonimmune populations from low infectious areas to high infectious areas. Behavior patterns, such as unprotected sex, multiple partners, and intravenous drug usage, are other factors that contribute to the spread of infectious diseases.

- **Technology.** Technology will greatly facilitate the detection, diagnosis, and control of certain infectious pathogens, although it also introduces new dangers in developing countries. Globalization of food supplies tends to introduce nonhygienic food production, preparation, and handling practices in originating countries.

- **Economic Development.** Changes in land and water use patterns will remain major factors in the spread of infectious diseases. Human encroachment on tropical forests will bring populations into closer proximity with insects and animals carrying diseases. Close contact between humans and animals will increase the incidence of zoonitic diseases—those transmitted from animals to humans.

- **International Travel.** The increase in international air travel, trade, and tourism will increase the spread of infectious pathogens endemic in one population or geographical area to another. The cross-border movement of more than two million people daily, including one million between developed and developing countries, weekly, will remain key factors in the spread of infectious diseases.

- **Microbial Adaptation.** Infectious disease microbes are constantly evolving. Oftentimes new strains are resistant to current antibiotics. Pathogens, such as Tuberculosis and Malaria, will remain difficult to treat due to their evolving strains. Domestic livestock are saturated daily with antibiotics to prevent sickness and increase maturation. Currently, first-line drugs used to prevent malaria are no longer effective in 80 of the 92 countries where the disease is a major problem. Low-cost, first-choice antibiotics have lost their power to clear infections, thus increasing the cost and length of treatment.

- **Public Health.** Many factors have led to a breakdown in the delivery of health care and the subsequent rise of infectious diseases. In developing countries, war, natural disasters, economic collapse, and the migration of population have overwhelmed basic health care services, leaving countries unable to care for their people. Funding for adequate infection control, sanitation, and water purification has been cut as economic problems become evident.

- **Climate changes.** Warmer temperatures and increased rainfall already have expanded the geographical range of mosquito-borne diseases, such as malaria. Many water-borne diseases are associated with temperature-sensitive environments. Global warming and increased ocean temperature will significantly affect the spread of infectious pathogens.

8. Several biologic pathogens have been used against civil and military populations by rogue states and terrorist organizations over the past 20 years. Diseases highly exportable are:

HIV/AIDS: At the end of the year 2000, 40 million people were living with the HIV virus. To date, more than 14 million have died from complications of this infectious disease. In an area where one-tenth of the world's population lives, 12 million deaths due to HIV/AIDS have occurred. The worst affected region is sub-Saharan Africa, accounting for nearly 95 percent of the world's deaths. By the year 2020, HIV/AIDS will be the leading cause of infectious disease death in the world.

Tuberculosis: Mycobacterium Tuberculosis is the caustic, viral agent spread exclusively by small-particle aerosols to a susceptible host not previously infected with the organism. In 1993, the World Health Organization called the Tuberculosis pandemic a global emergency. Its dramatic resurgence is due to the rise of primary infectious disease killers, such as HIV/AIDS and malaria, the breakdown of health services, and growing drug resistance. This disease is one of the biggest infectious killers of adolescents and adults, affecting more than two million people a year and serving as the world's largest potential reservoir—two billion people have the latent Tuberculosis infection. Currently, drug resistance is a growing problem. Approximately 50 percent of deaths occur despite treatment with current medications. Tuberculosis will be the second leading cause of death in the year 2020.

Malaria: This mosquito-borne tropical parasitic disease is the second leading cause of death from infectious disease. Since the 1970s, malaria infection rates have increased by 40 percent per year throughout the world. In 1998, 300 to 500 million people were infected with this disease, and 1.1 million people die yearly as a result. Malaria is endemic to more than 101 countries and territories.

Diarrhea: Enteropathogenic E. Coli is the bacterial agent found in food and water supplies of developing nations. Each year, more than two million people die from this disease. In developing countries, epidemics of diarrhea diseases caused by cholera, typhoid fever, and rotavirus cause severe dehydration. Causes of this disease are due to poor sanitation, inadequate hygiene, and unsafe drinking water.

Pneumonia: Myoplasma Pneumoniae is the agent responsible for acute respiratory infections leading to pneumonia. Pneumonia takes a toll of 3.5 million deaths per year. This virulent organism gains access through the endobronchial tree where it begins to multiply.

Measles: Measles is the most contagious disease known to man. The measles virus kills approximately one million people yearly. The measles virus is responsible for more deaths than any other single microbe.

Anthrax: A Category A disease, this is an acute infectious disease caused by the spore-forming bacteria Bacillus anthraces. Humans generally acquire the disease directly or indirectly from infected animals or occupational exposure to infected or contaminated animal products. Anthrax spores have the ability to survive in the environment for years or decades, awaiting uptake by the next host.

Smallpox: A Category A disease almost completely eradicated in 1977, the virus Variola is spread from one person to another or by infected droplets of saliva that expose a susceptible person having face-to-face contact with the ill person.

Plague: A Category A disease caused by the infectious bacterium Yersinia Pestis, plague is spread by rodents and fleas around the world and through direct contact with infected animal tissue. This disease is capable of killing 50 to 60 percent of all latent carriers if left untreated. Several variations of this infectious disease cause pneumonic, septic shock, and death within four days.

9. Infectious diseases are an unfortunate reality of this world. Found in every country, environment, and activity in which animals and humans coexist, deadly diseases are on the rise and will compromise every nation's health, economy, and national security. Without international controls or oversight, the spread of disease and the inability of researchers to cost-effectively cure new diseases scould create a bleak and troublesome future.

18. Infectious diseases account for what percentage of mortality in the world each year?

   (A) One-quarter
   (B) One-third
   (C) One-half
   (D) Two-thirds
   (E) Not enough information is provided in the passage.

19. Classification of biological and infectious agents can be based on morbidity, mortality, speed, and geographical area they affect!

   (A) The statement is true.
   (B) The statement is false.
   (C) Biological agents are classified on the speed and geographical area they affect.
   (D) Infectious agents are classified based on the rates of morbidity only.
   (E) Not enough information is provided in the passage.

20. Which factor poses the most significant risk for transmission of infectious agents into the United States?

   (A) Business travel and tourism
   (B) Illegal immigration
   (C) Returning military forces
   (D) Bioengineering of the nation's food supplies
   (E) All of the above

21. Based on the passage, should the United States expect an increase in infectious diseases throughout the 20th century?

   (A) Yes, due to increasing world population and financial incentives to cure diseases
   (B) No, due to current U.S. policy, restriction of trade will be the hallmark of the 21st century business.
   (C) No, the rates of HIV and cancer are decreasing due to increased funding and research.
   (D) No, rogue nations and terrorist organizations will suspend the use of infectious agents.
   (E) Not enough information is provided in the passage.

22. Typhus fever is any of several similar diseases caused by Rickettsia bacteria. The Greek word "typhos" describes the state of mind of those affected. What category is this disease considered?

(A) Category A
(B) Category B
(C) Category C
(D) Category D
(E) Not listed

23. Based on current military operations overseas, one could infer that the National Guard or reserve soldiers would have a higher incidence of disease prevalence than active duty.

(A) The statement is true.
(B) The statement is false.
(C) The percentage of prevalence would be exactly the same.
(D) Soldiers conducting military operations overseas should not have any infectious diseases.
(E) Not enough information is provided in the passage.

24. Based on the information in the passage, why is the United States concerned about rogue nations?

(A) U.S. cities are within a 36-hour commercial flight of any area in the world.
(B) Replication and mass production of infectious agents are easy to accomplish.
(C) Packaging and delivery of biological agents can be delivered with pinpoint accuracy.
(D) Recent terrorist attacks have promoted widespread and justified societal concerns.
(E) All of the above

25. Pathogens with low mortality rates and which are moderately easy to disseminate can be categorized as

(A) Category A.
(B) Category B.
(C) Category C.
(D) Category D.
(E) Not listed

26. In 1976, approximately 48 million people in the United States were immunized against the swine flu. This outbreak would be considered a

(A) pandemic.
(B) endemic.
(C) national tragedy.
(D) epidemic.
(E) syndemic.

27. Based on the information in the passage, the Center for Disease Control would be most concerned about the spread of what type of disease?

(A) Endemics
(B) Epidemic
(C) Pandemic
(D) Epidemic
(E) Syndemic

28. In 1998, infectious disease was the leading cause of death globally. What percentage of deaths could be attributed to infectious diseases?

(A) 15 percent
(B) 20 to 33 percent
(C) 50 percent
(D) 66 percent
(E) 75 percent

29. Globalization of the world food supply has had deleterious effects on our nation's population. What actions could you infer would slow down food-borne illnesses?

    (A) Increase border testing of all fresh fruits and vegetables entering the United States
    (B) Certifying international growers
    (C) Preventing importation of foods that have potentially pathogenic microorganisms
    (D) Restricting fresh imported vegetables based on previous seasons of high infectious disease occurrence
    (E) All of the above

30. Category C threats include which of the following?

    (A) They are difficult to produce.
    (B) They have low morbidity and mortality rates.
    (C) There is no health impact.
    (D) They are engineered for mass dissemination.
    (E) They are difficult to disseminate.

31. Based on the 1980 infectious disease rate in the United States, one could extrapolate the expected deaths per 100,000 in the year 1990 to be

    (A) 89.66.
    (B) 94.14.
    (C) 98.80.
    (D) 103.8.
    (E) 108.98.

32. According to the passage, what is the United States doing to prevent rogue nations from gathering biological and chemical munitions?

    (A) Increasing security measure to protect infectious pathogens
    (B) Decreasing financial incentives to pharmaceutical companies to suspend research
    (C) Reducing the ability to replicate and mass produce infectious pathogens
    (D) Stopping experimentation of only the nation's most serious, Category A pathogens
    (E) No inference can be made about what the United States is doing to prevent rogue nations from gathering infectious agents.

33. Which of the following diseases does the World Health Organization call a "global disease?

    (A) HIV/AIDS
    (B) Malaria
    (C) Anthrax
    (D) Smallpox
    (E) Tuberculosis

34. How is Plague (Category A) spread?

    (A) By infected droplets of saliva
    (B) By poor sanitation and inadequate hygiene
    (C) By rodents and fleas in direct contact with infected animal tissue
    (D) By mosquitos
    (E) By small-particle aerosols

Question 35 through 50 are based on the following passage.

1. Dental occlusion is a foundational principle in understanding and practicing clinical dentistry. Fraught with controversy and fear, many dental practitioners view this subject with attitudes ranging from obsession to misunderstanding and bewilderment. Every procedure performed in the mouth requires the dental practitioner to have a basic understanding of the effects occlusion has on the jaw, supporting structures, and the neuromuscular system. Occlusion affects every dental specialty, from the oral surgeon who through surgery modifies the teeth, jaw bones, and the temporomandibular joint, the restorative dentist who removes tooth decay, fills cavities, and repairs fractured teeth, the prosthodontist who treats dental and facial problems that involve restoring missing tooth and jaw structures, and the orthodontist who treats malocclusions. The risk of failing to understand basic occlusal concepts that dental practitioners approach in restoring damaged teeth may lead to inappropriate levels of care, thus causing patients to suffer from either over treatment or lack of treatment.

2. Controversy over occlusion exists because of a lack of thorough understanding of gnathology: confusing dental terminology; complex mandibular movements that require neuromuscular function; various philosophies of occlusion and their impact on dentate, partially edentulous and edentulous patients and practitioner's level of knowledge of occlusal morphology and the lack of clinical studies to support evidence-based dentistry.

3. Dental occlusion simply refers to the way the occlusal surfaces of the mandibular teeth occlude or slide over the maxillary occlusal surfaces in all moving and static relationships. These movements include chewing food, speaking, parafunctional habits including clenching, grinding, bruxing, or simply the position of the teeth when the mandible is at rest. These sliding movements occur when the mandible moves in a protrusive (forward), a retrusive (backward), to the left (left working, right balancing), right (right working, left balancing), and straight up and down (centric relation or

centric occlusion) relationship. All of these movements are extremely complex and are carefully orchestrated by the brain. What complicates dental occlusion is that no two individuals have the exact same mandibular movements.

4. An overwhelming amount of information and misinformation exists on this subject. Recent research on a popular search engine reveals that the word "occlusion" has greater than 11.4 million hits and that "dental occlusion" has almost 1 million hits. The majority of these sites are individual practitioners' views, opinions and websites, educational presentations, historical literature, journal publications, and dental insurance advertisements. These websites espouse a particular belief or attitude that may or may not be grounded in evidence-based dentistry. A MEDLINE peer-reviewed search of all English language publications using keyword "dental occlusion" listed more than 14,500 titles.

5. Mastery of dental occlusion requires a thorough understanding of the anatomy and physiology of the muscles of the masticatory system that includes the muscles, occluding teeth, and components of the temporomandibular joint. The remainder of this article describes why dental occlusion is often a challenging and difficult concept to understand and requires basic skills, education, and a thorough understanding of the movements of the mandible.

Complicated Terminology

6. The Gnathology Society was started in the early 1900's by a group of dental pioneers with the intention of defining how the anatomy and physiology and histology and pathology of the mouth, jaws, and closely associated structures work together and how they can be treated. The society's early-published reports described the principles of mandibular movement and the development of an articulator that could replicate all of the jaw's movements. The results of these findings established the development of terminology and improvements to articulator designs that could replicate mandibular movement. One of the most important and useful definitions in dentistry is the term centric relation (CR). Since 1940, CR has been defined and redefined at least 14 times. Glossary of Prosthodontic Terms (GPT) defines CR as:

1: the maxilla-mandibular relationship in which the condyles articulate with the thinnest avascular portion of their respective disks with the complex in the anterior-superior position against the shapes of the articular eminencies. This position is independent of tooth contact. This position is clinically discernible when the mandible is directed superior and anteriorly. It is restricted to a purely rotary movement about the transverse horizontal axis (GPT-5) **2**: the most retruded physiologic relation of the mandible to the maxillae to and from which the individual can make lateral movements. It is a condition that can exist at various degrees of jaw separation. It occurs around the terminal hinge axis (GPT-3) **3**: the most retruded relation of the mandible to the maxillae when the condyles are in the most posterior unstrained position in the glenoid fossae from which lateral movement can be made at any given degree of jaw separation (GPT-1) **4**: The most posterior relation of the lower to the upper jaw from which lateral movements can be made at a given vertical dimension (Boucher) **5**: a maxilla to mandible relationship in which the condyles and disks are thought to be in the midmost, uppermost position. The position has been difficult to define anatomically but is determined clinically by assessing when the jaw can hinge on a fixed terminal axis (up to 25 mm). It is a clinically determined relationship of the mandible to the maxilla when the condyle disk assemblies are positioned in their most superior position in the mandibular fossae and against the distal slope of the articular eminence (Ash) **6**: the relation of the mandible to the maxillae when the condyles are in the uppermost and rearmost position in the glenoid fossae. This position may not be able to be recorded in the presence of dysfunction of the masticatory system **7**: a clinically determined position of the mandible placing both condyles into their anterior uppermost position. This can be determined in patients without pain or derangement in the TMJ (Ramsfjord) Boucher CO. Occlusion in prosthodontics. The Glossary of Prosthodontic Terms, July 2005 J PROSTHET DENT 1953; 3:633-56. Ash MM. Personal communication, July 1993.Lang BR, Kelsey CC. International prosthodontic workshop on complete denture occlusion. Ann Arbor: The University of Michigan School of Dentistry, 1973. Ramsfjord SP. Personal communication, July 1993.

7. In another instance of confusing terminology, several words can be used to define the complete intercuspation of the opposing teeth independent of condylar position or "best fit" of the teeth. The GPT refers to this position as centric occlusion (CO), maximum intercuspation (MI), intercuspation position (ICP), or habitual state.

Complex Mandibular Movements

8. In 1952, Dr. Posselt described the movement of the mandible in three dimensions: sagittal, horizontal, and frontal planes. These movements vary depending on the condition of the temporomandibular joints, neuromuscular system, and occlusal surfaces of the permanent teeth. The following diagram depicts the mandibular opening around the hinge axis. The sagittal plane provides the following distinct positions of the mandible: motion of the mandible that occurs around an axis-A; maximum opening of the mandible on the hinge-B; centric relation-C; centric occlusion-D; rest position-E; and maximum protrusion-F.

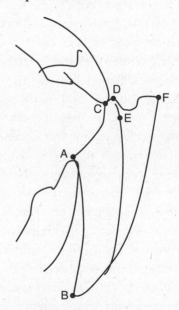

Figure 1. (Posselt's diagram)

9. The neuromuscular system is responsible for movement of the mandible. There are several muscle groups involved in movement of the posterior neck, supra, and infrahyoid muscles. The primary muscles

of mastication include the Temporalis, which elevates the jaw, retracts, and positions the mandibles and clenches teeth; the Masseter muscle, which elevates the jaw and clenches the teeth; the medial pterygoid, which protracts and elevates the mandible, assists lateral movements of the mandible; and the lateral pterygoid which aids in protrusion of the mandible, pulls the articulator disc forward, and assists in lateral movements of the mandible.

10. The teeth are an important part of occlusion since they are the structures that cut, chew, and incise food once placed in the mouth. The number, shape, and condition of the teeth are extremely important to overall balance of the occlusal function. Missing, broken, and carious teeth can severely affect the temporomandibular joint.

Philosophy of Occlusion

11. Through dental education, lectures, continuing education, and clinical experience, dentists develop a method or philosophy for treating patients requiring the reshaping, building, or fabricating the occlusal surfaces of broken, damaged, badly worn, or attrited teeth. Many dentists tend to follow the teachings of specialists, such as prosthodontists, orthodontists, or restorative dentists, who have extensive clinical skills and research. Occlusal philosophies include: Bioesthetics, which is the intimate relationship of form and function through esthetics and tooth morphology; Conformative occlusion, which does not change the existing occlusion for fear of temporomandibular dysfunction; Gnathology, which dictates that posterior occlusal anatomy should replicate condylar motion; the Pankey/Dawson philosophy, which utilizes simultaneous contacts of the canine and posterior teeth during a working excursion and only anterior contact during protrusive excursive movement; Neuromuscular occlusion, which uses myomonitor stimulation to develop the rest position for the myocentric point; and the Orthocranial concept, which results in flexure of cranial sutures, which impacts systemic health.

Occlusal Schemes

12. With the number of occlusal schemes and treatments available, it is not surprising that general practitioners are often confused. Misunderstanding prevails as to the best way to treat complex dental occlusal needs. Even among experts, consensus as to the best type of treatment is rare. For the patients who have physiological occlusion and maintain all or most of their natural teeth with no dental prosthesis, the three occlusal schemes are: canine guidance, which concentrate lateral gliding forces on the canines in working relationships; group function, which tries to stabilize lateral gliding forces over several teeth on the same side; or a full balanced occlusion with bilateral simultaneous anterior and posterior contact of teeth in centric and eccentric positions.

13. For edentulous or partially edentulous patients with missing or deficient teeth and or oral structures and who require some type of biocompatible, the three occlusal schemes are: bilateral balanced occlusion, the simultaneously contacting of the maxillary and mandibular teeth on the right and left side and in posterior and anterior areas in centric and eccentric positions; lingualized occlusion, the arrangement of posterior teeth so that only the maxillary palatal cusps occlude with the mandibular central fossa in all excursions of the mandible; or monoplane, flat plane teeth with no cusps angles to prevent deflection of the teeth or prosthesis.

Dental Education

14. The Commission of Dental Accreditation (CODA) requires every dental school in the United States to teach basic occlusal concepts in the first year of dental education. An understanding of basic occlusal concepts are tested in the National Board part I examination. The attending, clinic specialist teaches additional training and education that students receive for the remaining of their dental education experience or, as a resident, may have been taught years earlier.

15. In summary, no definitive scientific study has determined the correct occlusal philosophy or scheme for dentate, partially edentulous, or totally edentulous patients. Dentistry continues to deliver uncalibrated occlusal treatment, which is not based on scientific evidence.

35. The author's purpose for writing this passage is to

    I. address future dental needs of the United States population.
    II. describe why patients are often overtreated when seeking dental care.
    III. describe why a dentist's clinical experience, not necessarily scientific evidence, guides the practice of dentistry in the United States.

    (A) I only
    (B) II only
    (C) III only
    (D) I and II only
    (E) I and III only

36. Based on the information in the passage, the mastery of dental occlusion requires a thorough understanding of

    (A) the anatomy of the head and neck.
    (B) teeth and structures supporting teeth.
    (C) the components that comprise the temporomandibular joint.
    (D) the muscles of the head, neck, and upper torso.
    (E) All of the above

37. In Posselt's diagram describing protrusive movement of the maxillary and mandibular teeth, "the most important term in dentistry" can be located as what point?

    (A) Point A
    (B) Point B
    (C) Point C
    (D) Point D
    (E) Point E

38. In the occlusal scheme termed "group function," what is the primary role of the teeth?

    (A) The bilateral simultaneous anterior and posterior contact of teeth in centric and eccentric positions
    (B) Concentration of lateral gliding forces on the canine in working relationships
    (C) Stabilizing lateral gliding forces over several teeth on the same side
    (D) The bilateral nonsimultaneous contact of the teeth in eccentric positions
    (E) Concentration of the lateral forces on the premolar teeth in nonworking relationships

39. Based on Posselt's analysis of mandibular movements from the sagittal plane, one could reasonably conclude that mandibular movement from point C to point B involves

    I. simple rotation movement of the condyle with the glenoid fossa.
    II. translational movement of the condyle down the articular eminence.
    III. the neuromuscular system.
    IV. permanent dentition.

    (A) I only
    (B) II only
    (C) III only
    (D) I, II and III only
    (E) All of the above

40. Based on the number of Internet hits for "dental occlusion" compared to the MEDLINE peer-reviewed articles, what could you infer about the large difference in numbers?

  I. There are more personal clinical experiences written on the Internet than in peer-reviewed, evidenced-based articles.
  II. Advertisements and journal publications may not be grounded in evidenced-based dentistry.
  III. Internet postings under the heading "Dental Occlusion" does not require a D.M.D. or D.D.S. degree.

  (A) I only
  (B) I and II only
  (C) III only
  (D) I and III only
  (E) All of the above

41. Which is the most appropriate title for this passage?

  (A) The Dental Practitioners Guide to Understanding Patient's Occlusion
  (B) Dental Occlusion and Functional Disturbances
  (C) The Complexities Involved in Diagnosing Occlusal Disease
  (D) How the Lack of Permanent Teeth Can Affect Dental Occlusion
  (E) Dental Occlusion and the Need for Evidence-Based Science

42. According to the article, what group was responsible for describing the principles of mandibular movement?

  (A) Glossary of Prosthodontic Terms (GPT)
  (B) Commission of Dental Accreditation (CODA)
  (C) Gnathology Society
  (D) American Dental Association (ADA)
  (E) MEDLINE

43. According to the diagram, the reader could infer that the relationship of the maxillary and mandibular teeth at point F on the graph would relate to

  (A) protrusion.
  (B) retrusion.
  (C) a working relationship.
  (D) a balancing relationship.
  (E) a rest position.

44. What muscle is responsible for pulling the articulator disc forward and assisting in lateral movements?

  (A) Lateral pterygoid
  (B) Medial pterygoid
  (C) Masseter
  (D) Temporalis
  (E) Infrahyoids

45. Which of the following terms is used to describe the closing of teeth together?

  (A) Maximum intercuspation
  (B) Complete intercuspation
  (C) Intercuspation position
  (D) Habitual state
  (E) All of the above

46. CODA is the organization that requires all dental schools to have a formal, structured teaching methodology. Dental students are tested on basic occlusal concepts through what testing examination?

  (A) NERB
  (B) SERB
  (C) WERB
  (D) National Boards, part I
  (E) National Boards, part II

47. When making an impression for a bruxing guard, Dr. Dash noticed that his patient was missing five posterior mandibular teeth and two anterior teeth were broken. Based on information in the passage, you could conclude that

(A) overall balance of occlusion could be improved with fewer teeth.
(B) the temporomandibular joint would be healthier.
(C) missing teeth or damaged teeth do not affect dental occlusion.
(D) occlusal philosophy would remain the same regardless of the missing teeth.
(E) None of the above

48. The sliding and gliding movements of the mandibular and maxillary teeth can be viewed from other planes of reference. What shape would you expect the anterior teeth to scribe in a horizontal plane, as the patient moved from protrusive, right working (mandible shifts to the right), retrusive and left working (mandible shifts to the left), and back to protrusive?

(A) ◇
(B) □
(C) ○
(D) ×
(E) ▢

49. The philosophy of occlusion that does not change the existing occlusion for fear of temporomandibular dysfunction would be termed

(A) bioesthetics.
(B) gnathology.
(C) Pankey/Dawson.
(D) conformative.
(E) neuromuscular.

50. Based on information in the passage, what dental practitioner is responsible for treating complicated dental and facial problems that involve restoring missing teeth and jaw structures?

(A) Restorative dentist
(B) Oral surgeon
(C) Prosthodontist
(D) Orthodontist
(E) Endodontist

TIME LIMIT: 45 MINUTES

PRACTICE TEST 1

> **Directions:** The following items are questions or incomplete statements. Read each item carefully, and then choose the best answer or completion. Blacken the corresponding space on the answer sheet. This section contains 40 items.

1. 30% of the group likes scones, and 50% likes donuts. If 20% likes both, what percentage likes scones, donuts, or both?

   (A) 80%
   (B) 70%
   (C) 60%
   (D) 50%
   (E) 40%

2. A fair coin is flipped three times. What is the probability that at least one tails will appear?

   (A) $\frac{1}{8}$

   (B) $\frac{1}{4}$

   (C) $\frac{1}{2}$

   (D) $\frac{2}{3}$

   (E) $\frac{7}{8}$

3. The volume of a cone is given by $\frac{1}{3}\pi r^2 h$, where r is the length of the radius of the base of the cone and h is the height of the cone. If the radius has its length increased by 50% and the height is increased 50%, by what percent is the volume increased?

   (A) 100%
   (B) 237.5%
   (C) 250%
   (D) 337.5%
   (E) 350%

4.

Column A	Column B
The area of a square inscribed in a circle of radius 1	The area of a square circumscribed around a circle of radius $\frac{\sqrt{2}}{2}$

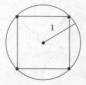

   (A) Column A is greater.
   (B) Column B is greater.
   (C) Columns A and B are equal.
   (D) Cannot be determined

5. The mean of a population of scores does which of the following if each score is doubled and then has 3 added to it?

   (A) It remains the same.
   (B) It increases by 3.
   (C) It doubles.
   (D) It quadruples and then increases by 3.
   (E) It doubles and then increases by 3.

6. The average of 7 scores (set A) is 50, and the average of 8 scores (set B) is 60. It is determined that two of the scores in the set of 7 are identical to 2 of the scores in the set of 8. If these scores are removed, the new average for set B is 70. What is the average for the set of all scores combined once these scores have been removed from both sets?

   (A) 47.33
   (B) 51.33
   (C) 64.55
   (D) 70
   (E) 75.45

7. Rila can make 120 hot dogs in 70 minutes, and Jennifer can make 180 hot dogs in 50 minutes. How long will it take them to make 3,720 hot dogs?

   (A) 350 minutes
   (B) 525 minutes
   (C) 700 minutes
   (D) 1,050 minutes
   (E) 1,488 minutes

8. A solution of $x^3 - 15x - 4 = 0$ is

   (A) −4.
   (B) −2.
   (C) 0.
   (D) 2.
   (E) 4.

9. The speed of light is 3×10^8 m/s. If galaxy α is 2.15×10^{20} km away, approximately how long will it take light to reach galaxy α?

   (A) 1.5×10^{-12} s
   (B) 6.7×10^9 s
   (C) 6.7×10^{11} s
   (D) 1.5×10^{13} s
   (E) 6.7×10^{14} s

10. Which line best fits the data below?

x	y
1	7.5
2	8
3	8.5
4	9
5	9.5

   (A) $y = \dfrac{1}{2}x + 7$
   (B) $y = 2x + 3$
   (C) $y = 3x + 5$
   (D) $y = -2x + 5$
   (E) $y = -3x + 7$

11. In $PV = nRT$, if n is increased by 25% and T is increased by 100%, but R remains the same, what percent increase occurs for the product PV?

   (A) 150%
   (B) 125%
   (C) 112.5%
   (D) 62.5%
   (E) 25%

12. Which of the following describes an ellipse with semimajor axis length 3, which has its center at (1, 5)?

   (A) $\dfrac{x-1}{3} + \dfrac{y-5}{1} = 1$

   (B) $\dfrac{(x-1)^2}{3^2} + \dfrac{(y-2)^2}{2^2} = 1$

   (C) $\dfrac{(x-1)^2}{3^2} + \dfrac{(y-5)^2}{10^2} = 1$

   (D) $\dfrac{(x-1)^2}{9^2} + \dfrac{(y-5)^2}{10^2} = 1$

   (E) $\dfrac{(x-5)^2}{9^2} + \dfrac{(y-1)^2}{10^2} = 1$

13. A train travels 50 miles in 3 hours and must travel 250 additional miles. If the average rate for the entire journey must be 50 miles per hour, how fast must the train travel the last 250 miles?

   (A) 41.33 mph
   (B) 55 mph
   (C) 60 mph
   (D) 76.67 mph
   (E) 83.33 mph

14. Note: Compare sector area and area length by magnitudes (for the units given).

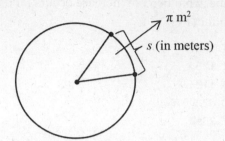

Column A	Colum B
Area of a sector of the circle	The distance s

(A) Column A is greater.
(B) Column B is greater.
(C) Columns A and B are equal.
(D) Cannot be determined

15. The sum of three consecutive numbers is 330. What is the greatest value of the three numbers?

(A) 103
(B) 110
(C) 111
(D) 112
(E) 120

16.

Study Periods

12:53

15:27

17:30

18:35

23:10

19:45

The study period times are listed in minutes and seconds. What was the total study time logged?

(A) 1 hr, 47 min, 20 s
(B) 1 hr, 45 min, 20 s
(C) 1 hr, 30 min, 10 s
(D) 47 min, 20 s
(E) 40 min, 10 s

17. Solve for y: $2^y = 16^{y-15}$

(A) 5
(B) 10
(C) 20
(D) 30
(E) 40

18. How many ways can 3 freshmen, 2 juniors, and 2 seniors sit at a table from left to right if all students of the same year must sit together?

(A) 12
(B) 24
(C) 144
(D) 1,680
(E) 5,040

19. A fair six-sided die is rolled twice. What is the probability that 11 or greater is rolled given that the first roll resulted in a 5 or 6?

(A) $\frac{1}{3}$

(B) $\frac{1}{4}$

(C) $\frac{1}{5}$

(D) $\frac{2}{13}$

(E) $\frac{1}{18}$

20. From a group of five people, two are chosen to be on a committee, and one of the two is chosen to be president. How many ways can this be done?

(A) 10
(B) 20
(C) 40
(D) 120
(E) 240

21. What is the probability of picking a chocolate cookie?

    (1) The probability of picking a chocolate cookie given that the cookie picked was from store A.
    (2) The probability of picking a cookie from store A given that it is a chocolate.

    (A) Statement (1) alone is sufficient, but statement (2) alone is not sufficient.
    (B) Statement (2) alone is sufficient, but statement (1) alone is not sufficient.
    (C) Both statements together are sufficient, but neither statement alone is sufficient.
    (D) Each statement alone is sufficient.
    (E) Statements (1) and (2) together are not sufficient.

22. $\dfrac{2y - 3\alpha}{2\alpha} = 3y + 5$. What is y in terms of α?

    (A) $\dfrac{13\alpha}{2 - 6\alpha}$

    (B) $\dfrac{7\alpha}{2 - 6\alpha}$

    (C) $\dfrac{3\alpha}{10}$

    (D) $\dfrac{3\alpha + 5}{10}$

    (E) $\dfrac{3\alpha + 10}{10}$

23. A cylindrical can is painted on its side, outside only, while the circular top and circular bottom of the can are left unpainted. If the radius of the top and bottom is 3 cm, and the height of the can is 10 cm, what is the cost of painting the can if paint costs $1.00 per cm^2?

    (A) 18π
    (B) 30π
    (C) 60π
    (D) 100π
    (E) 108π

24. 350% of what number is $\dfrac{35}{13}$?

    (A) $\dfrac{20}{26}$

    (B) $\dfrac{15}{26}$

    (C) $\dfrac{5}{26}$

    (D) $\dfrac{15}{39}$

    (E) $\dfrac{30}{39}$

25.
Column A	Column B
$\sqrt[3]{21,600} - \sqrt[3]{6,400}$	$\sqrt[3]{800}$

    (A) Column A is greater.
    (B) Column B is greater.
    (C) Columns A and B are equal.
    (D) Cannot be determined

26. Every 5 s a pebble is placed in container A, and every 15 s a pebble is removed from container A. One pebble is added every

    (A) 3 s
    (B) 5 s
    (C) $\dfrac{15}{2}$ s
    (D) $\dfrac{19}{2}$ s
    (E) $\dfrac{25}{2}$ s

27. Let a and b be positive integers both greater than 3. If $5(a - 3) = (b - 3)7$, what is the smallest possible sum for $a + b$?

    (A) 5
    (B) 12
    (C) 18
    (D) 21
    (E) 24

28. $\dfrac{y}{y-5}+\dfrac{2y}{y-7}=$

   (A) $\dfrac{y(3y-17)}{(y-5)(y-7)}$

   (B) $\dfrac{(3y-35)}{(y-7)(y-5)}$

   (C) $\dfrac{y-2y}{(y-5)(y-7)}$

   (D) $\dfrac{y}{(y-7)}$

   (E) $\dfrac{3y}{(y-7)}$

29. The average of three numbers is α. If the lowest number is y, and the middle number is δ, what is the largest number?

   (A) $3\alpha-3\gamma-3\beta$
   (B) $3\alpha-\gamma-\beta$
   (C) $3\alpha-\gamma$
   (D) $\alpha-\gamma-3\beta$
   (E) $3\gamma-3\beta-3\alpha$

30. A 20% percent raise followed by a 30% raise for Kiroi results in what percent increase from the original pay received?

   (A) 50%
   (B) 56%
   (C) 60%
   (D) 70%
   (E) 80%

31. For $ax-y=b$ and the line perpendicular to it at $(1,1)$, given by $Ax+y=B$, what is the product aA?

   (A) -1
   (B) 0
   (C) 1
   (D) $\dfrac{1}{\sqrt{2}}$

   (E) $\dfrac{2}{\sqrt{2}}$

32. If a glass contains 350 mL of orange juice, then how many liters of orange juice are there on a rack that contains 15 glasses?

   (A) 5,250
   (B) 52.5
   (C) 5.25
   (D) .525
   (E) .0525

33. $\dfrac{1}{\frac{1}{3}}+\dfrac{\frac{12}{12}}{1}+\dfrac{\frac{5}{5}}{2}+\dfrac{\frac{12}{6}}{14}+\dfrac{\frac{2}{2}}{31}=$

   (A) 51
   (B) 65
   (C) 72
   (D) 91
   (E) 144

34. If $|x-3|<5$, then

   (A) $-5<x<5$
   (B) $-8<x<2$
   (C) $-2<x<8$
   (D) $-5<x$ or $x>5$
   (E) $-8<x$ or $x>2$

35. $a=3\times15\times25\times16\times19$. Which of the following is NOT an integer?

   (A) $\dfrac{a}{75}$

   (B) $\dfrac{a}{13}$

   (C) $\dfrac{a}{57}$

   (D) $\dfrac{a}{30}$

   (E) $\dfrac{a}{285}$

36. The probability of getting a ticket during any given hour is $\frac{2}{3}$. If getting a ticket in any given hour is independent, what is the probability that exactly three tickets are given if a car is parked for five hours?

(A) $\frac{2}{3}$

(B) $\frac{8}{243}$

(C) $\frac{80}{243}$

(D) $\frac{16}{81}$

(E) $\frac{32}{81}$

37. Five black balls and five red balls are placed in an urn with one unnumbered green ball. The red balls are numbered 1–5, and the black balls are numbered 1–5. If five balls are picked without replacement, and one of them is the green ball, how many ways can the remaining four balls be picked such that no number is picked twice? (Assume that the order in which the balls are selected does not matter.)

(A) 10
(B) 50
(C) 80
(D) 100
(E) 120

38. $xy = 10,000$

$$\frac{1}{\log x} + \frac{1}{\log y} = \frac{4}{3}$$

$(\log x)(\log y) = ?$

(A) 3

(B) 2

(C) 1

(D) $\frac{1}{2}$

(E) $\frac{1}{3}$

39. From the data shown below (Group A and Group B), the variance is 75, and the mean is 30. What would be the new variance if a score of 30 were added? (Assume that Group A and Group B account for the entire population under study and are not used as a sample to estimate variance for the population.)

Group A	Group B
20	30
25	30
30	30
40	20
25	50

(A) 68.18
(B) 70
(C) 75
(D) 80
(E) 85.25

40. An urn has three red balls and two black balls. If two are chosen without replacement, what is the probability that both are black?

(A) $\frac{1}{20}$

(B) $\frac{1}{10}$

(C) $\frac{1}{5}$

(D) $\frac{1}{4}$

(E) $\frac{1}{3}$

ANSWER KEY
Practice Test 1

Survey of the Natural Sciences Test

1.	D	26.	A	51.	B	76.	E
2.	C	27.	D	52.	A	77.	C
3.	B	28.	B	53.	D	78.	D
4.	E	29.	E	54.	A	79.	C
5.	A	30.	A	55.	E	80.	B
6.	E	31.	B	56.	B	81.	B
7.	C	32.	E	57.	C	82.	B
8.	D	33.	A	58.	D	83.	A
9.	C	34.	D	59.	A	84.	B
10.	E	35.	B	60.	D	85.	B
11.	B	36.	E	61.	C	86.	B
12.	A	37.	C	62.	D	87.	A
13.	A	38.	B	63.	B	88.	B
14.	E	39.	E	64.	E	89.	C
15.	A	40.	C	65.	E	90.	D
16.	B	41.	E	66.	D	91.	A
17.	C	42.	C	67.	E	92.	E
18.	B	43.	B	68.	D	93.	C
19.	D	44.	D	69.	E	94.	A
20.	A	45.	D	70.	A	95.	B
21.	C	46.	D	71.	C	96.	D
22.	A	47.	A	72.	D	97.	D
23.	E	48.	B	73.	A	98.	D
24.	B	49.	D	74.	D	99.	E
25.	C	50.	E	75.	D	100.	C

ANSWER KEY
Practice Test 1

Perceptual Ability Test

1.	C	24.	D	47.	E	70.	B
2.	B	25.	C	48.	B	71.	E
3.	C	26.	C	49.	E	72.	D
4.	E	27.	D	50.	D	73.	E
5.	A	28.	B	51.	B	74.	E
6.	D	29.	A	52.	D	75.	E
7.	A	30.	B	53.	D	76.	B
8.	B	31.	B	54.	E	77.	C
9.	B	32.	C	55.	B	78.	C
10.	D	33.	B	56.	A	79.	D
11.	E	34.	A	57.	C	80.	D
12.	C	35.	C	58.	C	81.	C
13.	A	36.	C	59.	C	82.	B
14.	D	37.	B	60.	A	83.	B
15.	E	38.	A	61.	B	84.	A
16.	D	39.	D	62.	B	85.	D
17.	B	40.	D	63.	C	86.	B
18.	A	41.	C	64.	B	87.	A
19.	B	42.	D	65.	A	88.	A
20.	B	43.	B	66.	C	89.	B
21.	C	44.	A	67.	D	90.	A
22.	A	45.	D	68.	B		
23.	D	46.	C	69.	A		

ANSWER KEY
Practice Test 1

Reading Comprehension Test

1.	C	14.	E	27.	C	40.	E
2.	A	15.	C	28.	B	41.	E
3.	D	16.	D	29.	E	42.	C
4.	D	17.	E	30.	D	43.	A
5.	E	18.	B	31.	C	44.	A
6.	D	19.	A	32.	E	45.	E
7.	C	20.	A	33.	E	46.	D
8.	E	21.	A	34.	C	47.	E
9.	E	22.	B	35.	C	48.	A
10.	C	23.	A	36.	E	49.	D
11.	B	24.	E	37.	C	50.	C
12.	C	25.	B	38.	C		
13.	C	26.	D	39.	D		

Quantitative Reasoning Test

1.	C	11.	A	21.	E	31.	C
2.	E	12.	C	22.	A	32.	C
3.	B	13.	E	23.	C	33.	B
4.	C	14.	C	24.	A	34.	C
5.	E	15.	C	25.	C	35.	B
6.	C	16.	A	26.	C	36.	C
7.	C	17.	C	27.	C	37.	C
8.	E	18.	C	28.	A	38.	A
9.	E	19.	B	29.	B	39.	A
10.	A	20.	B	30.	B	40.	B

ANSWER EXPLANATIONS

Survey of the Natural Sciences Test

1. **D** The common elements necessary for life are C, O, H, N, P, and S. Arsenic is a semimetal and a metabolic poison. (Chapter 2 and Appendix, Figure A.1)

2. **C** Allosteric enzymes have a special configuration, which includes a substrate binding site and another "effector" site. Binding of an effector molecule, such as the end product of a metabolic pathway, will change the configuration of the enzyme so that it can no longer bind the substrate. This mode of activity allows allosteric enzymes to function in feedback inhibition type mechanisms. Coenzymes, such as NAD and FAD, participate in reactions in glycolysis and the electron transport chain. However, they function as electron donors and acceptors and are not typical enzymes. (Chapter 2)

3. **B** Phospholipids have a cylindrical shape that naturally forms a symmetrical bilayer with the polar hydrophilic head groups facing the outside and fatty acids on the inside. Since the cell membrane houses various cell functions, it also contains proteins that float free in the lipid bilayer in an arrangement defined in the fluid mosaic model. Photosynthesis requires a specific organelle, the chloroplast, which has a membranous structure. (Chapter 2 and Figure 2.12)

4. **E** The concentration of solutes (salts) naturally equilibrates against a gradient on both sides of a semipermeable membrane, such as the cell membrane. However, this equilibration is achieved by the movement of water molecules across the membrane. Water molecules will move from the side containing the highest concentration to solutes to the side, which has the lowest. An isotonic solution contains a physiological concentration of solute or salt so it is the same concentration both inside and outside the cell. (Chapter 2 and Figure 2.13).

5. **A** A hallmark of prokaryotic cells is that they lack a nuclear membrane. (Chapter 3 and Figure 3.1)

6. **E** Bacterial viruses are known as bacteriophages. Plasmids and transposons are other extrachromosomal genetic elements found in prokaryotic cells. However, they are composed entirely of DNA. (Chapter 3)

7. **C** Ribosomes in both prokaryotic and eukaryotic cells are composed of two protein subunits. Lipids are not part of the ribosome structure. (Chapter 3 and Appendix, Figure A.2)

8. **D** Mitochondria are the energy producing organelle in eukaryotic cells. There is an electron transport chain in the membrane of mitochondria. According to the endosymbiotic theory and molecular data, mitochondria represent an early prokaryotic cell that lost its ability to live autonomously. ATP is made in the cytoplasmic membrane of prokaryotic cells. Prokaryotic cells or bacteria do not contain mitochondria. (Chapter 3)

9. **C** Based on the metabolism of one mole of glucose or sugar, the Embden-Meyerhof-Parnas pathway requires two moles of ATP to make phosphorylated intermediates early in the pathway. Two moles of ADP are used in these reactions. Four moles of ATP are made in reactions later in the pathway because of a splitting reaction that occurs when a 6-carbon intermediate is converted to two 3-carbon molecules. This results in a net

synthesis of 2 moles of ATP. Only two moles of NAD are reduced to NADH during these reactions. (Chapter 3 and Figure 3.8)

10. **E** The goal of fermentation is to further metabolize the pyruvic acid, a 3-carbon molecule, which is made during glycolysis when the cells are growing anaerobically. Typically smaller carbon molecules are made due to the removal of carbon in the form of CO_2 from the pyruvic acid during these reactions. The Krebs cycle and electron transport chain are typically functional during aerobic respiration. No ATP is made during either the Krebs cycle or Calvin cycle, the dark reaction in photosynthesis. (Chapter 3 and Figure 3.8)

11. **B** The chemiosmotic hypothesis explains how ATP synthesis in aerobic respiration is coupled to the flow of electrons through the electron transport chain. Ideally, 38 moles of ATP are made per mole of glucose. There is only a net synthesis of two moles of ATP in the reactions in the Embden-Meyerhof-Parnas pathway. No additional ATP, or very small amounts (one mole per mole of glucose), is made in most fermentation reactions. Some intermediates made in the Krebs cycle are used by cells to make amino acids. Oxygen is the usual terminal electron acceptor in aerobic respiration. Glucose is made from carbon dioxide in photosynthesis. (Chapter 3 and Figure 3.8)

12. **A** The chemiosmotic theory explains how the flow of electrons through the electron transport chain creates a proton gradient across the membrane. The flow of protons back across the membrane through a proton channel drives the activity of ATP synthase, which converts ADP to ATP. (Chapter 3 and Figure 3.8)

13. **A** Chloroplasts are required for photosynthesis because the light and dark reactions take place within the structure of the chloroplast membrane. An electron transport chain is coupled to photosystem II in the chloroplast membrane. Coupled oxidation-reduction reactions, not substrate level phosphorylation reactions, are a hallmark of the electron transport chain. Only autotrophs, not heterotrophs, can use carbon dioxide as the sole source of carbon. (Chapter 13 and Figure 3.10)

14. **E** The eukaryotic cell cycle contains four phases of growth. These include two gap phases, a DNA synthesis phase, and mitosis. There is no division phase. Cell division, or cytokinesis, takes place after mitosis and is separate from the cell cycle. (Chapter 3 and Figure 3.11)

15. **A** There are four stages of mitosis (prophase, metaphase, anaphase, and telophase) following interphase. Nucleophase is not a real phase. (Chapter 3 and Figure 3.12)

16. **B** In "The Origin of Mitosing Eukaryotic Cells," Lynn Margulis proposed that mitochondria and chloroplasts evolved from once living prokaryotic cells. (Chapter 5)

17. **C** Alteration of generations is a reproductive process in which an organism switches between a haploid, multicellular gametophyte stage and a diploid, multicellular sporophyte stage. Members of the kingdom Chromista and the embryophytes in the Plantae kingdom use this method of reproduction. (Chapter 5 and Table 5.2)

18. **B** Among the answers listed, only the members of the phylum chordata have a notochord or vertebral column. (Chapter 7 and Figure 3.8, Figure 5.3, and Table 5.3)

19. **D** The Hardy-Weinberg principle mathematically explains the connection between genetic equilibrium and evolution in a population and is represented by the equation: $p^2 + 2pq + q^2 = 1$. (Chapter 6)

20. **A** There are three outcomes of evolution: adaptation, speciation, and extinction. The other answers are events or processes that contribute to evolution. (Chapter 6)

21. **C** Brown eye color is a dominant trait that can be expressed by either a pair of homozygous (BB) or heterozygous (Bb) alleles. Blue eye color is a recessive trait requiring a pair of homozygous (bb) alleles. Therefore, a genetic cross would potentially yield offspring that have brown eyes (Bb and Bb) and blue eyes (bb and bb). (Chapter 7 and Figure 7.4)

22. **A** Since male offspring obtain their X chromosome from the female parent, all X-linked genes are inherited from the mother. Therefore, recessive X-linked traits usually affect the phenotype of male offspring. X-linked traits cannot be obtained by male offspring from the father because the Y chromosome is only obtained from the male parent. Since males only have a single X chromosome, they cannot be carriers for recessive X-linked traits. (Chapter 7)

23. **E** Development of the zygote in animals goes through three ordered stages: blastula, gastrula, and organogeneis. The blastula develops into a gastrula to allow the formation of the germ layers (ectoderm, mesoderm, and endoderm) of the embryo. Gastrulation exhibits five basic types of cell movements: invagination, involution, ingression, delamination, and epiboly (Chapter 7 and Figure 7.2)

24. **B** The lymphatic system removes lymph, primarily interstitial fluid, by filtering out waste products and returning important plasma components back to the blood. (Chapter 7 and Figure 7.16)

25. **C** Myosin and actin are fibrous proteins present in the sarcomeres of muscle cells. Actin, activated by the binding of calcium, binds to myosin leading to a contraction. Relaxation occurs when ATP binds to myosin causing these fibrils to release the bound actin. (Chapter 7 and Figure 7.10)

26. **A** An erythrocyte is a red blood cell. (Chapter 7)

27. **D** Erythrocytes, or red blood cells, are the most abundant type of cell in blood. Erythrocytes contain heme which is an iron (Fe^{2+})-containing cofactor. (Chapter 7 and Figure 7.13)

28. **B** Bile is made in the liver and stored in the gallbladder. It is released into the duodenum when chyme enters that part of the small intestine. Bile acts as a surfactant that facilitates the emulsification of fats in the chyme. Bilirubin is a pigment in bile, and amylase is an enzyme in saliva that breaks down carbohydrates. (Chapter 7 and Figure 7.22)

29. **E** Antibodies, or immunoglobulins, bind to unique epitopes in antigens via the variable regions of the light and heavy chains. The various isotypes are composed of 1 (IgD, IGE, IgG), 2 (IgA), or 5 (IgM) pairs of identical light and heavy chains. (Chapter 7 and Figure 7.21)

30. **A** The parasympathetic nervous system originates in the spinal cord and medulla and controls "resting" activities of the body, such as salivation, lacrimation, urination, and digestion. (Chapter 7 and Figure 7.25)

31. **B** Action potentials are created by a type of voltage-gated ion channel present in the cell membrane. The channels are closed when the membrane potential is close to the resting potential (–70 mV) of the cell. The channels begin to open when the membrane potential

increases to a defined threshold value. There is an influx of sodium ions when the channels open resulting in a change in the electrochemical gradient. This leads to a greater increase in the membrane potential causing additional channels to open further, increasing the electric current across the membrane. The process continues until all available ion channels are open and maximum membrane potential is reached at +40 mV. Glial cells, or neuroglia, are non-neuronal structural and metabolic support cells found in the nervous system. (Chapter 7 and Figure 7.27)

32. **E** Luteinizing hormone (LH) is made in the pituitary gland. Insulin, estrogen, melatonin, and calcitonin are made in the pancreas, ovaries, pineal body, and thyroid gland, respectively. (Chapter 7 and Figure 7.28 and Table 7.3)

33. **A** When a sperm and egg join during fertilization, the zygote needs to end up with two sets of each chromosome, one set donated by the father and one by the mother. The primary oocyte is diploid ($2n$) at the start of oogenesis. Therefore, the ovum must end up with one set of chromosomes before fertilization can occur. (Chapter 7 and Figure 7.30B)

34. **D** Plants cannot metabolize the gaseous form of nitrogen (N_2), which is the most abundant form of nitrogen in the atmosphere. Some species of soil bacteria can "fix" gaseous nitrogen in organic nitrogen compounds. Plants can take up the organic nitrogen from the soil. Animals eat the plants and secrete organic nitrogen as part of their waste. (Chapter 8 and Figure 8.3)

35. **B** Plants, which convert sunlight to energy during photosynthesis, are autotrophs because they can use carbon dioxide as their only source of carbon for growth. (Chapter 8 and Figure 8.4A)

36. **E** The Loop of Henle, which is a U-shaped tube containing descending and ascending branches, is a major part of the renal tubule. The Loop of Henle is connected to Bowman's capsule by the proximal tubule and is surrounded by the vasa recta renis, which is a series of capillaries. The primary function of this loop is to concentrate the salt in the surrounding tissue. (Chapter 7 and Figure 7.23)

37. **C** The menstruation cycle is regulated by the endocrine system. At the start of ovulation, around the midpoint of the menstrual cycle, the luteinizing hormone (LH), produced by the pituitary gland, induces the mature follicle to release an ovum into the oviduct. The rapid increase in the level of LH is thought to be controlled by the stimulation of the hypothalamus, by estrogen, to secrete the gonadotropin-releasing hormone (GnRH). Estradiol, a human sex hormone, is also thought to be involved in the regulation of LH production. (Chapter 7 and Figure 7.30A)

38. **B** When a sperm and egg join during fertilization, the zygote needs to end up with two sets of each chromosome, one set donated by the father and one by the mother. The primary oocyte is diploid ($2n$) at the start of oogenesis. Therefore, the ovum and sperm each must end up with one set of chromosomes before fertilization can occur. (Chapter 7 and Figure 7.31 and Question 33)

39. **E** Species in a community can exhibit various types of interactions including competition, predation, parasitism, mutualism, and commensalism. When interactions between organisms are beneficial to both species, the relationship is known as mutualism. (Chapter 8)

40. **C** Kin selection is an altruistic behavior that ensures the reproductive success of an animal's relatives over that of the individual. The altruistic individual endures a fitness loss, and the receiving individual experiences a fitness gain in this behavior. This sacrifice of one individual to benefit the other is common among insects, such as ants, bees, and wasps, because colonies of these species contain male drones that are genetically identical. (Chapter 8)

41. **E** Choice (B) is incorrect because it gives the moles of nitrate (NO_3) in one mole of $Ca(NO_3)_2$ and not specifically the moles of oxygen. Choice (C) is the number of moles of oxygen in one nitrate, but it doesn't consider the fact there are 2 moles of nitrate $(NO_3)_2$ in the compound and is, therefore, incorrect. Choice (D) does include that there are 2 moles of nitrate, meaning there are 3×2 moles of oxygen, but did not include that there are 2 moles of $Ca(NO_3)_2$. The correct answer is choice (E), where there are 3 moles of oxygen in each nitrate (NO_3) → there are 2 nitrates $(NO_3)_2$, and, therefore, 6 moles of oxygen AND there are 2 moles of the entire compound (2 moles $Ca(NO_3)_2$), $3 \times 2 \times 2 = 12$ moles of oxygen.

42. **C** Notice that polyatomic ions (SO_4^{2-} and OH^-) did not split up in this reaction, so keep them together to help make balancing easier. Sometimes it's easier to think of water as H–OH to keep track of which hydrogen is coming from where (the H is coming from the acid, and the OH is coming from the base). Now, start balancing atoms. There is one Na on the reactant side and two on the product side. Place a 2 in front of NaOH. There is one SO_4 on the reactant side and one on the product side. This is balanced. Now, all that is left is to balance the OH on the reactant side with the OH in the water (H–OH). There is now 2OH on the reactant side since a 2 has been placed in front of NaOH, which means there needs to be a 2 in front of H_2O (H–<u>OH</u>). There are 2 H atoms in H_2SO_4, and now there are 2 "acidic" H's in water ($2H_2O \rightarrow 2\underline{H}$–OH). That means the correct order of coefficients is 2, 1, 1, 2. Choice (A) is incorrect because this is not the lowest ratio possible, and choice (D) is incorrect because it should be whole number ratios.

43. **B** Recall that

Mass percent of element X = $\dfrac{\text{mass of element X in one mole of compound}}{\text{molecular mass of one mole of compound}} \times 100$

First, calculate the mass due to just oxygen:

O: 4×16.00 g/mol = 64.00 g/mol

Second, determine the total mass of H_2SO_4.

H: 2×1.008 g/mol = 2.016 g/mol

S: 1×32.07 g/mol = 32.07 g/mol

O: 4×16.00 g/mol = 64.00 g/mol

$(2.016 + 32.07 + 64.00)$ g/mol = 98.09 g/mol

% composition of O = $64.00/98.09 * 100 = 65.24\%$

Choice (A) is incorrect because it is the percent composition of hydrogen. Choice (C) is incorrect because it is the percent composition of sulfur. Choice (D) is incorrect because it only accounts for 1 mole of oxygen instead of the 4 moles in H_2SO_4. Choice (E) is the mass percent of oxygen subtracted from 100, or the mass percent that is NOT oxygen.

44. **D** Choice (D) is false because the kinetic molecular theory of gases states that gas molecules collide, but that these collisions are elastic.

45. **D** This is an example using Charles's Law, where $\frac{V_1}{T_1} = \frac{V_2}{T_2}$.

$$V_2 = \frac{T_2 V_1}{T_1} = \frac{315K * 19.9L}{298K} = 19.9\underline{8} \text{ L} = 20.0 \text{ L}$$

Choice (A) is incorrect because it is calculated without converting the temperature to Kelvin. Choice (B) is incorrect because the temperatures are swapped or the *wrong* setup of $T_1 V_1 = T_2 V_2$ was used. Choice (C) is incorrect because the pressure was used in place of the volume. Choice (E) is the volume of one mole of gas at standard temperature and pressure.

46. **D** The ideal gas law assumes that gases behave ideally, which means they do not interact with each other. It also combines three laws, which is why choice (A) is incorrect. Using the gas law allows scientists to estimate that 1 mole of GAS takes up 22.4 L of volume (choice (B) is incorrect). The standard temperature is based on 0°C, which is 273K (choices (C) and (E) are incorrect).

47. **A** Atoms located at the corners of a unit cell only have $\frac{1}{8}$ of an atom INSIDE the unit cell.

$$\frac{1}{8} \times 8 = 1$$

48. **B** Choice (A) is an incorrect because as the boiling point increases, the less gas molecules escape and the lower the vapor pressure. Choices (C) and (D) are incorrect because as temperature increases, more molecules are able to escape into the gas phase, the higher the vapor pressure, and vice versa. Choice (E) is incorrect because the stronger the intermolecular forces, the higher the boiling point, and the lower the vapor pressure.

49. **D** When a salt dissolves, each ion on the crystal surface attracts the oppositely charged end of the water molecule. As each ion is separated from the crystal surface, it becomes surrounded by a sphere of hydration. Therefore, an ion is interacting with a polar compound (water), which is an ion-dipole interaction.

50. **E** Molality is moles of solute divided by kg of solvent.

First, find number of moles of solute: $40.0 \text{ g NaOH} \cdot \frac{1 \text{ mol NaOH}}{40.0 \text{ g NaOH}} = 1 \text{ mol NaOH}$

Then, convert mL of solvent to kg:

$$500 \text{ mL ethanol} \cdot \frac{0.789 \text{ g}}{1 \text{ mL}} \cdot \frac{1 \text{ kg}}{100 \text{ g}} = 0.3945 \text{ kg ethanol}$$

Then, divide moles of NaOH by kg of ethanol: $\frac{1 \text{ mol NaOH}}{0.3945 \text{ kg}} = 2.53 \text{ m}$

Choice (A) is simply the number of grams divided by the volume in mL. Choice (B) is moles of NaOH divided by 500 mL. Choice (C) is molarity (mol/L) instead of molality. Choice (D) is moles of solute divided by kg of both solute and solvent (0.4345 kg) instead of just solvent.

51. **B** Write a balanced chemical reaction and NOTE THE STOICHIOMETRY.

$$HClO_4 + KOH \rightarrow H_2O + K^+ + ClO_4^-$$

For every one mole of KOH, it titrates one mole of acid. At the equivalence point, equal moles of acid and base must be combined. Therefore, $V_{acid}C_{acid} = V_{base}C_{base}$. There is no need to convert the volume unit from mL to L because it will cancel on the two sides as long as the SAME unit is used. The calculation can be set up as:

$$(50.00 \text{ mL})(C_{acid}) = (43.91 \text{ mL})(0.08775 \text{ M}), \text{ where } C_{acid} = 0.07706 \text{ M}$$

False answers arise from these errors: putting both volumes on one side and both concentrations on the other side (choice (D)), dividing volume by concentration instead of taking the product of them (choice (A)). A common mistake is using the 1 : 1 mole ratio, when stoichiometry is 2:1 *in other cases*.

52. **A** Recall the rules for equilibrium constants, when reactions are (1) multiplied by a factor and (2) added together. Looking at the first reaction, it needs to be multiplied by 3 to get the 3A's needed for the overall reaction. This means the new

$$K_{1(3A \rightarrow 6D)} = \frac{[A]^3}{[D]^6} = (K_1)^3$$

For reaction 2, it needs to be reversed and halved. When a reaction is reversed, the

new $K_{2(4D \rightarrow 4B + 2C)} = \frac{[B]^4[C]^2}{[D]^4} = \left(\frac{1}{K_2}\right)$. Then, the reaction was halved, which means

$K_{2(2D \rightarrow 2B + 1C)} = \frac{[B]^2[C]^1}{[D]^2} = \left(\frac{1}{K_2}\right)^{\frac{1}{2}} = \sqrt{\frac{1}{K_2}}$. For equilibrium constants, when the reac-

tions are added together, the K_{eq}s are multiplied. Therefore, the K_{eq} of the overall reaction

is: $K_{eq(overall)} = (K_1)^3 \cdot \left(\frac{1}{K_2}\right)^{\frac{1}{2}} = (1.2)^3 \cdot \left(\frac{1}{4.4}\right)^{\frac{1}{2}}$. Do not confuse these rules with Hess's law

with ΔH.

53. **D** The K_a value is smaller than the K_a for H_3O^+ of water for a neutral solution at 25°C ($K_w = (H_3O^+)(OH^-)] = 1 \times 10^{-7} \cdot 1 \times 10^{-7}$). This means the concentration of acid is low, and, therefore, the pH is higher. The only pH that is basic (high) is choice (D).

54. **A** The key to answering this question revolves around two concepts: (1) knowing what EDTA does, and (2) recognizing that this is a Le Chatelier's principle problem. EDTA binds to metals, which means it will bind to Fe^{3+}. This decreases the concentration of Fe^{3+}. In order to go back to equilibrium, more Fe^{3+} will need to be made to make up for that loss, resulting in a shift toward reactants.

55. **E** Hess's law states that if the sum of multiple reaction steps equals the overall reaction, then the sum of each individual ΔH_{rxn} will equal the overall ΔH_{rxn}. Reaction 1 (ΔH_1) has to be multiplied by 2 and reversed to match with the overall reaction. If the reaction is reversed, the sign is changed ($-\Delta H_1$), and if the reaction is multiplied by 2, so is (ΔH_1). Therefore, for reaction 1, the new $\Delta H_{1_{new}} = -2(\Delta H_1)$. Reaction 2 is already set up correctly

to match with the overall reaction. The ΔH_{total} is the sum of $\Delta H_{1_{new}}$ and ΔH_2, which is –87.0 kJ, as shown below:

$$2Fe(s) + 2Cl_2(g) \rightarrow 2FeCl_2(s) \qquad \Delta H_{1_{new}} = -2(25.6)\ kJ$$

$$2FeCl_2(s) + Cl_2(g) \rightarrow 2FeCl_3(s) \qquad \Delta H_2 = -35.8\ kJ$$

$$\overline{2Fe(s) + 3Cl_2(g) \rightarrow 2FeCl_3(g) \qquad \Delta H_{total} = -2(25.6\ kJ) + (-35.8\ kJ) = -87.9\ kJ}$$

56. **B** A basic definition of entropy is the measure of disorder in a system. Melting, mixing two solutions, and sublimation (solid → gas) all increase randomness. Choice (E) produces more gas molecules, which also increases disorder. These are examples of an increase in entropy. Condensation occurs when a gas turns into a liquid, which decreases disorder, and, therefore, decreases entropy.

57. **C** The activation energy is the minimum amount of energy needed for reactants to overcome the transition state and become products. Choices (A) and (D) in the picture show only the energy associated with reactants (choice (A)) and products (choice (D)). Choice (E) represents the overall change in breaking and forming bonds (ΔH), which is the same as determining if the reaction is endothermic or exothermic. This leaves choices (B) and (C). Choice (B) is the activation energy going in the forward direction, but choice (C) is the activation energy if products are turned into reactants [(D) to (A)], the reverse reaction.

58. **D** This question is testing the definition of half-lives. How many times does it take for 24 g to be divided by 2 until it reaches 0.75 g? A mathematical representation for this question is: $24\ g \cdot \left(\frac{1}{2}\right)^x = 0.75\ g$. Another way is to calculate the mass after each half-life and count the number of half-lives it underwent to reach 0.75 g: $24\ g\frac{1}{2} = 12\ g$, $12\ g\frac{1}{2} = 6\ g$, $6\ g\frac{1}{2} = 3\ g$, $3\ g\frac{1}{2} = 1.5\ g$, $1.5\ g\frac{1}{2} = 0.75\ g$. Count the number of times, one-half was used, and it is 5 half-lives.

59. **A** The key concepts to answer this question are assigning oxidation numbers and definitions. The reducing and oxidizing agents have to be on the reactant side. MnO_2 is a reactant, so the next step is to assign oxidation numbers. The oxidation number for oxygen doesn't typically change, so start on Mn first. The oxidation number for Mn in MnO_2 is 4+, which is reduced to 2+ on the product side (Mn^{2+}). Since Mn was reduced, it is the oxidizing agent. Therefore, choice (A) is a false statement. Redox reactions can occur under acidic and basic conditions, where the presence of H^+ ions does indicate that the reaction occurred under acidic condition. This statement is correct. Cl on the reactant side has an oxidation state of –1 (Cl^-), and on the product side it is 0 (Cl_2). That means Cl lost electrons and became oxidized. This statement is correct. The oxidation state of a single element is equal to the overall charge, which means the oxidation number for Mn^{2+} is 2+. This statement is correct.

60. **D** First, match the half-reactions to the overall reaction. The electrode potential for Ag will have to be multiplied by three since there are 3 Ag's in the overall reaction ($0.80 \times 3 = 2.40$). The half-reaction for Fe matches with the overall reaction already, so it doesn't have to be altered. To calculate the E°_{cell}, recall that $E^\circ_{cell} = E_{cath} - E_{an} = 2.40 - (-0.04) = +2.44$. (Recall that the cathode is the electrode with the higher/more positive potential.)

61. **C** Isotopes of an element will have the same number of protons but a different number of neutrons. Carbon usually has 6 protons and 6 neutrons and an atomic mass of 12. Carbon-13 has one additional neutron. Choice (A) is the atomic mass (protons + neutrons) for carbon-13. Choice (B) is the typical atomic mass of carbon as shown on the periodic table. Choice (D) subtracted a neutron instead of adding a neutron, and choice (E) is the number of additional neutrons, but not the total number of neutrons.

62. **D** The Pauli exclusion principle states that ELECTRONS with the *same* spin (m_s) cannot occupy the same orbital; one is spin up, and the other is spin down.

63. **B** Start with the least electronegative atom in the middle, unless it is H, which can only make 1 bond. In this example, choice (B) is the least electronegative, so it should go in the middle (this eliminates choices (A), (C), and (D)). Then, add in the correct number of valence electrons around each atom. Have each atom obey the octet rule, unless the atom is in the 1st, 2nd, or 3rd column. In this example, choice (B) is in the 3rd column and only wants to make 3 bonds (this eliminates choice (E)). If needed, assign formal charges to see if the Lewis dot structure is the most stable configuration.

64. **E** Fluorine is the most electronegative element, and the trend is that electronegativity increases up a group ($\uparrow$) and going left to right across a row ($\rightarrow$).

65. **E** Group I elements are very reactive, and reactivity increases down within the group.

66. **D** Covalent compounds are nonmetals bound to other nonmetals, which eliminates choices (A) and (B). Choices (C) and (E) are polyatomic ions, which means these form ionic compounds even though they are made up of nonmetals. Choice (D) is CO_3 (*not* $CO_3{}^{2-}$), which is a nonmetal bound to another nonmetal and has an overall charge of zero. Covalent compounds also use mono, di, tri, etc., in their naming, and choice (D) is the only one that uses that naming system.

67. **E** Alpha decay can be represented with the Greek letter α, which is the same as ^4_2He. Using the law of conservation of mass, the atomic mass and atomic number on the product side has to equal the atomic mass and atomic number on the reactant side. Using this, the A and Z in ^A_ZX is $^{206}_{82}\text{X}$ ($210 - 4 = 206$ and $84 - 2 = 82$). Looking at the periodic table, element 82 is Pb. Be careful not to pick choice (C) because that is adding ^4_2He to the wrong side $\left(^{210}_{84}\text{PO} + ^4_2\text{He} \rightarrow ^{214}_{86}\text{Rn}\right)$. Choice (A) is the result if the reaction underwent gamma emission $\left(^0_0\gamma\right)$. Choice (D) is the result if the reaction underwent beta decay (β or $^0_{-1}\text{e}$).

68. **D** Random errors cannot be predicted and, therefore, are unavoidable.

69. **E** A radiation suit would only be needed under certain circumstances.

70. **A** Choices (B), (D), and (E) are all lower in concentration than the working solution and therefore cannot be used to make a 100 mM (or 0.100 M) stock solution. Between choices (A) and (C), choice (A) is more appropriate because 500 M is too concentrated.

71. **C** Producing the stereochemistry shown in the product (thiol compound) requires two successive stereochemical inversions at the chirality center. The reagents shown in choice (C) are the only ones that can affect this. First, to make the hydroxyl group a better leaving group, it is converted to a tosilate. Next, 2-iodopentane is formed by S_N2 reaction (first stereochemical inversion –I⁻ nucleophile), and finally, the thiol product is produced by another S_N2 reaction (second stereochemical inversion –HS⁻ nucleophile).

72. **D** The first set of reagents in the sequence will produce a resonance-stabilized enolate (a strong base will remove a proton from the methylene between the two carbonyl groups) followed by nucleophilic attack on the methyl iodide by the enolate to add a two-carbon chain to the carbon between the carbonyl groups. The next set of conditions will first hydrolyze the ester group to a carboxylic acid (the reagent H_3O^+), and then the elevated temperature (heat) will cause decarboxylation of the acid (loss of CO_2) to produce the ketone product. Choice (D) is the only product that can be produced from the given reagents/conditions.

73. **A** The first three choices are all carboxylic acids and will have pK_a's of less than 5. This makes all of these compounds considerably more acidic than choices (D) and (E), which are phenols with pK_a's generally above 10. Of the carboxylic acids, choice (A) will be the most acidic. In addition to being able to stabilize its carboxylate anion by resonance, the attached fluorine atom (the most electronegative element) will stabilize the anion by induction.

74. **D** The best term for this special type of structural isomerization, which involves an equilibrium between a ketone and an enol, is *tautomerization*. It should be remembered that the equilibrium between these two species *heavily* favors the ketone isomer form. This process is also sometimes referred to as enolization.

75. **D** Choice (D) is not true. Alkenes are more reactive and more polarizable than alkanes due to the π component of their double bonds. π-bond electrons are more delocalized than σ-electrons and can act as nucleophiles under the right conditions to form bonding interactions with other compounds (addition reactions). Choices (A), (B), (C), and (E) are all true. The heats of combustion of *trans* alkenes are lower than those of *cis* alkenes. This difference is due to steric strain. Alkyl groups attached to double bonds can only avoid steric interactions when they are in the *trans* configuration. The transition state in an E2 reaction, leading to an alkene that is lower in energy when it assumes an *anti*-periplaner geometry. If there is only a single proton on the carbon β to the leaving group, a *stereospecific* alkene product results. However, if there is an additional β proton present, the reaction is *stereoselective* (it produces more than one stereoisomer with a preference for one). The product that predominates will be the more thermodynamically stable isomer. *Cis* alkenes are indeed usually more polar than *trans* isomers. This is an electronic effect where substituent dipoles on the same side of the double bond add and those on opposite sides subtract. Many different types of low molar mass alkenes can be polymerized by addition polymerization (free radical, anionic addition, cationic addition, etc.) to produce numerous types of synthetic polymers. Just a few examples are: polyethylene (a number of different types), polypropylene, polyvinyl chloride (PVC), polystyrene, and polytetrafluoroethylene (Teflon).

76. **E** This reaction is an example of an aldol condensation. The aldol term is referring to an aldehyde or ketone enolate bonding to the carbonyl carbon of another aldehyde or ketone group—in this case in the *same* molecule as in "intermolecular." The addition is followed by dehydration (loss of water) to give an α, β unsaturated aldehyde or ketone. One of the other choices (B) involves a similar intermolecular addition process, the Claisen condensation, but it occurs with *ester* enolates and electrophiles.

77. **C** The reagent sequence shown will first involve nitration (HNO_3/H_2SO_4) of the toluene (methyl benzene) reactant through an electrophilic aromatic substitution process. The

methyl group on the benzene ring is activating (this will speed up the reaction) and an ortho-para director (controls the regiochemical outcome of the reaction). As such, the nitration will be predominately at the ortho and para position of the ring relative to the methyl group and produce a mixture. The second set of reagents (H$_2$/Pt) will reduce the nitro groups to amino groups. The final result is a mixture of ortho and para methyl aniline.

78. **D** Based on the given molecular formula, there are six possible isomers (this includes both structural isomers and stereoisomers) as follows:

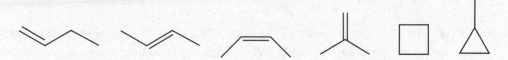

These are the only possible structural isomers without breaking the octet rule.

79. **C** Using the Cahn-Ingold-Prelog (C-I-P) protocol for prioritizing attachments and assigning the absolute stereochemistry of a chirality center as either R (where the substituents progress from high to low priority in a clockwise direction) or S (where the substituents progress from high to low priority in a counterclockwise direction), the assignments for the given structure are as follows: chirality center 1–R; chirality center 2–R; and chirality center 3–S.

80. **B** The given reaction conditions (ozonolysis) will result in the oxidative cleavage of an alkene functional group to form ketone and/or aldehyde functional groups. Reactant (C) contains seven carbons, which is one too many to form the six carbon chain of the product, so it can immediately be eliminated. When the double bonds associated with reactants (A) and (D) are cleaved, two or more products will be formed. The given reaction only produces one product, so those choices can be eliminated. Cleavage of the cyclohexene ring (choice (E)) will produce a single product, but it will be terminated on both ends by aldehyde groups separated by four carbons as shown below.

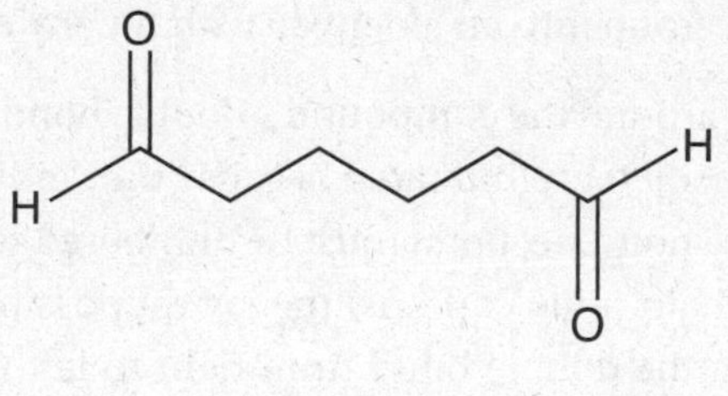

Only reactant (B), upon cleavage of its double bond, will give the single six carbon keto-aldehyde product shown.

81. **B** The oxidation state of the carbon in the carbonyl group (as hydrogen is added by the reagents) of cyclohexanone goes from +2 to 0 when the alcohol product (cyclohexanol) is formed. It can be seen that the oxidation state of carbon is *reduced*, and thus the reaction process is termed a "reduction."

82. **B** A significant factor that affects both the rate and thermodynamics of the interaction between a nucleophile and an electrophile is steric hindrance. Of the electrophile substrates to choose from, structure B's carbonyl carbon in the aldehyde group is the least hindered and is the most open to nucleophilic attack.

83. **A** All the choices except (A), which is an aromatic amide, are aromatic or aliphatic amines. Aromatic amines are always weaker bases than aliphatic amines due to lone pair delocalization into the benzene ring. Amides are always less basic than amines because of *extreme* nitrogen lone pair delocalized by resonance (see the diagram below).

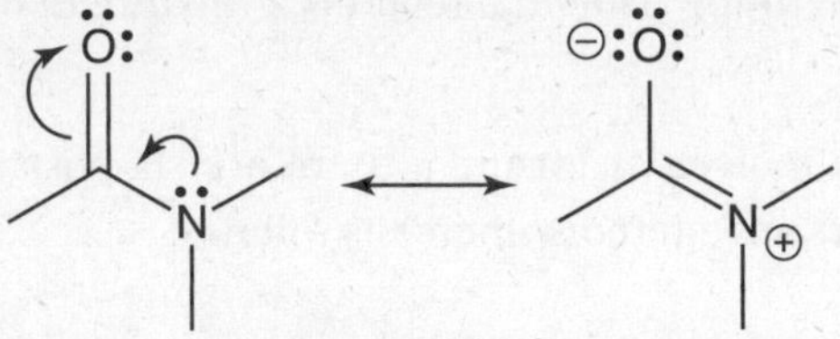

84. **B** The pK_a's of alcohols are generally between ~15 and 20. They are not strong enough acids to react with common hydroxide and alkoxide bases. Much stronger bases are need to deprotonate them—only sodium hydride (choice (B)) falls into this category.

85. **B** The two compounds have the same molecular formula ($C_1N_1O_1$), but different connectivity. As such, they are structural (or constitutional) isomers. Choices (A) and (D) can be eliminated because resonance forms of compounds must have identical σ bond connectivity, and the two compounds shown don't. The compounds can't be stereoisomers of each other because nether contains a chirality center or sp^2 carbon atoms)—choice (E) is eliminated. Since the compounds *are* structural isomers, choice (C) can be eliminated.

86. **B** The hydrogens attached to the indicated (arrow) methyl group have only one neighboring hydrogen (attached to the carbon α to the carbonyl group). Using the $n + 1$ splitting rule for ¹H NMR, where n is the number of hydrogen neighbors, $1 + 1 = 2$. So the indicated methyl hydrogen atoms' signal should be split into a doublet (2 peaks).

87. **A** The reaction shown is the oxidation of a primary alcohol. All the reagents shown are oxidizing agents. Some will tend to either transform the hydroxyl group into a carboxylic acid ($KMnO_4$ and $Na_2Cr_2O_7/H_2SO_4$) or react with the double bond in the compound to make a diol (OsO_4) or cleave it completely to produce ketone and aldehyde fragments. Only PCC (pyridinium chlorochromate—choice (A)) is selective and mild enough to transform the hydroxyl group into an aldehyde without any effect on the double bond.

88. **B** The stereochemistry around the compound's double bond is "*E*." As such, choices (A), (C), and (E) can be immediately eliminated because they indicate incorrect stereochemistry. The compound is a non-ene, but it must be numbered so as to give the double bond in the longest carbon chain (nine carbons) the lowest possible number. Numbering the nine-carbon chain with the double bond from right to left (choice (B)) gives the lower number for the double bond position—non-4-ene (correct). Numbering from left to right (choice (D)) gives a higher number—non-5-ene (incorrect).

89. **C** In the gauche conformation of butane (shown below as a Newman projection), it can be seen that the front and rear methyl groups attached to the two central carbons approach each other rather closely.

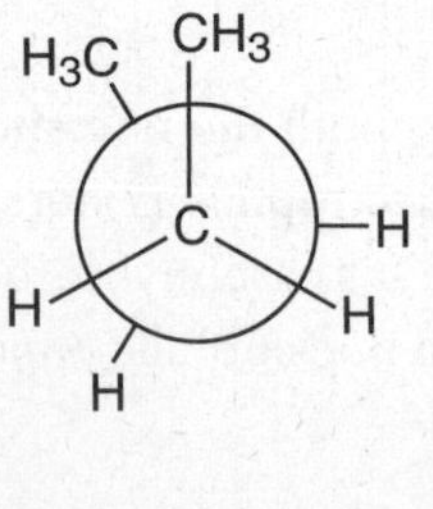

The result of this interaction is primarily *steric* strain. Steric strain is associated with an increase in energy caused by bulky electron clouds in close proximity repelling each other. Torsional strain is associated with the energy differences between staggered (more stable) and eclipsed (much less stable) conformations; although, some eclipsed conformations also result in steric strain. Angle strain is almost always found only in cyclic compounds (those with carbon-carbon rings).

90. **D** The positions of the chlorine, methyl, and ethyl groups for the lowest energy conformation of the compound can be seen in the structure below (when this type of question is encountered on the DAT, it is best to draw the chair form of the compound to do the analysis). Note that the two largest substituents (the methyl and ethyl groups—on the top of the ring) are in equatorial positions and the smallest substituent, the chloro group is axial (on the bottom of the ring). If possible, large substituents should always be placed in equatorial positions.

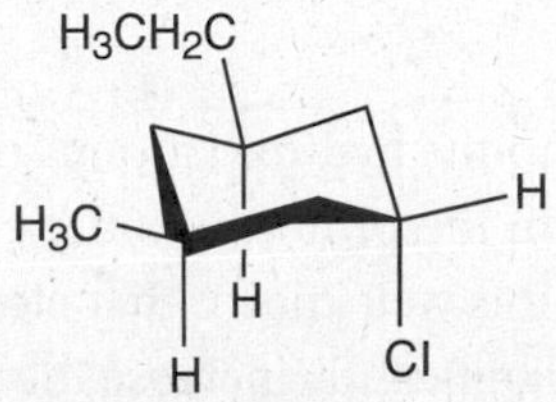

91. **A** In order for a compound to be aromatic, it must possess $4n + 2\pi$ electrons (where n is a positive whole integer). In addition to this criteria, the compound's π bonding system must be *cyclic*, *conjugated* (the double bonds must alternate with single bonds), and in a planar conformation. Only compound (A) meets all these requirements. It has 6π electrons (in this case $n = 1$)—a six-membered carbon ring with three conjugated double bonds (all the carbons in the ring are sp^2 hybridized) resulting in a ring where each of the carbon centers has a trigonal planar geometry (the ring is flat).

92. **E** One of the most characteristic absorption bands seen in IR spectroscopy is the carbonyl stretch (C=O). This absorption produces a strong band and generally ranges from ~1,780 to 1,680 cm^{-1}. The only choice that references carbonyl-containing compounds is (E). It's possible that a carbon-carbon double bond (choice (D) alkene) absorption band might appear on the lower fringe of the carbonyl absorption range, but it would be *much* weaker.

93. **C** The ammonium ions (conjugate acids) of heterocyclic amines are generally weak acids. The lower the pK_a value for a compound, the more acidic it is and the weaker its conjugate base. In this case, the ammonium ion of pyrrole is much more acidic than the same ion of pyridine. As such, the free amine of pyrrole is a much weaker base than the free amine of pyridine—choice (C) is true.

94. **A** Only primary and secondary alcohols can be oxidized to carbonyl-containing functional groups (aldehydes, ketones, and carboxylic acids). Tertiary alcohols (choice (A)) are unreactive toward oxidizing reagents because they have no protons α to the hydroxyl group. The carbonyl group is formed by an E2 mechanism, where an α hydrogen atom is abstracted by a weak base (usually water)—no α hydrogens, no oxidation.

95. **B** The primary products for this reaction are shown below:

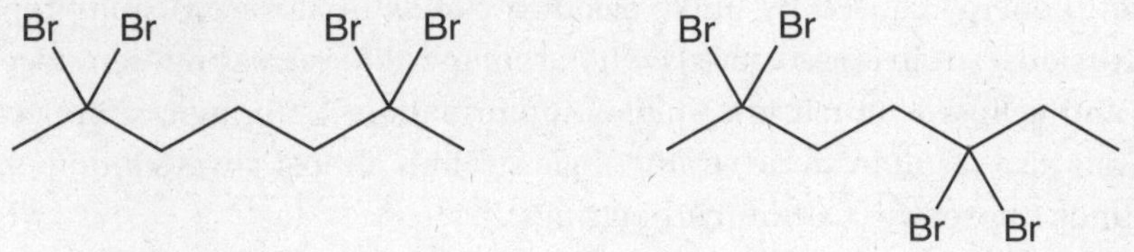

The dialkyne reactant contains both a terminal and internal triple bond. The HBr will add to a terminal alkyne group in a Markovnikov-like fashion producing a germinal dibromide (shown on the left side of the above molecules). There is no major preference for the regiochemical addition of the HBr to the internal alkyne group. This results in approximately equal amounts of addition to either side of the internal alkyne group (shown on the right side of the molecules—bromide ion addition is either to the second or third carbon from the right end of the molecule)—only the above two products (choice (B)) would be expected.

96. **D** All of the protons attached to the hydroxyl groups of the carboxylic acids in the compound will be more acidic than the proton α to the carboxylic acid carbonyl group, so choice (A) can be eliminated. It is well known that electronegative substituents α to the carboxylic acid carbonyl can significantly increase the acidity of the functional group. Of the α substituents present on the carboxylic acid groups in the compounds shown, the chloro groups are by far the most electronegative. Thus, proton 4 (choice (D)), which is attached to this group, will be by far the most acidic ($pK_a \sim 1.3$).

97. **D** Ordinary hydrocarbons (in this case pentane) are not reactive under Grignard reagent formation reaction conditions, so choices (A), (B), and (E) can be eliminated. Protic solvents (those that can hydrogen bond) are too acidic and immediately react with the extremely basic Grignard complex and can't be used for this process (choice (C)). Only the conditions shown in choice (D) will produce the desired result—the formation of a Grignard reagent. Ether solvents are usually used for these processes because they are aprotic and help stabilize the reaction transition state.

98. **D** The best mechanistic explanation from the formation of an intermediate carbocation for this process is the protonation of the alcohol's hydroxyl group (choice(D)). This makes the hydroxyl group a better "leaving group," and it is ultimately lost as water (dehydration) with the formation of an alkene (see the mechanistic steps shown below):

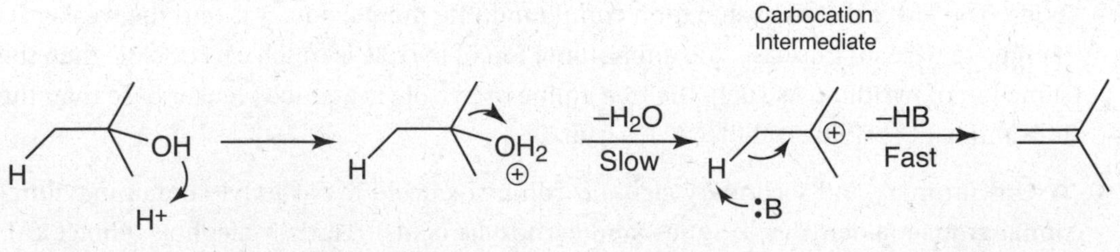

Choices (B) (hydroxyl groups are very bad leaving groups) and (E) (acids are electrophiles not nucleophiles) are particularly poor explanations.

99. **E** Esters are derivatives of carboxylic acids. Choices (A) and (D) are not derivatives of a carboxylic acid and generally can't be used to make esters, so they can be eliminated. In theory, a carboxylic acid (choice (C)), an amide (choice (B)), an acid chloride (choice (E)) could all be converted into an ester, but of these choices, the best by far would be choice (E), the acid chloride. This carboxylic acid derivative (choice (E)) is even more reactive than an anhydride because, when reacted with an alcohol (nucleophilic attack of the carbonyl carbon, also known as nucleophilic acyl substitution), it loses the very stable chloride anion (Cl^-—an excellent leaving group).

100. **C** The products from each step, in sequence, of the reactions shown are as follows:

- The reactant carboxylic acid with thionyl chloride ($SOCl_2$) will produce an acid chloride.
- The acid chloride will react with ethanol to produce an ethyl ester of the original carboxylic acid (choice (D)) (the pyridine solvent serves to trap HCl gas, which is lost as a byproduct).
- Last, the methyl Grignard reagent, by nucleophilic acyl addition, will produce the product shown as choice (C) (an ether alcohol).

Choice (B) is the starting reactant, so it doesn't work. Products (A) and (D) (an intermediate product) are not consistent with the reaction sequence shown.

Perceptual Ability Test

1. **C** Entry-1, top/bottom, as viewed in the diagram.
2. **B** Entry-2, after object rotated 90 degrees to counterclockwise.
3. **C** Entry-2, after object rotated 180 degrees clockwise.
4. **E** Entry-3, after object rotated 180 degrees clockwise.
5. **A** Entry-3, as seen in diagram, after object rotated 180 degrees clockwise.
6. **D** Entry-2, toward right, as viewed.
7. **A** Entry-2, after object rotated 180 degrees clockwise.
8. **B** Entry-2, after object rotated 90 degrees counterclockwise.
9. **B** Entry-2, after object rotated 180 degrees.
10. **D** Entry-2, after object rotated 90 degrees clockwise.
11. **E** Entry-2, after object rotated 90 degrees. Note object proportions.
12. **C** Entry-3, toward right, as viewed.
13. **A** Entry-2, after object rotated 90 degrees counterclockwise.
14. **D** Entry-3, after object rotated 180 degrees clockwise.
15. **E** Entry-2, after object rotated 180 degrees counterclockwise.
16. **D** Note front view (6 solid lines), side view (4 solid lines), lower hidden.
17. **B** Note end view, 6 total lines (2 hidden) on lower edge, 1 hidden to upper.
18. **A** Note front view, 7 total lines (2 hidden), end view (3 solid lines) (2 hidden).

19. **B** Note 6 lines from all views.

20. **B** Note top view, 6 lines (4 hidden), end view (2 hidden).

21. **C** Note top view, 6 lines (none hidden), front view, hidden box at top.

22. **A** Note front view, 6 lines, end view (5 lines) (2 hidden). Note small projection.

23. **D** Front view shows a hidden box open to top (hidden lines). Note proportions.

24. **D** Note top view, 6 lines (2 hidden), 2 hidden lines at lower front to back.

25. **C** Note top and side view positions of 5 lines.

26. **C** Note side view, 3 lines (1 hidden), front view (4 lines) (2 hidden).

27. **D** Note top view, position of 2 solid lines and 2 hidden.

28. **B** Note all proportions and all solid lines from the front view.

29. **A** Note front view, vertical, 3 solid lines.

30. **B** Note front view, 7 lines and 4 hidden.

31. **B** 4 appears smallest (omit A, D), 3 appears smaller than 1 (omit C).

32. **C** 2 appears largest (omit B), 3 appears smallest (omit A, D).

33. **B** 2 appears smallest (omit A, C, D).

34. **A** 4 appears largest (omit B, C, D).

35. **C** 4 appears smallest, 1 appears largest (omit A, B, D).

36. **C** 3 appears smallest, 4 appears largest (omit A, B, D).

37. **B** 4 appears largest (omit A, D), 1 appears smaller than 3 (omit C).

38. **A** 4 appears smallest (omit B, C, D).

39. **D** 1 appears smallest (omit B, C), 3 appears smaller than 4 (omit A).

40. **D** 3 appears largest (omit A, C), 4 appears larger than 1 (omit B).

41. **C** 4 appears smallest (omit A, B), 2 appears smaller than 1 (omit D).

42. **D** 2 appears smallest (omit A, B, C).

43. **B** 4 appears largest (omit A, D), 1 appears smaller than 3 (omit C).

44. **A** 4 appears smallest (omit B), 3 appears largest (omit C, D).

45. **D** 3 appears smallest (omit B, C), 4 appears smaller than 2 (omit A).

46. **C** 4 folds at final position (omit A, B), 1 unfold identifies E.

47. **E** 4 folds at final position (omit A, C, D), 1 unfold identifies E.

48. **B** 4 folds at final position (omit A, D, E), 2 unfolds identifies B.

49. **E** 1 fold at final position (omit A, B, C, D).

50. **D** 2 folds at final position (omit A, B, E), 1 unfold identifies D.

51. **B** 6 folds at final position (omit A, C, D, E).

52. **D** 4 folds at final position (omit A, C, E), 1 unfold identifies D.

53. **D** 8 folds at final position (omit A, B, C, E).

54. **E** 2 folds at final position (omit A, B, C, D).

55. **B** 4 folds at final position (omit A, D), 1 unfold identifies B.

56. **A** 8 folds at final position (omit E), 2 unfolds identifies A.

57. **C** 3 folds at final position (omit A, D), 1 unfold (omit E), 2 unfolds identifies C.

58. **C** 3 folds at final position (omit B, E), 1 unfold identifies C.

59. **C** 6 folds at final position (omit A, D, E), 1 unfold identifies C.

60. **A** 2 folds at final position (omit B, C, E), 1 unfold isolates A.

61. **B** Note 1 partially hidden cube (2 painted sides).

62. **B** Note 1 partially hidden cube (2 painted sides).

63. **C** Note 1 partially hidden cube (2 painted sides).

64. **B** Note 1 partially hidden cube (2 painted sides).

65. **A** Note 1 partially hidden cube, 1 fully hidden cube (3 & 2 painted sides).

66. **C** Note 1 partially hidden cube, 1 fully hidden cube (3 & 2 painted sides).

67. **D** Note 3 hidden cubes (1, 2, 2 painted sides).

68. **B** Note 3 hidden cubes (1, 2, 2 painted sides).

69. **A** Note 3 hidden cubes (1, 2, 2 painted sides).

70. **B** Note 1 hidden cube, 1 partially hidden cube (3, 3 painted sides).

71. **E** Note 1 hidden cube, 1 partially hidden cube (3, 3 painted sides).

72. **D** Note 1 hidden cube, 1 partially hidden cube (3, 3 painted sides).

73. **E** Note 3 hidden cubes, 1 partially hidden cube (2, 0, 3, 3 painted sides).

74. **E** Note 3 hidden cubes, 1 partially hidden cube (2, 0, 3, 3 painted sides).

75. **E** Note 3 hidden cubes, 1 partially hidden cube (2, 0, 3, 3 painted sides).

76. **B** Focus on the position of the circle and adjacent sides.

77. **C** Focus on the line and adjacent sides.

78. **C** Focus on solid square and adjacent sides.

79. **D** Focus on planes of points and positions of shaded area.

80. **D** Note sizes and shapes of base and top.

81. **C** Note relative positions and shapes of sides and top.

82. **B** Note relative positions of dots.

83. **B** Note shapes and positions of pointed objects.

84. **A** Note relative sizes of notches on notched sides.

85. **D** Note positions of larger triangular surfaces, note relative positions and sizes.

86. **B** Note relative positions of objects and planes.

87. **A** Note relative positions of all triangles, no rectangles.

88. **A** Focus on relative positions of clear square and shaded areas.

89. **B** Note relative size of angle surface.

90. **A** Focus on shaded areas and relative positions of extensions.

Reading Comprehension Test

1. **C** This question is an extrapolation question that involves basic mathematics to solve. The question asks you to compare and analyze the 18–34 year age groups between the years 2000 and 2020. Table 1 describes the population projection by year and age group. To answer this question, add up the two age group columns for the years 2000 and 2020

Age Group	1991	2000	2010	2020
18–24	26,351,000	26,258,000[1]	30,138,000	29,919,000
25–34	42,889,000	37,233,000	30,138,000	29,919,000
		63,491,000		59,838,000

Calculate the difference between the 2 columns: –3,653,000

Divide: –3,653,000 ÷ 59,838,000

Result: 6.1% (negative)

Choices (A) and (E) could be eliminated immediately since the population number is decreasing, not increasing.

2. **A** This question is a retrieval question that requires you to locate the part of the passage that describes the polymerization information. Remember that the question is asking you what would NOT be a reason for polymerization failure. Paragraph 3 describes why polymerization fails to go to completion and lists a number of reasons.

"Polymerization often fails to complete itself for four main reasons. First, several reactive groups may not participate in the process. Second, the surface layer exposed to oxygen/air is polymerized incompletely. Third, the dental acrylic lacks adequate chemical and physical properties, and last, many operators fail to follow the recommended manufacturer's instructions."

Again, remember the question asks for reasons a polymerization reaction fails to go to completion and NOT reasons that determine the percentage of residual monomer. The correct answer, "thickness of the oxygen-inhibited layer that is unpolymerized determines the percentage of residual monomer. No other paragraph addresses unpolymerized methyl methacrylate.

3. **D** This question is a retrieval question that requires you to locate the part of the passage that describes actions taken by the Federal Drug Administration (FDA) to regulate dental materials. Paragraph 5 describes the 1984 FDA's efforts to establish a system for individuals to report side effects of restorative materials. No other paragraphs in the passage address the FDA's actions.

4. **D** This question is a retrieval question that asks you to locate a definition (hence the word "termed") in the passage. Only paragraphs 2 and 5 list definitions for a process or term. The question addresses the process described as "chain transfer" from paragraph 2.

5. **E** This question is an inference question that asks you to interpret the intent of American Dental Association Specification #41 and apply that intent to the possible responses to determine the answer. After reading the ADA Specification #41 located in paragraph 4, you should infer that this specification is meant to protect individuals handling acrylic components.

"The American Dental Association (ADA), for example, mandates that ideal dental materials should be harmless to all oral tissues—gingival, mucosa, pulp, and bone. Materials should not be toxic, leachable, or diffusible into the circulatory system where they could cause systemic toxic responses that could elicit sensitization or an allergic response in a sensitized patient."

The other responses are definitions in paragraph 5 that clarify immune responses of the human body due to reported residual methyl methylacrylate allergic responses.

6. **D** This question is an inference question that requires you to review the entire passage and summarize its content. Keys to answering this question can usually be found in the introduction or closing paragraphs. As you evaluate each response, eliminate those choices that focus only on individual paragraphs.

Responses:

(A) The passage describes the history of methyl methacrylate; although, it does goes beyond that to describe past, present, and future edentulous rates.

(B) The projected increase in the edentulous population is stated in the form of surveys and studies, but fails to address the first 5 paragraphs.

(C) Higher edentulous rates for the lower socioeconomic population is a result of an increase in unemployment and slower economic growth.

(D) The passage begins by stating the history and polymerization process of methyl methacrylate and reviews surveys and studies indicating how edentulism affects this nation.

(E) This response is not addressed in the passage.

7. **C** This question is a retrieval question that asks you to locate the corresponding study that refers to the question, "What study was responsible for reporting an 11.2% edentulism rate in the United States?" After reviewing each possible response, paragraph 6 reports "The National Health Interview Survey (NHIS) is responsible for reporting estimated national rates of edentulism in the United States. The edentulous rates in the United States in 1957 and 1971 were 13 and 11.2 percent, respectively, for all ages."

8. **E** This question is an inference question. The passage does not specifically address the main benefits of wearing a complete denture, but paragraph 1 best describes the esthetic and functional advantages of dentures fabricated in dental acrylic. All responses are reviewed in the passage.

9. **E** This question is a retrieval question that asks you to locate the conclusions of the NHANES III study and select the best possible response. Paragraph 7 summarizes the results of the study.

10. **C** This question is an extrapolation question that asks you to locate the table, compare select age groups between the years 2000 and 2020, and identify the group with the highest percentage of growth.

Age Group	1991	2000	2010	2020
25–34		37,233,000		29,919,000
35–44		44,659,000		39,612,000
55–64		23,962,000		41,714,000
75–84		12,315,000		15,375,000
85+		4,259,000		6,460,000

Choice (A) indicates negative growth from the years 2000 to 2020. This response can be eliminated.

Choice (B) indicates negative growth from the years 2000 to 2020. This response can be eliminated.

Choice (C) indicates a positive growth and requires you to calculate the difference.

Calculate the difference between the two columns: $41,714,000 - 23,962,000 = 17,752,000$ (an increase).

Divide: $17,752,000 \div 41,714,000$

Result: +42.55%

Choice (D) indicates a positive growth and requires you to calculate the difference.

Calculate the difference between the two columns: $15,375,000 - 12,315,000 = 3,060,000$ (an increase).

Divide: $3,060,000 \div 15,375,000$

Result: +19.9%

Choice (E) indicates a positive growth and requires you to calculate the difference.

Calculate the difference between the two columns: $6,460,000 - 4,259,000 = 2,201,000$ (an increase).

Divide: $2,201,000 \div 6,460,000$

Result: +34.1%

The answer choice can be made quickly by eliminating the two negative trends and estimating the remaining choices as a percentage.

11. **B** This question is a tone or attitude question. The intent of the question is for you to interpret the author's tone or attitude in his word choice describing the passage. Understanding the definition of each response is important to answering this type of question correctly. Standard definitions are:

alarming—being worried or disturbing

concerned—being troubled, anxious, uneasy, or apprehensive

confused—being unable to think clearly

optimistic—being hopeful and confident about the future

apathetic—showing no feeling or interest

12. **C** This question is an inference question. The confusion in answering this question can be "which table do I use." Table 1 addresses the population projections, and Table 2 addresses the number of U.S. adults who need one or two dentures. Most of the responses are summarized in Table 2 findings, although minor changes are made that negate many of the responses.

Chioce (A) The edentulous rates are higher for lower socioeconomic groups according to the passage.

Choice (B) Members of the Armed Forces requiring dentures is actually underreported.

Choice (C) This response is a correct statement based on the published data.

Choice (D) The number of adults requiring future dentures does not include lost, broken, or worn-out dentures.

Choice (E) The summarized data states institutionalized elderly and homebound people have greater needs for complete dentures and tend to be underreported.

13. **C** This question is an inference question. The author is asking you to use the findings from Table 2 and infer the results of what happens in a slowed economy with high unemployment. The passage states "with a slowdown in the economy and increase in unemployment rates, there may be a rise in the edentulous rate."

14. **E** This question is a retrieval question that requires you to review the entire passage and determine if responses I, II and III were discussed by the author. Paragraphs 1 through 5 discuss the history and adverse reactions of methyl methacrylate after the polymerization process is complete. Paragraphs 6 through 8 discuss the edentulism rates and population growth. No information in the passage is provided about the history of vulcanite dentures or the population groups by ethnicity.

15. **C** This question is a retrieval question that requires you to identify the paragraph and understand the details that describe the polymerization process. Paragraph 2 outlines the polymerization process.

Choice (A) The polymerization process involves covalently bonded molecules, not ionically bonded.

Choice (B) The polymerization process involves linear chains, not branched or cross-linked.

Choice (D) van der Waals forces are not described in the passage and form indefinite lengths.

Choice (E) Negated due to choice (C).

16. **D** This question is a retrieval question that requires you to locate specifics about the polymerization reaction. The question does not ask about the process of polymerization, only what initiates the reaction. Paragraph 3 states the components involved in the reaction.

Choice (A) Accelerators are used to speed up the reaction.

Choice (B) Explains why the reaction is incomplete.

Choice (C) Refers to activators of the reaction.

Choice (E) Inhibitor to the reaction process.

17. **E** This question asks you to draw a conclusion based on information in the passage. The study is described in paragraph 3 and indicates that chemical-activated acrylic resin has a much higher amount of residual monomer than heated-activated resin. With this information, you must associate unreacted or higher residual monomer with incomplete polymerization as also described in the paragraph. Lastly, the paragraph lists four reasons why polymerization fails to go to completion. Reason number two lists the surface area exposed to oxygen/air is polymerized incompletely. Therefore, having a lower content of residual monomer leads to more complete polymerization and thinner surface area exposed to the oxygen/air.

18. **B** Paragraph 1 states "54 million per year or one-third of all mortality."

19. **A** Paragraph 5 states that "United States Public Health System classifies biological and infectious agents based on rates of morbidity and mortality. In addition, infectious diseases can be classified based on the speed and geographical area they affect." Only infectious agents can be classified based on the speed and geographical area they affect.

20. **A** Paragraph 1 lists four factors causing the increase in infectious diseases in the United States. By far, international travel has the highest susceptibility to spreading infectious diseases.

21. **A** Paragraphs 2 and 3 state "well-known illnesses thought to be under control are reemerging and pose a serious global health threat" and "mortality rates associated with infectious diseases in the United States have increased by approximately 5 percent yearly, since 1980." No other information is provided to substantiate the remaining responses.

22. **B** This disease is listed under Category B in paragraph 5.

23. **A** Paragraph 6 states "Soldiers are immunized against many infectious diseases and are sensitized to detecting any symptoms before or after their return. Unfortunately, Reserve and National Guard soldiers must rely on the civilian health care system to diagnosis and treat postdeployment infections and illnesses." The civilian health care providers are immune to the threats that soldiers are subjected to in austere combat conditions overseas.

24. **E** Paragraph 3 explains a rogue nation's objectives in using an infectious agent to target population centers in the United States.

25. **B** Paragraph 6 identifies the three categories of threats. Category B states "these diseases are moderately easy to disseminate, result in moderate morbidity rates and low mortality rates, and require specific enhancements of CDC's diagnostic disease surveillance."

26. **D** Paragraph 6 explains the differences between endemic, pandemic, and epidemic—"the emergence of the swine flu in the United States several years ago led to an epidemic."

27. **C** Paragraph 6 explains the differences between endemic, pandemic, and epidemic—"A pandemic is a worldwide epidemic affecting an exceptionally high proportion of the global population. An example is HIV/AIDS. Pandemics are becoming increasingly common due to the ease of travel, flow of imports/exports, and large numbers of continuously moving refugees and displaced persons throughout the world.

28. **B** Paragraph 2 states, "Infectious disease is the leading cause of death globally, accounting for a quarter to one-third of the estimated deaths in 1998."

29. **E** Paragraph 4 addresses globalization of the nation's food supply. All the above actions would reduce infectious disease from the importation of fruits and vegetables.

30. **D** Paragraph 6 discusses emerging pathogens and states "Category C agents are emerging pathogens that could be engineered for mass dissemination in the future due to availability and ease of production and dissemination and potential for high morbidity and mortality rates."

31. **C** Paragraph 3 addresses the mortality rate in the United States due to infectious diseases to be 59 deaths per 100,000. A five percent yearly increase would place the 1990 infectious disease rate at 98.80 deaths per 100,000.

32. **E** Paragraph 4 cites reasons for misuse of offensive biological agents, but does not discuss avoidance measures employed by the United States government.

33. **E** Paragraph 8 talks about "highly exportable" disease. Of those listed is Mycobacterium Tuberculosis which is the caustic, viral agent spread exclusively by small-particle aerosols to a susceptible host not previously infected with the organism.

34. **C** Paragraph 8 reviews the biological pathogens and their mode of transmission. It describes that infectious bacterium Yersinia Pestis plaque is spread by rodents and fleas around the world and through direct contact with infected animals.

35. **C** This question is a retrieval question that requires you to review the entire passage and determine if any of the responses were discussed by the author. This article does not mention specific dental needs of the American population, nor does it discuss why patients are sometimes overtreated. Paragraph 15 summarizes the article and states, "no definitive scientific study has determined the correct occlusal philosophy or scheme for dentate, partially or totally edentulous patients. Dentistry continues to deliver uncalibrated occlusal treatment, which is not based on scientific evidence."

36. **E** This question is a retrieval question that requires you to review paragraph 5. This article states that to have a thorough understanding of occlusion, the dental practitioner must understand how teeth, temporomandibular joint, muscles, and the neuromuscular anatomy work together. Each response is correct, but mastery level requires an understanding of all the components.

37. **C** This question is a retrieval question that requires you to locate the part of the passage that describes the most important term in dentistry. Paragraph 6 discusses why dental occlusion is often challenging and difficult to understand. The first subparagraph on complicated terminology states that the most important and useful definition in dentistry is the term centric relation (CR). This should be the dental practitioner's starting point for any occlusal restoration or replacement of missing teeth. The other choices are definition for positions along Posselt's diagram in a sagittal plane.

38. **C** This question is a retrieval question that requires you to locate the part of the passage that describes occlusal schemes. Paragraph 12 states, "group function, which tries to stabilize lateral gliding forces over several teeth on the same side." This relationship reduces

the occlusal forces on the canine teeth during eccentric movements. No other response is appropriate for this definition.

39. **D** This question asks you to draw a conclusion based on information in the passage. Paragraph 8 "Complex Mandibular Movements" defines point A as the motion of the mandible around an axis or hinge. Point B is the maximum opening of the mandible due to translation or gliding of the condyles down the eminence. The neuromuscular system is responsible for all muscle movements. The teeth are not involved in this movement.

40. **E** This question asks you to draw a conclusion based on information in the passage. It is hard to believe that some things on the Internet are NOT true. The large difference between the hits on the Internet and peer-reviewed, evidence-based articles indicates that dentistry lacks the scientific research and studies to prescribe one treatment for similar patient diagnosis.

41. **E** This question is an inference question that requires you to review the entire passage and summarize its content. Keys to answering this question can usually be found in the introduction or closing paragraphs. As you evaluate each response, eliminate those choices that focus on just individual paragraphs. This article addresses every possible response.

42. **C** This is a retrieval question that asks you to locate the person or organization responsible for defining mandibular movements. Paragraph 6 describes accomplishments of the Gnathology Society and the development of the dental articulator in the early 1900's as important in defining and relating the mandibular movements outside the mouth.

43. **A** This question is an inference question that requires you to review the basic movements of the mandible from Figure 1. Paragraph 8 states that position F is the maximum protrusion. No other points on the graph are correct.

44. **A** This question is a retrieval question that requires you to locate the part of the passage that describes the neuromuscular process. The question is the definition for lateral pterygoid. No other response is appropriate for this question.

45. **E** This question is a retrieval question that requires you to locate the part of the passage that describes complicated terminology. Several words can be used to describe the closing of teeth together.

46. **D** This question is a retrieval question that requires you to locate the part of the passage that describes dental education, paragraph 14. CODA is the accreditation organization and, the National Boards, part I is the test dental students must pass to move to next phase clinical and preclinical training.

47. **E** This question requires you to understand how the teeth, neuromuscular system, temporomandibular joint, and anatomy affect occlusion. The permanent teeth are an important part of occlusion since they are the only structures that can cut, chew, and incise food.

48. **A** This question is a conceptual question. Paragraph 8 describes movement in three dimensions, but does not diagram the motion from the horizontal plane. This question asks you to IMAGINE moving your mandibular teeth forward, right, back, left, forward, and describe what that motion would look like. Motion in this plane would look like a square rotated 90 degrees.

49. **D** This question is a retrieval question that requires you to locate the part of the passage that describes philosophy of occlusion, paragraph 11. The question being asked is the definition of conformative philosophy. All the other choices would not apply to this definition.

50. **C** This question is a retrieval question that requires you to locate the part of the passage that describes dental specialist, paragraph 1. The question being asked is the definition of the duties and responsibilities of a prosthodontist.

Quantitative Reasoning Test

1. **C** We are looking for the union of "scones" and "donuts." So,

P(scones ∪ donuts) = P(scones) + P(donuts) − P(scones ∩ donuts) = 0.3 + 0.5 − 0.2 = 0.6 = 60%.

2. **E** This is easiest to compute using the complement. The probability that no "tails" appears is the complement of at least one "tails" appears. The probability that no "tails" appears is the probability that all "heads" appears: $P(HHH) = \left(\frac{1}{2}\right)\left(\frac{1}{2}\right)\left(\frac{1}{2}\right) = \frac{1}{8}$. Here, we assume that the coin flips are independent as is usual for coin flipping. So, the probability of our intended event "at least one tails" is $1 - P(\text{no tails}) = 1 - \frac{1}{8} = \frac{7}{8}$.

3. **B** Let's pick numbers. Let $r = 2$, and $h = 2$. The original volume is

$$\frac{1}{3}\pi r^2 h = \frac{1}{3}\pi(2)^2 2 = \frac{1}{3}\pi(8)$$

The new r is $2 + 1 = 3$, and the new $h = 2 + 1 = 3$. The new volume is $\frac{1}{3}\pi(3)^2 3 = \frac{1}{3}\pi(27)$.

The percent change is

$$\frac{\text{find} - \text{initial}}{\text{initial}} \times 100\% = \frac{\frac{27}{3}\pi - \frac{8}{3}\pi}{\frac{8}{3}\pi} \times 100\% = \frac{\frac{19}{3}}{\frac{8}{3}} \times 100\% = \frac{19}{8} \times 100\% = 2.375 \times 100\% = 237.5\%$$

See *www.youtube.com/user/Swartwoodprep* for video version as well as an alternate explanation.

4. **C**

Column A:

The diagonal of the square is the diameter of the circle. The length of the diagonal must then be 2(1) = 2. The square is cut into two right triangles by any given diagonal. Since the triangles cut out are 45-45-90 right triangles, the length of the diagonal is $s\sqrt{2}$, where s is the length of either side. $2 = s\sqrt{2}$, so $s = \frac{2}{\sqrt{2}}$. The area of the square is then $s^2 = \left(\frac{2}{\sqrt{2}}\right)^2 = \frac{4}{\left(\sqrt{2}\right)^2} = \frac{4}{2} = 2$. This can also be noticed directly from the fact that the length of the diagonal comes from the Pythagorean theorem, and that the lengths of the sides are the same.

Column B:

The diameter of the circle is $2\left(\dfrac{\sqrt{2}}{2}\right) = \sqrt{2}$. But the diameter of the circle is the length of the side of the square. Thus, the area of the square is $\left(\sqrt{2}\right)^2 = 2$.

The columns are equal.

5. **E** This is basically a test of rules. When you get problems like this on the DAT, they are basically giving you points, so you should take them. Make sure you are comfortable with the "manipulation of mean and variance." Since each score is doubled, and then has three added to it, the mean will also double and then have 3 added to it.

6. **C** Organization is key to making this problem simpler:

(1) The average at the end will come from $\dfrac{\text{total}}{\text{\# scores}}$. The total number of scores is

$$(7 - 2) + (8 - 2) = 11$$

(2) We go after the total points. From Set A, we know that the original total was:

$$\frac{\text{total}}{\text{\# scores}} = \frac{\text{total}}{7} = 50 \rightarrow \text{total} = 50(7) = 350$$

The original total from Set B was:

$$\frac{\text{total}}{\text{\# scores}} = \frac{\text{total}}{8} = 60 \rightarrow \text{total} = 60(8) = 480$$

(3) After the two scores are removed from Set B, we have:

$$\frac{\text{total}}{\text{\# scores}} = \frac{\text{total}}{6} = 70 \rightarrow 70(6) = 420$$

(4) The difference between the old total for Set B and the new total is $480 - 420 = 60$. So, the two scores add up to 60.

(5) We now find the total when we place all the scores together, minus the four scores we have removed.

420 (total from Set B after two of the scores have been removed) + 350 – 60 (total from Set A after the two scores have been deleted) = 710.

Back to (1) $\dfrac{\text{total}}{\text{\# scores}} = \dfrac{\text{total}}{11} = \dfrac{710}{11}$. Here, it is easy to see that the average is over 60 but less than 70. You can, of course, just use the calculator.

7. **C** This can be solved as a system of equations or a rate problem. For example, D = RT.

$$120 = R_{\text{Rila}}\,(70) \rightarrow R_{\text{Rila}} = \frac{120}{70}\,.\ 180 = R_{\text{Jennifer}}\,(50) \rightarrow R_{\text{Jennifer}} = \frac{180}{50}$$

$$R_{\text{Total}} = \frac{12}{7} + \frac{18}{5} = \frac{186}{35}\,.\ D_{\text{Total}} = R_{\text{Total}} T_{\text{Total}} \rightarrow 3720 = \left(\frac{186}{35}\right)(T_{\text{Total}})$$

$$T_{\text{Total}} = 700$$

There is a much slicker solution shown at *www.youtube.com/user/Swartwoodprep*.

8. **E** While this can be factored and solved, plugging in is a good option. 0 gives $0^3 - 15(0) - 4 \neq 0$, so choice (C) is out. 2 gives $2^2 - 15(2) - 4 = 0$, so choice (D) is out. 4 gives $4^3 - 15(4) - 4 = 0$, so choice (E) is the winner. In case you tried choices (A) or (B), –4 gives $(-4)^3 - 15(-4) - 4 \neq 0$ and –2 gives $(-2)^3 - 15(-2) - 4 \neq 0$.

9. **E** This is a distance problem. D = RT. Don't forget to convert from km to m.

2.15×10^{20} km is 2.15×10^{23} m. This is approximately 2×10^{23} m.

Then, $2 \times 10^{23} = (3 \times 10^8 \text{ m/s})(T)$

$T = 0.67 \times 10^{15}$ s

$T = 6.7 \times 10^{14}$ s

10. **A** You can plug in any set of numbers to verify. If more than one equation works, make sure to try another set of numbers. (This will not happen in this question, but may in others.) But the easiest way is to notice that y increases as x increases, so the slope must be positive. Additionally, x must increase more than one point for y to increase one point, so the slope must be less than one.

11. **A** Picking 10 and 20 leads to a quick solution. Let T = 10, R = 1, and $n = 20$.

Then, PV = 200. If T increases by 100%, then T = 20. (10 + 10)

If n increases by 25%, then $n = 20 + 5 = 25$. (We choose 20 since 25% of 20 is easy to calculate.) So, PV = 25(1)(20) = 500. The percent increase is

$$\frac{\text{final} - \text{initial}}{\text{initial}} = \frac{500 - 200}{200} = \frac{300}{200} = 150\%$$

12. **C** Recall that the general equation for an ellipse is $\dfrac{(x-h)^2}{a^2} + \dfrac{(y-k)^2}{b^2} = 1$. a *is* the semi-major axis length, so choices (B) and (C) are the only real options. Since the center is (h, k), $h = 1$ and $k = 5$.

13. **E** We can plug in answer choices, but here the straightforward computation is effective.

Total travel is 50 + 250 = 300. D = R(T). 300 = 50(T).

$T = 6 \to$ T for the second part = $6 - 3 = 3$.

$\text{Dist}_{\text{second}} = RT$

$250 = R(3)$

$R = \dfrac{250}{3} = 83.33$

14. **C** Since the area of the sector is π, the angle enclosed must be 90°.

$$\frac{\text{sec}}{\text{area of circle}} = \frac{\pi}{4\pi} \to \text{area of } \frac{\text{sec}}{\text{area of circle}} = \frac{1}{4} \to \frac{1}{4} = \frac{\theta}{360} \to \theta = 90$$

Here, sec refers to the area of the sector (see the geometry section of your Barron's book

for a refresher).

$$\text{Circumference} = \frac{\theta}{360} = \frac{90}{360} = \frac{1}{4}$$

$$\text{Circumference} = \frac{\text{arc } s}{4\pi} = \frac{1}{4} \to s = \pi$$

15. **C** You can plug in answer choices or try:

$$a + (a + 1) + (a + 2) = 3a + 3 = 330$$

$$3a = 327$$

$$a = 109$$

So, $a + 2 = 111$.

16. **A** There are many ways to add the times. Just remember that once the total for sec hits 60, 1 minute has passed. Likewise 60 min = 1 hr.

$$
\begin{array}{r}
12:53 \\
15:27 \\
17:30 \\
18:35 \\
23:10 \\
\underline{19:45} \\
104:200
\end{array}
$$

1 hr, 44 min, 3 min 20s

1 hr, 47 min, 20s

17. **C**

$$2^y = (2^4)^{y-15}$$

$$2^y = 2^{4y-60}$$

$$y = 4y - 60$$

$$3y = 60$$

$$y = 20$$

18. **C** The easiest way (maybe) to think of this problem is to imagine 3 blocks: Freshmen, Juniors, and Seniors. We can permute them 3! = 6 ways. We must then place the 3 freshmen in 3! = 6 ways, the 2 juniors in 2! = 2 ways, and the 2 seniors in 2! = 2 ways. There are then $6 \times 6 \times 2 \times 2 = 144$ ways to do this.

19. **B** Here, looking at only the "given" cases results in 12 options:

5, 1

…

5, 6

6, 1

…

6, 6

Of these 12 options, only 3 give 11 or higher:

5, 6

6, 5

6, 6

So, $\dfrac{3}{12}$ is the answer.

20. **B** Although the numbers are small and you can write out the possibilities, it is not that hard to see that you have $\begin{pmatrix} 5 \\ 2 \end{pmatrix} = \dfrac{5!}{2!3!} = 10$ ways of choosing the 2 people, and 2 ways of choosing the president from the 2. This gives $10(2) = 20$.

21. **E** (1) is not sufficient since we do not know the probability of a cookie being picked from store A, and since we do not know the probabilities of the other cases (store B, etc.).

(2) is not sufficient since knowing the probability that a cookie is from store A given that it is chocolate, does not even give us the probability of getting a chocolate cookie given that the store was store A (without more information), much less a chocolate cookie regardless of the store.

Even combined, the statements are not enough. We need something like:

(1) + the probability of ending up at store A [P(A)] + the probability of picking a chocolate cookie if the store chosen is not A [P(C/A^c)]. Then, we could say

$$P(C) = P(C/A)P(A) + P(C/A^c)P(A)^c$$

22. **A** $\quad \dfrac{2y - 3\alpha}{2\alpha} = 3y + 5 \rightarrow 2y - 3\alpha = (3y + 5)2\alpha \rightarrow 2y - 3\alpha = 6y\alpha + 10\alpha)$

$$\rightarrow y(2 - 6\alpha) = 13\alpha \rightarrow y = \dfrac{13\alpha}{(2 - 6\alpha)}$$

23. **C** The surface area of the side of the can is $2\pi rh = 2\pi(3)(10) = 60\pi$. Since paint costs $1.00 per cm^2, the cost is 60π.

24. **A** While this can be done directly as $y(3.5) = \dfrac{35}{13}$, a quicker way might be to reduce the fractions so that the denominators are all 13. Then, just compare the numerators. For choice (A), $\dfrac{10}{13}$ increased by a factor of 3.5—350%—gives $\dfrac{35}{13}$. Note that 50% of 10 is 5, and 300% of 10 is 30, so 350% of 10 is $5 + 30 = 35$ (fairly fast).

Traditionally: $y(3.5) = \dfrac{35}{13} \rightarrow y = \dfrac{10}{13}$.

25. **C** Make things look alike:

Column A

$$\sqrt[3]{21600} - \sqrt[3]{6400} = \sqrt[3]{6^3(100)} - \sqrt[3]{4^3(100)}$$
$$\sqrt[3]{6^3}\sqrt[3]{100} - \sqrt[3]{4^3}\sqrt[3]{100}$$
$$6\sqrt[3]{100} - 4\sqrt[3]{100} = 2\sqrt[3]{100}$$

Column B

$$\sqrt[3]{800} = \sqrt[3]{2^3(100)} = \sqrt[3]{2^3}\sqrt[3]{(100)}$$
$$2\sqrt[3]{(100)}$$

Clearly, $2\sqrt[3]{(100)} = 2\sqrt[3]{(100)}$.

26. **C** Since every 5 seconds a pebble is placed in, and every 15 seconds a pebble is removed, every 15 seconds we have 3 pebbles added and 1 removed. (We chose 15 s to give both the rate of addition and subtraction common ground.) This gives $3 - 1 = 2$ pebbles per 15 s. The rate is $\dfrac{2}{15}$ pebbles/sec.

$$\dfrac{2 \text{ pebbles}}{15 \text{ s}} \Rightarrow \dfrac{15 \text{ s}}{2 \text{ pebbles}}$$

Divide the top and bottom by 2 to get $\dfrac{\frac{15}{2} \text{ s}}{1 \text{ pebble}}$, so that it is easy to see that the s per pebble is $\dfrac{15}{2}$.

27. **C** One thing to do is eliminate choice (A) since both a, b must each be bigger than 3. Since 5 and 7 are prime, any number that has both as factors must contain 5 and 7. The smallest of these is 35. So, set $5(a-3) = 35$. $a = 10$. $(b-3)7 = 35$ gives $b = 8$

$$a + b = 18$$

28. **A** Here, combining is the fastest way to solve this problem.

$$\frac{y}{y-5} + \frac{2y}{y-7} = \frac{y(y-7) + 2y(y-5)}{(y-5)(y-7)} = \frac{y^2 - 7y + 2y^2 - 10y}{(y-5)(y-7)} = \frac{3y^2 - 17y}{(y-5)(y-7)} = \frac{y(3y-17)}{(y-5)(y-7)}$$

29. **B** Call the other number a.

$$\alpha = \frac{a + \gamma + \beta}{3}$$
$$3\alpha = a + \gamma + \beta$$
$$a = 3\alpha - \gamma - \beta$$

30. **B** Pick 100.

$100 + 20 = 120$ after first raise

$120 + 120(0.3) = 156$ after second raise

Percent increase $= \dfrac{\text{final} - \text{initial}}{\text{initial}} = \dfrac{156 - 100}{100} = .56$

56%

31. **C** We examine the slope-intercept form of both lines.

$$y = ax - b$$
$$y = -Ax + B$$

Since the lines are perpendicular, $a = 1/A$. So, $Aa = A(1/A) = 1$.

32. **C** $350 \times 15 = 5{,}250$ mL. 1 L = 1,000 mL. 5.25 L are contained.

33. **B** Rather than run this on the calculator, remember that dividing by a fraction is multiplying by the reciprocal.

$$\frac{1}{\frac{1}{3}} + \frac{12}{\frac{12}{1}} + \frac{5}{\frac{5}{2}} + \frac{12}{\frac{6}{14}} + \frac{2}{\frac{2}{31}}$$

Only $\dfrac{12}{\frac{6}{14}} = 12\left(\dfrac{14}{6}\right) = 28$ involves some computation.

$3 + 1 + 2 + 28 + 31$

65

34. **C** $\qquad |x-3| < 5 \rightarrow x - 3 < 5 \text{ or } -(x-3) < 5 \rightarrow x < 8 \text{ and } x > -2$

Shortcut: $|x-3| < 5 \rightarrow -5 < x - 3 < 5 \rightarrow -2 < x < 8$

35. **B** Rather than try out all the numbers, we can notice that 13 is prime, and that it is not a factor of any of the given factors: $3 \times 15 \times 25 \times 16 \times 19$.

36. **C** The probability that a ticket is given is $\frac{2}{3}$. The probability that a ticket is not given is $\frac{1}{3}$. Thus, since the events are independent, the probability TTTNN happens [T = ticket, N = no ticket] is $\frac{2}{3} \cdot \frac{2}{3} \cdot \frac{2}{3} \cdot \frac{1}{3} \cdot \frac{1}{3} = \frac{8}{243}$.

But, TTNTN, TNTTN, etc. also work. There are $\binom{5}{3} = 10$ ways 3Ts and 2Ns can be chosen (picture the "spots" labeled 1–5 and pick any three of them to be the tickets). See the probability section for a refresher. In total, the probability is $\frac{8}{243}(10) = \frac{80}{243}$.

37. **C** If you do not like these sorts of problems, skip them. If you chose to do this or come back to do the question, you might want to think of the problem as:

(1) One ball must be green so ignore it. Consider 4 balls to be picked from the remaining ten.

(2) If we choose all 4 balls from the red group, no number can be picked twice. There are $\binom{5}{4} = 5$ ways to do this. (Alternately, think of discarding one ball from the five to get 4. This can be done 5 ways.) The same is true if all of the balls are black $\binom{5}{4} = 5$. So, there are 10 ways if the balls are all the same color.

(3) Imagine we choose 3 to be red and 1 to be black. Pick the black one first. There are 5 ways to do this. Whatever number the black ball is, that number must be excluded from the red balls picked. So, there are $\binom{4}{3} = 4$ ways to do this. There are $5 \times 4 = 20$ ways. The same holds if we choose 3 black/1 red as our choice. There are $20 + 20 = 40$ ways this can happen.

(4) If we choose 2 red balls and 2 black balls, there are $\binom{5}{2} = 10$ ways to pick the red ball. But, the ball picked must be excluded from the list of options for choosing the black balls from, so there are $\binom{3}{2} = 3$ ways to pick the black balls. Hence, there are $10(3) = 30$ ways to do this.

(5) Picking 1 red and 3 black and vice versa has been done (see 3). Picking 0 red and 4 black and vice versa has been done (see 1).

So, altogether, there are $10 + 40 + 30 = 80$ ways.

38. **A**

$$\frac{1}{\log x} + \frac{1}{\log y} = \frac{4}{3}$$

$$\frac{\log y}{(\log x)(\log y)} + \frac{\log x}{(\log y)(\log x)}$$

$$\frac{\log y + \log x}{(\log y)(\log x)} = \frac{\log(yx)}{(\log y)(\log x)} = \frac{4}{(\log y)(\log x)} = \frac{4}{3}$$

$$\frac{4}{(\log y)(\log x)} = \frac{4}{3}$$

$$\frac{1}{(\log y)(\log x)} = \frac{1}{3}$$

$$(\log y)(\log x) = 3$$

39. **A** The note in parentheses advises that the scores represent the entire population, so the

$$\text{variance} = \frac{\displaystyle\sum_{i=1}^{N}(x_i - avg)^2}{N}.$$

$$\frac{\displaystyle\sum_{i=1}^{N}(x_i - avg)^2}{10} = 75$$

$$\sum_{i=1}^{N}(x_i - avg)^2 = 750$$

Since 30 is the average (compute it), it does not contribute to $\displaystyle\sum_{i=1}^{N}(x_i - avg)^2$, but it increases N from 10 to 11.

$$\frac{\displaystyle\sum_{i=1}^{N}(x_i - avg)^2}{11}$$

$$\frac{750}{11}$$

$$68.18$$

40. **B** You were rewarded with this easier version of 37 if you skipped 37 and pushed on. The probability the first ball is black is $\frac{2}{5}$. The probability that the second ball is black given that the first is black is $\frac{1}{4}$. The probability that both events occur is $\frac{2}{5} \cdot \frac{1}{4} = \frac{1}{10}$

Alternate approach:

$$\frac{\dbinom{2}{2}\dbinom{3}{0}}{\dbinom{5}{2}} = \frac{1}{10}$$

Top: Choose 2 black from 2 black; pick 0 red from the red.

Bottom: Take out 2 balls from all 5.

ANSWER SHEET
Practice Test 2

Survey of the Natural Sciences Test

1. Ⓐ Ⓑ Ⓒ Ⓓ Ⓔ
2. Ⓐ Ⓑ Ⓒ Ⓓ Ⓔ
3. Ⓐ Ⓑ Ⓒ Ⓓ Ⓔ
4. Ⓐ Ⓑ Ⓒ Ⓓ Ⓔ
5. Ⓐ Ⓑ Ⓒ Ⓓ Ⓔ
6. Ⓐ Ⓑ Ⓒ Ⓓ Ⓔ
7. Ⓐ Ⓑ Ⓒ Ⓓ Ⓔ
8. Ⓐ Ⓑ Ⓒ Ⓓ Ⓔ
9. Ⓐ Ⓑ Ⓒ Ⓓ Ⓔ
10. Ⓐ Ⓑ Ⓒ Ⓓ Ⓔ
11. Ⓐ Ⓑ Ⓒ Ⓓ Ⓔ
12. Ⓐ Ⓑ Ⓒ Ⓓ Ⓔ
13. Ⓐ Ⓑ Ⓒ Ⓓ Ⓔ
14. Ⓐ Ⓑ Ⓒ Ⓓ Ⓔ
15. Ⓐ Ⓑ Ⓒ Ⓓ Ⓔ
16. Ⓐ Ⓑ Ⓒ Ⓓ Ⓔ
17. Ⓐ Ⓑ Ⓒ Ⓓ Ⓔ
18. Ⓐ Ⓑ Ⓒ Ⓓ Ⓔ
19. Ⓐ Ⓑ Ⓒ Ⓓ Ⓔ
20. Ⓐ Ⓑ Ⓒ Ⓓ Ⓔ
21. Ⓐ Ⓑ Ⓒ Ⓓ Ⓔ
22. Ⓐ Ⓑ Ⓒ Ⓓ Ⓔ
23. Ⓐ Ⓑ Ⓒ Ⓓ Ⓔ
24. Ⓐ Ⓑ Ⓒ Ⓓ Ⓔ
25. Ⓐ Ⓑ Ⓒ Ⓓ Ⓔ

26. Ⓐ Ⓑ Ⓒ Ⓓ Ⓕ
27. Ⓐ Ⓑ Ⓒ Ⓓ Ⓔ
28. Ⓐ Ⓑ Ⓒ Ⓓ Ⓔ
29. Ⓐ Ⓑ Ⓒ Ⓓ Ⓔ
30. Ⓐ Ⓑ Ⓒ Ⓓ Ⓔ
31. Ⓐ Ⓑ Ⓒ Ⓓ Ⓔ
32. Ⓐ Ⓑ Ⓒ Ⓓ Ⓔ
33. Ⓐ Ⓑ Ⓒ Ⓓ Ⓔ
34. Ⓐ Ⓑ Ⓒ Ⓓ Ⓔ
35. Ⓐ Ⓑ Ⓒ Ⓓ Ⓔ
36. Ⓐ Ⓑ Ⓒ Ⓓ Ⓔ
37. Ⓐ Ⓑ Ⓒ Ⓓ Ⓔ
38. Ⓐ Ⓑ Ⓒ Ⓓ Ⓔ
39. Ⓐ Ⓑ Ⓒ Ⓓ Ⓔ
40. Ⓐ Ⓑ Ⓒ Ⓓ Ⓔ
41. Ⓐ Ⓑ Ⓒ Ⓓ Ⓔ
42. Ⓐ Ⓑ Ⓒ Ⓓ Ⓔ
43. Ⓐ Ⓑ Ⓒ Ⓓ Ⓔ
44. Ⓐ Ⓑ Ⓒ Ⓓ Ⓔ
45. Ⓐ Ⓑ Ⓒ Ⓓ Ⓔ
46. Ⓐ Ⓑ Ⓒ Ⓓ Ⓔ
47. Ⓐ Ⓑ Ⓒ Ⓓ Ⓔ
48. Ⓐ Ⓑ Ⓒ Ⓓ Ⓔ
49. Ⓐ Ⓑ Ⓒ Ⓓ Ⓔ
50. Ⓐ Ⓑ Ⓒ Ⓓ Ⓔ

51. Ⓐ Ⓑ Ⓒ Ⓓ Ⓔ
52. Ⓐ Ⓑ Ⓒ Ⓓ Ⓔ
53. Ⓐ Ⓑ Ⓒ Ⓓ Ⓔ
54. Ⓐ Ⓑ Ⓒ Ⓓ Ⓔ
55. Ⓐ Ⓑ Ⓒ Ⓓ Ⓔ
56. Ⓐ Ⓑ Ⓒ Ⓓ Ⓔ
57. Ⓐ Ⓑ Ⓒ Ⓓ Ⓔ
58. Ⓐ Ⓑ Ⓒ Ⓓ Ⓔ
59. Ⓐ Ⓑ Ⓒ Ⓓ Ⓔ
60. Ⓐ Ⓑ Ⓒ Ⓓ Ⓔ
61. Ⓐ Ⓑ Ⓒ Ⓓ Ⓔ
62. Ⓐ Ⓑ Ⓒ Ⓓ Ⓔ
63. Ⓐ Ⓑ Ⓒ Ⓓ Ⓔ
64. Ⓐ Ⓑ Ⓒ Ⓓ Ⓔ
65. Ⓐ Ⓑ Ⓒ Ⓓ Ⓔ
66. Ⓐ Ⓑ Ⓒ Ⓓ Ⓔ
67. Ⓐ Ⓑ Ⓒ Ⓓ Ⓔ
68. Ⓐ Ⓑ Ⓒ Ⓓ Ⓔ
69. Ⓐ Ⓑ Ⓒ Ⓓ Ⓔ
70. Ⓐ Ⓑ Ⓒ Ⓓ Ⓔ
71. Ⓐ Ⓑ Ⓒ Ⓓ Ⓔ
72. Ⓐ Ⓑ Ⓒ Ⓓ Ⓔ
73. Ⓐ Ⓑ Ⓒ Ⓓ Ⓔ
74. Ⓐ Ⓑ Ⓒ Ⓓ Ⓔ
75. Ⓐ Ⓑ Ⓒ Ⓓ Ⓔ

76. Ⓐ Ⓑ Ⓒ Ⓓ Ⓔ
77. Ⓐ Ⓑ Ⓒ Ⓓ Ⓔ
78. Ⓐ Ⓑ Ⓒ Ⓓ Ⓔ
79. Ⓐ Ⓑ Ⓒ Ⓓ Ⓔ
80. Ⓐ Ⓑ Ⓒ Ⓓ Ⓔ
81. Ⓐ Ⓑ Ⓒ Ⓓ Ⓔ
82. Ⓐ Ⓑ Ⓒ Ⓓ Ⓔ
83. Ⓐ Ⓑ Ⓒ Ⓓ Ⓔ
84. Ⓐ Ⓑ Ⓒ Ⓓ Ⓔ
85. Ⓐ Ⓑ Ⓒ Ⓓ Ⓔ
86. Ⓐ Ⓑ Ⓒ Ⓓ Ⓔ
87. Ⓐ Ⓑ Ⓒ Ⓓ Ⓔ
88. Ⓐ Ⓑ Ⓒ Ⓓ Ⓔ
89. Ⓐ Ⓑ Ⓒ Ⓓ Ⓔ
90. Ⓐ Ⓑ Ⓒ Ⓓ Ⓔ
91. Ⓐ Ⓑ Ⓒ Ⓓ Ⓔ
92. Ⓐ Ⓑ Ⓒ Ⓓ Ⓔ
93. Ⓐ Ⓑ Ⓒ Ⓓ Ⓔ
94. Ⓐ Ⓑ Ⓒ Ⓓ Ⓔ
95. Ⓐ Ⓑ Ⓒ Ⓓ Ⓔ
96. Ⓐ Ⓑ Ⓒ Ⓓ Ⓔ
97. Ⓐ Ⓑ Ⓒ Ⓓ Ⓔ
98. Ⓐ Ⓑ Ⓒ Ⓓ Ⓔ
99. Ⓐ Ⓑ Ⓒ Ⓓ Ⓔ
100. Ⓐ Ⓑ Ⓒ Ⓓ Ⓔ

Perceptual Ability Test

Part 1: Aperture Passing

1. Ⓐ Ⓑ Ⓒ Ⓓ Ⓔ   5. Ⓐ Ⓑ Ⓒ Ⓓ Ⓔ   9. Ⓐ Ⓑ Ⓒ Ⓓ Ⓔ   13. Ⓐ Ⓑ Ⓒ Ⓓ Ⓔ
2. Ⓐ Ⓑ Ⓒ Ⓓ Ⓔ   6. Ⓐ Ⓑ Ⓒ Ⓓ Ⓔ   10. Ⓐ Ⓑ Ⓒ Ⓓ Ⓔ   14. Ⓐ Ⓑ Ⓒ Ⓓ Ⓔ
3. Ⓐ Ⓑ Ⓒ Ⓓ Ⓔ   7. Ⓐ Ⓑ Ⓒ Ⓓ Ⓔ   11. Ⓐ Ⓑ Ⓒ Ⓓ Ⓔ   15. Ⓐ Ⓑ Ⓒ Ⓓ Ⓔ
4. Ⓐ Ⓑ Ⓒ Ⓓ Ⓔ   8. Ⓐ Ⓑ Ⓒ Ⓓ Ⓔ   12. Ⓐ Ⓑ Ⓒ Ⓓ Ⓔ

Part 2: Orthographic Projections

16. Ⓐ Ⓑ Ⓒ Ⓓ   20. Ⓐ Ⓑ Ⓒ Ⓓ   24. Ⓐ Ⓑ Ⓒ Ⓓ   28. Ⓐ Ⓑ Ⓒ Ⓓ
17. Ⓐ Ⓑ Ⓒ Ⓓ   21. Ⓐ Ⓑ Ⓒ Ⓓ   25. Ⓐ Ⓑ Ⓒ Ⓓ   29. Ⓐ Ⓑ Ⓒ Ⓓ
18. Ⓐ Ⓑ Ⓒ Ⓓ   22. Ⓐ Ⓑ Ⓒ Ⓓ   26. Ⓐ Ⓑ Ⓒ Ⓓ   30. Ⓐ Ⓑ Ⓒ Ⓓ
19. Ⓐ Ⓑ Ⓒ Ⓓ   23. Ⓐ Ⓑ Ⓒ Ⓓ   27. Ⓐ Ⓑ Ⓒ Ⓓ

Part 3: Angle Discrimination

31. Ⓐ Ⓑ Ⓒ Ⓓ   35. Ⓐ Ⓑ Ⓒ Ⓓ   39. Ⓐ Ⓑ Ⓒ Ⓓ   43. Ⓐ Ⓑ Ⓒ Ⓓ
32. Ⓐ Ⓑ Ⓒ Ⓓ   36. Ⓐ Ⓑ Ⓒ Ⓓ   40. Ⓐ Ⓑ Ⓒ Ⓓ   44. Ⓐ Ⓑ Ⓒ Ⓓ
33. Ⓐ Ⓑ Ⓒ Ⓓ   37. Ⓐ Ⓑ Ⓒ Ⓓ   41. Ⓐ Ⓑ Ⓒ Ⓓ   45. Ⓐ Ⓑ Ⓒ Ⓓ
34. Ⓐ Ⓑ Ⓒ Ⓓ   38. Ⓐ Ⓑ Ⓒ Ⓓ   42. Ⓐ Ⓑ Ⓒ Ⓓ

Part 4: Paper Folding

46. Ⓐ Ⓑ Ⓒ Ⓓ Ⓔ   50. Ⓐ Ⓑ Ⓒ Ⓓ Ⓔ   54. Ⓐ Ⓑ Ⓒ Ⓓ Ⓔ   58. Ⓐ Ⓑ Ⓒ Ⓓ Ⓔ
47. Ⓐ Ⓑ Ⓒ Ⓓ Ⓔ   51. Ⓐ Ⓑ Ⓒ Ⓓ Ⓔ   55. Ⓐ Ⓑ Ⓒ Ⓓ Ⓔ   59. Ⓐ Ⓑ Ⓒ Ⓓ Ⓔ
48. Ⓐ Ⓑ Ⓒ Ⓓ Ⓔ   52. Ⓐ Ⓑ Ⓒ Ⓓ Ⓔ   56. Ⓐ Ⓑ Ⓒ Ⓓ Ⓔ   60. Ⓐ Ⓑ Ⓒ Ⓓ Ⓔ
49. Ⓐ Ⓑ Ⓒ Ⓓ Ⓔ   53. Ⓐ Ⓑ Ⓒ Ⓓ Ⓔ   57. Ⓐ Ⓑ Ⓒ Ⓓ Ⓔ

Part 5: Cubes

61. Ⓐ Ⓑ Ⓒ Ⓓ Ⓔ   65. Ⓐ Ⓑ Ⓒ Ⓓ Ⓔ   69. Ⓐ Ⓑ Ⓒ Ⓓ Ⓔ   73. Ⓐ Ⓑ Ⓒ Ⓓ Ⓔ
62. Ⓐ Ⓑ Ⓒ Ⓓ Ⓔ   66. Ⓐ Ⓑ Ⓒ Ⓓ Ⓔ   70. Ⓐ Ⓑ Ⓒ Ⓓ Ⓔ   74. Ⓐ Ⓑ Ⓒ Ⓓ Ⓔ
63. Ⓐ Ⓑ Ⓒ Ⓓ Ⓔ   67. Ⓐ Ⓑ Ⓒ Ⓓ Ⓔ   71. Ⓐ Ⓑ Ⓒ Ⓓ Ⓔ   75. Ⓐ Ⓑ Ⓒ Ⓓ Ⓔ
64. Ⓐ Ⓑ Ⓒ Ⓓ Ⓔ   68. Ⓐ Ⓑ Ⓒ Ⓓ Ⓔ   72. Ⓐ Ⓑ Ⓒ Ⓓ Ⓔ

ANSWER SHEET
Practice Test 2

Part 6: Form Development

76. Ⓐ Ⓑ Ⓒ Ⓓ   80. Ⓐ Ⓑ Ⓒ Ⓓ   84. Ⓐ Ⓑ Ⓒ Ⓓ   88. Ⓐ Ⓓ Ⓒ Ⓓ

77. Ⓐ Ⓑ Ⓒ Ⓓ   81. Ⓐ Ⓑ Ⓒ Ⓓ   85. Ⓐ Ⓑ Ⓒ Ⓓ   89. Ⓐ Ⓑ Ⓒ Ⓓ

78. Ⓐ Ⓑ Ⓒ Ⓓ   82. Ⓐ Ⓑ Ⓒ Ⓓ   86. Ⓐ Ⓑ Ⓒ Ⓓ   90. Ⓐ Ⓑ Ⓒ Ⓓ

79. Ⓐ Ⓑ Ⓒ Ⓓ   83. Ⓐ Ⓑ Ⓒ Ⓓ   87. Ⓐ Ⓑ Ⓒ Ⓓ

Reading Comprehension Test

1. Ⓐ Ⓑ Ⓒ Ⓓ Ⓔ   14. Ⓐ Ⓑ Ⓒ Ⓓ Ⓔ   27. Ⓐ Ⓑ Ⓒ Ⓓ Ⓔ   40. Ⓐ Ⓑ Ⓒ Ⓓ Ⓔ

2. Ⓐ Ⓑ Ⓒ Ⓓ Ⓔ   15. Ⓐ Ⓑ Ⓒ Ⓓ Ⓔ   28. Ⓐ Ⓑ Ⓒ Ⓓ Ⓔ   41. Ⓐ Ⓑ Ⓒ Ⓓ Ⓔ

3. Ⓐ Ⓑ Ⓒ Ⓓ Ⓔ   16. Ⓐ Ⓑ Ⓒ Ⓓ Ⓔ   29. Ⓐ Ⓑ Ⓒ Ⓓ Ⓔ   42. Ⓐ Ⓑ Ⓒ Ⓓ Ⓔ

4. Ⓐ Ⓑ Ⓒ Ⓓ Ⓔ   17. Ⓐ Ⓑ Ⓒ Ⓓ Ⓔ   30. Ⓐ Ⓑ Ⓒ Ⓓ Ⓔ   43. Ⓐ Ⓑ Ⓒ Ⓓ Ⓔ

5. Ⓐ Ⓑ Ⓒ Ⓓ Ⓔ   18. Ⓐ Ⓑ Ⓒ Ⓓ Ⓔ   31. Ⓐ Ⓑ Ⓒ Ⓓ Ⓔ   44. Ⓐ Ⓑ Ⓒ Ⓓ Ⓔ

6. Ⓐ Ⓑ Ⓒ Ⓓ Ⓔ   19. Ⓐ Ⓑ Ⓒ Ⓓ Ⓔ   32. Ⓐ Ⓑ Ⓒ Ⓓ Ⓔ   45. Ⓐ Ⓑ Ⓒ Ⓓ Ⓔ

7. Ⓐ Ⓑ Ⓒ Ⓓ Ⓔ   20. Ⓐ Ⓑ Ⓒ Ⓓ Ⓔ   33. Ⓐ Ⓑ Ⓒ Ⓓ Ⓔ   46. Ⓐ Ⓑ Ⓒ Ⓓ Ⓔ

8. Ⓐ Ⓑ Ⓒ Ⓓ Ⓔ   21. Ⓐ Ⓑ Ⓒ Ⓓ Ⓔ   34. Ⓐ Ⓑ Ⓒ Ⓓ Ⓔ   47. Ⓐ Ⓑ Ⓒ Ⓓ Ⓔ

9. Ⓐ Ⓑ Ⓒ Ⓓ Ⓔ   22. Ⓐ Ⓑ Ⓒ Ⓓ Ⓔ   35. Ⓐ Ⓑ Ⓒ Ⓓ Ⓔ   48. Ⓐ Ⓑ Ⓒ Ⓓ Ⓔ

10. Ⓐ Ⓑ Ⓒ Ⓓ Ⓔ   23. Ⓐ Ⓑ Ⓒ Ⓓ Ⓔ   36. Ⓐ Ⓑ Ⓒ Ⓓ Ⓔ   49. Ⓐ Ⓑ Ⓒ Ⓓ Ⓔ

11. Ⓐ Ⓑ Ⓒ Ⓓ Ⓔ   24. Ⓐ Ⓑ Ⓒ Ⓓ Ⓔ   37. Ⓐ Ⓑ Ⓒ Ⓓ Ⓔ   50. Ⓐ Ⓑ Ⓒ Ⓓ Ⓔ

12. Ⓐ Ⓑ Ⓒ Ⓓ Ⓔ   25. Ⓐ Ⓑ Ⓒ Ⓓ Ⓔ   38. Ⓐ Ⓑ Ⓒ Ⓓ Ⓔ

13. Ⓐ Ⓑ Ⓒ Ⓓ Ⓔ   26. Ⓐ Ⓑ Ⓒ Ⓓ Ⓔ   39. Ⓐ Ⓑ Ⓒ Ⓓ Ⓔ

Quantitative Reasoning Test

1. Ⓐ Ⓑ Ⓒ Ⓓ Ⓔ   11. Ⓐ Ⓑ Ⓒ Ⓓ Ⓔ   21. Ⓐ Ⓑ Ⓒ Ⓓ Ⓔ   31. Ⓐ Ⓑ Ⓒ Ⓓ Ⓔ

2. Ⓐ Ⓑ Ⓒ Ⓓ Ⓔ   12. Ⓐ Ⓑ Ⓒ Ⓓ Ⓔ   22. Ⓐ Ⓑ Ⓒ Ⓓ Ⓔ   32. Ⓐ Ⓑ Ⓒ Ⓓ Ⓔ

3. Ⓐ Ⓑ Ⓒ Ⓓ Ⓔ   13. Ⓐ Ⓑ Ⓒ Ⓓ   23. Ⓐ Ⓑ Ⓒ Ⓓ Ⓔ   33. Ⓐ Ⓑ Ⓒ Ⓓ Ⓔ

4. Ⓐ Ⓑ Ⓒ Ⓓ Ⓔ   14. Ⓐ Ⓑ Ⓒ Ⓓ Ⓔ   24. Ⓐ Ⓑ Ⓒ Ⓓ Ⓔ   34. Ⓐ Ⓑ Ⓒ Ⓓ Ⓔ

5. Ⓐ Ⓑ Ⓒ Ⓓ   15. Ⓐ Ⓑ Ⓒ Ⓓ Ⓔ   25. Ⓐ Ⓑ Ⓒ Ⓓ Ⓔ   35. Ⓐ Ⓑ Ⓒ Ⓓ Ⓔ

6. Ⓐ Ⓑ Ⓒ Ⓓ Ⓔ   16. Ⓐ Ⓑ Ⓒ Ⓓ Ⓔ   26. Ⓐ Ⓑ Ⓒ Ⓓ Ⓔ   36. Ⓐ Ⓑ Ⓒ Ⓓ Ⓔ

7. Ⓐ Ⓑ Ⓒ Ⓓ Ⓔ   17. Ⓐ Ⓑ Ⓒ Ⓓ   27. Ⓐ Ⓑ Ⓒ Ⓓ Ⓔ   37. Ⓐ Ⓑ Ⓒ Ⓓ Ⓔ

8. Ⓐ Ⓑ Ⓒ Ⓓ Ⓔ   18. Ⓐ Ⓑ Ⓒ Ⓓ   28. Ⓐ Ⓑ Ⓒ Ⓓ Ⓔ   38. Ⓐ Ⓑ Ⓒ Ⓓ Ⓔ

9. Ⓐ Ⓑ Ⓒ Ⓓ Ⓔ   19. Ⓐ Ⓑ Ⓒ Ⓓ Ⓔ   29. Ⓐ Ⓑ Ⓒ Ⓓ Ⓔ   39. Ⓐ Ⓑ Ⓒ Ⓓ Ⓔ

10. Ⓐ Ⓑ Ⓒ Ⓓ Ⓔ   20. Ⓐ Ⓑ Ⓒ Ⓓ Ⓔ   30. Ⓐ Ⓑ Ⓒ Ⓓ Ⓔ   40. Ⓐ Ⓑ Ⓒ Ⓓ Ⓔ

Practice Test 2

TIME LIMIT: 90 MINUTES

Directions: The following items are questions or incomplete statements. Read each item carefully, and then choose the best answer. Blacken the corresponding space on the answer sheet.

1. Which one of the following statements best describes the difference between the nucleotide sequences
   (1) ATAAAGTCCAAAATTGTT and
   (2) GCUUAGGGGCUACCGA?

   (A) Sequence 1 is RNA.
   (B) Sequence 2 is more stable than sequence 1.
   (C) Sequence 2 is DNA.
   (D) Sequence 1 is more stable than sequence 2.
   (E) Sequence 2 contains more purines than sequence 1.

2. What is the difference between transcription and translation?

   (A) In transcription, a polypeptide is made from DNA. In translation, mRNA is made from DNA.
   (B) In transcription, the template sequence is RNA. In translation, the addition of amino acids is based on codons.
   (C) In transcription, mRNA is made from DNA. In translation, the template is DNA.
   (D) In transcription, anticodons specify the mRNA sequence. In translation, ribosomes move along a DNA template.
   (E) In transcription, mRNA is made from DNA. In translation, a polypeptide is made from mRNA.

3. The secondary structure of a protein is defined by its

   (A) combination of α-helixes and β-pleated sheets.
   (B) sequence of amino acids.
   (C) number of subunits.
   (D) enzymatic activity.
   (E) folding.

4. An important role of kinases in biological reactions is to

   (A) add carbohydrate to a protein.
   (B) add phosphate to a protein.
   (C) add phosphate to DNA.
   (D) remove phosphate from a protein.
   (E) add an amino group to a protein.

5. Two coenzymes nicotinamide adenine dinucleotide (NAD^+) and flavin adenine dinucleotide (FAD^+) are essential for glycolysis and respiration because they

   (A) function as terminal electron donors.
   (B) regulate the fixation of carbon dioxide (CO_2).
   (C) catalyze the synthesis of ATP.
   (D) function as electron acceptors.
   (E) facilitate the uptake of glucose.

6. Energy or ATP is produced in fungi by which one of the following structures?

(A) Spores
(B) Chloroplasts
(C) Mitochondria
(D) Peroxisomes
(E) Phosphosomes

7. Members of the domain Archaea typically live in habitats suitable for the growth of

(A) thermophiles.
(B) pathogens.
(C) symbionts.
(D) endosymbionts.
(E) angiosperms.

8. Cladistics is the

(A) description, classification, identification, and naming of organisms.
(B) process by which populations of organisms become altered over relatively long periods of time.
(C) study of evolutionary relationships among organisms by comparing gene sequencing data.
(D) classification of organisms based on the phylogenetic relationships of groups of organisms.
(E) study of the interactions between organisms and their environments.

9. By the end of mitosis and cytokinesis, two daughter cells are formed. Which one of the following statements best describes the state of the chromosomes in each of the daughter cells?

(A) Each has double the number of chromosomes as the parent cell.
(B) Each has half the number of chromosomes as the parent cell.
(C) Each has the same number of chromosomes as the parent cell.
(D) Each has the same number of chromosomes as the parent cell when it is in anaphase.
(E) The two daughter cells have an unequal number of chromosomes.

10. Which one of the following is not a polymer of glucose?

(A) Glycogen
(B) Starch
(C) Cellulose
(D) Amylose
(E) Insulin

11. A major difference between prokaryotic and eukaryotic ribosomes is the

(A) lipid composition of the membrane.
(B) number of chromosomes.
(C) size of the large subunit.
(D) length of the mRNA.
(E) amount of ATP that is made.

12. If a red blood cell is placed in a hypotonic solution, the cell will

(A) burst because water enters the cell to balance the internal and external salt concentrations.
(B) shrink because water enters the cell to balance the internal and external salt concentrations.
(C) burst because salt enters the cell to balance the internal and external salt concentrations.
(D) swell because water leaves the cell to balance the internal and external salt concentrations.
(E) do nothing.

13. The first law of thermodynamics states that

    (A) the capacity to do work is based on a relationship between time and temperature.
    (B) no natural process can occur unless it is accompanied by an increase in the entropy or degree of disorder of the universe.
    (C) the production of energy is inversely proportional to the amount of glucose available.
    (D) energy can be changed from one form to another but neither be created nor destroyed.
    (E) the conversion of energy that occurs in cells and structures is dependent on the type of biochemical reaction.

14. The hydronium ion (H_3O^+) concentration, as measured on a standard scale of 1–14, of an environment has important consequences in biology because

    (A) many types of cells require pH values around 10.0 for growth.
    (B) pH values that deviate significantly above and below 7.0 can denature enzymes.
    (C) fermentation reactions are optimal at a pH value of 2.0.
    (D) ATP synthesis cannot occur at pH 7.0.
    (E) pathogens are more aggressive at pH values in the range of 9.0–12.0.

15. Each of the following statements describes a difference between asexual and sexual reproduction EXCEPT one. Which one is the EXCEPTION?

    (A) Ability of offspring to pass on genetic information
    (B) Number of parents needed
    (C) Time required to complete the process
    (D) Fusion of gametes
    (E) Same number of offspring

16. The most common method of reproduction in "yeast" is

    (A) formation of hyphae.
    (B) formation of gametes.
    (C) binary fission.
    (D) conjugation.
    (E) budding.

17. DNA polymerase functions in DNA synthesis by

    (A) separating the two DNA strands to create a replication fork.
    (B) directing the synthesis of new DNA strands in a 5′ to 3′ direction.
    (C) attaching the RNA primer to the 5′ strand template.
    (D) separating the sister chromatids to chromosomes during anaphase.
    (E) dissolving the nuclear membrane.

18. Another name for flowering plants is

    (A) monera.
    (B) bryophytes.
    (C) angiosperms.
    (D) conifers.
    (E) gymnosperms.

19. All of the following statements about alleles are true EXCEPT one. Which one is the EXCEPTION?

    (A) Alleles make up the phenotype of an organism.
    (B) New alleles can be produced by mutation.
    (C) Alleles are found on different chromosomes.
    (D) Alleles are inherited.
    (E) Alleles represent different copies of the same gene.

20. Organisms that contain one set of chromosomes

    (A) reproduce by mitosis.
    (B) are haploid.
    (C) are eukaryotes.
    (D) have one pair of sex chromosomes.
    (E) exhibit X-linked inheritance.

21. In the respiratory system carbon dioxide (CO_2) is

    (A) exchanged with oxygen on white blood cells.
    (B) recycled to produce glycogen.
    (C) circulated through capillaries for delivery to the tissues of the body.
    (D) oxidized to form acetyl CoA.
    (E) transferred from hemoglobin to the alveoli.

22. In the first stage of a human heartbeat,

    (A) the atria contract, forcing blood from the atria to the ventricles.
    (B) the semilunar valves close to start a new cardiac cycle.
    (C) the semilunar valves (pulmonary and aortic) close and the atrioventricular valves (mitral and tricuspid) open to draw blood into the atria.
    (D) the semilunar valves open and the blood leaves the ventricles.
    (E) the ventricles contract and the atrioventricular and semilunar valves close.

23. Blood clots because

    (A) platelets and proteins in the blood are activated during an injury.
    (B) red blood cells eventually die and must be removed as waste.
    (C) oxygen levels in the blood reach a plateau.
    (D) white blood cells become activated in response to some diseases.
    (E) of oxidation.

24. A person that has an O blood type is considered to be a "universal" blood donor because

    (A) people having an O blood type make up almost half of the human population.
    (B) this person's red blood cells contain both A and B antigens.
    (C) people having an O blood type have a relatively high percentage of white blood cells.
    (D) this person's red blood cells lack all typing antigens.
    (E) O type blood is rich in red blood cells.

25. Salivary glands are part of the digestive system. Which one of the following is a salivary gland?

    (A) Pineal body
    (B) Parotid
    (C) Pituitary
    (D) Adrenal
    (E) Subaceous

26. The green algae

    (A) are endosymbionts.
    (B) produce seeds as part of the alteration of generations reproduction cycle.
    (C) have an asexual budding reproductive stage.
    (D) belong to the protozoa (protista).
    (E) belong to the kingdom chromista (protista).

27. A primary function of the lymphatic system is to

    (A) maintain the balance of body fluids.
    (B) manufacture red blood cells.
    (C) manufacture antibodies.
    (D) store excess glycogen.
    (E) store excess fatty acids.

28. The main difference between endocrine and exocrine glands is

   (A) endocrine glands contain a lumen but exocrine glands do not.
   (B) exocrine glands but secrete hormones into the bloodstream not endocrine glands do not.
   (C) endocrine glands are typically more vascular than exocrine glands and do not contain ducts.
   (D) endocrine glands are typically larger than exocrine glands and secrete enzymes.
   (E) endocrine glands typically have rapid response times while exocrine glands have slow response times.

29. Which one of the following is a primary layer of human skin that is made up of keratinocytes?

   (A) Epidermis
   (B) Mesoderm
   (C) Ectoderm
   (D) Notochord
   (E) Myelin

30. Teeth develop in the embryo from which one of the following germ layers?

   (A) Endoderm
   (B) Ectoderm
   (C) Mesoderm
   (D) Gastrula
   (E) Archenteron

31. Which one of the following statements is true about the gallbladder?

   (A) The gallbladder aids the digestion of complex carbohydrates.
   (B) The gallbladder delivers bile to the large intestine.
   (C) The gallbladder is part of the endocrine system.
   (D) Bile is stored in the gallbladder.
   (E) Bile is made in the gallbladder.

32. Which one of the following statements is true about bone marrow?

   (A) Blood cells are produced in the red bone marrow of long bones.
   (B) Lymphocytes are produced in the yellow marrow of long bones.
   (C) Sesamoid cells contain more yellow bone marrow than long bones.
   (D) Bone marrow is an essential component of the cardiovascular system.
   (E) Platelets are the only component of blood that is not made in bone marrow.

33. Synarthrosis joints

   (A) require synovial fluid to properly function.
   (B) are a type of ball-and-socket joint.
   (C) are found in the human cranium.
   (D) are structured to permit significant lateral movement.
   (E) are found in the adult vertebral column.

34. All of the following statements about cartilage are true EXCEPT one. Which one is the EXCEPTION?

   (A) In the developing embryo, cartilage is made from mesoderm.
   (B) Cartilage is part of the musculoskeletal system.
   (C) Cartilage, along with ligaments and tendons, supports bones in joints.
   (D) The skeleton of some vertebrates is made of cartilage rather than of bone.
   (E) Cartilage is harder and more rigid than bone.

35. One of the features that distinguishes the vertebrates from the invertebrates

   (A) is a notochord.
   (B) is a chambered heart.
   (C) is gills.
   (D) is teeth.
   (E) is wings.

36. According to the fossil record, vertebrates began to evolve during which geological period?

   (A) Cambrian
   (B) Devonian
   (C) Triassic
   (D) Jurassic
   (E) Cretaceous

37. Glial cells

   (A) are key signal transducing cells in the parasympathetic nervous system.
   (B) are responsible for the creation of action potentials in the musculoskeletal system.
   (C) release neurotransmitters during electrical impulses.
   (D) are metabolic support cells in the nervous system.
   (E) make up the body of motor neurons.

38. An important process performed by energy producers in the carbon cycle is

   (A) predation.
   (B) decomposition.
   (C) photosynthesis.
   (D) nitrogen fixation.
   (E) fossilization.

39. Instinctive behavioral responses that occur in animals due to the action of "sign" or "releasing" stimuli are known as

   (A) fixed action patterns.
   (B) kinesis.
   (C) tropism.
   (D) imprinting.
   (E) observational learning.

40. An example of an aquatic ecosystem is a

   (A) tundra.
   (B) grassland.
   (C) desert.
   (D) wetland.
   (E) tropical rain forest.

41. What are the correct coefficients for the reaction of magnesium with oxygen?

   $$\_\_\_ \ Mg(s) + \_\_\_ \ O_2(g) \rightarrow \_\_\_ \ MgO(s)$$

   (A) 1, 2, 1
   (B) 2, 1, 1
   (C) 2, 2, 2
   (D) 2, 1, 2
   (E) 1, 1, 1

42. How many oxygen atoms are in a formula unit of aluminum sulfate, $Al_2(SO_4)_3$?

   (A) 2
   (B) 4
   (C) 3
   (D) 7
   (E) 12

43. What is the percent mass composition of carbon in calcium acetate, $Ca(CH_3COO)_2$ (MW = 158.17 g/mol)?

   (A) 15.19%
   (B) 30.04%
   (C) 7.594%
   (D) 25.34%
   (E) 25.00%

44. What is the volume of 25.0 grams of oxygen gas (MW = 32.00 g/mol) at STP?

   (A) 35.7 L
   (B) 17.5 L
   (C) 560. L
   (D) 611. L
   (E) 19.1 L

45. The kinetic molecular theory of gases allows us to make assumptions about gases. Which of the following is NOT an assumption based off the kinetic molecular theory?

(A) Gases are compressible.
(B) Gases change to fill the shape and volume of the container.
(C) Gases have low densities.
(D) The average kinetic energy of a gas molecule depends on the absolute temperature of the system.
(E) Gas molecules have inelastic collisions.

46. A balloon containing an unknown gas was filled to 1.5 L at STP. The balloon was then released and ended at a pressure of 0.67 atm and a temperature of 18.3°C. What is the correct set up to find the volume of the balloon at the new pressure and temperature?

(A) $\dfrac{(0.67)(1.5)}{(0.0821)(18.3)}$

(B) $\dfrac{(0.67)(1.5)}{(0.0821)(291.45)}$

(C) $\dfrac{(1.5)(1)(273.15)}{(291.45)(0.67)}$

(D) $\dfrac{(1.5)(1)(291.45)}{(273.15)(0.67)}$

(E) $\dfrac{(1)(1.5)(18.3)}{(25)(0.67)}$

47. What is the empirical formula if the corner atoms are S and the face atoms are O:

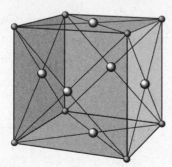

(A) S_8O_6
(B) SO_2
(C) S_3O
(D) S_2O_3
(E) SO_3

48. An unknown compound does not conduct electricity below its melting point, but does conduct electricity above its melting point. The unknown compound can best be classified as

(A) molecular.
(B) binary.
(C) covalent.
(D) polymeric.
(E) ionic.

49. Which of the following compounds could NOT participate in hydrogen bonding with itself?

(A) CH_3F
(B) H_2O
(C) HF
(D) CH_3OH
(E) NH_3

50. Which of the following will decrease the solubility of $BaCrO_4(s)$? The K_{sp} for barium chromate is 1.17×10^{-10}.

(A) Increasing temperature
(B) Decreasing pressure
(C) Adding salt
(D) Removing salt
(E) Adding calcium chromate

51. What is the molality of a solution prepared by dissolving 2.3 moles of sodium hydroxide (40.0 g/mol) into 500. mL of ethanol ($d = 0.789$ g/mL)?

(A) $\dfrac{2.3}{500}$

(B) $\dfrac{2.3}{0.5}$

(C) $\dfrac{\left(2.3 \times \dfrac{40}{1} \times \dfrac{1}{1,000}\right)}{0.5}$

(D) $\dfrac{2.3}{\left(500 \times \dfrac{0.789}{1} \times \dfrac{1}{1,000}\right)}$

(E) $\dfrac{2.3}{\left(500 \times \dfrac{0.789}{1}\right)}$

52. What is the correct setup to calculate the pH of a 0.1257 M HIO solution that has a K_a of 2.29×10^{-11}?

(A) $-\log\left(\sqrt{(0.1257)(2.29 \times 10^{-11})}\right)$

(B) $[IO^-][H^+]/[HIO]$

(C) $\sqrt{(0.1257)(2.29 \times 10^{-11})}$

(D) $-\log(0.1257)$

(E) $14 - \log(0.1257)$

53. Which of the following statements is *true* about a neutral solution at 40°C?

(A) pH = 7.00

(B) pOH = 7.00

(C) $K_w = 1.00 \times 10^{-14}$

(D) All of the above are true.

(E) None of the above are true.

54. Which of the following has the best conditions to make a buffer solution?

(A) 0.1 M HCl, 0.1 M NaOH

(B) 3 M CH_3COOH, 2 M NH_4Br

(C) 10 M NH_4Cl, 0.1 M NH_3

(D) 0.5 M CH_3COONa, 0.5 M CH_3COOH

(E) 5 M H_2SO_4, 5 M $Ca(OH)_2$

55. Which of the following statements is *true* regarding the reaction at equilibrium?

$$N_2O_2(g) \rightleftharpoons 2NO(g) \quad K_{eq} = 1.23 \times 10^{-5}$$

(A) $[N_2O_2] = [NO]$

(B) $[N_2O_2] = [NO]_2$

(C) $k_{fwd}[N_2O_2] = k_{rev}[NO]^2$

(D) $K_{eq} = [2NO]^2/[N_2O_2]$

(E) Products are favored.

56. Based on the given K's, what is the K_{eq} for $A_2 + 2Bf \rightleftharpoons 2C$?

$$A_2f \rightleftharpoons 2A \quad K_1$$
$$A + Bf \rightleftharpoons C \quad K_2$$

(A) $K_{eq} = K_1 + K_2$

(B) $K_{eq} = K_2 - K_1$

(C) $K_{eq} = (2K_2)(K_1)$

(D) $K_{eq} = 2K_2 + K_1$

(E) $K_{eq} = (K_2)^2(K_1)$

57. Which of the following statements can be concluded from the given information?

$$2XY_3 \rightarrow X_2 + 3Y_2 \quad \Delta H = -93 \text{ kJ/mol}$$
$$\Delta S = +198 \text{ J/mol} \cdot \text{K}$$

(A) The reaction is spontaneous at high temperatures and nonspontaneous at low temperatures.

(B) The reaction is spontaneous at low temperatures and nonspontaneous at high temperatures.

(C) The reaction is spontaneous at all temperatures.

(D) The reaction is nonspontaneous at all temperatures.

(E) Gibbs free energy is zero at 215K.

58. Which of the following is an example of a decrease in entropy?

(A) $X^{2+}(aq) + Y^{2-}(aq) \rightarrow XY(s)$

(B) $H_2O(s) \rightarrow H_2O(g)$

(C) $2H_2O(g) \rightarrow 2H_2(g) + O_2(g)$

(D) Melting ice

(E) $\Delta S = +$

59. What are the units for the rate constant, k, for the given rate law: Rate = $k[NO_2][F_2]^2$?

(A) $M \ s^{-1}$

(B) $M^{-2} \ s^{-1}$

(C) s^{-1}

(D) M^3

(E) M^{-3}

60. Which of the following is a *correct* way to represent the rate of the reaction:

$$2NO(g) + O_2(g) \rightarrow 2NO_2(g)$$

(A) Rate = $-\dfrac{\Delta[NO]}{2\Delta t}$

(B) Rate = $\dfrac{\Delta[NO]}{2\Delta t}$

(C) Rate = $-\dfrac{\Delta[NO_2]}{\Delta t}$

(D) Rate = $\dfrac{\Delta[O_2]}{\Delta t}$

(E) Rate = $k[NO]^2[O_2]$

61. What is the oxidation state for S in SO_2^{2-}?

(A) 2–
(B) 2+
(C) 4–
(D) 4+
(E) 0

62. Which compound is oxidized in the following reaction:

$$MnO_2 + 4HCl \rightarrow MnCl_2 + Cl_2 + 2H_2O$$

(A) MnO_2
(B) HCl
(C) $MnCl_2$
(D) Cl_2
(E) H_2O

63. Which of the statements below is *true*?

(A) Isotopes are atoms that have the same number of neutrons.
(B) Most ions are formed when an atom gains a proton.
(C) Isotopes have different mass but are the same type of element.
(D) Ions differ only in the number of neutrons they have.
(E) All of the above are true.

64. What is the change in molecular geometry around the oxygen when water gains an H atom and becomes a hydronium ion?

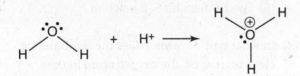

(A) Bent → trigonal pyramidal
(B) Tetrahedral → bent
(C) Bent → planar
(D) Tetrahedral → tetrahedral
(E) Bent → trigonal planar

65. Zn^+ ion has how many valence electrons?

(A) 1
(B) 9
(C) 10
(D) 2
(E) 29

66. Decide if the following statements are true (T) or false (F):

I. All elements can be classified as either metals, metalloids, or nonmetals.
II. Elements in a group have similar chemical properties.
III. Vanadium is a halogen.
IV. In the modern periodic table, elements are arranged in the order of increasing atomic number.

(A) T, T, F, T
(B) F, F, T, F
(C) T, T, T, T
(D) T, F, T, F
(E) F, F, T, T

67. Which statement about periodic trends is *correct*?

(A) Electron affinity is the energy change that occurs when an atom loses an electron.
(B) The atomic radius of an anion is smaller than the neutral atom from which it is formed.
(C) The smallest neutral atom is F.
(D) The neutral atomic radius decreases from left to right in the same row due to a higher attraction between protons and electrons.
(E) The most electronegative atom is C.

68. What element is missing in this beta decay:

$$^{230}_{90}Th \rightarrow {}^{A}_{Z}X + \beta$$

(A) $^{230}_{90}Th$
(B) $^{234}_{92}U$
(C) $^{230}_{89}Ac$
(D) $^{226}_{88}Ra$
(E) $^{230}_{91}Pa$

69. What is the concentration of a 2.1 M solution after a 1:7 dilution?

(A) 3.0 M
(B) 0.3 M
(C) 1.5 M
(D) 0.21 M
(E) 0.26 M

70. Which of the following statements is false?

(A) Systematic errors shift all measurements, so their mean value is displaced.
(B) Systematic errors may be due to incorrect calibration of equipment.
(C) Random errors fluctuate from one measurement to the next.
(D) Random errors can occur from lack of sensitivity and noise.
(E) Some random errors can be eliminated, but systematic errors are unavoidable.

71. S_N1 reactions are characterized by

(A) second-order kinetics and approximate racemization of chirality centers.
(B) first-order kinetics and approximate racemization of chirality centers.
(C) first-order kinetics and inversion of chirality centers.
(D) second-order kinetics and inversion of chirality centers.
(E) a one-step concerted reaction mechanism.

72. Which of the following structures would have a formal charge greater than zero:

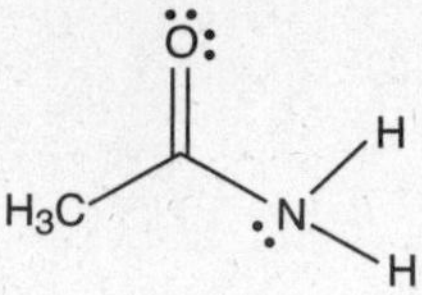

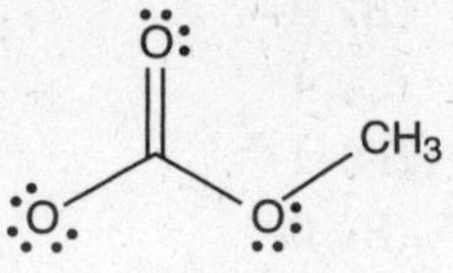

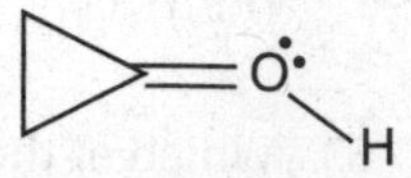

(A) 1
(B) 2
(C) 3
(D) 4
(E) 3 and 5

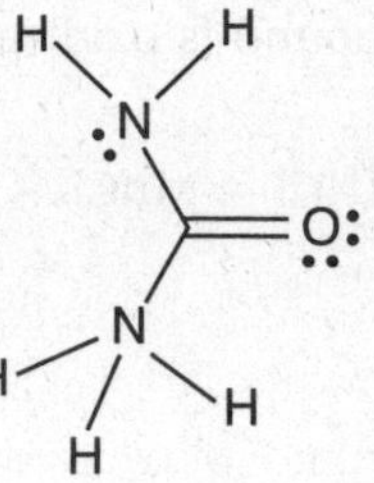

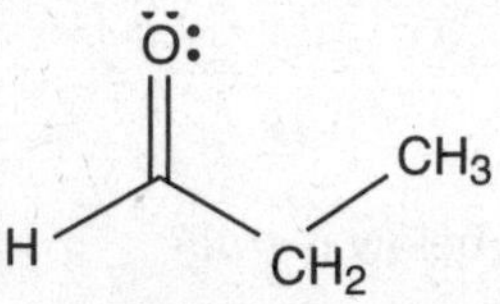

73. The synthesis of epoxides by treating halohydrins with a base is an example of a/an

(A) intramolecular E2 reaction.
(B) hydrolysis reaction.
(C) intramolecular S_N1 reaction.
(D) intramolecular S_N2 reaction.
(E) intermolecular S_N2 reaction.

74. In what type of orbital does the nonbonding electron pair on the oxygen atom in the triethyloxonium ion (shown below) reside?

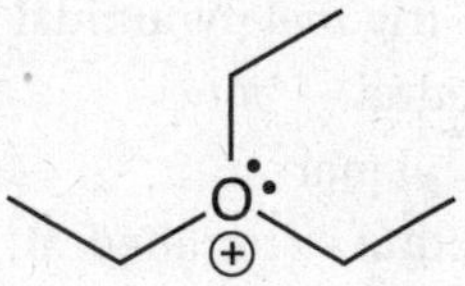

(A) s
(B) p
(C) sp
(D) sp^2
(E) sp^3

75. The process depicted in the reaction energy diagram shown below can best be described as

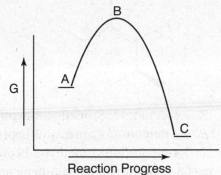

Reaction Progress

(A) nonspontaneous.
(B) fast and exergonic.
(C) slow and endergonic.
(D) slow and exergonic.
(E) fast and endergonic.

76. Predict the *major* product of the following reaction.

HCl → ?

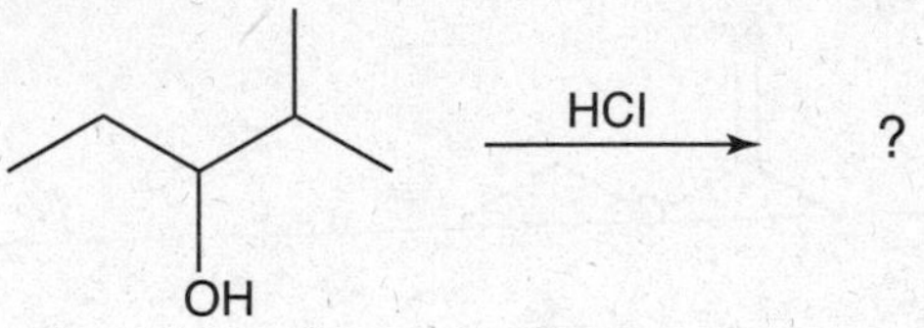

(A)

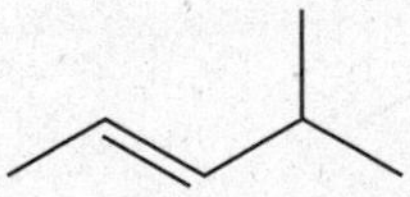

(B)

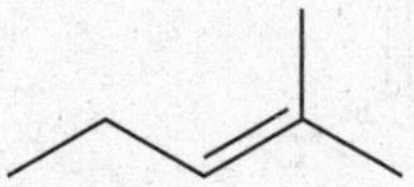

(C)

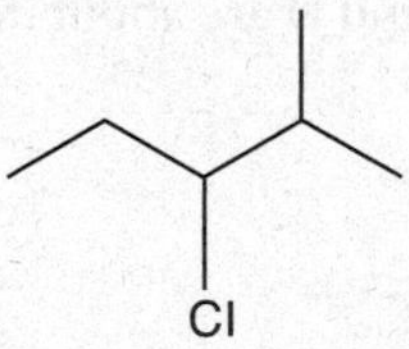

(D)

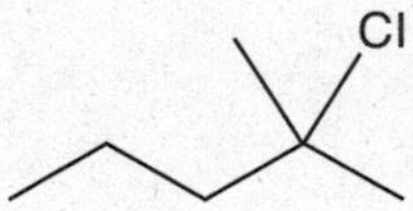

(E) None of the above

77. A decoupled ^{13}C NMR spectrum was acquired for the compound shown below. How many individual signals appear in the spectrum?

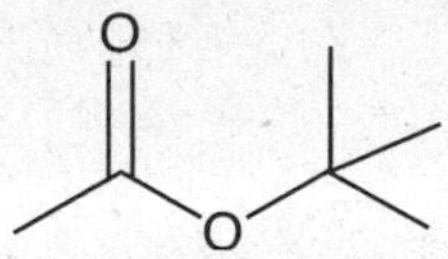

(A) 2
(B) 3
(C) 4
(D) 5
(E) 6

78. Predict the *major* product of the following reaction.

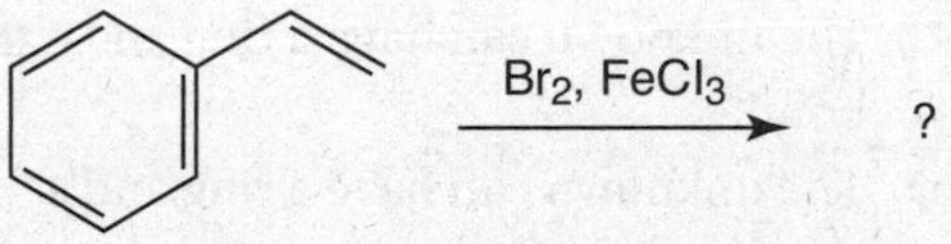

Br$_2$, FeCl$_3$ → ?

(A)

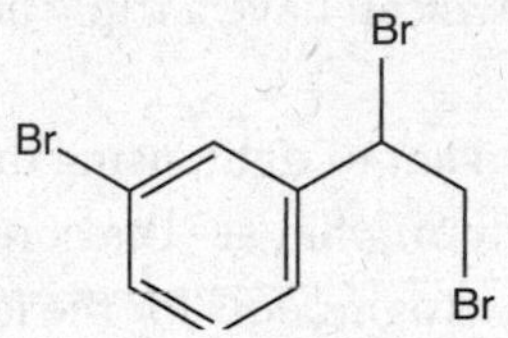

Br

Br

Br

(B)

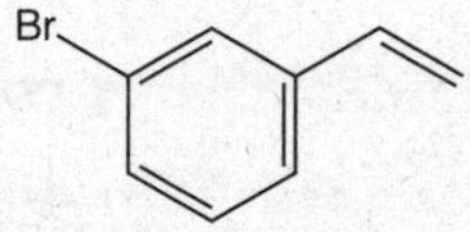

Br

(C)

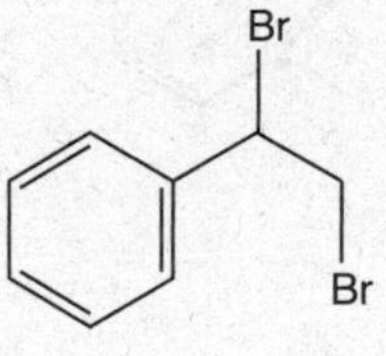

Br

Br

(D)

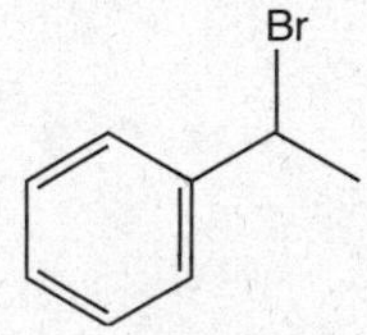

Br

(E) None of the above

79. How many pairs of enantiomers could exist for the compound 1-chloro-2-fluorocyclopentane?

(A) 1
(B) 2
(C) 3
(D) 4
(E) 5

80. An unknown compound has the molecular formula: C_6H_{10}

Which of the following is *incorrect*?

(A) The unknown can have two rings.
(B) The unknown can have two double bonds.
(C) The unknown can have a ring and a triple bond.
(D) The unknown can have a ring and a double bond.
(E) The unknown can have a triple bond.

81. Proceeding from left to right, using the *E/Z* designation system, what are the correct stereochemical assignments for the four double bonds in the compound shown below?

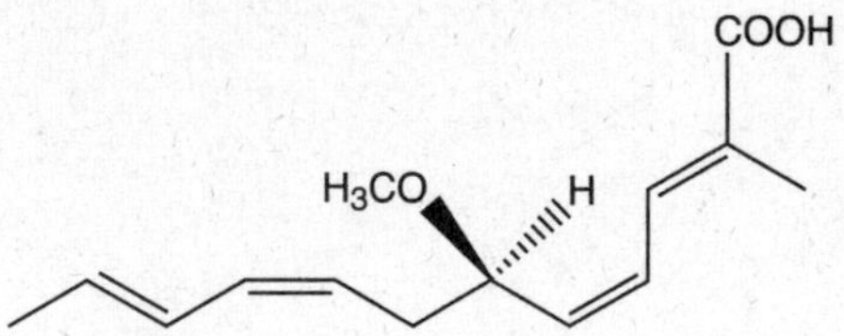

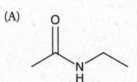

(A) *E, Z, Z, E*
(B) *Z, E, E, Z*
(C) *Z, Z, E, E*
(D) *Z, E, Z, E*
(E) *E, Z, E, Z*

82. What is the correct IUPAC name for the following structure?

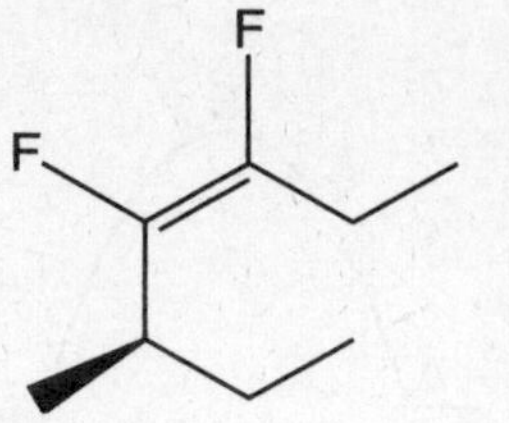

(A) (*Z*)-3,4-difluoro-(5*S*)-methyl-3-heptene
(B) (*E*)-3,4-difluoro-(5*R*)-methyl-3-heptene
(C) (*Z*)-3,4-difluoro-(5*R*)-methyl-3-heptene
(D) *cis*-4,5-difluoro-(4*S*)-ethyl-3-heptene
(E) *trans*-4,5-difluoro-(5*R*)-ethyl-3-heptene

83. Which of the following compounds would be the most susceptible to hydrolysis by water?

(A)

(B)

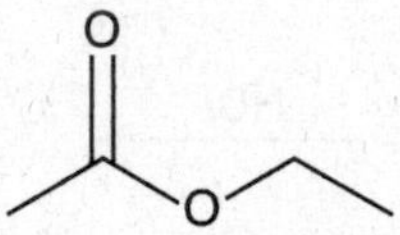

(C)

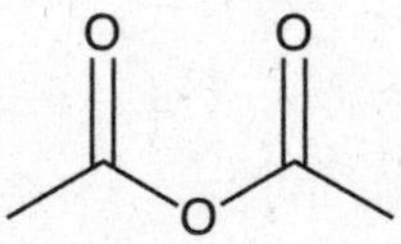

(D)

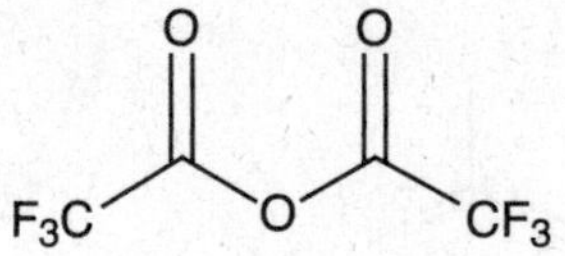

(E) Compounds C and D are about the same.

84. Which of the following compounds absorbs the lowest energy (longest wavelength) radiation?

(A)

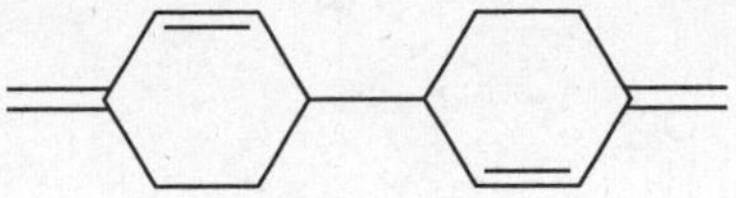

(B)

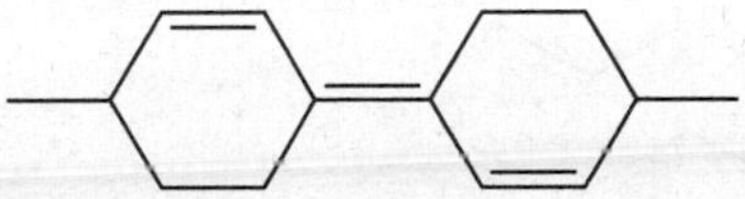

(C)

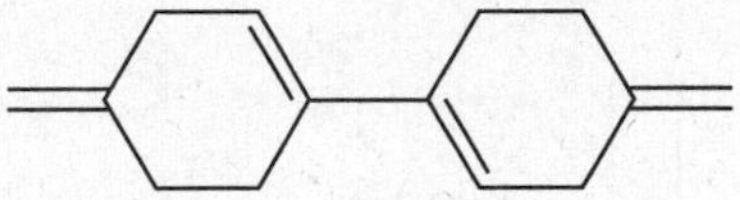

(D)

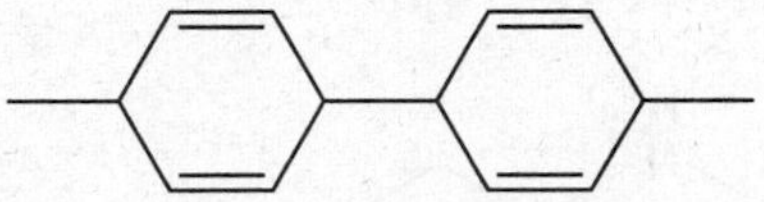

(E)

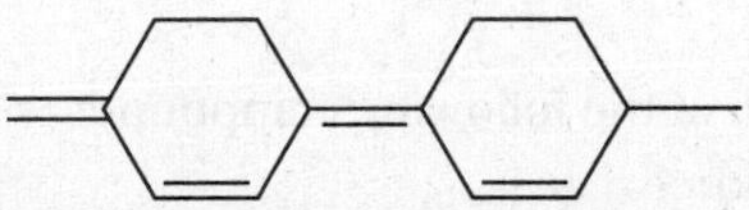

85. Predict the *major* product of the following reaction.

$$\xrightarrow[\text{2) NaHCO}_3]{\text{1) H}_3\text{O}^+}$$?

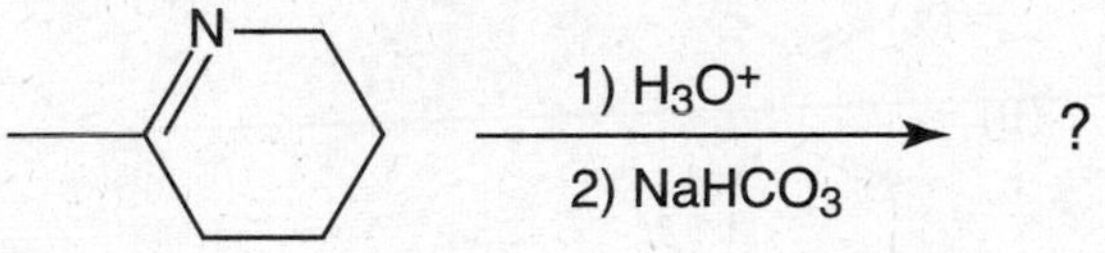

(A)

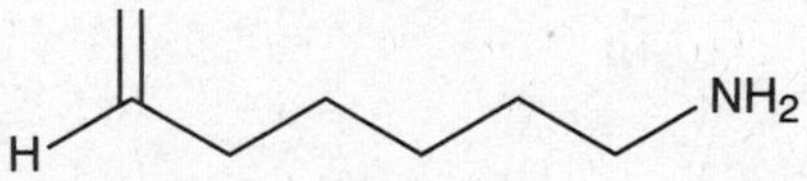

(B)

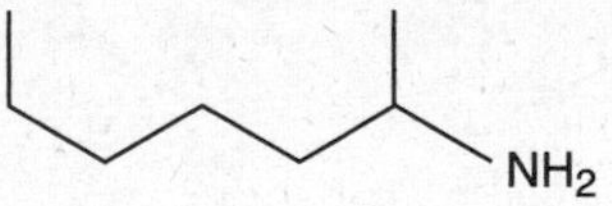

(C)

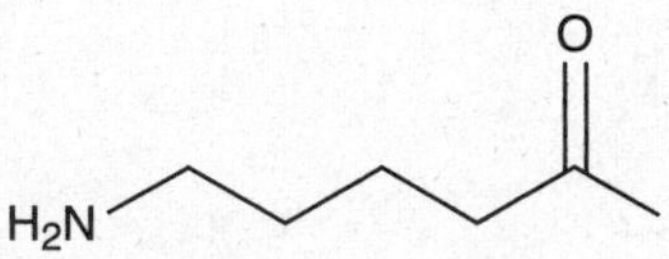

(D)

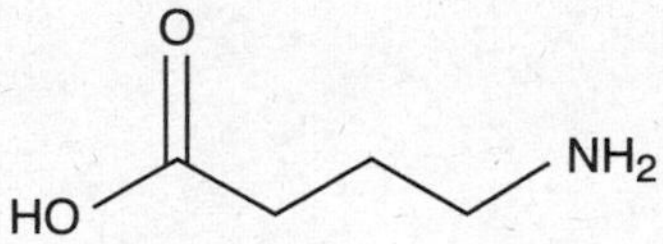

(E)

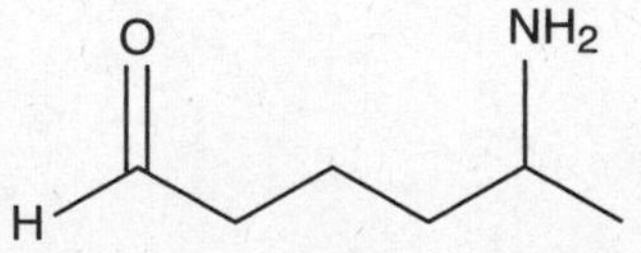

86. The amoxicillin molecule is shown below. How many stereoisomers of this compound are possible?

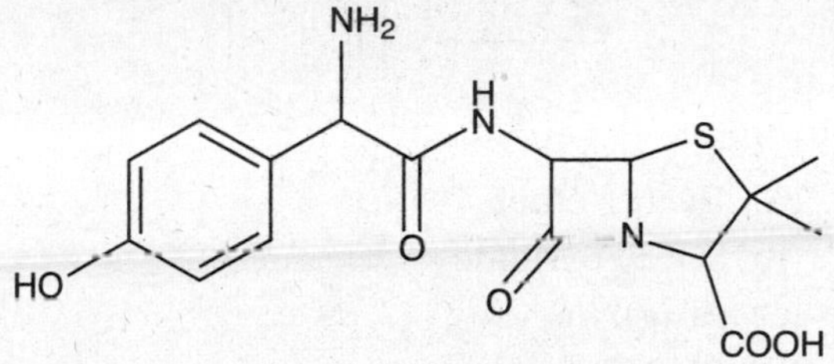

(A) 2
(B) 4
(C) 8
(D) 16
(E) 32

87. Which pair of reactants could be used to produce the product shown in the following reaction scheme?

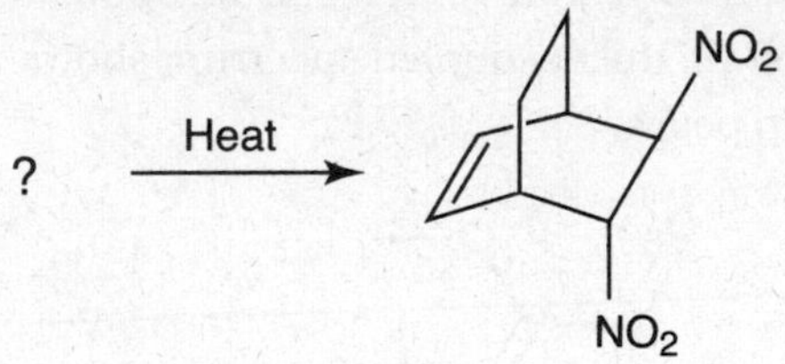

? $\xrightarrow{\text{Heat}}$

(A)

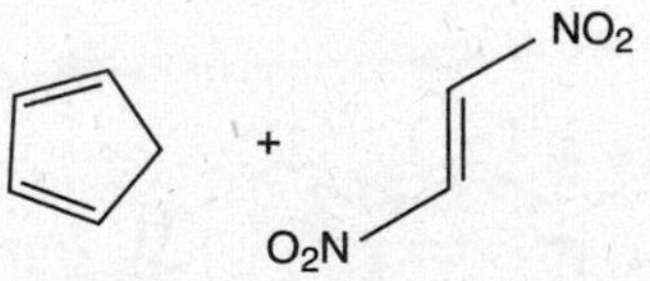

(B)

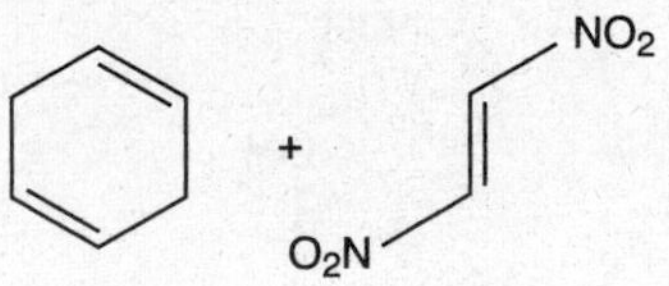

(C)

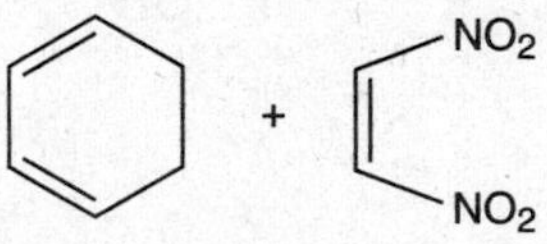

(D)

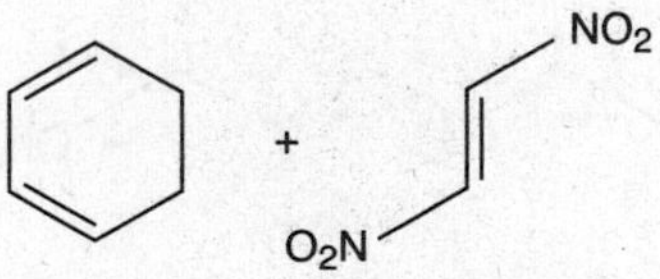

(E)

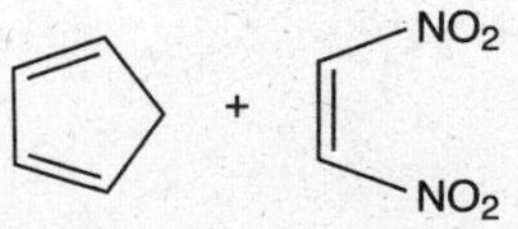

88. Select the *best* reagent combination (reliable and mild) for the following transformation.

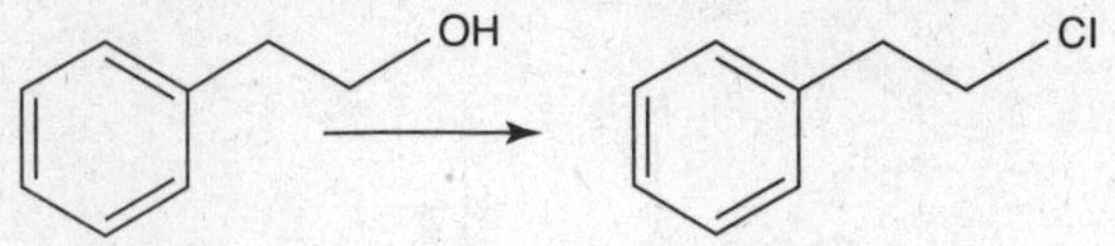

(A) HCl(g)/ether
(B) SOCl$_2$/pyridine
(C) Cl$_2$(g)/hv
(D) Cl$_2$/CCl$_4$
(E) KCl(aq)/methanol

89. Which of the following compounds is consistent with the provided characterization data?

Molecular formula: C$_4$H$_6$O$_4$
IR: 3,600 cm^{-1} – 2,500 cm^{-1} (very broad, strong band) and 1,770 cm^{-1} (sharp, strong band)
^{1}H NMR: 2.45 ppm (s, 4H) and 12.1 ppm (s, 2H)
^{13}C NMR: the decoupled spectrum shows two peaks

(A)

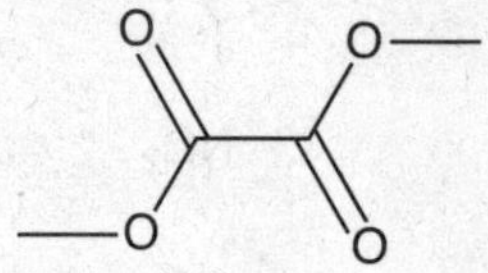

(B)

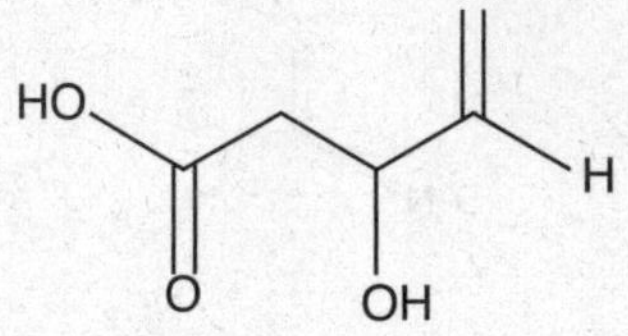

(C)

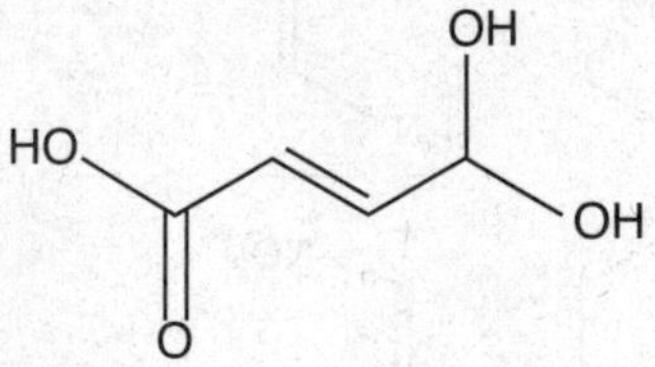

(D)

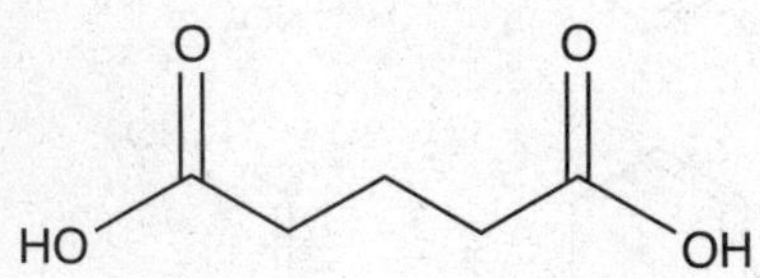

(E)

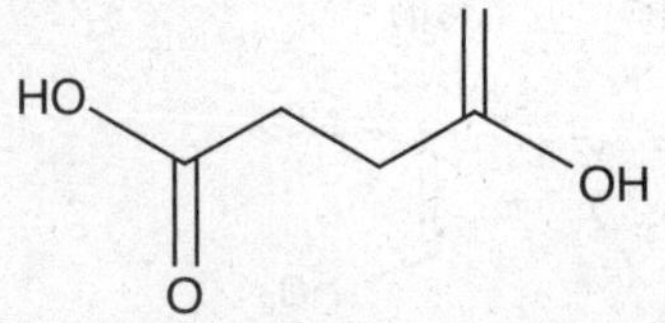

90. Which compound has the highest boiling point?

(A)

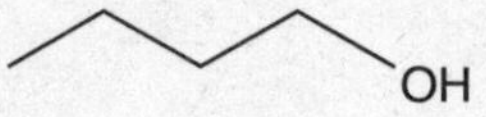

(B)

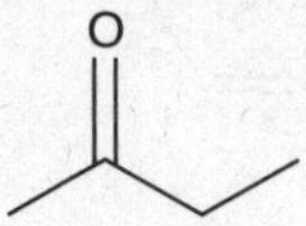

(C)

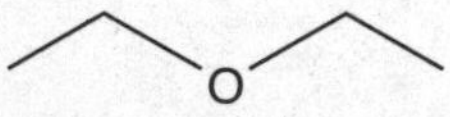

(D)

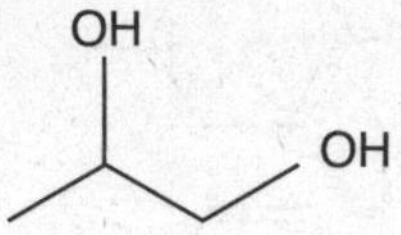

(E)

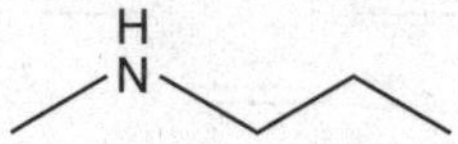

91. Which of the following compounds is not aromatic?

(A)

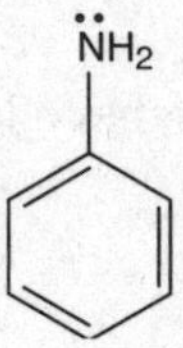

(B)

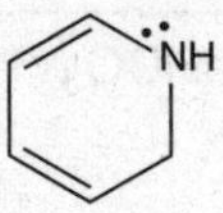

(C)

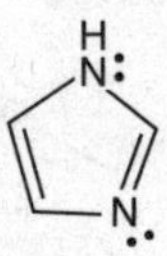

(D)

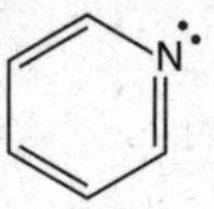

(E)

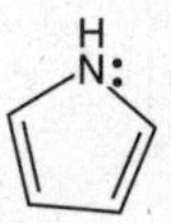

92. Which of the following structures represents the most stable (lowest energy) conformation of 2,3-dimethylbutane?

(A)

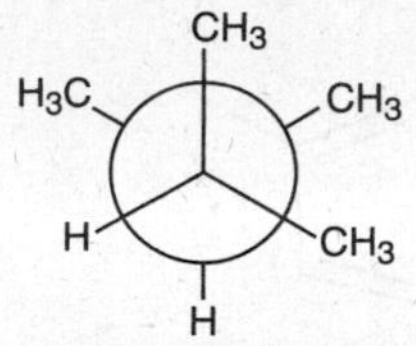

(B)

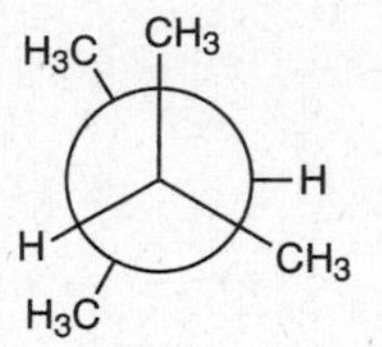

(C)

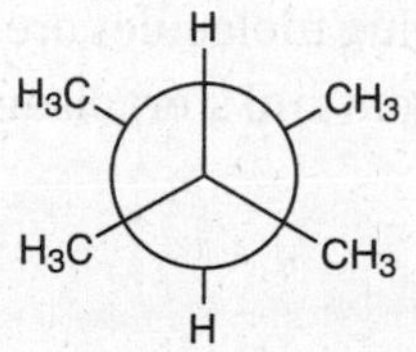

(D)

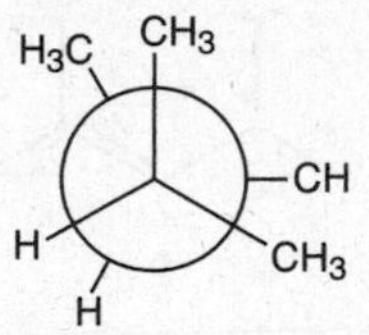

(E)

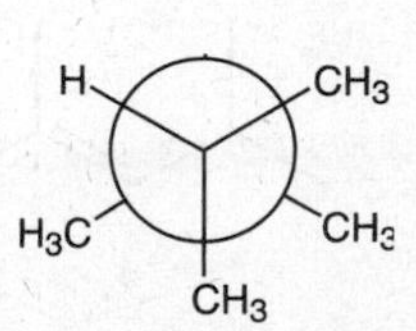

93. Proceeding from left to right, what types of hybrid orbitals do each of the *five* carbon atoms in the following molecule use for bonding?

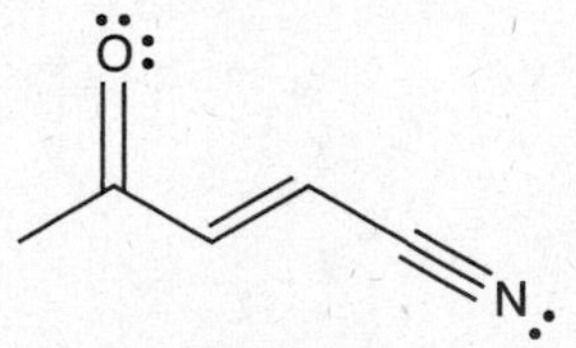

(A) $sp, sp^2, sp^2, sp^2, sp^3$
(B) $sp^3, sp^3, sp^2, sp^2, sp$
(C) $sp^3, sp^2, sp^2, sp^2, sp$
(D) $sp^3, sp^2, sp^2 \ sp^2, sp^2$
(E) sp^3, sp^3, sp, sp, sp

94. *All* the bond angles in the ethene molecule are

(A) 90°.
(B) 109.5°.
(C) 120°.
(D) 180°.
(E) They are not all the same.

95. Predict the *major* product from the following reaction sequence.

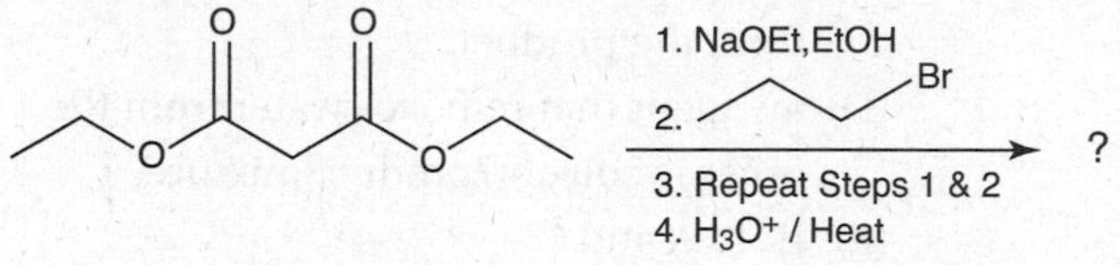

(A)

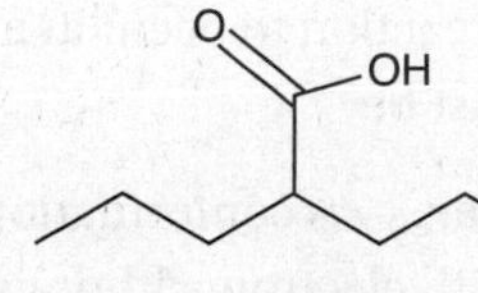

(B)

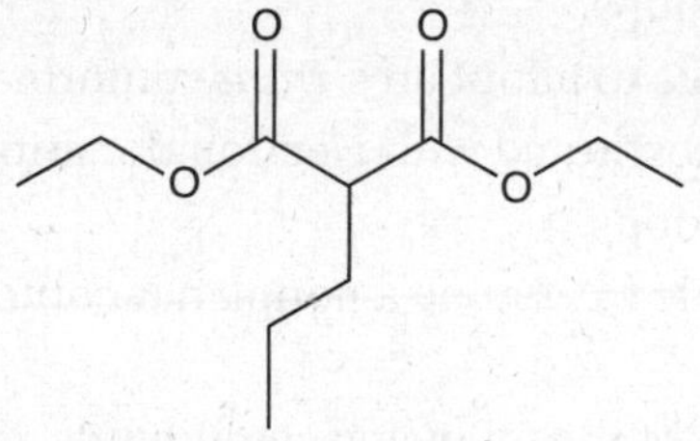

(C)

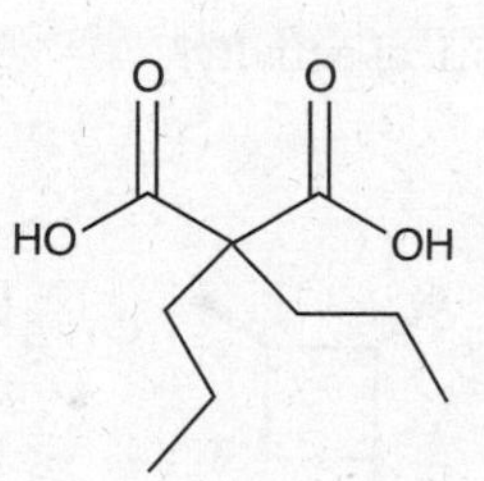

(D)

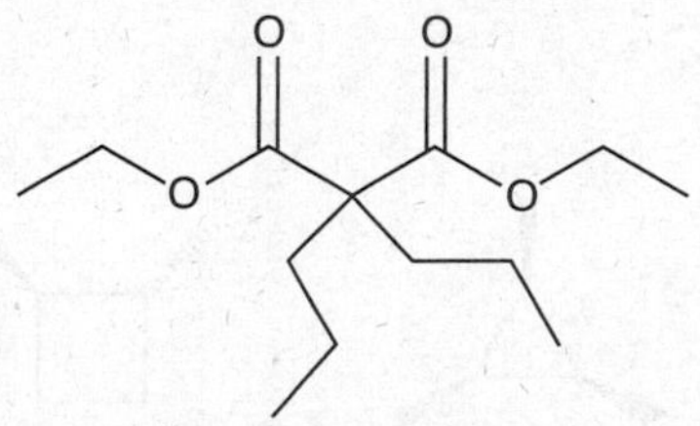

(E)

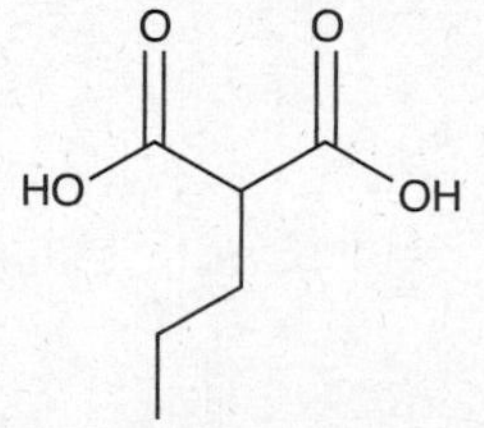

96. When performing an aqueous/organic two-phase liquid extraction, Na_2SO_4 or $MgSO_4$ is often added to the combined organic fractions prior to evaporation of the solvent and isolation of the product. The Na_2SO_4 or $MgSO_4$ functions as

(A) a preliminary solvent-removing step.
(B) a reactant that forms a complex with the product.
(C) an agent that removes colored impurities from the product.
(D) an agent that removes water from the organic solvent/product mixture.
(E) Both A and C

97. For a Diels-Alder reaction to occur at a viable rate, the diene must be

(A) able to adopt an s-*cis* conformation.
(B) substituted with electron withdrawing groups.
(C) able to adopt an s-*trans* conformation.
(D) substituted with electron donating groups.
(E) able to assume a nonplanar conformation.

98. Which of the following compounds, if tested, would exhibit optical activity?

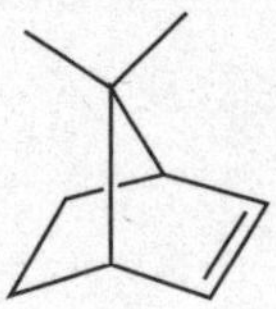

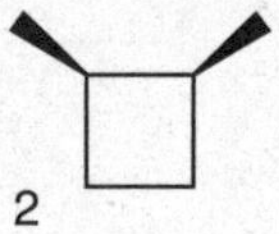

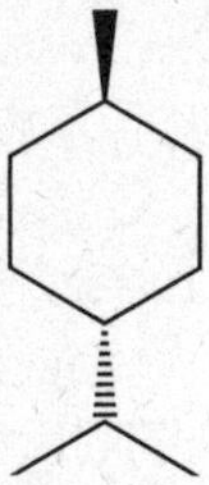

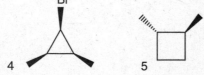

(A) 1
(B) 2
(C) 3
(D) 4
(E) 5

99. How many *pairs* of enantiomers would be expected to form when the following conjugated diene is reacted with hydrobromic acid?

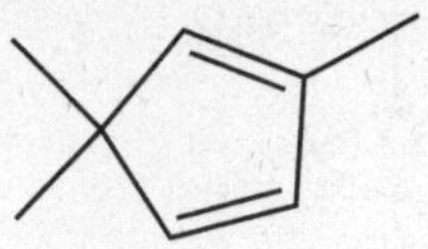

(A) 1
(B) 2
(C) 3
(D) 4
(E) 5

100. Which of the following molecules are both constitutional isomers and stereoisomers of each other?

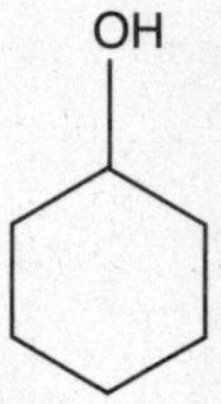

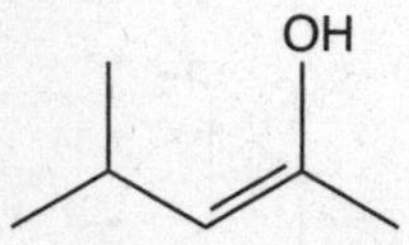

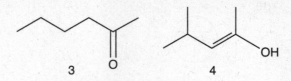

(A) 1 and 2
(B) 1 and 3
(C) 1 and 4
(D) 2 and 3
(E) 2 and 4

TIME LIMIT: 60 MINUTES

Part 1: Aperture Passing

Directions: For questions 1 through 15:

This section of the exam consists of 15 items similar to the example below. In each item, a three-dimensional object is shown on the left, followed by outlines of five apertures to its right.

The task is the same for each item. Conceptualize how the three-dimensional object looks from each possible side (in addition to the side shown). Then, pick the outline in which the three-dimensional object could pass if the proper side were inserted. Choose the letter corresponding to the correct aperture.

Here are rules for Part 1, the aperture section:

1. The irregular solid three-dimensional object on the left can be rotated in any direction prior to passing through the aperture.

2. The object may not be twisted or rotated in any way once it has started to be passed through the aperture. The correct answer is the exact representation of the external outline of the object viewed from the appropriate side.

3. The objects and the outlines are drawn to the same scale.

4. There are no irregularities in hidden portions of the objects. If the figure has symmetric indentations, it is assumed that the hidden portion is symmetric with the portion shown.

5. There is only one correct answer.

EXAMPLE

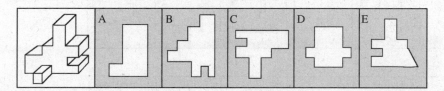

The correct answer is C.

1.

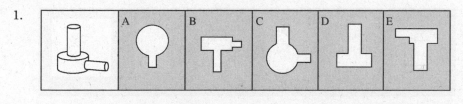

2.

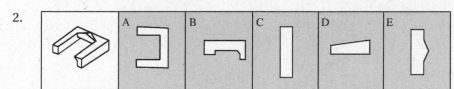

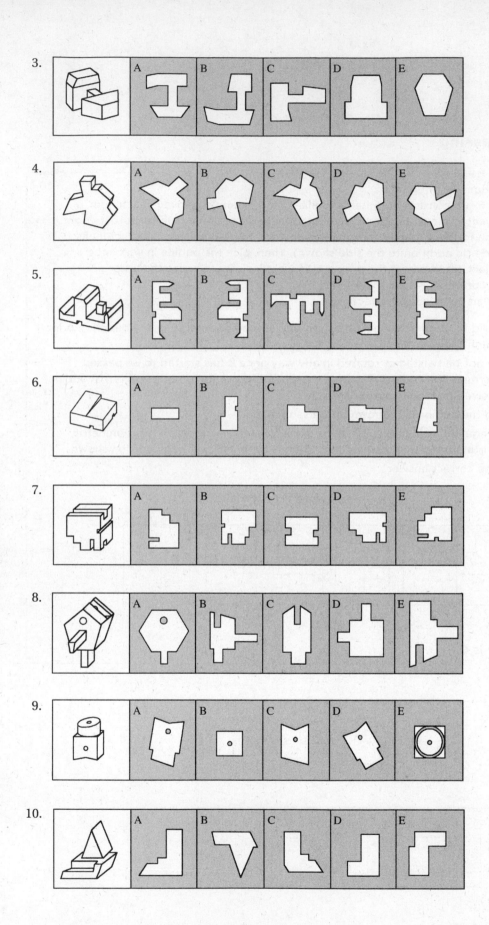

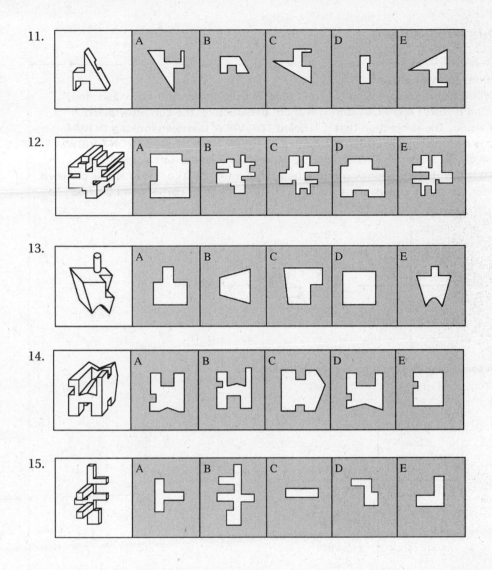

11.

12.

13.

14.

15.

Part 2: Orthographic Projections

Directions: For questions 16 through 30:

The pictures that follow are representations of solid objects from three different views: top, front, and end views. The pictures are views drawn without perspective: the surface viewed is along parallel lines of vision. The projection that is labeled TOP VIEW is shown looking DOWN on its top surface and is pictured in the upper-left corner. The projection labeled FRONT VIEW is shown looking at the object from the FRONT and is pictured in the lower-left corner. The projection labeled END VIEW is shown looking at the object from the END (or side) and is pictured in the lower-right corner. These three views are always in their respective corners and labeled accordingly.

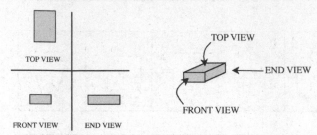

If there were a hole in the figure, it would be represented like this:

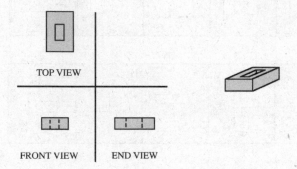

DOTTED lines indicate lines that exist but cannot be seen in the perspective shown.

In the following problems, TWO of the previous three views discussed will be shown with four alternatives to the right. Choose the correct letter that represents the correct view that completes the set.

EXAMPLE

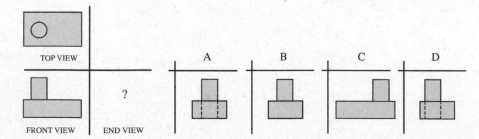

The FRONT VIEW shows that there is a smaller block on top of a larger block and there is no hole. The TOP VIEW shows that the top block is round and is centered on a rectangular block. From this information gathered in the two views given, the correct answer must be B.

In the following problems, one of the three views will be omitted; it is not always the END VIEW as shown in the example.

16. Choose the correct TOP VIEW.

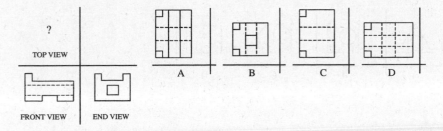

17. Choose the correct END VIEW.

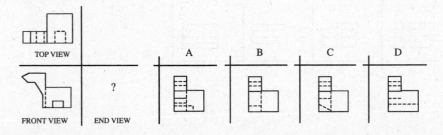

18. Choose the correct FRONT VIEW.

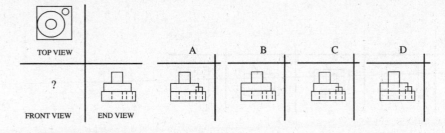

19. Choose the correct FRONT VIEW.

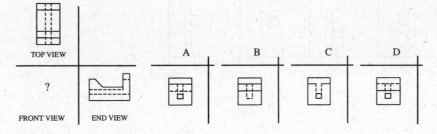

20. Choose the correct END VIEW.

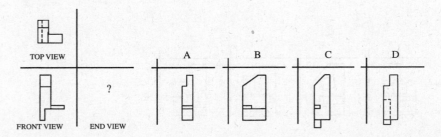

21. Choose the correct TOP VIEW.

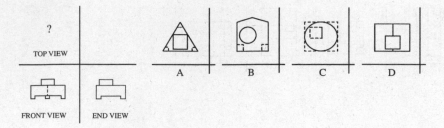

22. Choose the correct TOP VIEW.

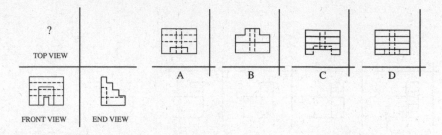

23. Choose the correct END VIEW.

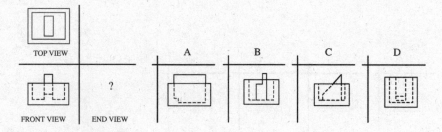

24. Choose the correct TOP VIEW.

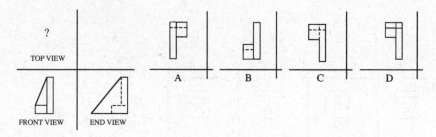

25. Choose the correct FRONT VIEW.

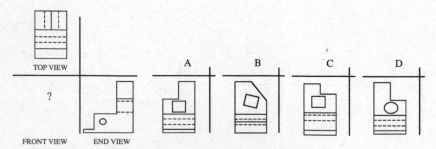

26. Choose the correct END VIEW.

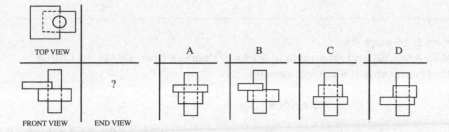

27. Choose the correct TOP VIEW.

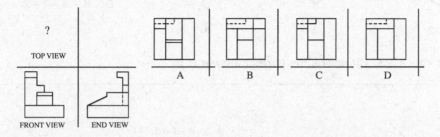

28. Choose the correct FRONT VIEW.

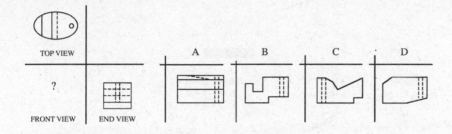

29. Choose the correct TOP VIEW.

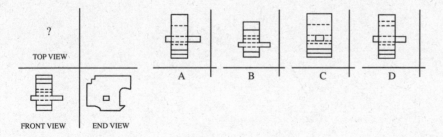

30. Choose the correct FRONT VIEW.

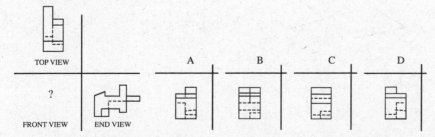

Part 3: Angle Discrimination

Directions: For questions 31 through 45:
Examine the INTERNAL ANGLES and rank them in terms of degrees from SMALL to LARGE. Select the alternative that represents the correct ranking.

EXAMPLE

1   2   3   4

A. 1 – 2 – 4 – 3
B. 2 – 1 – 4 – 3
C. 3 – 4 – 2 – 1
D. 3 – 4 – 1 – 2

The correct ranking is 2 – 1 – 4 – 3. Therefore, the correct answer is B.

31.

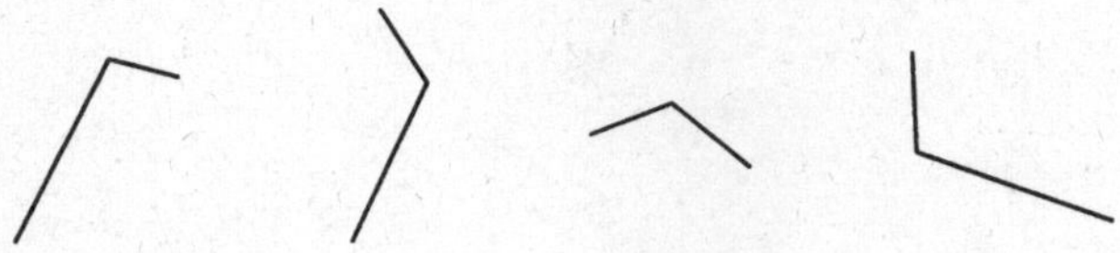

1   2   3   4

A. 3 – 4 – 1 – 2
B. 1 – 4 – 3 – 2
C. 3 – 1 – 4 – 2
D. 1 – 3 – 4 – 2

32.

1   2   3   4

A. 4 – 2 – 3 – 1
B. 4 – 1 – 2 – 3
C. 2 – 4 – 1 – 2
D. 4 – 2 – 1 – 3

33.

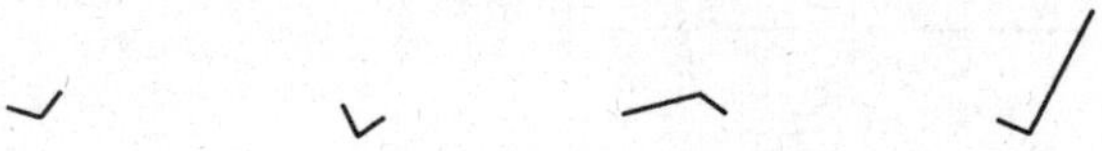

1   2   3   4

A. 2 – 1 – 4 – 3
B. 1 – 2 – 4 – 3
C. 2 – 4 – 1 – 3
D. 4 – 2 – 3 – 1

34.

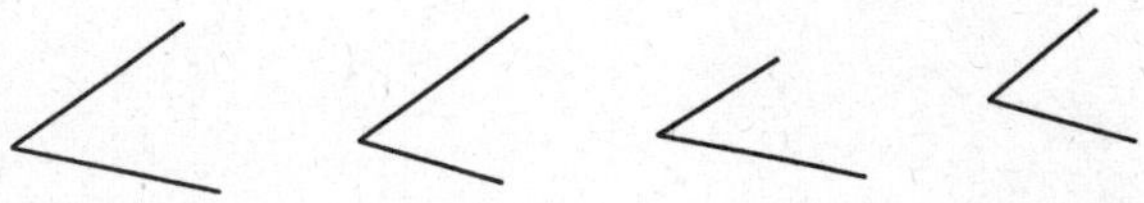

1   2   3   4

A. 3 – 1 – 2 – 4
B. 1 – 3 – 2 – 4
C. 3 – 1 – 4 – 2
D. 1 – 3 – 4 – 2

35.

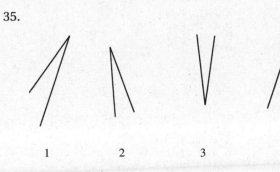

1 2 3 4

A. 3 – 2 – 1 – 4
B. 3 – 1 – 2 – 4
C. 2 – 4 – 1 – 3
D. 4 – 3 – 2 – 1

36.

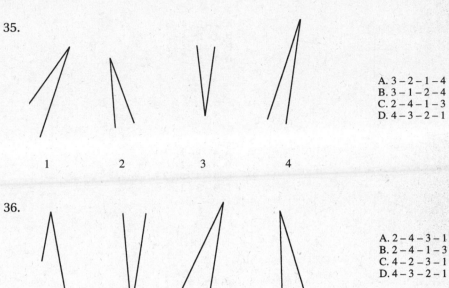

1 2 3 4

A. 2 – 4 – 3 – 1
B. 2 – 4 – 1 – 3
C. 4 – 2 – 3 – 1
D. 4 – 3 – 2 – 1

37.

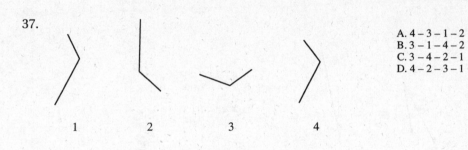

1 2 3 4

A. 4 – 3 – 1 – 2
B. 3 – 1 – 4 – 2
C. 3 – 4 – 2 – 1
D. 4 – 2 – 3 – 1

38.

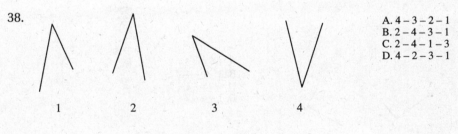

1 2 3 4

A. 4 – 3 – 2 – 1
B. 2 – 4 – 3 – 1
C. 2 – 4 – 1 – 3
D. 4 – 2 – 3 – 1

39.

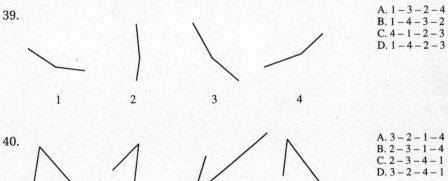

1 2 3 4

A. 1 – 3 – 2 – 4
B. 1 – 4 – 3 – 2
C. 4 – 1 – 2 – 3
D. 1 – 4 – 2 – 3

40.

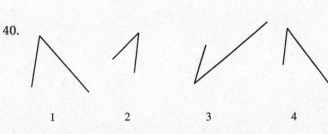

1 2 3 4

A. 3 – 2 – 1 – 4
B. 2 – 3 – 1 – 4
C. 2 – 3 – 4 – 1
D. 3 – 2 – 4 – 1

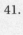

41.

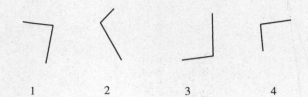

1   2   3   4

A. 1 – 2 – 4 – 3
B. 4 – 1 – 3 – 2
C. 1 – 4 – 3 – 2
D. 4 – 1 – 2 – 3

42.

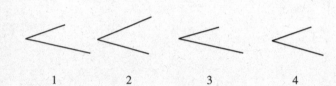

1   2   3   4

A. 4 – 1 – 3 – 2
B. 4 – 1 – 2 – 3
C. 1 – 4 – 3 – 2
D. 4 – 3 – 2 – 1

43.

1   2   3   4

A. 1 – 2 – 3 – 4
B. 3 – 1 – 4 – 2
C. 1 – 3 – 4 – 2
D. 4 – 3 – 1 – 2

44.

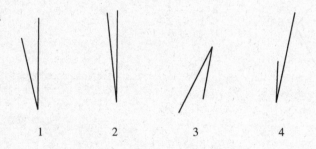

1   2   3   4

A. 4 – 2 – 3 – 1
B. 2 – 4 – 1 – 3
C. 2 – 4 – 3 – 1
D. 4 – 2 – 1 – 3

45.

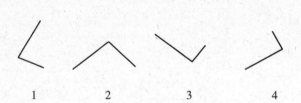

1   2   3   4

A. 1 – 4 – 3 – 2
B. 3 – 1 – 4 – 2
C. 4 – 3 – 1 – 2
D. 1 – 4 – 2 – 3

Part 4: Paper Folding

Directions: For questions 46 through 60:

A flat, square piece of paper is folded one or more times starting from the left, proceeding stepwise to the illustrations to the right. The original position of the paper is represented by broken lines. The solid line indicates edges of the folded paper. The piece of paper is never twisted or turned and always remains within the outline of the original square. There may be ONE FOLD, TWO FOLDS, or THREE FOLDS in each item. After the last fold, a hole is punched in the paper. Your task is to unfold the paper in your mind and determine the placement of the holes on the original flat, square piece of paper. There is only one correct pattern of hole punches for each item. The black circles indicate hole punches. Choose the pattern that indicates the correct pattern of hole punches in the unfolded paper.

PRACTICE ILLUSTRATIONS:

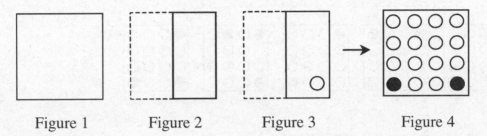

Figure 1   Figure 2   Figure 3   Figure 4

In this example, Figure 1 shows the original flat, square piece of paper. Figure 2 shows the first fold. Figure 3 shows the location of the hole punch in the folded paper. The black circles in Figure 4 show the pattern of the hole punches on the unfolded paper. The answer has two holes since the paper was two layers thick in the position where the hole was punched.

EXAMPLE

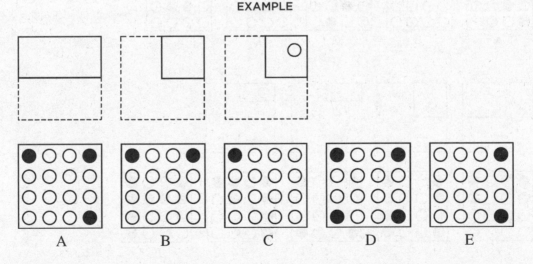

A   B   C   D   E

The correct answer is D. The paper was four thicknesses and, therefore, has four hole punches. The punch was made in the corner, so the four hole punches in the four corners are shown in black in the correct pattern.

46.

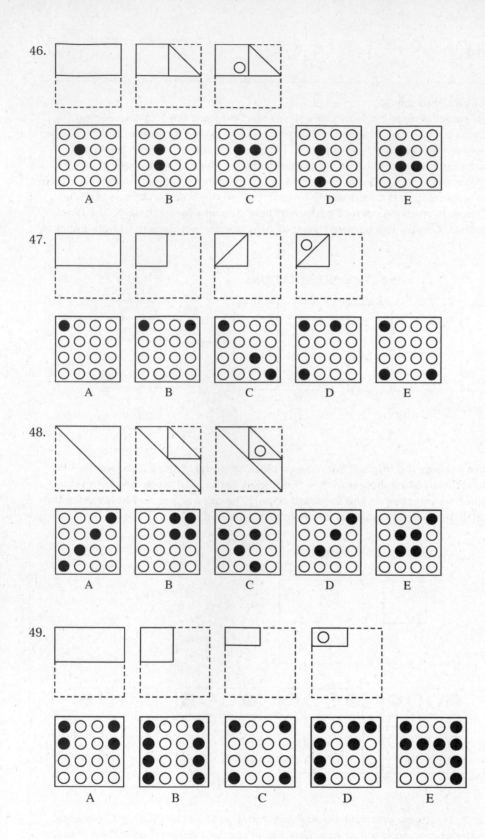

47.

48.

49.

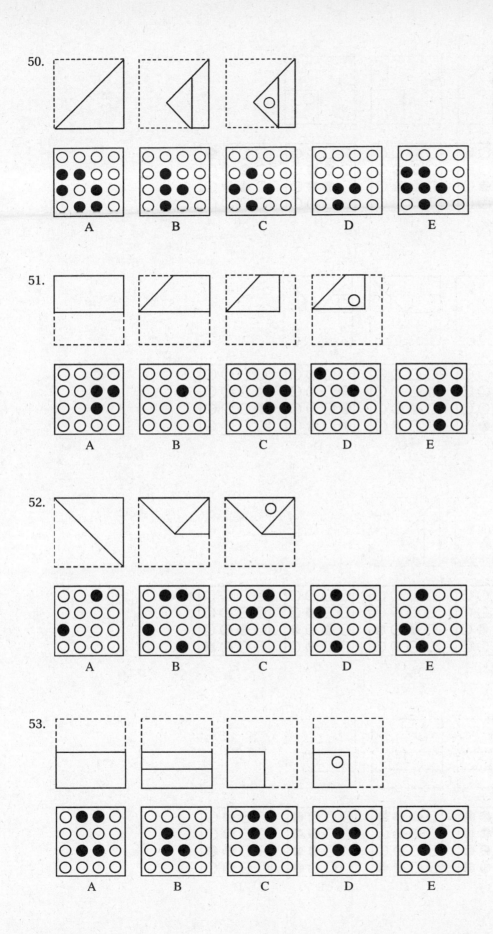

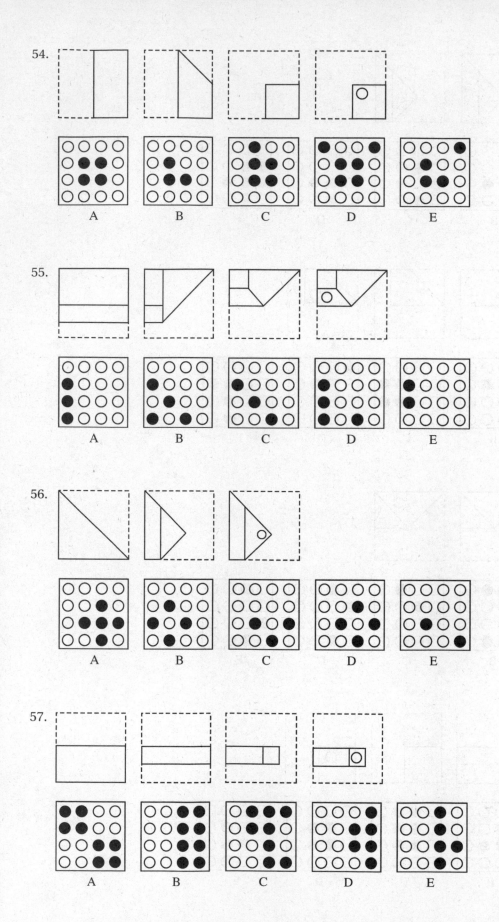

54.

55.

56.

57.

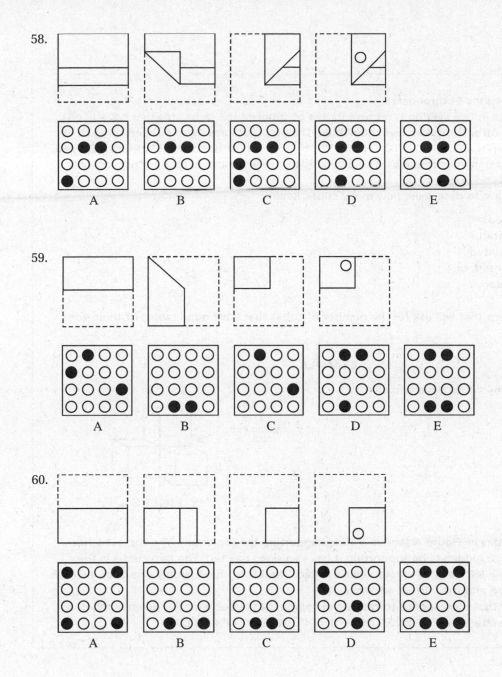

58.

59.

60.

Part 5: Cubes

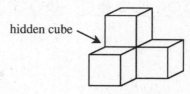
61. In Figure A, how many cubes have one of their exposed sides painted?

(A) 1 cube
(B) 2 cubes
(C) 3 cubes
(D) 4 cubes
(E) 5 cubes

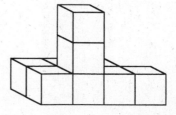

FIGURE A

62. In Figure A, how many cubes have two of their exposed sides painted?

(A) 1 cube
(B) 2 cubes
(C) 3 cubes
(D) 4 cubes
(E) 5 cubes

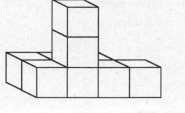

FIGURE A

63. In Figure A, how many cubes have three of their exposed sides painted?

(A) 1 cube
(B) 2 cubes
(C) 3 cubes
(D) 4 cubes
(E) 5 cubes

64. In Figure A, how many cubes have four of their exposed sides painted?

(A) 1 cube
(B) 2 cubes
(C) 3 cubes
(D) 4 cubes
(E) 5 cubes

65. In Figure B, how many cubes have two of their exposed sides painted?

(A) 1 cube
(B) 2 cubes
(C) 3 cubes
(D) 4 cubes
(E) 5 cubes

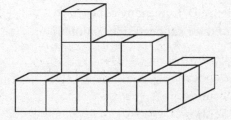

FIGURE B

66. In Figure B, how many cubes have three of their exposed sides painted?

(A) 1 cube
(B) 2 cubes
(C) 3 cubes
(D) 4 cubes
(E) 5 cubes

67. In Figure C, how many cubes have one of their exposed sides painted?

(A) 1 cube
(B) 2 cubes
(C) 3 cubes
(D) 4 cubes
(E) 5 cubes

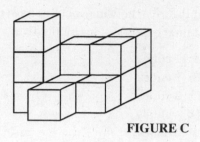

FIGURE C

68. In Figure C, how many cubes have two of their exposed sides painted?

(A) 1 cube
(B) 2 cubes
(C) 3 cubes
(D) 4 cubes
(E) 5 cubes

69. In Figure C, how many cubes have four of their exposed sides painted?

(A) 1 cube
(B) 2 cubes
(C) 3 cubes
(D) 4 cubes
(E) 5 cubes

70. In Figure D, how many cubes have two of their exposed sides painted?

(A) 1 cube
(B) 2 cubes
(C) 3 cubes
(D) 4 cubes
(E) 5 cubes

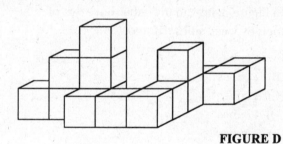

FIGURE D

71. In Figure D, how many cubes have four of their exposed sides painted?

(A) 1 cube
(B) 2 cubes
(C) 3 cubes
(D) 4 cubes
(E) 5 cubes

72. In Figure D, how many cubes have five of their exposed sides painted?

(A) 1 cube
(B) 2 cubes
(C) 3 cubes
(D) 4 cubes
(E) 5 cubes

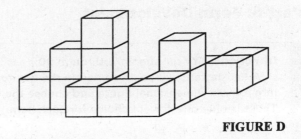

FIGURE D

73. In Figure E, how many cubes have one of their exposed sides painted?

(A) 1 cube
(B) 2 cubes
(C) 3 cubes
(D) 4 cubes
(E) 5 cubes

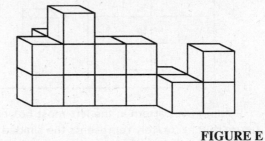

FIGURE E

74. In Figure E, how many cubes have two of their exposed sides painted?

(A) 1 cube
(B) 2 cubes
(C) 3 cubes
(D) 4 cubes
(E) 5 cubes

75. In Figure E, how many cubes have four of their exposed sides painted?

(A) 1 cube
(B) 2 cubes
(C) 3 cubes
(D) 4 cubes
(E) 5 cubes

Part 6: Form Development

Directions: For questions 76 through 90:

A flat pattern will be presented in the box to the left. Your task is to mentally fold this pattern into a three-dimensional figure and choose the correct representation from the choices to the right. There is only one correct choice for each item.

EXAMPLE

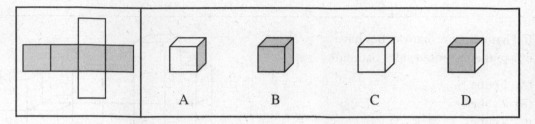

Folding the pattern in the left-most box can form only one of the figures to the right. The only figure that accurately represents the shaded areas once the pattern is folded is D.

Choose the letter that represents the three-dimensional object that correctly represents the folded pattern.

76.

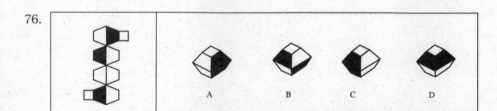

77.

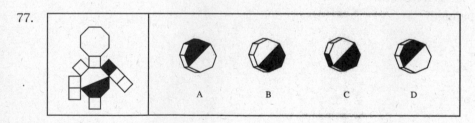

78.

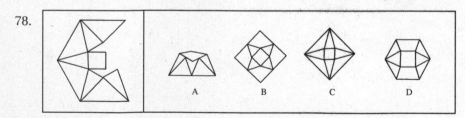

79.

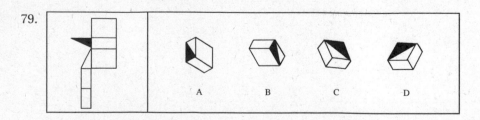

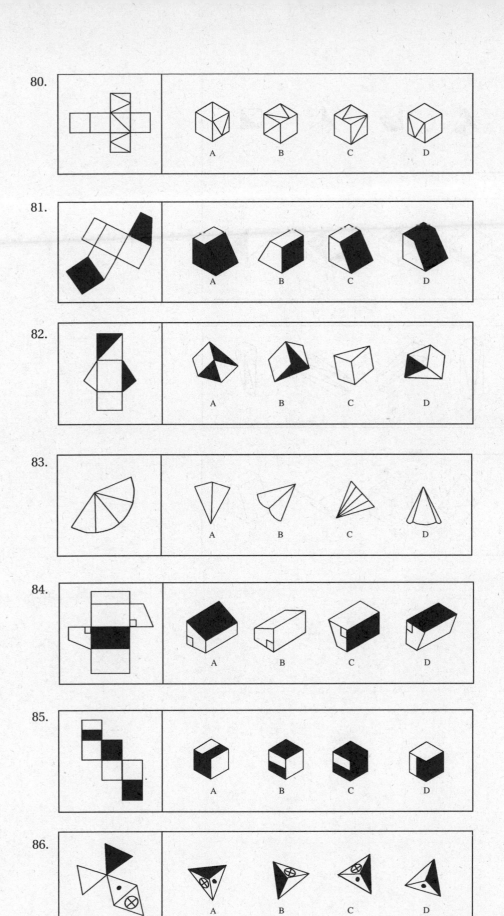

87.

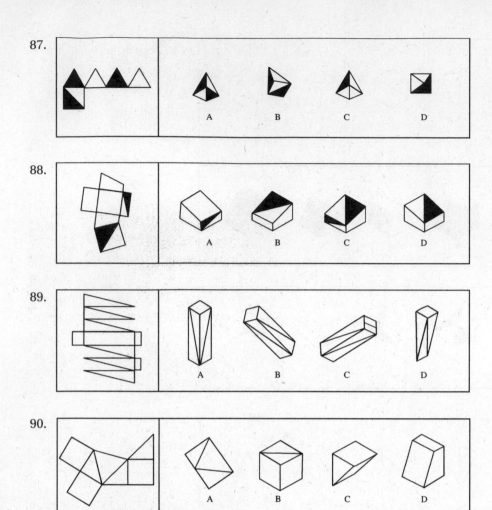

88.

89.

90.

TIME LIMIT: 60 MINUTES

Directions: This section consists of three passages, with questions and/or incomplete statements following each passage. Read each passage; then read the questions and/or incomplete statements and answer choices carefully. For each question and/or incomplete statement, choose the best answer and blacken the corresponding space on the answer sheet. This section contains 50 items.

Questions 1 through 18 are based on the following passage.

1. Three-dimensional printing of dental crowns, removable partial frameworks, and complete dentures is revolutionizing the dental profession and becoming a mainstay in dental offices and laboratories. Rapid prototyping is a combination of technologies used together to fabricate a part, model, or subassembly through computer-aided design (CAD) and computer-aided manufacturing (CAM) processes. Implementing this technology in dentistry provides dentists the tools to scan, design, and fabricate dental prostheses that would normally take weeks to complete, and they can be easily delivered in-office at a fraction of the time and cost.

2. The revolution in prototyping is due to advancements in scanning devices, three-dimensional computer software, and printers capable of fabricating polymers, ceramics, and metal prostheses. Currently, dental impressions, gypsum models, or structures of the head and neck are scanned using desktop or hand-held intraoral scanner cone beam computed tomography (CT). Depending on the resolution, scanners vary in price and are available in fixed or portable units. User-friendly computer-aided design (CAD) software interprets scanner data and provides readable language that describes the surface geometry of a 3D object allowing the dental technician to sculpt or modify scanning results on the computer. Each dental prosthesis is unique and custom made to individual specifications, and no two prostheses have the same fit, contour, or shape.

With simple adjustments to the design, the dental professional or technician can change the surface of the occlusal anatomy, the size or characteristics of the tooth, and save it as a stereolithography (.stl) file format. This type of file format, developed in 1987, describes surface geometry through triangulated surfaces of an object (Figure 1).

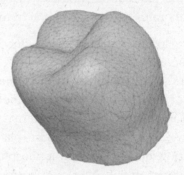

Figure 1

3. Three-dimensional computer-aided manufacturing (CAM) printers use data sets to develop a useful product. With recent prototyping advancements, materials have been developed that are stronger, harder, and capable of being milled on a machine. Cements have now also been produced with higher bond strengths allowing teeth to withstand the forces of parafunctional habits. This combination of technologies allows the fabrication process to be pushed from the traditional dental laboratory to the dental operatory.

4. In the field of maxilla-facial prosthodontics, impression materials used to fabricate ears, eyes, and palatal lift devices, such as alginate, polyvinyl

siloxane, and specialty waxes, are being replaced by intra/extra oral scanners and materials that allow the dental professional to digitally sculpt prostheses. The use of new materials, techniques, and three-dimensional printing of dental prostheses using a variety of biocompatible materials ultimately saves patients time and money.

5. Additive and subtractive technologies were developed and tested in the dental profession to fabricate prostheses. The additive manufacturing technique relies on successively layering material on top of each other until the model is complete. This approach reduces time and preserves material with little to no waste. Subtractive manufacturing, as the name implies, removes unwanted material from a solid block until the model is complete. This technique requires more time, more raw materials, and longer machining times. A significant portion, approximately 50 to 90 percent of the initial block, is cut away to create the dental restoration. Below are several fabrication methods that are used in dental laboratories to make dental restorations:

a. The lost-wax casting technique of fabricating a dental restoration was used for more than 200 years. This technique involves making a wax pattern of the prepared or missing tooth structure (enamel and dentin). The wax pattern is then placed on a sprue, waxed to a sprue base, placed inside a casting ring, and invested in a phosphate bonded investment material. After curing, the sprue base is removed, the casting ring is set in a furnace to burn out the wax pattern, and biocompatible molten metal is centrifuged through the sprue base and into the investment pattern or burned-out wax pattern. After cooling, the investment material is broken and sectioned, and the metal casting is finished and polished. The accuracy of the completed model is dependent on the technique used, the type of wax and metal used, and the ability to balance the expansion and contraction of materials before and after the casting procedure.

b. Stereolithography (SLA) is the method of creating a dental prosthesis through photopolymerization from a computer-aided drawing. This technology uses ultraviolet lasers to scan the surface of photosensitive polymers and selectively hardens the material in successive thin layers. After one layer is polymerized, the build plate moves to accommodate each successive layer until the model is constructed. This technique was developed in 1970 as a method of prototyping models used in preoperative planning, design, and manufacturing of medical or dental prostheses. This method of fabrication requires supports for overhangs and cavities that can be removed. This method is accurate but requires a minimum thickness of 0.8 mm.

c. Selective laser sintering (SLS) printing is an additive manufacturing process that can fabricate strong, durable, highly complex models with excellent surface finishes. This method uses a lens and a laser light source to fuse together small polymers, plastics, and nonmetal particles spread across the build plate to create the fabricated 3D computer-aided drawing model. SLS printing works best with nonmetal powder distributed on the build plate, rolled to compress the powder, lasered to a fused or semifused state, and then lowered by one thickness of material to allow the next layer to be added and lasered. The material is usually preheated and requires no support structure, but models do need to be assembled and finished in postproduction.

d. Selective laser melting (SLM) is an additive manufacturing process involving the use of atomized fine metal powder evenly distributed on a movable build plate in an enclosed chamber using inert gases. After each layer is distributed on the build plate, a high power laser beam directed in the x- and y-axis fuses, or melts, the powder particles together and no additional sintering is required. This process continues until the model is fabricated. This process is used to fabricate single component metal models that have complex geometries, hidden voids, or thin walls.

e. Binder jet printing (BJP) is an additive manufacturing technique that requires a computer-aided drawing in stereolithography file format. The printer uses a print head nozzle that distributes a thin, cross-sectional layer of metal powder across the build plate, followed by a liquid binding material, selectively placed to join the layered powder particles to each. As the printing bed lowers, the layering process continues, with each layer of powder followed by a roller to lightly compact and smooth the surface until the model is complete. Since the particles of the completed model are lightly bonded, the model is placed in a sintering oven to densify at a temperature that is material dependent. Unbound powder falls away, and the liquid binding material evaporates. This is a fast, low-cost printing method that enables stress-free structures with complex internal and external geometries, and, since no heat or residual stresses are built into the fabricated part, the final product is extremely accurate.

f. Fused deposition (FDM) is the most common and economical method for prototyping models using various types and colors of materials. Developed approximately 30 years ago, FDM uses layering of plastic filament or wire across a movable bed. This additive manufacturing method requires a scanned or computer-aided design model in a stereolithography file format. The model is fabricated by ejecting heated plastic filament through a nozzle or extrusion head onto a controlled moving table. As it cools and hardens, successive layers are added. Typically, the extrusion head is capable of moving in the x- and y-axis to complete the layer and will move up to start a new layer, while the table moves in a z-axis. The bed can be heated or cooled to prevent the model from sticking to the base plate. The disadvantages of FDM are lack of accuracy, visible layering of lines, and lack of speed depending on the density.

6. The advantages of rapid prototyping are the time and money saved and the quality of the final dental prostheses. The adage "good technique pays off" is imperative in the dental profession. Traditional methods of fabrication require numerous steps that include impression making, model fabrication, transporting models back and forth to the dental laboratory, casting metal, adding porcelain, finishing, polishing, and storage of casts. Every step in the fabrication process requires a thorough understanding of the coefficient of thermal expansion and manipulation of materials to avoid ill-fitting prostheses. Whether it is contraction of impression materials, expansion of gypsum, contraction of molten metal or zirconia, or contrac-

tion of dental polymers, good technique dictates success or failure. Digital scanning and fabrication methods eliminate many of the changes metals, porcelain, and impression materials undergo.

7. In order to meet the growing expectations and patient demands in the United States population, dental professionals will need to make prostheses faster and more economical, and use materials that arc less expensive and lighter weight. The future dental professional must be able to use a hand-held or cone beam tomography scanner on patients requiring prostheses, modify and design the prosthesis on a computer, fabricate by printing, and adjust the prostheses before the patient leaves the operatory. Scanning and computer-aided design and manufacturing techniques must be introduced early on in the dental curriculum, so students move from beginner to novice to competent clinicians and meet the future needs and requirements of this profession. Prototyping through additive and subtractive manufacturing allows the dental profession to treat diseased and missing teeth in an efficient, productive manner, while reducing cost.

1. The primary purpose of this passage is to

   (A) discuss materials used in the field of dentistry and maxilla prosthetics.
   (B) discuss rapid prototyping methods used in the dental profession.
   (C) summarize the capabilities of rapid prototyping technology.
   (D) discuss the disadvantages of the lost-wax casting technique.
   (E) discuss three-dimensional software for rapid prototyping.

2. According to the passage, does the author indicate which method of three-dimensional printing will revolutionize the dental profession?

   (A) Yes, the author favors FDM and BJP to fabricate metal frameworks.
   (B) Yes, the author favors the lost-wax casting technique to give the most favorable results.
   (C) Yes, all the manufacturing technologies can produce acceptable prosthesis.
   (D) No, the article only discusses fabrication methods using current technologies.
   (E) Yes, the SLA method is becoming the printer of choice in dentistry.

3. What can you infer from the passage about each printing method?

   (A) Each method of manufacturing requires a stereolithography file format.
   (B) A scanned or CAD model design may be used with any manufacturing process.
   (C) Each fabrication method requires certain metal powders or filaments.
   (D) A basic understanding of the advantages and disadvantages is important in deciding the type of machine to use.
   (E) All of the above

4. Name a component of three-dimensional printing technology.

   (A) Understanding the coefficient of thermal expansions of dental materials
   (B) Knowledge and understanding of computer-aided software and formats
   (C) The build plate axis as it moves in relationship to the other two axes
   (D) Understanding how "good technique" relates to model construction
   (E) Removing and finishing the final product from the build plate

5. Which type of manufacturing method conserves material and is more expedient?

   (A) Additive manufacturing using the lost-wax casting technique
   (B) Subtractive manufacturing using FDM
   (C) Additive manufacturing using SLA
   (D) Subtractive manufacturing using SLS
   (E) Subtractive manufacturing using GLS technology

6. How do the SLA and FDM methods of printing differ?

   (A) Type of material used to construct the model
   (B) Curing/processing of material to form a solid model
   (C) Movement of the build plate
   (D) Postprocessing of the material at the end of the build
   (E) All of the above

7. The author conveys the idea that "good technique pays off." What manufacturing method requires the greatest time commitment and degree of accuracy?

   (A) Lost-wax casting technique
   (B) Stereolithography
   (C) Selective laser melting
   (D) Selective laser sintering
   (E) Fused deposition

8. Which printing method requires heated plastic filament placed in successive layers?

   (A) Fused deposition model
   (B) Stereolithography
   (C) Selective laser melting
   (D) Selective laser sintering
   (E) Lost-wax casting technique

9. How does the author describe the future educational requirements for dentists?

(A) Understanding how to manipulate and design from cone beam tomography scans
(B) Focus on didactic and hands-on training with prototyping technologies
(C) The need to see more patients that require fabrication of complicated dental prostheses
(D) Dental educators and manufacturing engineers working together to develop protocols and industry standards
(E) Understanding variations in dental tooth morphology, form, and function

10. What can you infer from the passage about the physical and mechanical properties of BJP manufactured models?

(A) Placing metal powder particles in layers can reduce the effects of internal and external stresses.
(B) The metal powder is manufactured to prevent changes due to heat and pressure.
(C) Liquid binding material prevents changes of physical properties.
(D) In the absence of heat and pressure, internal stresses can be reduced.
(E) Internal stresses would be increased due to the cross-sectional layer of metal powder.

11. How does SLS printing differ from SLM printing?

(A) The type of inert gas used in production is different.
(B) The type of roller used to compress the material is different.
(C) The type of laser used to fuse the particles is different.
(D) SLS requires postproduction and sintering.
(E) The quality and quantity of resin required is different.

12. What is one disadvantage of subtractive manufacturing?

(A) Sintering the fabricated model
(B) The need for a .stl file format
(C) Additional manufacturing and resource costs
(D) Price per unit model produced
(E) Additional time required to manufacture the final product

13. What would happen during a BJP printing cycle if resin binder was not placed on the next layer of material?

(A) Metal powder particles would bind together during densification.
(B) Metal powder particles would be held loosely bound until sintering and then fuse.
(C) Metal powder particles would be tightly bound before sintering and then fuse.
(D) Metal powder particles would not adhere to the next layer and after sintering the particles would not fuse together.
(E) The metal powder particles would fuse after removal from the sintering oven.

14. Which if the following is the recommended scanning method for fabricating head and neck structures?

(A) Hand-held scanner
(B) Cone beam computed tomography
(C) Desktop scanner
(D) The author does not recommend one method over the other.
(E) Positron-emission tomography

15. According to the passage, what is the function of the *z*-axis in a three-dimensional printer?

(A) It supports the vertical component of model fabrication.
(B) It supports the horizontal component of model fabrication.
(C) It is the measurement when *x* and *z* are equal to zero.
(D) It supports the dependent/independent variable.
(E) It serves as a reference point for calibrating the printer.

16. What material is used to form the inside perimeter of a restoration using the lost-wax casting technique?

(A) Casting ring
(B) Phosphate bonded investment material
(C) Polymer coating surrounding the waxed model
(D) Sprue base
(E) Paper liner

17. What is unique about the stereolithography file format?

(A) It describes the color, texture, and other attributes of the model.
(B) It uses a particular scale calibrated in millimeters.
(C) It describes the surface geometry of the three-dimensional object.
(D) It can be interpreted by five software programs.
(E) It has limited use due to its *x*, *y*, and *z* constraints.

18. What type of file format is described in Figure 1?

(A) TIFF—Tag Image File Format
(B) JPEG—File Interchange Format
(C) STL—Stereolithography File Format
(D) PNG—Portable Network Graphics Format
(E) GIF—Graphics Interchange Format

Question 19 through 34 are based on the following passage.

1. The first week at this military installation was spent processing and transitioning into active duty, a career that I left just fifteen years earlier. The days were long, as approximately four hundred essential personnel were processed through human resources, medical and dental screening, weapons training, basic tactics, and loads of Power Point presentations on things that will get you killed if you failed to pay attention. After receiving immunizations for smallpox, tetanus, anthrax, tuberculosis, and several others, and drawing three hundred pounds of standard issue uniforms, boots, hot and cold weather garments, protective suits and masks, helmets, weapons, and protective body armor, they told us we were ready. We learned rudimentary movement techniques and tactics to survive in a combat environment. The three-to-five-second rushes were a movement technique used to eliminate a threat that required one to stand up, move at a fast pace, and get back down in a prone position. Unfortunately, the training manual was not updated to reflect the aging population of essential personnel—three to five seconds translated into ten to fifteen seconds. By the end of week, we were all mentally, emotionally, and somewhat physically prepared for what laid ahead, and most of us boarded contracted airplanes to go to different regions of the world.

2. I remember seeing the outside of the airplane before boarding and feeling disheartened that I never heard of the airline, and I wondered who was flying this enormous aircraft and if a safety briefing was part of the contract. The plane was configured to seat as many personnel as possible, with no upgrades, no frequent flier miles, and a decor that stated the year was 1960. The plane landed somewhere across the Atlantic Ocean to refuel. At touchdown, two of the aircraft's landing tires decided that 1,200 duffle bags and 330 personnel were more than they could handle and blew out on landing. We agreed that the aircraft was simply saying that it needed more time to recover, and the one-hour stop turned into four hours of refueling—tire rotation,

routine maintenance, and, for us, a few hours of shut-eye. After flying through seven time zones and more than twenty-four hours of intimate relaxation in an upright, uncomfortable airline seat, and being fed every two hours by the lowest bidder airline, we were closer to our final destination. When the doors opened, we all looked at each other and agreed this was not part of the training. Deplaning wearing 30 pounds of battle armor, feeling weary and tired, and carrying very expensive, sensitive items on our person and the blast of one 110-degree heat, we felt like we were entering a blast furnace full of molten steel. To make things worse, the baggage conveyor broke, and 1,200 duffle bags had to be offloaded by hand from the belly of the beast that just brought us thousands of miles to this inhospitable location. The cruel and unusual punishment was just starting.

3. Commercial buses were used to transport us to our next location. With heightened security, we could feel the anxiety and nervousness of traveling under the cover of darkness on a moonless night in the middle of nowhere. We took no comfort in knowing there were other people on the bus for *our* protection. The diesel fumes kept us awake and alert for the next sixty minutes. The lack of undulating terrain and penetrating darkness made us all aware that hell was just around the corner. When the vibrations stopped, the artificial lighting penetrated the darkened window alerting us that we arrived somewhere. We picked up all our worldly possessions in the form of four olive drab duffle bags from the back end of a tractor-trailer. At this point, I realized that this was all I could count on for the next twelve months.

4. It was a Sunday at high noon, and the sky was cloudless. The temperature at the barren outpost was 141 degrees Fahrenheit—shorts and tee shirts were not an option. I remember drinking quarts of water every hour. Even after drinking two gallons of water in less than four hours, my urine would still not even fill a shot glass. The training lasted several more days. The focus this time was on insects, animals, and other things you do not want to touch or step on in the desert. We received additional classes and training on survival tactics, weapons firing, how to recognize mines and impoverished explosive

devices, and how to keep hydrated in order to prevent your vital organs from turning into a delicacy.

5. It was the end of the second week; we manifested this time on a dark-gray-colored military transport airplane. It was time to suit up and wait again. When putting on a five-pound helmet with a sweaty helmet band for the umpteenth time, looking through scratched protective goggles, with body armor stuck between soaking layers of uniform, a rucksack containing all the immediate emergency needs, and flying into the middle of nowhere, it makes you suddenly realize you'd better believe in something quickly, in case your plane has to make an emergency landing in the sky. With over 250 combat-ready personnel, duffle bags, and a basic issue of live ammunition locked and loaded, we departed. The taxpayers would have been proud that this flight had no food or beverage service or fancy amenities like toilet paper. The seats amounted to stained, worn webbing that literally supported just parts of your body, while the remaining parts slumped just inches from the floor of the aircraft. Sitting in the cockpit at 32,000 feet felt like looking at Heaven and realizing Dante's Inferno was just below, and there was no runway in Heaven yet. Suddenly the plane made a rapid descent, with plenty of instruction coming from someone on the ground about where to turn, at what speed, and if we were in an acceptable glide path and approach. We touched down in a controlled movement, grabbed our duffle bags at the rear of the plane, and ran for cover and protection at concrete bunkers that lined the runway.

6. After a two-hour rest, the journey continued, but this time on a helicopter. At times, I became angry and disappointed about carrying four bags that represented safety and security from place to place and still not having a home. The word came that helicopters were coming, and we were ordered to go to the flight line. Suited up, we had fifteen seconds to load, enter, and buckle in before this machine went airborne. The crew chief instructed all the passengers that things might get "dicey" in the air and to hang on. Flying at lower elevations made us susceptible to direct fire. We noticed patches of trees dotting the sandscape. The pilots

and gunner made us believe that we should be prepared for anything. The helicopters flew up and over the hilltops and down into valleys at a maddening pace that made our skin pasty colored and our stomachs squeamish. Whether it was the powdered eggs, the grits, or the greasy S.O.S served just hours earlier, it wanted to just come out. By the end of this free, magical roller coaster experience, all six of us disembarked with just one casualty to clean up on the floor of the helicopter. We all looked around and tried to guess what continent we touched down on, or if *National Geographic* ever photographed this part of our new world.

7. My greeter showed up at the airfield to welcome me to a year of anguish! I carried misery on my right shoulder and despair on my left. I placed my four olive drab duffle bags in the back of a civilian vehicle. While driving down a dusty, hot, insect invested, and bumpy, washed-out road, we made some interesting conversation with the driver. His recommendation for a successful stay was, "just get used to it." Driving to our final destination at just ten miles an hour felt like I was only six hours into a twelve-hour airplane ride. The unique sights and smells, and the intense sun clearly told me I was far, far away from the east coast of the United States. When I asked my driver about the weather for the next few days, he remarked that there are many things you can predict in this county. For instance, the mess hall WILL serve you S.O.S. every morning, bugs will bite you, people will die, and the sun will rise and set. The weather forecast yesterday was very hot and dusty, today's weather forecast is very hot and dusty, tomorrow the weather will be very hot and dusty, and next week the weather will be very hot and dusty.

8. The base camp was austere, with no luxuries or amenities. The fortunate ones got a mattress instead of a cot, some got a trailer, and others got a tent, but everyone used the dreaded porta-potties to take care of their business. It was a challenge when you REALLY had to go. You had to remove all your battle armor, weapons, ammunition, and helmet, and have a good aim into a European toilet as the sand flies, mosquitoes, and other insects looked on with envy. Since nothing is paved in this coun-

try, the fine dust remains like a cloud. The sand gets in your underwear, the bright sun wakes you up regardless of how tired you are, and at the far corner of the post the smell of burning human feces from the porta-potties was suffocating. There was a small exchange if you wanted to buy incidentals, although the ordering clerk clearly had mistaken priorities. The shelves were barren except for quarts of transmission fluid, fancy steering wheel covers, protein shake powder, and outdated electronic equipment—most expired four years ago. There were plenty of T-shirts that said, "My boyfriend loves me and sent me this T-shirt from _____." We learned that tax-free money is spent quicker on merchandise that you really don't need. Since time goes slowly and everyday seems like the one before, no calendars hang on any walls. You might see a picture of a wife, husband, or boyfriend or girlfriend as a reminder that loved ones are waiting for you back home, but everyone tries to compartmentalize the good from the bad. Work started before the sun rose, ended four hours after sunset, seven days a week without overtime or holidays. Since everyone had the same schedule, time went by quickly.

9. The medical clinic, my final destination, was in sight. I only had to motivate myself to carry 30 pounds of personal equipment and my 160-pound frame, and lift and carry four dreaded olive-green duffle bags 200 yards. Welcome to my journey!

19. The author's attitude for most of his journey can best be described as

(A) alarming.
(B) concerned.
(C) concerned and confused.
(D) concerned and optimistic.
(E) apathetic.

20. According to the passage, which of the following can you infer would most likely be true?

    (A) The individual equipment assigned was needed and required.
    (B) A travel agency established the movement overseas for this individual.
    (C) Getting to the final destination was extremely important to the entire operation.
    (D) If an airplane was not able to fly, other contingencies were established,
    (E) Meals were served between transportation segments.

21. The author's purpose for writing this passage is to

    (A) describe the process of overseas travel.
    (B) describe the medical and training requirements to travel overseas.
    (C) describe the comfort and conveniences available of several modes of transportation.
    (D) travel overseas.
    (E) describe the equipment personnel are required to carry when traveling.
    (F) describe the need to be physically, mentally, and emotionally prepared for traveling to a foreign country for an extended stay.

22. Based on the passage, one could easily conclude that

    (A) significant time and preparation were required for overseas travel.
    (B) being physically and mentally prepared is important to adjust to changing situations.
    (C) it is important to understand one's strengths and weaknesses.
    (D) it is important to have a clear understanding of your mission.
    (E) All of the above

23. From the passage, how would you sense the importance of security of personnel and equipment through this journey?

    (A) The security of personnel and equipment was given the highest priority.
    (B) The security of personnel and equipment was not discussed in the passage.
    (C) Only select individuals were responsible for security.
    (D) The security of personnel and equipment was not important.
    (E) The security of personnel and equipment was only important when arriving at the final destination.

24. What did the four duffle bags represent to the author?

    (A) Change of clothing and personal essentials
    (B) Gifts and food items for other personnel
    (C) Gifts and food items for family at home
    (D) Equipment to be used in the medical clinic
    (E) Essential clothing and protective garments for the next twelve months

25. What can the reader infer about the types of training that took place at the processing and transition station?

    (A) It was basic and rudimentary.
    (B) It was detailed and focused.
    (C) It was not relevant.
    (D) It was not required for essential personnel.
    (E) It was only required for security personnel.

26. According to the passage, what was the driver referring to when he stated, "just get used to it"?

    (A) The dusty environment
    (B) The temperature
    (C) The insects
    (D) The poor road conditions
    (E) All of the above

27. How does the author describe the present weather conditions?

    (A) Cloudy
    (B) Sunny and hot
    (C) Hot and dusty
    (D) Dusty and humid
    (E) Rainy and humid

28. What was the sequence of travel for the soldier?

    (A) Airplane, foot, automobile, helicopter, airplane
    (B) Airplane, automobile, airplane, helicopter, foot
    (C) Airplane, helicopter, bus, airplane, foot, automobile
    (D) Airplane, airplane, helicopter, bus, foot, automobile
    (E) Airplane, bus, airplane, helicopter, automobile, foot

29. What is the author's attitude toward carrying and moving four duffle bags through the country?

    (A) Parsimonious
    (B) Overwhelmed
    (C) Exasperated
    (D) Ambivalent
    (E) Frustrated

30. At what point did the author become concerned about his security?

    I. When departing the processing and transition installation
    II. When departing the airfield on a commercial bus
    III. When departing the airfield on a helicopter

    (A) I only
    (B) II only
    (C) III only
    (D) I and II only
    (E) II and III only

31. What was the author's final destination?

    (A) Base camp
    (B) Airport
    (C) Medical clinic
    (D) Base exchange
    (E) Mess hall

32. What form of transportation caused soldiers to feel sick?

    (A) Airplane
    (B) Automobile
    (C) Helicopter
    (D) Commercial bus
    (E) Military bus

33. The author states that the helmet weighs approximately how many pounds?

    (A) 3 pounds
    (B) 5 pounds
    (C) 7 pounds
    (D) 9 pounds
    (E) 30 pounds

34. Calculate the weight of personnel and equipment on the departing aircraft, if each duffle bag weighs 75 pounds and the average soldier with body armor weighs 190 pounds.

    (A) 47,500 pounds
    (B) 62,700 pounds
    (C) 97,400 pounds
    (D) 141,700 pounds
    (E) 152,700 pounds

Questions 35 through 50 are based on the following passage.

1. When asked to describe cement, most people would say it is a hard substance found almost everywhere: sidewalks, roads, building, and bridges. The product is environmentally friendly, inexpensive, and plentiful. The components are simple: sand, gravel, cement powder, water, and air when mixed together produces a flowable mass that hardens when set. The physical properties of cement make it extremely strong and durable, and it can withstand tremendous compressive forces and extreme weather and temperature differences. The purpose of cement is to act as a binder material that sets and hardens other materials together.

2. The components used and percentage of the components in the mixture is important in the production of the five types or categories of Portland cement. The types of cement reflect the requirements for sulfate resistance in wet environments, setting times, and property and strength requirements. Altering the components changes the type and usage. The basic components are:

a. Lime is calcium oxide and accounts for 60 to 65 percent of the mixture. Controlling the percent of lime in a cement mixture is important since too much lime causes expansion and will ultimately lead to cracking and disintegration, while too little lime reduces the strength and increases the setting time.

b. Silica (SiO_2) is the second-most important ingredient at 17 to 25 percent and serves to provide strength to the cement through the formation of dicalcium and tricalcium silicates. Too much silica increases the strength of the cement and increases setting time.

c. Alumina (Al_2O_3) accounts for 3 to 8 percent of the mixture and provides the quick setting properties to cement. Its purpose is to reduce the sintering temperature of the raw materials alumina and iron oxide. Excess alumina reduces the strength.

d. Magnesia (MgO) is 1 to 3 percent of the mixture and imparts hardness and color to the cement. Excess magnesia causes large changes in volume due to expansion after it sets.

e. Sulfur (SO_3), at 1 to 3 percent, helps control the expansion of setting cement.

f. Iron oxide (FeO) in trace amounts of 0.5 to 0.6 percent imparts color, hardness, and strength to cement.

g. Calcium sulfate ($CaSO_4$) in trace amounts of 0.1 to 0.5 percent functions to increase the initial setting of the cement.

tricalcium silicate + water → calcium silicate hydrate + calcium hydroxide + heat

$$2Ca_3SiO_5 + 7H_2O \rightarrow$$
$$3CaO_2SiO_2 + 4H_2O + 3Ca(OH)_2 + 173.6 \text{ kJ}$$

3. While the connection between Portland cement and dental cement might not be immediately apparent, both cements are used to describe a material that hardens through a chemical reaction to firmly attach two substances together. In dentistry, this is the dental crown to remaining tooth structure. Similar to Portland cement, the dental profession uses the term cement or "luting agent" to provide retention of the restoration placed over the tooth structure and seal the margin around the crown. The retention and sealing of the restoration is accomplished by a combination of the tooth preparation and type of luting agent.

4. Tooth preparation is probably the most important requirement for the restoration's long-term success. The practitioner must possess skill, attention to detail, and the ability to visualize the final restoration before picking up a hand piece to remove any diseased tooth structure. Like an artist carving a statue from a block of stone, the dentist must understand how retention form, the preparations ability to impede removal of the restoration along its path of insertion, is dependent on taper, surface area, texture, and location of the tooth in the mouth. In addition, resistance form is defined as the ability of the preparation to prevent dislodgement of the restoration by forces directed in a horizontal, oblique, or apical direction. This requires an understanding of a patient's parafunctional habits, tooth taper, diameter, height of the restoration, and coverage area. In the above examples, a molar tooth having a large surface area, primarily one that accepts compressive forces along the long axis

of the tooth, would be designed differently from a mandibular, anterior tooth, which is shorter with shear forces acting on the incisal surface.

5. Types of luting agents affect the resistance and retention form of the restoration and are classified by their chemical reaction with the tooth structure. Most luting agents are powder-liquid or liquid-liquid that when mixed manually or when dispensed together, form a solid mass.

a. Water-based cements rely on an acid-base reaction. This category includes glass ionomer and resin-modified glass ionomer cements, zinc polyacrylate, and zinc phosphate. The classic acid-base reaction of zinc phosphate cement is the oldest and most widely used cement in dentistry. This cement requires the addition of zinc and magnesium oxide powder and phosphoric acid liquid mixed over several minutes to dissipate the heat of the reaction. The mixture and placement of this cement is critical to the life of the tooth since raising the internal temperature of the tooth beyond 6°F could heat the pulp of the tooth and eventually cause it to die. The powder is divided up in 6 equal amounts and placed on one side of a "cooled" glass slab. The phosphoric acid and water mixture is dispensed in droplet form on the opposite side. Slowly, a small amount of powder is mixed into the liquid with a stainless steel spatula and spread over a large surface area to cool the reaction. This process continues for up to 2 minutes and stops when the cement droops 1 inch off the mixing spatula. This cement has been the "gold standard" to which all cements are measured against due to a film thickness of less than 25 microns. If mixed improperly, the cement may cause hypersensitivity due to the exothermic reaction.

$$\text{zinc oxide} + \text{phosphoric acid} \rightarrow$$
$$\text{amorphous zinc phosphate} + \text{water} + \text{heat}$$

$$ZnO + H_3PO_4 \rightarrow Zn_2(PO_4)_2 + H_2O + \text{heat}$$

b. Resin cements involve a polymerization reaction. The characteristics of this cement are high bond strengths, technique sensitivity, separate monomer and polymer components, and multiple clinical purposes. This category of cement includes composites, adhesive resins, and com-

pomers. Developed as an alternative for luting zirconia, cast alloys, and all other ceramic restorations, resin cements have the advantage of being self-cured, light cured, or dual cured. The polymer powder is methyl methacrylate containing the initiator benzoyl peroxide, along with other pigments and coloring agents. The liquid monomer is a methyl methacrylate containing an anime accelerator. As the monomer dissolves and softens the polymer particles, the reaction goes through three distinct stages: initiation, propagation, and termination. The polymer forms through the action of free radicals from the peroxide amine interaction. The available systems range from very simple to relatively complex kits designed for esthetic restorations. Specific coupling agents are available to bond to dentin, silica-based substrates, and noble metals. Without the specific bonding agents, the resin cements are considered very strong luting media, which have only modest bond strengths to dentin. The use of bonding agents and primers is, therefore, essential in obtaining optimal results.

c. Oil based represents the oldest category of acid-based reaction cements that, when two components are combined, set in a hard biocompatible mass. This category of cements includes zinc oxide-eugenol and noneugenol zinc oxide and is primarily used for the temporary cementation of provisional restorations, surgical dressing, and sealing root canals where strength is not important. The main ingredients of the powder are zinc oxide and white rosin used to reduce the brittleness of the set cement. The liquid component is primarily eugenol with olive oil and the reaction takes place with the formation of zinc eugenolate chelate.

6. Dental cement, along with resistance and retention form of the tooth, seal and retain the crown to the remaining tooth structure. Other forces help supply additional strength to the tooth and crown, such as:

a. Mechanical retention—due to small undercuts or irregular surface on the tooth from the bur that prepared the tooth surface and small grooves from the fabrication of the inside of the restoration. The cement layer fills in and conforms to the space inside the crown and outside tooth. When the cement hardens, it provides retention and seals the margin.

b. Micromechanical retention—due to microscopic undercuts as a result of the effects of etching the remaining tooth structure. The tooth is etched with phosphoric acid to provide irregular surfaces on the outside of the tooth, in addition to the mechanical retention efforts by the bur. Similar to mechanical retention, the cement fills in and conforms to the space between the crown and tooth structure.

c. Chemical reaction—through chemical attraction of the carboxyl group of the cement with the calcium ions remaining in the tooth structure. For these cements, the bond to dentin is obtained by a link to the calcium ion in dentin. Because calcium is a divalent ion, cross-linking of the acid chains occurs.

35. According to the passage, what is the purpose of dental cement?

   I. To seal the margin of the restoration
   II. To retain the restoration over the tooth structure
   III. To reduce the number of microorganisms growing on the tooth

   (A) I only
   (B) II only
   (C) III only
   (D) I and II only
   (E) I and III only

36. The author's purpose in writing the passage is to

   (A) describe the components of Portland cement.
   (B) identify the percentage and types of Portland cement.
   (C) describe the most important requirements to tooth preparation.
   (D) understand that all cements are components of various materials that act to seal, bind, and harden materials together.
   (E) identify how additional retentive features can aid in the restoration of a tooth.

37. How does the author describe the chemical retention of a restoration to tooth structure?

   (A) Surface area, texture, and taper
   (B) Carboxyl group with the calcium ions
   (C) Polymerization reaction
   (D) Microscopic undercuts in the tooth
   (E) Small undercuts from the bur

38. What cement is considered the "gold standard" in dentistry?

   (A) Water-based cements
   (B) Glass ionomer cements
   (C) Resin-modified glass ionomer cements
   (D) Cements having a film thickness of 25 microns or less
   (E) All of the above

39. Long-term success of a dental restoration is dependent on which of the following criteria?

   (A) Type of material used for the dental restoration
   (B) Tooth preparation
   (C) Condition of the tooth
   (D) Type of cement
   (E) The use of additional factors, such as mechanical, chemical, and micro-mechanical retention

40. What can the reader infer about the chemical reaction of an acid-base dental cement?

   (A) The restoration can be removed only one time after cementation.
   (B) The reaction can be reversed in certain situations.
   (C) The reaction proceeds due to the action of free radicals from the peroxide amine interaction.
   (D) Heat is a byproduct of the reaction.
   (E) It is used as temporary cement for provisional restorations.

41. What type of cement reaction proceeds with the formation of zinc eugenolate chelate?

(A) Luting agents
(B) Water-based cements
(C) Acid-base cements
(D) Resin cements
(E) Oil-based cements

42. What is the function of sulfur in the production of Portland cement?

(A) It increases the initial setting time.
(B) It controls expansion of the setting cement.
(C) It imparts hardness and color to the cement.
(D) It reduces strength.
(E) It causes expansion.

43. Which is the most appropriate title for this passage?

(A) The Function and Components of Dental Cement
(B) Understanding the Microscopic and Macroscopic Properties of Cement
(C) The Minimum Requirements for Long-Term Restoration Success
(D) The Effects of Self-Cured, Light-Cured, and Dual-Cured Cements
(E) How the Practitioner's Skill, Attention to Detail, and Visualization Affect the Long-Term Success of a Dental Restoration

44. What can the reader infer from the author's detailed description of mixing water-based cements?

(A) The mixing technique has a long established history.
(B) Proper use of mixing components is extremely important to the overall success of the tooth.
(C) Removal of heat using a cold glass slab helps distribute heat over a large surface area.
(D) The consistency of cement is important to insertion of the restoration.
(E) All of the above

45. Which of the following is not a characteristic of resin cement?

(A) Low bond strength
(B) Technique sensitivity
(C) Serves multiple purposes
(D) Has a polymer component
(E) Self-cured

46. According to the passage, how does the author describe the use of small grooves inside the restoration?

(A) Chemical attraction
(B) Micromechanical retention
(C) Mechanical retention
(D) Retention form
(E) Resistance form

47. What components are used in the production of cements?

(A) Cement powder, gravel, sand, air, and liquid polymer
(B) Lime, sulfur, calcium hydroxide, heat, and air
(C) Water, gravel, sand, cement powder, and air
(D) Zinc oxide, water, powder, air, and phosphoric acid
(E) Zinc oxide, eugenol, water, air, and olive oil

48. The passage describes techniques used for successful cementation of dental restorations. Which cement requires the use of bonding agents and primers for optimal results?

   (A) Luting agents
   (B) Water-based cements
   (C) Acid-base cements
   (D) Resin cements
   (E) Oil-based cements

49. Retention and resistance forces are important factors for retaining a dental restoration. Which cement provides additional strength through mechanical, chemical, and micro-mechanical forces to the restoration?

   (A) Resin cements
   (B) Oil-based cements
   (C) Acid-base cements
   (D) Luting agents
   (E) Water-based cements

50. Five types of Portland cement can be produced by which of the following modifications?

   (A) Removing magnesia, sulfur, and iron oxide from the basic components
   (B) Changing the percentage of silica as the primary component
   (C) The addition or subtraction of sand, gravel, cement powder, and water
   (D) Changing the components and percentage of the basic components
   (E) None of the above

TIME LIMIT: 45 MINUTES

Directions: The following items are questions or incomplete statements. Read each item carefully, and then choose the best answer or completion. Blacken the corresponding space on the answer sheet. This section contains 40 items.

1. The ratio of historians to anthropologists is 1 : 2. If the number of historians is doubled and the number of anthropologists is tripled, which of the following is the possible number of historians and anthropologists attending?

   (A) 6
   (B) 7
   (C) 8
   (D) 9
   (E) 10

2. The probability of winning a game is $\frac{1}{5}$.

   If games are independent, what is the probability of winning three times in a row if one win has already occurred?

   (A) $\frac{1}{5}$

   (B) $\frac{1}{25}$

   (C) $\frac{4}{5}$

   (D) $\frac{16}{25}$

   (E) $\frac{24}{25}$

3. Every hour a population of bacteria containing R plasmids increases by an amount that is $\frac{2}{5}$ the population present. After three hours, what fraction of bacteria containing R plasmids is present relative to the initial population?

   (A) $\frac{4}{125}$

   (B) $\frac{8}{125}$

   (C) $\frac{117}{125}$

   (D) $\frac{49}{25}$

   (E) $\frac{343}{125}$

4. Given $K_{eq} = \frac{[C]^2[D]^1}{[A]^2[B]^3}$, if somehow C increases by 50% and A decreases by 20%, but all other quantities remain the same, what is the percent increase in K_{eq}?

   (A) 251.56%
   (B) 195.34%
   (C) 70%
   (D) 50%
   (E) 20%

5. | Column A | Column B |
   |---|---|

   $x > 2$

   x^2 $4x - 4$

   (A) Column A is greater.
   (B) Column B is greater.
   (C) Columns A and B are equal.
   (D) Cannot be determined

6. If $\alpha = 3$, what is the value of the units digit of $2^{25\alpha} + 5$?

   (A) 1
   (B) 3
   (C) 7
   (D) 9
   (E) 13

7. $S = k_B \ln w$. If $S_1 = k_B \ln a^b$ and $S_2 = k_B \ln y^b$, where k_B is a constant, then what is $S_1 + S_2$?

   (A) $k_B \ln a^b$
   (B) $b(k_B \ln ay)$
   (C) $y(k_B \ln b^a)$
   (D) $k_B \ln ab$
   (E) $k_B \ln yb$

8. A six-sided die is rolled twice. What is the probability of getting a sum of 10 given that the first roll was a 5—assuming that the die is fair?

   (A) $\dfrac{1}{12}$
   (B) $\dfrac{1}{6}$
   (C) $\dfrac{1}{4}$
   (D) $\dfrac{1}{3}$
   (E) $\dfrac{1}{2}$

9. $14y + 7x = 3$; $10y + 4x = 7$. What is $6y + x$?

   (A) 10
   (B) 11
   (C) 12
   (D) 13
   (E) 14

10. A container holds 3 red balls, numbered 1–3, and 3 green balls, numbered 1–3. If three balls are picked one after the other without replacement, how many ways can this be done if the balls are lined up left to right, and the first ball must have an even number?

    (A) 10
    (B) 20
    (C) 40
    (D) 120
    (E) 360

11. How many ways can the letters in "TOOTH" be arranged?

    (A) 15
    (B) 30
    (C) 60
    (D) 150
    (E) 285

12. If the probability of selecting green tea is 30%, the probability of selecting black tea is 20%, and the probability of selecting both is 5%, what is the probability of selecting green tea, black tea, or both?

    (A) 0.05
    (B) 0.10
    (C) 0.20
    (D) 0.25
    (E) 0.45

13. | Column A | | Column B |
    |---|---|---|
    | | $0 \le \theta \le \dfrac{\pi}{2}$ | |
    | $\cos \theta$ | in radians. | $\tan \theta$ |
    | | $\sin \theta = \dfrac{3}{5}$ | |

    (A) Column A is greater.
    (B) Column B is greater.
    (C) Columns A and B are equal.
    (D) Cannot be determined

14. The probability of winning a local raffle is $\frac{3}{10}$. If each raffle is independent of the rest, what is the probability that a person who played twice won both given that she won at least once?

(A) $\frac{3}{10}$

(B) $\frac{9}{51}$

(C) $\frac{42}{51}$

(D) $\frac{10}{20}$

(E) $\frac{12}{20}$

15. A cube has each of its sides lengthened. What is the percent increase in volume?

(1) The length of each side is increased by 15%.
(2) The initial volume is 20 L.

(A) Statement (1) alone is sufficient, but statement (2) alone is not sufficient.
(B) Statement (2) alone is sufficient, but statement (1) alone is not sufficient.
(C) Both statements together are sufficient, but neither statement alone is sufficient.
(D) Each statement alone is sufficient.
(E) Statements (1) and (2) together are not sufficient.

16. 3 red books and 2 blue books are placed on a shelf from left to right. If books of the same color are indistinguishable, how many arrangements of the books can be achieved?

(A) 5
(B) 6
(C) 10
(D) 60
(E) 120

17. A 15 ft ladder leans against a wall. The foot of the ladder is 9 ft from the wall.

Column A	Column B
9 ft	Height of the top of the ladder as it leans against the wall

(A) Column A is greater.
(B) Column B is greater.
(C) Columns A and B are equal.
(D) Cannot be determined

18.

Column A	Column B

A is between $10 and $1,000.

59% of 35% of A	35% of 59% of A

(A) Column A is greater.
(B) Column B is greater.
(C) Columns A and B are equal.
(D) Cannot be determined

19. 5 books are arranged on a shelf. If three books are picked with one designated to become a special edition, how many ways can this be done? (Assume that the order in which the books are picked is irrelevant.)

(A) 6
(B) 15
(C) 30
(D) 45
(E) 60

20. A 10 L solution is 80% apple juice and 20% orange juice. Another solution is 20 L and 20% apple juice and 80% orange juice by volume. What fraction is apple juice when both solutions are put together?

(A) $\frac{6}{15}$

(B) $\frac{8}{15}$

(C) $\frac{9}{15}$

(D) $\frac{12}{15}$

(E) $\frac{13}{15}$

21. What is the probability of picking a code with an even number from codes made up of 3 digits 0–9 and 7 letters from the letters A and B with repetition allowed?

(A) $\dfrac{1}{8}$

(B) $\dfrac{3}{8}$

(C) $\dfrac{7}{8}$

(D) $\dfrac{7}{9}$

(E) $\dfrac{8}{9}$

22. If the speed of light in a vacuum is 3×10^8 m/s, how long will it take light to traverse 1.2×10^{20} m through the vacuum?

(A) 4×10^{-12} s
(B) 4×10^{-11} s
(C) 6.6×10^{9} s
(D) 6.6×10^{10} s
(E) 4×10^{11} s

23. The sum of three consecutive, positive even numbers is $10y$. If the numbers are $a < b < c$, what is b in terms of y?

(A) $5y$

(B) $\dfrac{5y}{3}$

(C) $\dfrac{10y}{3}$

(D) $\dfrac{10y + 3}{3}$

(E) $\dfrac{10y + 6}{3}$

24. If $n \otimes m = \dfrac{n + m}{n - m}$, then what is $(2 \otimes 3) \otimes 1$ assuming that parentheses work in the standard way? (Operations in parentheses are carried out first.)

(A) $\dfrac{2}{3}$

(B) $\dfrac{-5}{4}$

(C) $\dfrac{5}{4}$

(D) $\dfrac{-6}{5}$

(E) $\dfrac{6}{5}$

25. Three scores have an average of 70 and a variance of 250. If each score is doubled, and then has ten added to it, what are the new average and variance, respectively?

(A) 150, 1,010
(B) 150, 1,000
(C) 150, 510
(D) 150, 500
(E) 140, 1,000

26. 250% of $\dfrac{2}{8}$ is

(A) $\dfrac{1}{8}$

(B) $\dfrac{3}{8}$

(C) $\dfrac{5}{8}$

(D) $\dfrac{6}{8}$

(E) $\dfrac{7}{8}$

27. The probability of getting a red ball is 0.20, and the probability of getting a green ball is 0.8. The probability of a ball being made of ebonite given that it is red is 0.8, but the probability of a ball being made of ebonite given that it is green is 0.9. What is the probability that a randomly picked ball is made of ebonite?

(A) 0.16
(B) 0.72
(C) 0.88
(D) 0.96
(E) 0.99

28. A dentist systematically checks fillings until he finds a faulty one. If the probability that a given filling is faulty is 0.1, and if fillings being faulty are independent events, then what is the probability that the first faulty filling found is on the third tooth inspected?

(A) 0.081
(B) 0.09
(C) 0.2
(D) 0.3
(E) 0.4

29. The mass of a container with its solution is 235 g. If the container has a mass of 135 g, what is the density of the solution? The total volume of the solution and the container is 200 mL, and the density of the container is 27 g/mL.

Density is given as $\dfrac{\text{mass}}{\text{volume}}$.

(A) $\dfrac{9}{13}$

(B) $\dfrac{1}{2}$

(C) $\dfrac{20}{39}$

(D) $\dfrac{47}{40}$

(E) $\dfrac{47}{39}$

30. Water pours into a cylindrical tank at 20 gal/min. If water empties at 5 gal/min, how long will it take to fill a 40 gal tank?

(A) 2 min
(B) $2\dfrac{2}{3}$ min
(C) $2\dfrac{6}{7}$ min
(D) 3 min
(E) $3\dfrac{6}{7}$ min

31. Which of the following is the new value of S, S_{new}, as I is increased by a factor of 1,000 in $S = k \log_{10} I$ in terms of the original S value, S_{old}?

(A) $3k + S_{\text{old}}$
(B) $3kS_{\text{old}}$
(C) $1{,}000k + 3S_{\text{old}}$
(D) $1{,}000k + S_{\text{old}}$
(E) $3{,}000kS_{\text{old}}$

32. A car increases its speed by 20% and then by 50%. What is its percent increase from its original speed?

(A) 35%
(B) 70%
(C) 80%
(D) 90%
(E) 100%

33. a and b are primes, with $a > b$. Which of the following is NOT possible?

(A) a^b is odd.
(B) b^a is odd.
(C) a^b is even.
(D) b^a is even.
(E) $a + b$ is even.

34. $k = Ae^{-\beta/RT}$. Note that e is a constant and that ln is the $\log_e$. What is β?

(A) $-\left(\ln \dfrac{A}{k}\right) = \beta$

(B) $\ln\left(\dfrac{A}{k}\right)^{RT} = \beta$

(C) $-\left(\ln \dfrac{A}{k}\right)^{RT} = \beta$

(D) $\left(\ln \dfrac{k}{A}\right)RT = \beta$

(E) $-(\ln k) = \beta$

35. How many ways can 3 identical balls (cannot be distinguished) be placed into 3 distinguishable urns?

(A) 6
(B) 9
(C) 10
(D) 30
(E) 45

36. The base and height of a rectangle are y and y^2, respectively. The area of the rectangle is given by base(height). If $y = 100$ cm, what is the area of the rectangle?

(A) $1\ \text{m}^2$
(B) $100\ \text{m}^2$
(C) $10{,}000\ \text{m}^2$
(D) $100{,}000\ \text{m}^2$
(E) $1{,}000{,}000\ \text{m}^2$

37. The average of 3 numbers is 30, and the average of 5 other numbers is 70. What is the new average when all 5 numbers are put together?

(A) 45
(B) 50
(C) 55
(D) 60
(E) 65

38. A circular table has 5 seats around it. How many different ways can 5 people be placed in the seats if the seats are indistinguishable?

(A) 24
(B) 120
(C) 720
(D) 725
(E) 730

39.
Column A	Column B

$$\alpha > 1$$

Column A	Column B
$\dfrac{\alpha}{1} + \dfrac{\alpha}{3} + \dfrac{\alpha}{5} + \dfrac{\alpha}{7}$	$\dfrac{15\alpha + 21\alpha + 35\alpha + 105\alpha}{103}$

(A) Column A is greater.
(B) Column B is greater.
(C) Columns A and B are equal.
(D) Cannot be determined

40.
Column A	Column B
The area of triangle $\triangle ABC$	The area of rectangle $ABCD$

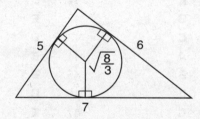

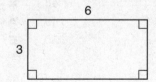

(A) Column A is greater.
(B) Column B is greater.
(C) Columns A and B are equal.
(D) Cannot be determined

Survey of the Natural Sciences Test

1.	B	26.	E	51.	D	76.	D
2.	E	27.	A	52.	A	77.	C
3.	A	28.	C	53.	E	78.	A
4.	B	29.	A	54.	D	79.	B
5.	D	30.	B	55.	C	80.	C
6.	C	31.	D	56.	E	81.	A
7.	A	32.	A	57.	C	82.	C
8.	D	33.	C	58.	A	83.	D
9.	C	34.	E	59.	B	84.	E
10.	E	35.	B	60.	A	85.	C
11.	C	36.	A	61.	B	86.	D
12.	A	37.	D	62.	B	87.	D
13.	D	38.	C	63.	C	88.	B
14.	B	39.	A	64.	A	89.	E
15.	A	40.	D	65.	A	90.	D
16.	E	41.	D	66.	A	91.	B
17.	B	42.	E	67.	D	92.	C
18.	C	43.	B	68.	E	93.	C
19.	A	44.	B	69.	B	94.	D
20.	B	45.	E	70.	E	95.	A
21.	E	46.	D	71.	B	96.	D
22.	C	47.	E	72.	E	97.	A
23.	A	48.	E	73.	D	98.	E
24.	D	49.	A	74.	E	99.	D
25.	B	50.	E	75.	D	100.	E

Perceptual Ability Test

1.	D	24.	D	47.	E	70.	C
2.	E	25.	D	48.	A	71.	C
3.	D	26.	A	49.	B	72.	B
4.	B	27.	C	50.	C	73.	B
5.	A	28.	B	51.	C	74.	B
6.	E	29.	D	52.	A	75.	D
7.	C	30.	A	53.	C	76.	B
8.	E	31.	B	54.	D	77.	B
9.	B	32.	A	55.	A	78.	C
10.	E	33.	C	56.	D	79.	B
11.	C	34.	A	57.	B	80.	D
12.	C	35.	D	58.	C	81.	A
13.	D	36.	A	59.	B	82.	A
14.	C	37.	A	60.	E	83.	B
15.	A	38.	C	61.	A	84.	D
16.	D	39.	B	62.	B	85.	A
17.	C	40.	D	63.	C	86.	D
18.	B	41.	C	64.	B	87.	B
19.	A	42.	B	65.	E	88.	C
20.	B	43.	B	66.	C	89.	C
21.	A	44.	B	67.	B	90.	A
22.	D	45.	A	68.	A		
23.	C	46.	B	69.	D		

ANSWER KEY
Practice Test 2

Reading Comprehension Test

1.	B	14.	D	27.	C	40.	D
2.	D	15.	A	28.	E	41.	E
3.	E	16.	B	29.	D	42.	B
4.	B	17.	C	30.	E	43.	B
5.	C	18.	C	31.	C	44.	E
6.	E	19.	D	32.	C	45.	A
7.	A	20.	C	33.	B	46.	C
8.	A	21.	E	34.	E	47.	C
9.	B	22.	E	35.	D	48.	D
10.	D	23.	A	36.	D	49.	A
11.	D	24.	E	37.	B	50.	D
12.	C	25.	A	38.	E		
13.	D	26.	E	39.	B		

Quantitative Reasoning Test

1.	C	11.	A	21.	C	31.	A
2.	B	12.	E	22.	E	32.	C
3.	E	13.	A	23.	C	33.	C
4.	A	14.	B	24.	A	34.	B
5.	A	15.	A	25.	B	35.	C
6.	B	16.	C	26.	C	36.	B
7.	B	17.	B	27.	C	37.	C
8.	B	18.	B	28.	A	38.	A
9.	B	19.	C	29.	C	39.	B
10.	C	20.	A	30.	B	40.	B

ANSWER EXPLANATIONS

Survey of the Natural Sciences Test

1. **B** A G–C pair has an additional hydrogen bond compared to an A–T pair and is, therefore, more stable. Sequence (1) is DNA and sequence (2) is RNA (U in place of T). (Chapter 2 and Figure 2.2)

2. **E** The synthesis of mRNA from a DNA template is called transcription. The synthesis of a polypeptide from an mRNA sequence is known as translation. Codons are sequences composed of three nucleotides that specify a specific amino acid (genetic code). Anticodons are the corresponding three nucleotides present in the amino acid specific tRNA. (Chapter 7 and Figure 2.4)

3. **A** The amino acid sequence of a protein makes up its primary structure. The secondary structure is made up of a combination of amino acids arranged in α-helixes and β-pleated sheets. The tertiary structure is defined by the way a protein folds. The quaternary structure is made up of the subunits (separate polypeptide chains) of the protein. (Chapter 7 and Figure 2.6)

4. **B** Kinases are enzymes that add a phosphate group to a protein using ATP as the phosphate donor. (Chapter 2 and Figure 2.7)

5. **D** NAD^+ and FAD^+ are coenzymes that function as electron donors and acceptors in oxidation-reduction reactions in metabolic and energy pathways. (Chapters 2 and 3 and Figure 3.8)

6. **C** ATP synthesis specifically takes place in mitochondria in all eukaryotic cells as described by the chemiosmotic theory. (Chapter 3 and Figure 3.8)

7. **A** Members of the domain Archaea are prokaryotic cells that contain proteins, enzymes, and cell components having properties not found in proteins, enzymes, and cell components of members of the domain Bacteria. The atypical properties of these Archaea products allow these cells to grow in environments that would inhibit the growth of many species of bacteria. (Chapter 3)

8. **D** The study of claudistics is the classification of organisms based on phylogenetic relationships. This method is different than those used in the study of taxonomy, phylogenetics, systematics, and evolution. (Chapter 5)

9. **C** The process of reproduction needs to ensure that offspring exhibit genetic fitness, that is, the ability to survive, reproduce, and expand the gene pool of the next generation. This means each offspring must receive a full complement of parental DNA. (Chapter 3)

10. **E** Insulin is a peptide hormone that regulates the metabolism of carbohydrates (glucose). (Chapter 7 and Figure 7.28)

11. **C** Ribosomes are composed of a large and small subunit, each composed of various proteins. The proteins and sizes of the subunits are different between prokaryotic- and eukaryotic-type ribosomes. (Appendix, Figure A.2)

12. **A** The salt gradient across a biological or semi-permeable membrane balances itself over time by the movement of water through the membrane (osmosis). If a balance of salt concentration inside and outside of the membrane is to be achieved, water

(solvent) flows from the side of lowest salt (solute) concentration to that of the highest. A hypertonic solution contains a high concentration of salt, a hypotonic solution contains a low concentration of salt, and an isotonic solution contains salt at a physiological concentration. If the salt concentration is higher inside of a cell than outside, water will rush out causing the cell to shrink or plasmolyze. If the salt concentration is lower inside of a cell than outside, water will rush in causing the cell to swell and eventually burst. If the salt concentration is equivalent inside and outside of the cell, water does not move to any great extent into or out of the cell. (Chapter 2 and Figure 2.13)

13. **D** There are four laws of thermodynamics that define the behavior of the fundamental physical quantities of temperature, energy, and entropy. The zero law of thermodynamics explains the quantity of temperature and states that if two systems are both in thermal equilibrium with a third, then they are in thermal equilibrium with each other. The first law of thermodynamics establishes that perpetual motion machines are not possible and states that energy can be neither created nor destroyed. However, energy can change forms and can flow from one place to another. The total energy of an isolated system does not change. The second law of thermodynamics states that the entropy of an isolated system not in equilibrium will tend to increase over time, approaching a maximum value at equilibrium. The third law of thermodynamics states that the entropy of a system approaches a constant value as the temperature approaches absolute zero. (Chapter 2)

14. **B** On the pH scale a value of 7.0 equals neutrality. Higher values (>7.0) designate basic conditions, and lower values (<7.0) signify acidic conditions. In general, proteins, enzymes, and cellular processes prefer conditions close to neutrality. Environmental conditions below and above this value can be denaturing. (Chapter 2)

15. **A** The ability of offspring to pass on their genetic information to new offspring is a fundamental concept in both asexual (no fusion of gametes) and sexual (fusion of gametes) reproduction. Asexual reproduction is a relatively rapid process that requires only a single parent cell and typically produces two diploid daughter cells. Sexual reproduction is a relatively slow process that requires male and female parent cells and typically produces four haploid daughter cells. (Chapter 3, Figure 3.12, and Figure 3.13)

16. **E** Budding is the most common method of reproduction (asexual) in yeast. Some yeast under certain conditions can reproduce by conjugation (sexual reproduction), but this is a more rare process. Some yeast can form pseudohyphae, but this is not part of the reproductive mechanism. Budding is distinct from binary fission. In the latter process, cells divide into two equal parts. Gametes are typical of sexual reproduction. (Chapter 5 and Figure 5.8)

17. **B** DNA polymerase, as part of the replisome complex, moves along the DNA template strand to create a complementary sequence. Helicase is the enzyme that unwinds the double-strand DNA. (Chapter 3 and Figure 3.3)

18. **C** Gymnosperms or conifers are another type of seed plant distinct from the flowering plants (angiosperms). Bryophytes are non-vascular plants, and monera is an older, commonly used name for the kingdom Bacteria. (Chapter 5, Figure 5.5, and Table 5.1)

19. **A** Alleles are variants or copies of the same gene present on different chromosomes. Therefore, they represent the genotype and not the phenotype of the organism. For example, an individual heterozygous for trait Xx has one dominant (X) and one recessive

(x) allele. Variations in genes can occur by mutation, and these mutated genes can be inherited. (Chapter 7)

20. **B** By definition, haploid and diploid mean one and two sets of chromosomes, respectively. Prokaryotic organisms, such as bacteria, are haploid. Eukaryotic cells are diploid. Organisms that are haploid do not have sex chromosomes and, therefore, cannot exhibit X-linked inheritance. (Chapters 3 and 7 and Figure 7.3)

21. **E** In the respiratory system, oxygen is picked up in the lungs by the heme on red blood cells that arrive via capillaries that are in close contact with the alveoli. The bound oxygen is carried to tissues and cells throughout the body. When oxygen is released, the red blood cells pick up carbon dioxide waste from the cells. The carbon dioxide is exchanged for oxygen when the red blood cells return to the alveoli. (Chapter 7 and Figure 7.8)

22. **C** There are five stages of each heartbeat. Stage 1: the semilunar valves (pulmonary and aortic) close, and the atrioventricular valves (mitral and tricuspid) open. Stage 2: the atria contract, forcing blood from the atria to the ventricles. Stage 3: the ventricles contract, and the atrioventricular and semilunar valves close. Stage 4: the semilunar valves open, and the blood leaves the ventricles. Stage 5: the semilunar valves close. (Chapter 7 and Figure 7.14)

23. **A** Blood clots to prevent excessive bleeding when a blood vessel is damaged. Platelet cells and specific proteins in the plasma of the blood initiate the formation of a fibrous network or clot to seal the injury and, thereby, prevent the leakage of blood. (Chapter 7 and Figure 7.13)

24. **D** Humans with a blood type designated "O" do not have serum antibodies against the red blood cell antigens A and B. Therefore, there is no adverse antibody-antigen reaction when O individuals receive blood from a type A, B, or AB individual. (Chapter 7 and Table 7.2)

25. **B** There are three primary salivary glands in the human oral cavity. They are the parotid, sublingual, and submandibular. (Chapter 7)

26. **E** The green algae are eukaryotic organisms and members of the kingdom Chromista (older terminology Protista). They carry out photosynthesis and reproduce by alteration of generations. (Chapter 5 and Figure 5.4)

27. **A** The role of the lymphatic system is to remove interstitial fluid from tissues, absorb and transport fatty acids and fats from the digestive system, transport white blood cells to and from the lymph nodes into the bones, and transport antigen-presenting cells (dendritic cells) to the lymph nodes to stimulate an immune response. Red blood cells are made in bone marrow, and antibodies are made by plasma cells. (Chapter 7 and Figure 7.16)

28. **C** Endocrine glands characteristically are vascular (containing vessels), store hormones in granules, and do not use ducts to transport hormones. Exocrine glands are less vascular than those of the endocrine system and contain ducts or a lumen (hollow area in a tube). Salivary, sweat, and prostate glands, and those in the gastrointestinal tract, are part of the exocrine system. (Chapter 7 and Table 7.3)

29. **A** There are three major layers of tissue in the human skin: epidermis, dermis, and hypodermis. The epidermis is the outermost layer and is the only layer composed primarily of keratinocytes or epithelial cells. The mesoderm and ectoderm are germ

layers that form during embryogenesis. Myelin is a nonconductive layer surrounding axons. (Chapter 7 and Figure 7.6)

30. **B** Human teeth arise from buds that form from the ectoderm germ layer during organogenesis. The endoderm, mesoderm, and ectoderm are germ layers that form following the gastrula stage of embryogenesis. The archenteron is a primitive digestive tube that forms during gastrulation. (Chapter 7 and Figure 7.2)

31. **D** The gallbladder resides under the liver. Bile, made in the liver, is stored in the gallbladder and released into the duodenum when chyme enters that part of the small intestine. (Chapter 7 and Figure 7.22)

32. **A** Yellow and red bone marrow are made in the long bones. Yellow marrow is made up of fatty connective tissue that serves as an energy source during times of starvation. Blood cells (leukocytes, erythrocytes) and platelets are produced in the red marrow. These cells migrate to the circulatory system from the bone marrow. Sesamoid is a type of bone that is found in joints. (Chapter 7 and Figure 7.8)

33. **C** A synarthrosis joint allows very little or no movement under normal conditions. The plates in the human cranium, which fuse by adulthood, are held together by synarthrosis joints. (Chapter 7 and Figure 7.11)

34. **E** Cartilage is a type of flexible connective tissue that is not as hard or as rigid as bone but is stiffer and less pliable than muscle. It is found between bones in the joints, the rib cage, the ear, the nose, the bronchial tubes, and the intervertebral discs. Members of the Chondrichthyes (cartilaginous fishes, such as sharks, rays, and skates) have a skeleton made of cartilage. (Chapter 7)

35. **B** Some members of the invertebrates and the vertebrates have a notochord, gills, teeth, and/or wings. However, vertebrates have a chambered heart (2–4 chambers), which is lacking in the invertebrates. (Chapter 5 and Table 5.3)

36. **A** Organisms with the basic vertebrate body plan are believed to have appeared approximately 500 million years ago during the Cambrian period. This is the oldest period among those provided as answers. (Chapter 7 and Figure 7.1)

37. **D** Glial cells or neuroglia are nonneuronal structural and metabolic support cells found in the nervous system. These cells support and hold neurons in place, supply nutrients and oxygen to neurons, electrically insulate neurons, destroy pathogens, and remove dead neurons. Glial cells wrap axons of the central nervous system with layers of myelin (a fatty mixture of lipids, cholesterol, and proteins) to electrically insulate them. (Chapter 7)

38. **C** Autotrophs are energy producing organisms that use photosynthesis to produce complex organic carbon compounds from the gaseous single carbon compound CO_2. Heterotrophs consume the complex organic carbon compounds through activities, such as predation, and cycle these compounds through decomposition and fossilization. Some bacteria can fix atmospheric nitrogen in organic nitrogen compounds, but this is not part of the carbon cycle. (Chapter 8 and Figure 8.2)

39. **A** Animal communication is thought to be influenced by instinctive behavioral responses that occur due to the action of "sign" or "releasing" stimuli. These instinctive responses

are known as fixed action patterns (FAPs) (behavioral patterns or acts). FAPs are the most simple kind of behavior in which a specific stimulus results in a "hard-wired" response that, once initiated, is not influenced by environment. FAPs are examples of instinctive or innate behavior. An animal's physical, nondirectional response to a stimulus is known as kinesis. A directional response or movement toward or away from a stimulus is taxis. A simple turning response, such as growth, is a tropism. Some animal species can identify or recognize members of their own species using a type of learning behavior, most commonly observed in birds, known as imprinting. Observational learning occurs through watching the behavior of others. (Chapter 8)

40. **D** An aquatic ecosystem is one that develops in a body of water. The other answers are examples of terrestrial ecosystems. (Chapter 8)

41. **D** For every one molecule of O_2, 2 molecules of Mg are required, which will react to form 2 molecules of MgO.

42. **E** There are 3 sulfate ions in the formula unit, and each sulfate ion contains 4 oxygen atoms. Therefore, there are 12 oxygen atoms in aluminum sulfate.

43. **B** To determine the percent mass composition, take the mass of carbon and multiply it by 4 (there are four carbons in calcium acetate). Then, take that mass and divide it by the total mass of calcium acetate, and then multiply by 100. Choice (A) is the mass percent based only on 2 moles of carbon instead of 4. Choice (C) is the mass percent based only on 1 mole of carbon instead of 4. Choice (D) is the percent mass composition of calcium.

44. **B** The volume of one mole of gas at STP is 22.4 L. Use this to convert moles of oxygen into liters of oxygen:

$$\frac{25 \text{ g } O_2}{1} \cdot \frac{1 \text{ mol } O_2}{32.00 \text{ g } O_2} \cdot \frac{22.4 \text{ L } O_2}{1 \text{ mol } O_2} = 17.5 \text{ L}$$

Choice (A) is a math error with multiplication and division. Choice (C) goes directly from mass to liters without converting to moles first. Choices (D) and (E) use PV = nRT instead of the shortcut (which can be used if done correctly), but choice (D) uses mass of oxygen instead of moles for the variable n, as well as using 298K instead of 273K. Choice (E) uses the wrong temperature (298K instead of 273K).

45. **E** The kinetic molecular theory makes the assumption that gas molecules will collide and have no loss of energy. Therefore, gas molecules have *elastic* collisions. Choices (A) and (C) are related to the kinetic molecular theory because the theory states that there is a lot of empty space between molecules, which allows them to be compressible and have low densities.

46. **D** This is using the combined gas law ($P_1V_1/T_1 = P_2V_2/T_2$) to solve for the new volume of the balloon. STP stands for standard pressure and temperature, which is 1 atm and 0°C (or 273.15K), respectively. To solve for V_2, rearrange the equation: $V_2 = \dfrac{P_1V_1T_1}{P_2T_1}$. Plugging in the numbers into the correct placement results in choice (D).

47. **E** Corner atoms have only $\dfrac{1}{8}$ of an atom inside the cell. There are 8 atoms for the 8 corners ($\dfrac{1}{8} * 8 = 1$ S atom). Face atoms have only $\dfrac{1}{2}$ of an atom inside the cell, and there

are 6 faces ($\frac{1}{2}$ * 6 = 3 O atoms). Therefore, the molecular formula is SO_3, which in this case is also the empirical formula.

48. **E** Ionic compounds cannot conduct electricity in their solid state, but will if melted. Binary compounds can be molecular or ionic, so choice (B) is not the best option.

49. **A** Hydrogen bonding occurs between an H and an N, O, or F. All five compounds have an H and an N, O, or F. However, the other requirement for hydrogen bonding is that the H involved with hydrogen bonding has to be ATTACHED to an N, O, or F as well. Choices (B) and (D) have an H attached to an O, choice (C) has an H attached to a F, and choice (E) has an H attached to an N. The only exception is choice (A), where all three H's are attached to the carbon and not to the F. Therefore, choice (A) cannot participate in hydrogen bonding.

50. **E** The solubility of a compound increases with increasing temperature, which eliminates choice (A). Increasing or decreasing pressure has a higher effect on gas molecules and not as much on solids, which eliminates choice (B). Adding or removing salt is not enough information to know if it would affect the solubility, if at all (i.e., adding or removing NaCl). Choice (E) is correct because adding common ions (such as CrO_4^{2-}) will decrease the solubility of a solid.

51. **D** *Molality*, not to be confused with *molarity*, is the moles of solute divided by the kg of solvent. NaOH is the solute, and ethanol is the solvent. NaOH is already in moles, so it stays as moles. The mL of ethanol needs to be converted to kg:

$$500 \text{ mL} \cdot \frac{0.789 \text{ g}}{1 \text{ mL}} \cdot \frac{1 \text{ kg}}{1{,}000 \text{ g}}$$

Then, take the moles of NaOH and divide it by the kg of ethanol:

$$\frac{2.3}{\frac{(500 \times 789 \times 1)}{1{,}000}}$$

52. **A** Choice (B) has the setup for writing the K_a expression. Choice (C) is the correct setup to calculate the approximate concentration of H^+ ions, which is not the pH. Choice (D) would be correct if HIO was a strong acid, but by looking at the K_a, HIO is a weak acid.

53. **E** Equilibrium constants depend on temperatures, which means the K_w will be different at 40°C instead of 25°C. Since K_w changes, the neutral value on the pH/pOH scale is also changed. Choice (D) would be the correct answer if the solution was at 25°C instead of 40°C.

54. **D** Strong acids and bases do NOT make good buffers, which eliminates choices (A) and (E). Choice (B) has two weak acids, AND they're not conjugate acid/base pairs. Choices (C) and (D) have conjugate acid/base pairs, but choice (C) has a lot more conjugate acid (10 M) than conjugate base (0.1 M). Therefore, choice (D) is the best option.

55. **C** When a reaction is at equilibrium, it does NOT mean the concentrations of products are equal to the concentrations of reactants. Since K_{eq} is small, this means the reactants are favored over the products. Equilibrium occurs when the rate of the forward reaction is equal to the rate of the reverse reaction (choice (C)).

56. **E** With equilibrium, when two equations are added together, the K's are multiplied. This eliminates choices (A), (B), and (D). When a reaction is multiplied by a factor, the K is now raised to that factor, which means it should be $(K_2)^2$, not $2K_2$. Do not get this confused with Hess's Law.

57. **C** The Gibbs free energy equation is: $\Delta G = \Delta H - T\Delta S$. If ΔH is negative, and ΔS is positive, then ΔG will be negative at all temperatures. A negative ΔG means the reaction is spontaneous. Therefore, the reaction is spontaneous at all temperatures.

58. **A** Entropy is a measure of disorder. When two compounds come together to form one, it decreases disorder, which means it decreases entropy. Choice (B) shows a solid becoming a gas, which increases entropy. Choice (C) shows 2 gas molecules separating into 3 gas molecules. Choice (D) increases entropy because melting ice means solid water is turning into liquid water. When entropy increases, ΔS is positive.

59. **B** Rate is measured in M/s or M s^{-1}. The brackets around NO_2 and F_2 stand for molarity (M). To determine the units for k, make sure the units cancel out appropriately:

$$\text{Rate} = k[NO_2][F_2]^2 \rightarrow \frac{M}{s} = (k)(M)(M)^2 = (k)M^3$$

Rearrange the equation to solve for k:

$$\frac{M}{M^3 s} = k = \frac{1}{M^2 s} = M^{-2}s^{-1}$$

60. **A** The rate of the reaction can be expressed in terms of product formation or reactant depletion: $\text{Rate} = -\dfrac{\Delta[NO]}{2\Delta t} = -\dfrac{\Delta[O_2]}{\Delta t} = +\dfrac{\Delta[NO_2]}{2\Delta t}$. Choice (E) is the rate law, and it cannot be determined from the data given if NO is raised to the 2nd power or if O_2 is raised to the first power.

61. **B** Oxygen has an oxidation state of 2−. There are two oxygens, which add up to 4−. The oxidation states of S and the two of O have to add up to the overall charge

$$(S + 2O = -2 \rightarrow S + 2(-2) = -2 \rightarrow S - 4 = -2 \rightarrow S = +2)$$

S has a 2+ oxidation state.

62. **B** Any answer with a product is automatically incorrect because these are the results AFTER the electrons have been transferred. This narrows it down to MnO_2 and HCl. The Mn in MnO_2 starts off with an oxidation state of +4 and goes to +2 in $MnCl_2$. That means Mn gained electrons and is reduced (recall GER/RIG). The Cl in HCl started as −1 for its oxidation state and some of it went to Cl_2 where the Cl has an oxidation state of 0. That means Cl lost electrons and became oxidized (recall LEO/OIL). Therefore, HCl was oxidized since this was the source of Cl atoms.

63. **C** Isotopes have the same number of protons, but a different number of neutrons. This means the type of element does not change (i.e., carbon stays as carbon), but because the number of neutrons changes, the mass changes. Recall that the mass of an atom is the number of protons plus the number of neutrons (electrons have mass, but it is negligible compared to the protons and neutrons). Ions are formed from atoms either gaining or losing electrons, not protons or neutrons.

64. **A** Water has a bent molecular geometry due to two H atoms branching off the oxygen and the two lone pairs. After the oxygen gains a proton, it now only has one lone pair, which gives it the trigonal pyramidal shape (same as NH_3).

65. **A** When Zn loses an electron to become Zn^+, the lost electron will come from the outermost shell. Therefore, the electron configuration of Zn^+ is $[Ar]4s^13d^{10}$. Valence electrons are the electrons in the outermost shell ($4s$), and the $4s$ orbital contains only one electron. Therefore, there is 1 valence electron.

66. **A** Vanadium is a transition metal and not a halogen. Statements I, II, and IV are all true.

67. **D** Electron affinity is the energy change that occurs when an atom *gains* an electron. Anions are *larger* than the neutral atoms from which they are formed. The smallest neutral atom is He. The most electronegative atom is F.

68. **E** Beta decay can be represented with the Greek letter β, which is the same as $_{1}^{0}e$. Using the law of conservation of mass, the atomic mass and atomic numbers on the product side has to equal the atomic mass and atomic number on the reactant side. Using this, the A and Z in $_{Z}^{A}X$ is $_{91}^{230}X(230 - 0 = 230$ and $90 - (-1) = 91)$. Looking at the Periodic Table, element 91 is Pa. Be careful not to pick choice (C) because that is adding $-_{1}^{0}e$ to the wrong side $\left(_{90}^{230}Th + _{-1}^{0}e \rightarrow _{89}^{230}Ac\right)$. Choice (A) is the result if the reaction underwent gamma emission $\left(_{0}^{0}\gamma\right)$. Choice (D) is the result if the reaction underwent alpha decay $\left(_{2}^{4}He\right)$.

69. **B** The dilution factor is represented as (1 : 7), "1 to 7," where 1 unit volume of solute is combined with 6 unit volumes of the solvent medium $(1 + 6 = 7)$. Using $C_1V_1 = C_2V_2$: $(2.1\ M)(1) = X(7)$, where $X = 0.3\ M$.

70. **E** A true statement for choice (E) would be, "Some *systematic* errors can be eliminated (or properly taken into account), but *random* errors are unavoidable."

71. **B** The S_N1 reaction mechanism involves two separate steps. In the first step, a "leaving group" is lost from the substrate and a carbocation forms. Solvent effects often stabilize this step's transition state, and the step is *slow* and rate determining. Thus, these reactions exhibit *first-order* kinetics. Next, in the second step, the carbocation intermediate reacts with a nucleophile to produce the product. This step is fast. If the substrate's leaving group is attached to a chiral carbon center, its loss results in a prochiral trigonal planer carbocation. The nucleophile can approach the flat carbocation, with almost equal access, from either side. This results in an approximately *racemic* product mixture. The only answer that meets these criteria is choice (D).

72. **E** As the structures shown below illustrate, both ions 3 and 5 have an overall formal charge of +1 (only charges greater than zero are shown).

Structures 1 and 4 have overall charges of zero, and the overall charge for structure 2 is −1.

73. **D** A halohydrin has a hydroxyl group attached to a carbon adjacent to a carbon with a halogen atom (usually a Cl or Br atom). The hydroxyl group is deprotonated with a strong base, and the resulting nucleophilic alkoxide anion attacks the back side (in S_N2 fashion) of the adjacent carbon with the halogen-leaving group (a halide ion is lost in the process). See this step of the mechanism below.

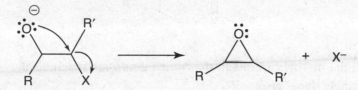

Because the process is concerted and occurs within the same molecule, it is described as being "intramolecular."

74. **E** The oxygen atom in the given compound has four electron groups surrounding it (a lone pair and three bonding pairs). To use these electron groups for bonding and nonbonding interactions, the oxygen atom must form four hybrid orbitals. It accomplishes this by combining a *p* and 3 *s* atomic orbitals to produce four sp^3 hybrid orbitals. The lone pair shown on the oxygen occupies one of these sp^3 orbitals. The correct answer is choice (E).

75. **D** The provided reaction energy diagram shows a rather steep increase in energy as reactant A reaches an energy maximum at point B (the energy of the reaction's transition state). The energy difference between the reactant and the transition state indicates that the reaction has a large activation energy (E_a), and, due to this barrier, will proceed to product *slowly*. The diagram also shows that relative to the reactant, the product's energy is much lower. Thus, the reaction's overall energy change is negative ($-\Delta G$), and energy is released during the process. Reaction processes with a ΔG of less than zero are described as *exergonic* and are spontaneous (choice (D)).

76. **D** Based on the given conditions, this reaction will proceed through an S_N1 mechanism. The strong acid (HCl) will protonate the hydroxyl group of the alcohol making it a better leaving group. In the next step, the loss of the leaving group as water will create a secondary carbocation. This will be followed by a hydride shift from the adjacent tertiary carbon to create the lower energy tertiary carbocation shown below.

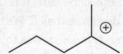

This species will next undergo nucleophilic attack by a chloride anion (left over from the ionization of HCl) to form the *major* product—choice (D). It should be noted that there might be some minor product formed from chloride anions reacting with the initial secondary carbocation (choice (C)).

77. **C** A decoupled ^{13}C NMR spectrum of the compound (*t*-butyl acetate) will show *four* peaks. As the numbered carbons on the structure shown below indicate, there are four magnetically nonequivalent carbons in the compound.

Note that all the methyl carbons in the *t*-butyl group are magnetically equivalent and appear as a single signal peak.

78. **A** Based on the given conditions, this reaction will produce primarily product (A). The bromine reactant will add to the double bond through the usual cyclic bromonium ion intermediate (anti-addition). The $FeCl_3$ will catalyze the bromination of the aromatic ring of the styrene reactant in the *meta* position (the alkene group attached to the benzene ring is a mild deactivator). This results in a tribrominated product (choice (A)).

79. **B** The compound, 1-chloro-2-fluorocyclopentane, contains two chirality centers and, thus, can exist as four stereoisomers ($2^2 = 4$). The possible configurations of these isomers are *RR*, *SS*, *RS*, and *SR*. This analysis shows *two* pairs of enantiomers are possible—the *RR*/*SS* pair and the *RS*/*SR* pair. All the other possible stereoisomer relationships are diastereomeric. As an example, the *RR* isomer is shown below.

80. **C** The given molecular formula (C_6H_{10}) indicates two degrees of unsaturation. This analysis makes choice (C) impossible because such a compound would require three degrees of unsaturation (*one* for the ring and *two* for the triple bond).

81. **A** The reader may recall that when a double bond has two high priority groups (using the C-I-P prioritization rules) on the same side, it is designated as *Z*, and when they are on opposite sides, the isomer is designated as *E*. With this in mind, the designations for the four double bonds in the given tetraene are as follows: *E, Z, Z, E* (choice (A)).

82. **C** The referenced structure contains a double bond, two fluoro groups, and a methyl substituent. The double bond has the highest priority, so the compound will be named as an alkene (suffix -ene). The longest carbon chain containing the double bond is seven carbons in length (hepta). Numbering the chain from *right to left* assigns the first carbon in the double bond the number "3" (numbering from the other direction gives the starting carbon in the double bond the number 4—the lower number must be used in the name). Thus, the root name of the compound will be 3-heptene. Using the numbering sequence described above, the two fluoro groups and the methyl substituent are assigned the numbers 3, 4, and 5, respectively. The molecule also contains a chirality center at carbon number 5. Its absolute stereochemical configuration is *R* (using the C-I-P rules). Finally, the double bond based on its configuration (both the higher priority fluoro

groups are on the same side) is designated as Z. Putting this all together gives choice (C): (Z)-3,4-difluoro-(5R)-methyl-3-heptene.

83. **D** Anhydrides, because the carboxylate anion is a very good leaving group, are easily hydrolyzed. Amides and esters are relatively stable toward this process, and thus choices (A) and (B) can be eliminated. The structures shown for choices (C) and (D) are both anhydrides, but trifluoroacetic anhydride's carboxylate anion will be more stabilized due to the electron withdrawing effect of the fluorine atoms attached to its methyl groups relative to acetic anhydride (choice (C)). Choice (D), trifluoroacetic anhydride, is the most reactive of the compounds shown and is the most susceptible to hydrolysis.

84. **E** Structure (E) has the largest number of conjugated double bonds (4). This long π system allows for significant electron delocalization and lower energy radiation absorption. This compound would be expected to absorb UV radiation around 300 nm. All the other compounds have shorter conjugated π systems.

85. **C** The reactant shown in this question is an "imine." Imines are hydrolyzed by acid to ammonium ions and ketones or aldehydes. In this case, the reaction will open the imine "bridge" in the six-membered ring to give a single product with a methyl ketone on one end and an ammonium ion on the other. In the second step, the ammonium ion is deprotonated with a weak base ($NaHCO_3$) to give the free amine. All the choices except for (C) can be eliminated, for among other reasons, they don't contain a methyl ketone group.

86. **D** The amoxicillin molecule contains *four* chirality centers (each is marked with an asterisk in the structure shown below).

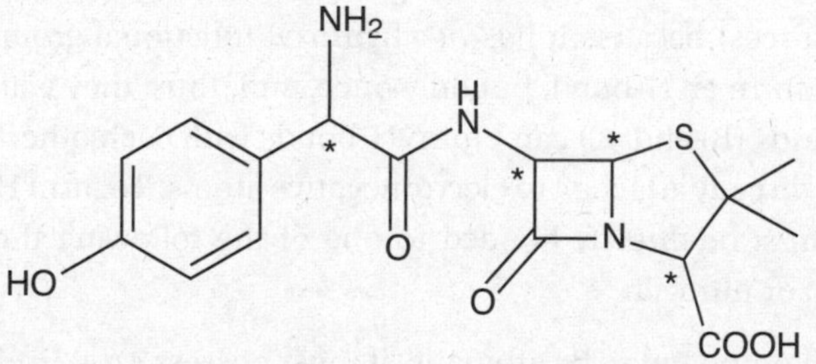

Using the formula, 2^n = the number of possible stereoisomers, where in this case $n = 4$, gives 16 possible isomers—choice (D).

87. **D** The most efficent way to produce the product shown for this reaction is by a Diels-Alder cycloaddition. The reactants required for this process are a diene and a dieneophile with attached electron withdrawing groups (in this case, nitro groups are present on all the dieneophiles). Only conjugated dienes (the two double bonds must alternate with a single bond) react with dieneophiles to form cyclic products. Choice (B) can be eliminated because the reactant diene is not conjugated. The product shown is bicyclic, and based on its structure, requires a cyclohexadiene reactant. This eliminates choices (A) and (E) because they show cyclopentadiene as a reactant. The *trans* configuration of the nitro groups in the product means the dieneophile must also be *trans*. Choice (C) can be eliminated on this basis—the nitro groups are *cis* in this dieneophile. That only leaves choice (D) (cyclohexa-1,3-diene + *trans*-1,2-dinitroethene) as the correct answer.

88. **B** The most commonly used combination of reagents to convert a hydroxyl group into an alkyl chloride is thionyl chloride ($SOCl_2$) and a basic solvent such as pyridine (choice (B)). Because the last step of this process involves an S_N2 mechanism, the reaction works best for primary and secondary alcohols. The pyridine is protonated in the reaction and combines with one of the chloride ions from the thionyl chloride to produce a pyridinium hydrochloride salt. Choices (C) and (D) will not produce the given product (they might produce a mixture of chlorinated alcohols in low yield). The rates of the reactions using the reagents show in choices (A) and (D) will be very slow. Both of these routes are not practical for producing the given product.

89. **E** The first thing the reader should note from a quick review of the given data is the small number of signals seen in the ^1H and ^{13}C NMR spectra—only two in each case. This information, along with the given molecular formula of the unknown, indicates a high degree of symmetry in the structure of the compound. On this basis alone, choices (B) and (C) can be eliminated. Planes of symmetry can be easily seen in the structures for choices (A), (D), and (E), so we move on to the IR data, which clearly indicate the presence of one or more carboxylic acid functional groups (both the O–H and C=O stretch bands are present in the spectrum). The structure for compound (A) is a diester and will not exhibit an O–H stretch band in the IR, so it can be eliminated. This leaves choices (D) and (E). The structure for compound (D) doesn't match the given molecular formula. The structure for choice (E) shows the required symmetry to match the NMR data, the carboxylic acid function group consistent with the IR, and it matches the given molecular formula—choice (E) is the clear winner.

90. **D** Of the compounds shown, structure (D), 1,2-propanediol, will have the highest boiling point. This molecule is capable of forming two hydrogen bonds (one of the strongest intermolecular forces) because it has *two* hydroxyl functional groups. Compounds (A) and (E) can also form an H-bond, but only once, and, thus, they will have lower boiling points. Compounds (B) and (C) can't form H-bonds with each other because they don't contain protons directly attached to electronegative atoms. To form H-bonds, hydrogens in a molecule *must* be directly bonded to one of the following three types of atoms: fluorine, oxygen, or nitrogen.

91. **B** In order for a compound to be aromatic, it must possess $4n + 2\pi$ electrons (where n is a positive whole integer). In addition to this criterion, the compound's π bonding system must be *cyclic, conjugated* (the double bonds must alternate with single bonds), and in a *planar* conformation. All the compounds shown *except* the structure for choice (B) meets these requirements. The compound shown for choice (B) does potentially have 6π electrons (if the lone pair on the nitrogen atom is included), but the ring's π system is broken up by an sp^3-hybridized carbon next to the nitrogen atom. This tetrahedral carbon distorts the required planer conformation of the ring—this compound is not aromatic.

92. **C** Of the Newman projections for choices (A) through (E), the projection shown for choice (C) would exhibit the lowest energy. The methyl groups in this projection are involved in two *gauche* interactions where methyl groups in the structure closely approach each other. This condition is energetically unfavorable and costs ~3.8 kJ/mol per interaction. Choices (B) and (D) show projections where methyl groups are starting to *eclipse* each other. This type of interaction is even more unfavorable than the gauche sited above

and each one costs ~11. kJ/mol. The projection shown in choice (D) has two eclipsed interactions making it the least stable of all the conformations shown. The projections for choices (A) and (E) both have three gauche interactions, making them equally stable, but they are both less stable than the projection shown for choice (C) with only two such interactions. It's a good idea for you to commit to memory the approximate energies associated with the gauche and eclipsed conformations. This allows for a quick way to judge the relative stabilities of different conformations of small alkane molecules.

93. **C** The easiest way to determine what hybrid orbitals are used for bonding by carbon centers is to count the electron groups around the center. Electron groups can be any bonding group (single, double, and triple bonds all count as one electron group) or nonbonding group (loan pairs and a single electron—as in a radical, each count as one group). The first carbon in the molecule starting from the left (as the instructions specify) has four electron groups around it and is thus sp^3 hybridized. The next three carbons, again from the left, have three electron groups and are all sp^2 hybridized. The last carbon on the far right in the triple bond has two electron groups and is sp hybridized. A summary of the hybridization of the carbon atoms in the molecule is shown below (choice (C)).

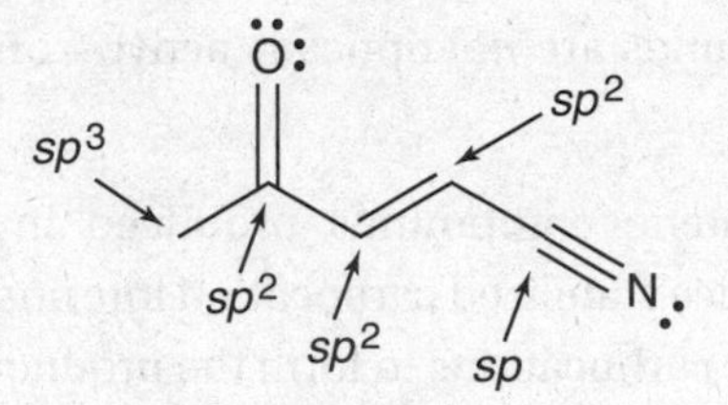

94. **D** The ethene molecule contains two central sp^2 hybridized carbon atoms as show in the structure below.

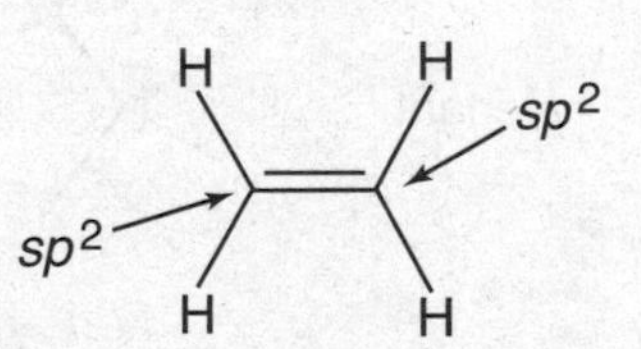

The bonding geometry around each of the carbons will be *trigonal planar*. The trigonal planar shape associated with each of the carbon atoms in the molecule will result in all the bond angles being ~120°.

95. **A** The reaction sequence shown is similar to the classic *acetoacetic ester synthesis* enol addition process. Except in this case, both of the carbonyl functional groups are esters. In the first three steps of the process, the base sodium ethoxide is use to deprotonate the methylene carbon in between the two carbonyl groups of the esters. This is followed by the nucleophilic attack of the anion produced in the first step via an S_N2 mechanism on the bromopropane reactant (shown in step 2). This gives an alkylated intermediate—a propyl chain is added to the central carbon in the starting diester. The reaction sequence is then repeated a second time to add another propyl chain (step 3). In step 4, acid is used to hydrolyze the ester groups and then is followed by heat, which causes one of the carboxylic acid groups to be lost as carbon dioxide (CO_2). This decarboxylation process is characteristic of 1,3-dicarboxylic acid compounds. The given reaction sequence

produces the carboxylic acid shown in choice (A). All the other choices show either dicarboxylic acid or ester functional groups, which aren't consistent with step four of the sequence—decarboxylation.

96. **D** Sodium sulfate and magnesium sulfate are drying agents used to remove water from a liquid organic phase. They are generally added and rapidly stirred with an organic phase to remove water prior to solvent removal and isolation of an organic compound after a reaction. The solid hydrate of these agents is generally removed by filtration just prior to solvent evaporation. None of the effects described in the other answer choices would be accomplished by adding these compounds to the reaction mixture.

97. **A** In order for a Diels-Alder reaction to proceed at a reasonable rate, the diene must have an s-*cis* conformation for the correct geometric overlap with the dieneophile's π system (choice (A)). Dienes with an s-*trans* conformation either react very slowly or not at all in Diels-Alder processes (choice (C) is eliminated). Choices (B) and (D) are references to the dieneophile and are not relevant to the question. To line up and correctly overlap with the dieneophile, the diene must be planar (choice (E) is eliminated).

98. **E** All the structures shown for the answer choices are *meso* compounds (they all contain an intramolecular reflective plane of symmetry), except for the structure shown for choice (E). Meso compounds are *not* optically active—only compound (E) will exhibit optical activity.

99. **D** The bromo-cyclopentene compounds produced in this addition reaction will proceed through resonance stabilized carbocation intermediates. Nucleophilic bromide anions will react with the carbocations to form the products. As shown below, four pairs of enantiomers will be formed (choice (D)).

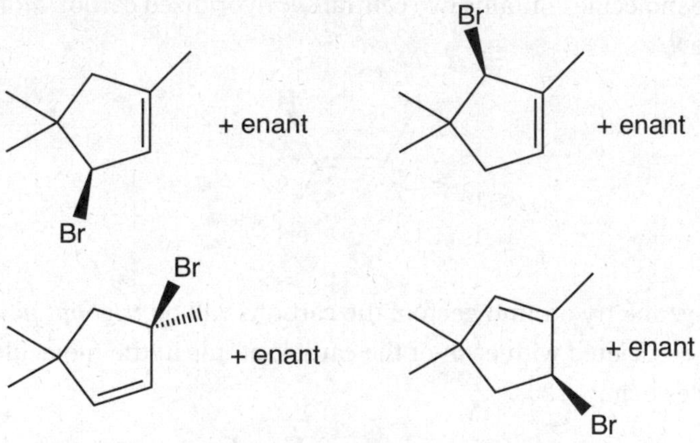

Each stereoisomer will contain one chirality center, and their respective *R* and *S* mirror images will be formed in equal amounts (a racemic mixture). All the compounds will be constitutional isomers of each other and cannot be expected to form in equal amounts (the carbocations they form from are *not* all equal in energy).

100. **E** *All* the structures for the answer choices have the same molecular formula ($C_6H_{12}O$) and are, thus, constitutional isomers of each other. Only structures 2 and 4, however, are also stereoisomers of each other (*Z* and *E* isomers, respectively). This makes choice (E) the only possible correct answer.

Perceptual Ability Test

1. **D** Entry-3.

2. **E** Entry-2.

3. **D** Entry-2.

4. **B** Entry-2, after 90 degree rotation counterclockwise.

5. **A** Entry-2, after 90 degree, counterclockwise, 180 degree rotation. Note small notch.

6. **E** Entry-3, after 90 degree clockwise and 180 degree rotation.

7. **C** Entry-3, rotated 90 degrees clockwise, 90 degree rotation. Note notches.

8. **E** Entry-2, note number of sides and position of side extrusions.

9. **B** Entry-1, note positions of angular surfaces.

10. **E** Entry-2, after 90 degree rotation clockwise.

11. **C** Entry-2, note thickness beneath notch.

12. **C** Entry-2, note relative positions of notches.

13. **D** Entry-3, note position of extension.

14. **C** Entry-2, note positions and sizes of notches.

15. **A** Entry-1, note relative sizes and positions (planes) of notches.

16. **D** Note front and end views show hidden lines.

17. **C** Note front view shows 6 lines (3 hidden), and partial enclosure.

18. **B** Note positions of circles relative to object sides and each other.

19. **A** Note end view shows 6 lines, 3 hidden above full-length enclosure.

20. **B** Note front view shows 5 solid lines. Note size of lower extension.

21. **A** Side shows extension toward front and 1 hidden line. Note hidden mid-line.

22. **D** End view shows 5 lines. Note the position of hidden lines.

23. **C** Front view shows 5 lines, 2 hidden.

24. **D** Front view shows 3 lines, all solid.

25. **D** End view shows 9 lines. Note positions of bottom lines, solid lines, and enclosure.

26. **A** Top view shows 6 lines, 2 hidden. Note relative positions.

27. **C** Front view shows 5 solid lines.

28. **B** Note omissions.

29. **D** Front and end views show 3 lines at top.

30. **A** End view shows 7 lines. Note position of hidden lines.

31. **B** 1 appears smallest (omit A, C), 4 appears smaller than 3 (omit D).

32. **A** 4 appears smallest (omit C), 1 appears largest (omit B, D).

33. **C** 2 appears smallest (omit B, D), 3 appears largest (omit A).

34. **A** 3 appears smallest (omit B, D), 2 appears smaller than 4 (omit C).

35. **D** 4 appears largest and 1 appears smallest (omit A, B, C).

36. **A** 2 appears smallest (omit C, D), 3 appears smaller than 1 (omit B).

37. **A** 4 appears smallest (omit B, C), 2 appears largest (omit D).

38. **C** 2 appears smallest (omit A, D), 3 appears largest (omit B).

39. **B** 1 appears smallest (omit C), 2 appears largest (omit A, D).

40. **D** 3 appears smallest (omit B, C), 1 appears largest (omit A).

41. **C** 1 appears smallest (omit B, D), 2 appears largest (omit A).

42. **B** 3 appears largest (omit A, C, D).

43. **B** 3 appears smallest (omit A, C, D).

44. **B** 3 appears largest (omit A, C), 4 appears smaller than 1 (omit D).

45. **A** 1 appears smallest (omit B, C), 3 appears smaller than 2 (omit D).

46. **B** 2 folds at final position (omit A, E), 1 unfold identifies B.

47. **E** 3 folds at final position (omit A, B), 2 unfolds identify E.

48. **A** 4 folds at final position (omit D, E), 2 unfolds identify A.

49. **B** 8 folds at final position (omit A, C, D), 2 unfolds identify B.

50. **C** 4 folds at final position (omit A, D, E), 2 unfolds identify C.

51. **C** 4 folds at final position (omit A, B, D), 2 unfolds identify C.

52. **A** 2 folds at final position (omit B, D, E), 2 unfolds identify A.

53. **C** 6 folds at final position (omit A, B, D, E).

54. **D** 6 folds at final position (omit A, B, C, E).

55. **A** 3 folds at final position (omit B, D, E), 1 unfold identifies A.

56. **D** 4 folds at final position (omit A, C, E), 1 unfold identifies D.

57. **B** 8 folds at final position (omit D, E), 2 unfolds identify B.

58. **C** 4 folds at final position (omit A, B, D, E).

59. **B** 2 folds at final position (omit A, D, E), 1 unfold identifies B.

60. **E** 6 folds at final position (omit A, B, C, D).

61. **A** Notice 2 partially hidden cubes (2, 3 painted surfaces).

62. **B** Notice 2 partially hidden cubes (2, 3 painted surfaces).

63. **C** Notice 2 partially hidden cubes (2, 3 painted surfaces).

64. **B** Notice 2 partially hidden cubes (2, 3 painted surfaces).

65. **E** Notice 3 fully hidden cubes (1, 1, 2 painted surfaces).

66. **C** Notice 3 fully hidden cubes (1, 1, 2 painted surfaces).

67. **B** Notice 1 fully hidden cube (2 painted surfaces).

68. **A** Notice 1 fully hidden cube (2 painted surfaces).

69. **D** Notice 1 fully hidden cube (2 painted surfaces).

70. **C** Notice 2 partially hidden cubes (3, 2 painted surfaces).

71. **C** Notice 2 partially hidden cubes (3, 2 painted surfaces).

72. **B** Notice 2 partially hidden cubes (3, 2 painted surfaces).

73. **B** Notice 2 partially hidden cubes, 1 fully hidden cube (4, 4, 3 painted surfaces).

74. **B** Notice 2 partially hidden cubes, 1 fully hidden cube (4, 4, 3 painted surfaces).

75. **D** Notice 2 partially hidden cubes, 1 fully hidden cube (4, 4, 3 painted surfaces).

76. **B** Focus on adjoining sides.

77. **B** Focus on adjoining sides of the eight-sided figure.

78. **C** Focus on all object shapes and proportions.

79. **B** Notice relative positions of the shaded and nonshaded three-sided figures.

80. **D** Focus on relative positions of the halved square.

81. **A** Focus on relative positions of the shaded side (nonsquare).

82. **A** Focus on the larger clear three-sided figure.

83. **B** Note number of sides and shape of shorter lines of three-sided figures.

84. **D** Focus on small squares relative to the shaded four-sided figure.

85. **A** Focus on relative positions of the shaded half-square and shaded squares.

86. **D** Focus on positions of the sides and joining point.

87. **B** Focus on the split square and adjoining shadowed three-sided figure.

88. **C** Focus on the split square, adjoining four-sided figure, and split small rectangle.

89. **C** Focus on the long rectangle, smaller "end-caps," and positions of "points."

90. **A** Notice the available shapes and number of these shapes.

Reading Comprehension Test

1. **B** The reader is being asked to describe the main idea or purpose of the passage. You can eliminate choices (A) and (D) since they are not mentioned at all. You can also eliminate choices (C) and (E) because they are only mentioned briefly. Choice (B) correctly summarizes the passage.

2. **D** This inference question asks the reader if the passage supports future printing choices. The informational passage discusses advancements, current technology, advantages, and the need to reduce cost and time. Every choice except (D) can be eliminated since only fabrication methods are reviewed, and the author provides no conclusions.

3. **E** This inference question asks the reader to identify similarities between printing methods. Choices (A) and (D) are described in the passage.

4. **B** This retrieval question asks the reader if a central theme exists between all the printing methods. Irrelevant of the method used to fabricate a prostetic, knowledge and understanding of computer software and file formats is mandatory for understanding any of the mentioned technologies.

5. **C** This retrieval question asks the reader to compare the printing methods and identify the most expedient one. Choice (A) requires wax-up time, spruing, and investing with excessive postprocessing. Choices (B) and (D) are not subtractive manufacturing methods; they are additive methods. No information is presented on GLS manufacturing.

6. **E** This retrieval question asks the reader to compare two printing methods. SLA and FDM differ by the type of material used to print (ABS filament versus photosensitive polymers), curing method (room temperature of air versus ultraviolet laser), movement of the build plate (x-y direction versus z direction), and accuracy.

7. **A** This retrieval question asks the reader to determine a manufacturing method that requires technique and accuracy. Paragraph 6 states that "Traditional methods of fabrication require numerous steps that include impression making, model fabrication, transporting models back and forth to the dental laboratory, casting metal, adding porcelain, finishing, polishing, and storage of casts. Every step in the fabrication process requires a thorough understanding of the coefficient of thermal expansion and manipulation of materials to avoid ill-fitting prostheses." The only manufacturing method discussed that requires numerous steps is the lost-wax casting technique.

8. **A** This retrieval question is discussed in paragraph 5(f). "The model is fabricated by ejecting heated plastic filament through a nozzle or extrusion head onto a controlled moving table. As it cools and hardens, successive layers are added."

9. **B** This retrieval question is discussed in paragraph 5. The author states that in order to meet growing expectations and patient demands, dental professionals will be required to understand new materials, techniques, and technologies. These technologies include cone beam tomography, modeling software, and postprocessing of prostheses.

10. **D** This inference question is discussed in paragraph 5(e). BJP is similar to other technologies, although the primary advantage is that "This is a fast, low-cost printing method that enables stress-free structures with complex internal and external geometries, and, since no heat or residual stresses are built into the fabricated part, the final product is extremely accurate."

11. **D** This retrieval question is discussed in paragraphs 5(c) and 5(d). Although the processes appear to be similar, metal powder used with a laser light source and a build plate, the difference is that SLS requires heating, sintering, and postproduction processing. Once the SLM laser fuses the atomized metal powder to the developing model, no postprocessing is required.

12. **C** This retrieval question is discussed in paragraph 5. The biggest disadvantage is the solid block of material and tooling required for successive removal of material layers. Most manufacturing methods require a .stl file to generate g-code to operate the control-

ler motors. The passage does not discuss the time or sintering requirements for subtractive manufacturing.

13. **D** This inference question is discussed in paragraph 5(e). With no resin binding the material layers together in the correct orientation on the build plate, the model would slump and have gross inaccuracies after the sintering process.

14. **D** This retrieval question is discussed in paragraph 2: "Currently, dental impressions, gypsum models, or structures of the head and neck are scanned using desktop or hand-held intraoral scanner cone beam computed tomography (CT). Depending on the resolution, scanners vary in price and are available in fixed or portable units." The quality of the prosthesis is dependent on the accuracy of the scanner, .stl file format software, and the printing method. All methods described produce acceptable results.

15. **A** This retrieval question is discussed in paragraph 5(f). "Typically, the extrusion head is capable of moving in the x- and y-axis to complete the layer and will move up to start a new layer, while the table moves in a z-axis." The z-axis is the vertical axis (up and down) component of the build plate.

16. **B** This retrieval question is discussed in paragraph 5(a). "The wax pattern is then placed on a sprue, waxed to a sprue base, placed inside a casting ring, and invested in a phosphate bonded investment material." The casting ring and paper liner hold the phosphate bonded investment material. There is no polymer coating surrounding the model.

17. **C** This is a retrieval question discussed in paragraph 2. The sterolithography file format describes triangulated surfaces that approximate the shape of the object. The triangles do not describe color or texture, or use a three-dimensional Cartesian coordinate system. The passage does not describe software programs that utilize this system.

18. **C** This retrieval question asks the reader to identify the file format used to fabricate the image shown in Figure 1. Paragraph 2 describes the stereolithography (.stl) file format and its use in 3D printing.

19. **D** This tone question asks the reader to identify the author's attitude or style during overseas travel. The word "concerned" refers to welfare, happiness, or interest of a person. Throughout the passage, the author describes a curious optimism and concern as the journey unfolds. Each transportation hub presents a new mode of movement and circumstances to overcome.

20. **C** This inference question asks the reader to describes the author's journey to a location critical to his unit's and his headquarter's overall strategic mission. The other responses were not described in the passage.

21. **E** The main idea of the passage is to understand the author's physical, mental, and emotion challenges while traveling overseas. From the arrival at the processing station to the final walk into the medical clinic, the author describes his five-day struggle of navigating his transformation from a civilian to a military health-care provider.

22. **E** This is an extrapolation question asking for the reader's opinion or judgment after reviewing the passage. After reviewing all the responses, the reader should infer that all the responses are reasonable and are supported by the passage.

23. **A** This inference question asks the reader if security of personnel and equipment was evident throughout the journey. The author describes classes, safety briefings, travel conditions, and time of travel to help the reader understand internal and external threats. Without security of personnel and equipment, the mission would be unachievable.

24. **E** This inference question asks the reader to describe the relationship of the duffle bag contents to the author's mission. Paragraph 1 describes the contents and wearing of some of the items during his journey. The items discussed were worn as protection for different possible scenarios.

25. **A** This inference question asks the reader to describe the quality and quantity of training for deploying personnel. The author makes light of the rudimentary movement techniques taught, but fails to reveal the personnel involved or any specific training for the essential personnel.

26. **E** This retrieval question is described in paragraph 7. The vehicle driver provides an insight into what the author will experience during his tour of service. All the responses are correct.

27. **C** This retrieval question is described in paragraph 7. The vehicle driver answers the author's question about weather in the statement "he weather forecast yesterday was very hot and dusty, today's weather forecast is very hot and dusty, tomorrow the weather will be very hot and dusty, and next week the weather will be very hot and dusty."

28. **E** This sequence question is described in paragraphs 2 through 9. The other responses are out of sequence.

29. **D** This tone question requires the reader to understand the definitions of the adjectives used to describe the author's attitude. *Parsimonious* means stingy or cheap; *overwhelmed* refers to being given too much; *exasperated* means being annoyed or irritated; and *frustrated* refers to the inability to change or achieve an outcome. To feel *ambivalent* means to have mixed feelings about a particular thing.

30. **E** This retrieval question asks the reader to identify the author's feelings during the processing, transition, and when departing the airfield on a bus and helicopter. Paragraphs 3 and 6 describe the author's uneasiness and uncertainty based on *personal* testimonies.

31. **C** This retrieval is described in paragraph 9. "I only had to motivate myself to carry 30 pounds of personal equipment and my 160-pound frame, and lift and carry four dreaded olive-green duffle bags 200 yards."

32. **C** This retrieval question asks the reader to describe what mode of transportation caused a sense of sickness or uneasiness for the passengers. Paragraph 6 describes helicopter maneuvers to prevent the engagement of direct fire from personnel on the ground. Based on the speed and maneuvers of the helicopter, motion sickness caused at least one casualty.

33. **B** This retrieval question is described in paragraph 5. "When putting on a five-pound helmet with a sweaty helmet band for the umpteenth time, looking through scratched protective goggles, with body armor stuck between soaking layers of uniform, a rucksack containing all the immediate emergency needs, and flying into the middle of nowhere, it makes you suddenly realize you'd better believe in something . . . ."

34. **E** This calculation question is described in paragraph 2. The total number of personnel on the aircraft is 330 and the total number of duffle bags is 1,200.

$$330 \times 190 = 62,700 \text{ pounds}$$

$$1,200 \times 75 = 90,000 \text{ pounds}$$

$$\text{TOTAL} = 152,700 \text{ pounds}$$

35. **D** This is a retrieval question discussed in paragraph 3. "Similar to Portland cement, the dental profession uses the term cement or 'luting agent' to provide retention of the restoration placed over the tooth structure and seal the margin around the crown. The retention and sealing of the restoration is accomplished by a combination of the tooth preparation and type of luting agent."

36. **D** This main idea question is asking the reader to summarize the passage. Two materials are presented—concrete and dental cement. The components of each are discussed and similarities are drawn. Choices (A), (B), (C), and (E) are discussed, but choice (D) best summarizes the author's purpose for the passage.

37. **B** This retrieval question is described in paragraph 6(c). There are several methods used to retain a restoration to tooth structure, but chemical retention requires the carboxyl group of the cement bonds with the calcium ions on the tooth structure. The calcium ions replace the hydrogen on the carboxyl group to make calcium polysalts.

38. **E** This retrieval question is described in paragraph 5(a). The "gold-standard" of cement refers to water-based cements having a film thickness of less than 25 microns. Choices (A), (B), (C), and (D) fit this description.

39. **B** This is a retrieval question described in paragraph 4. "Tooth preparation is probably the most important requirement for the restoration's long-term success." All other responses aid in retention, but tooth preparation is the primary requirement.

40. **D** This is an inference question described in paragraph 5(a). "This cement requires the addition of zinc and magnesium oxide powder and phosphoric acid liquid mixed over several minutes to dissipate the heat of the reaction." The other responses are not discussed in the passage.

41. **E** This is a retrieval question discussed in paragraph 5(c). "The liquid component is primarily eugenol with olive oil and the reaction takes place with the formation of zinc eugenolate chelate." The other responses have different mechanisms of reaction.

42. **B** This retrieval question is discussed in paragraph 2(e). "Sulfur (SO_3), at 1 to 3 percent, helps control the expansion of setting cement."

43. **B** This main idea question asks the reader to understand the relationship between cement and dental luting agents. The passage describes microscopic and macroscopic properties of cements to inform the reader of the components, chemical reactions, and methods of action. The other responses are briefly mentioned.

44. **E** This inference question is discussed in paragraph 5(c). All other choices are discussed and relevant to water-based cements.

45. **A** This retrieval question is described in paragraph 5(b). Choice (A) is not a characteristic of resin cement. "The characteristics of this cement are high bond strengths, technique sensitivity, separate monomer and polymer components, and multiple clinical purposes."

46. **C** This retrieval question is described in paragraph 6(a). "Mechanical retention depends on small undercuts or irregular surface on the tooth from the bur that prepared the tooth surface and small grooves from the fabrication of the inside of the restoration." All the other choices are incorrect.

47. **C** This is a retrieval question described in paragraph 1. "The components are simple: sand, gravel, cement powder, water, and air when mixed together produces a flowable mass that hardens when set." All the other choices are incorrect.

48. **D** This is a retrieval question described in paragraph 5(b). "Without the specific bonding agents, the resin cements are considered very strong luting media, which have only modest bond strengths to dentin. The use of bonding agents and primers is, therefore, essential in obtaining optimal results."

49. **A** This retrieval question is described in paragraphs 5(b) and 6. "Resin cements undergo a polymerization reaction. The characteristics of this cement are high bond strengths, technique sensitivity, separate monomer and polymer components, and multiple clinical purposes." In addition, "Dental cement, along with resistance and retention form of the tooth, seal and retain the crown to the remaining tooth structure. Other forces supply additional strength to the tooth and crown, such as mechanical, chemical, and micro-mechanical forces."

50. **D** This is a retrieval question described in paragraph 2. "The components and percentage of mixture is important in the production of the five types or categories of Portland cement. The types of cement reflect requirements for sulfate resistance in wet environments, setting times, properties, and strength requirements. Altering the components changes the cement type and usage." The other choices are not discussed in the passage.

Quantitative Reasoning Test

1. **C** If the number of historians is doubled, and the number of anthropologists is tripled, the ratio would become $(1 \times 2) : (2 \times 3) = 2 : 6 = 1 : 3$. Thus, the total number of people must be a multiple of 4 since you cannot have a part of a person attending. 8 is the only multiple of 4.

2. **B** The first win has already occurred, and the events are independent, so the probability of two more wins occurring is $\left(\frac{1}{5}\right)\left(\frac{1}{5}\right) = \frac{1}{25}$.

3. **E** You can pick numbers, such as 100. But, we will note that if a is the original population, then the population increases by $\frac{2}{5}a$ to give $\frac{2}{5}a + a = \frac{7}{5}a$. So, the population is at $\left(\frac{7}{5}\right)\left(\frac{7}{5}\right)\left(\frac{7}{5}\right)a = \frac{343}{125}a$. This is $\frac{343}{125}$ of the original population a.

4. **A** Please note that in actual G-chem, the K_{eq} would not change in many situations; the other concentrations would change. This looks like G-chem, but it is not. The equation and information are given to you.

Pick numbers. Set K_{eq} to be 100. Set [C] to be 100, [A] = 10, [D] = 1, and [B] = 1. Then,

$$100 = \frac{[100]^2[1]^1}{[10]^2[1]^3}$$ works. Increase [C] by 50% to 150, and decrease [A] by 20% to 8. Then,

$$\frac{[150]^2[1]^1}{[8]^2[1]^3} = \frac{22{,}500}{64}.$$

The percent increase is given by $\dfrac{final - initial}{initial} \times 100\%$.

$$\frac{\dfrac{22{,}500}{64} - \dfrac{6{,}400}{64}}{100}$$

$$\frac{\dfrac{16{,}100}{64}}{100} \times 100\% = \frac{16{,}100}{64} = 251.56$$

Although many DAT problems give you "nice" answers and problems that can be solved without a calculator, we wanted you to get a little practice in estimating.

Looking at the answers, you can see that no answer except choice (A) is over 200, and even without really calculating, it is clear that $\dfrac{16{,}100}{64} > 200$.

5. **A** You can pick numbers. Let $x = 3$. Then $3^2 = 9 > 8 = 4(3) - 4$. So, choice (A) wins. 0 and negative numbers (which are always good choices of numbers) are not tested since $x > 2$. So, let's try a "big" number like 1,000. $1{,}000^2 > 4(1{,}000) - 4$. It appears that (A) is bigger.

If you are not satisfied with that you can try pretending both sides are equal and see if anything reasonable occurs:

$$x^2 = 4x - 4$$

$$x^2 - 4x + 4 = 0$$

$$(x - 2)^2$$

But, this gets us to $(x - 2)^2 \geq 0$, which is always true.

So, $x^2 - 4x + 4 \geq 0$.

$x^2 \geq 4x - 4$.

Since $x > 2$, $x - 2$ cannot be zero, so $(x - 2)^2 > 0$. $x^2 > 4x - 4$.

6. **B** We notice that

$$2^1 = 2$$
$$2^2 = 4$$
$$2^3 = 8$$
$$2^4 = 16$$
$$2^5 = 32$$

So, the ones digit repeats on every fifth power; that is, it cycles through groups of four. This means that the ones digit cycles 2, 4, 8, 6, and so 2^{75} cycles 18 times with 3 left over ($\frac{75}{4}$ gives 18 with a remainder of 3). The 3 left over take us through "2," "4," and "8." So, the ones digit of $2^{25\alpha} + 5 \sim 8 + 5 \sim 13 \sim 3$.

7. **B**

$$k_B \ln a^b + k_B \ln y^b = k_B (\ln a^b + \ln y^b) = k_B (\ln a^b y^b) = k_B \ln (ay)^b = b(k_B \ln ay)$$

8. **B** This can be done with the "conditional probability formula," but a faster way might be to notice that if a 5 has been rolled, then the only way to get a 10 is to roll another 5. The likelihood that this will happen is $\frac{1}{6}$.

9. **B** Instead of going for y and x, attack $6y + x$.

$$2(10y + 4x = 7)$$
$$- (14y + 7x = 3)$$
$$\overline{\qquad\qquad\qquad}$$
$$6y + x = 11$$

10. **C** There are 2 ways to pick the first ball (since there are 2 even numbered balls). After first ball is chosen, there are 5 choices for the next ball. After the second one is chosen there are 4 choices for the third pick. This gives $2(5)(4) = 40$ ways. Note that each ball is distinguishable since any two with the same number have different colors.

11. **A** This is a multinomial. There are 5! ways to arrange the letters if they were all distinct. The overcount with the O's and T's is 2!(2!). So, the total count is $\frac{(5)(4)(3)(2)(1)}{(2)(1)(2)(1)}$.

12. **E** This is a straightforward application of $P(A \cup B) = P(A) + P(B) + P(A \cap B)$. P(green tea, black tea, or both) = P(green tea) + P(black tea) – P(green tea and black tea) = $0.3 + 0.2 - 0.05 = 0.45$. Don't forget that $P(A \cup B)$ indicates the probability of (A, B, or both).

13. **A** In the range given, sin, cos, and tan will all be positive. Let's construct a triangle with $0 \leq \theta \leq \frac{\pi}{2}$ and $\cos \theta = \frac{3}{5}$. Any right triangle that meets these requirements will do since all of the right triangles satisfying these conditions will be similar. Try the right triangle:

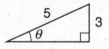

Remember that $\cos \theta = \dfrac{\text{adjacent}}{\text{hypotenuse}}$.

Using the Pythagorean theorem, we get that the other side is 4.

$$3^2 + b^2 = 5^2 \rightarrow b = 4$$

Since $\cos \theta = \dfrac{\text{adjacent}}{\text{hypotenuse}} = \dfrac{4}{5}$ and $\tan \theta = \dfrac{\text{opposite}}{\text{adjacent}} = \dfrac{3}{4}$, column A is bigger.

14. **B** This problem can be done in many ways, but students often actually find the "formulaic" solution easier: $P(A \mid B) = \dfrac{P(A \cap B)}{P(B)}$.

P(both are wins | at least 1 win) = P(both are wins AND at least 1 win)/P(at least 1 win).

We can make our lives easier by noticing that P(both wins AND at least 1 win) = P(both are wins) since having both tries be wins and also at least one win is equivalent to both tries being wins.

P(both are wins | at least 1 win) = P(both are wins)/P(at least 1 win)

P(both are wins) = $\dfrac{3}{10}\left(\dfrac{3}{10}\right) = \dfrac{9}{100}$

P(at least 1 win) = $1 - P$(no wins) = $1 - \dfrac{7}{10}\left(\dfrac{7}{10}\right) = \dfrac{51}{100} \rightarrow P$(at least 1 win) = $\dfrac{51}{100}$

P(both are wins)/P(at least 1 win) = $\dfrac{\frac{9}{100}}{\frac{51}{100}} = \dfrac{9}{51}$

15. **A** Let's look at statement (1). Since we have used the technique of picking numbers many times, especially in the context of percentages, we know that we can pick 100 as the starting amount in order to compute a percent increase. (See the Arithmetic Section—Percentages if you are rusty.) Following that procedure we know that we will get an answer. The whole point of data sufficiency is to NOT compute the actual answer whenever possible. For actual computations, see the Percentages section. So, (1) is sufficient.

Now, (2) is not sufficient by itself since knowing that the initial amount is 20 L gives us no clue as to the percent increase in volume.

(A) Statement (1) alone is sufficient, but statement (2) alone is not sufficient.

16. **C** A fast solution might be to code the colors as letters: R, R, R, B, B. The number of ways to arrange these is a multinomial computation: $\dfrac{5!}{3!2!} = 10$. Another way is to do the same thing but realize that we can think of the 5 "places" to place the letters as numbered 1–5 and that picking any 3 of them to be R would determine the sequence:

$$\binom{5}{3} = \dfrac{5!}{3!2!} = 10$$

Common mistakes: Students sometimes think 5! is the solution, forgetting that books of the same color are indistinguishable. Some students think that 3!2! works, but this would count the number of ways of arranging 3 distinguishable red books and 2 distinguishable blue books with blue books before red books. (In fact, this could count many such things: the number of ways of arranging 3 distinguishable red books and 2 distinguishable blue books with red books before blue books, etc.)

17. **B**

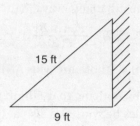

15 ft

9 ft

From the picture, we see that the length of the ladder is the hypotenuse of a right triangle and the distance from the wall is one side. We can use the Pythagorean theorem to get the height of the ladder above the ground. It might be faster to realize that this is, in fact, a Pythagorean triple: 3, 4, 5. Remember that multiples of triples work, too. So, we have 3×3, **something**, 5×3. Our "something" is $4 \times 3 = 12$.

18. **B** You can pick a number such as 10 since we are working with a percentage problem; however, 59% of 35% of $A = 0.59(0.35)(A)$ and $0.35(0.59)(A)$ are equal.

19. **C** One way to do this is to think of picking the special edition first. There are 5 ways to do this. Then, from the remaining four pick two. $\begin{pmatrix} 4 \\ 2 \end{pmatrix} = \dfrac{4!}{2!2!} = 6$. There are a total of $5(6) = 30$ ways to do this.

20. **A** The apple juice present is $0.8(10) + 0.2(20) = 12$ L. The total solution has $10\ L + 20\ L = 30\ L$. So, the fraction that is apple juice is $\dfrac{6}{15}$.

21. **C** We can ignore the letters D since, regardless of the letters chosen, the probability of getting an even number remains the same. Since we have a three digit code and are trying to get at least one even number, the easiest way is find the probability of the complement: (all odd) $= \dfrac{1}{2}\left(\dfrac{1}{2}\right)\left(\dfrac{1}{2}\right) = \dfrac{1}{8}$. The probability of getting at least one even number is $1 - \dfrac{1}{8} = \dfrac{7}{8}$.

22. **E** Distance = Rate(Time). Time $= \dfrac{\text{Distance}}{\text{Rate}}$. We divide 1.2×10^{20} m by 3×10^8 m/s to get 4×10^{11} s. You might want to think of this as 12×10^{19} divided by $3 \times 10^8 = 4 \times 10^{11}$.

23. **C** Let the three numbers be a, b, and c. Since the numbers are all consecutive, positive even numbers, the "middle" number is the average of the three. To compute the average, we add the numbers up and then divide by 3. The sum is already given to us as $10y$. So, the average is $\dfrac{10y}{3}$.

24. **A** For this sort of algebra problem, just remember that n and m are "place holders," in a sense, and plug in.

$$n \otimes m = \frac{n+m}{n-m} \ (2 \otimes 3) \otimes 1 = \left(\frac{2+3}{2-3}\right) \otimes 1 = \frac{5}{-1} \otimes 1 = -5 \otimes 1 = \frac{-5+1}{-5-1} = \frac{-4}{-6} = \frac{2}{3}$$

25. **B** The average behaves nicely: $2(70) + 10 = 150$. But, the variance changes by squaring the factor and is unaffected by addition: $2^2(250) = 1,000$.

26. **C** This can easily be done with a calculator, but the computation is fast if we look at the numerator. 250% of 2 is 5. (50% of 2 is 1, and 200% of 2 is 4.) So, the answer is $\frac{5}{8}$.

27. **C** This problem follows from the "sum rule."

$P(\text{ebonite}) = P(\text{ebonite/red})P(\text{red}) + P(\text{ebonite/green})P(\text{green})$

$P(\text{ebonite}) = 0.8(0.2) + 0.9(0.8) = .88$

Where does this come from?

$P(\text{ebonite}) = P(\text{ebonite and red}) + P(\text{ebonite and green})$

$P(\text{ebonite and red}) = P(\text{ebonite|red})P(\text{red})$

$P(\text{ebonite and green}) = P(\text{ebonite|green})P(\text{green})$

See example #9 in the Probability section for a refresher.

28. **A** Since the events are independent, the probability of finding GOOD, GOOD, FAULTY is $0.9(0.9)(0.1) = 0.081$. Note the $P(\text{GOOD}) = 1 - 0.1 = 0.9$.

29. **C** This is NOT a chemistry question. If it were, you would not be given the definition of density. Following the formula, we need $\frac{\text{mass}}{\text{volume}}$. The mass of the solution is the mass of the [solution + container] – the mass of the [container] = 235 g – 135 g = 100 g.

To get the volume of the container, we use the formula again. Density $= \frac{\text{mass}}{\text{volume}}$.

$$27\text{g/mL} = \frac{135}{\text{volume}} \rightarrow \text{volume} = 5 \text{ mL}$$

Volume of the solution = 200 mL – 5 mL = 195 mL.

Density of the solution $= \frac{100}{195} = \frac{20}{39}$ g/mL.

30. **B** Distance = Rate × Time

This is another rate problem. The rate is 20 gal/min – 5 gal/min = 15 gal/min, and the "distance" to be covered is 40 gal. The time is $\frac{40}{15} = 2\frac{2}{3}$.

31. **A** This is practice with logs. $S = k\log_{10}I \rightarrow$ if we increase I by a factor of 1,000,

$S_{\text{new}} = k\log_{10}1,000I = k\log_{10}((1,000)(I)) = k(\log_{10}1,000 + \log_{10}I) = k\log_{10}1,000 + k\log_{10}I = k(3) + S_{\text{old}}$

32. **C** Pick 100. Then, the increases lead to 100 + 20 = 120 followed by 120 + .5(120) = 180. The percent increase is then $\frac{\text{final} - \text{initial}}{\text{initial}} = \frac{180 - 100}{100} = 80\%$.

33. **C** Remember that primes are numbers that are only divisible by themselves and 1. So, 2 is the only even prime since all even numbers are divisible by 2. Let's use the strategy of picking numbers. Say $a = 5$ and $b = 3$. Then,

$$5^3 = 125$$
$$3^5 = 243$$
$$3 + 5 = 8$$

kills A, B, and E.

2 is the only even prime (and the smallest prime) and since $a > b$, a cannot be 2, but b can be 2. Let $a = 3$ and $b = 2$. $2^3 = 8$ kills b^a is even. But, $3^2 = 9$ shows why C is the right answer. Since a cannot be even, a must be odd. And, an odd number to any power is still odd. For more help with parity (odd and even) problems, see *www.youtube.com/user/Swartwoodprep*.

34. **B** This is a drill on log properties.

$$\frac{k}{A} = e^{-\beta/RT}$$

$$\ln \frac{k}{A} = -\beta/RT$$

$$\left(\ln \frac{k}{A}\right) R(T) = -\beta$$

$$-\left(\ln \frac{k}{A}\right)(RT) = \beta \rightarrow -RT\left(\ln \frac{k}{A}\right) = \beta \rightarrow \ln\left(\frac{k}{A}\right)^{-RT} = \beta \rightarrow \ln\left(\left(\frac{k}{A}\right)^{-1}\right)^{RT} = \beta \rightarrow \ln\left(\frac{A}{k}\right)^{RT} = \beta$$

35. **C** This is one of those DAT problems that can be solved by trying out cases. A quick way is to write out:

1. 1 way in which one ball is placed into each urn
2. 3 ways in which all three balls are placed in the same urn (urn 1, urn 2, or urn 3)
3. 6 ways to place 2 balls in one urn and 1 ball into another

Imagine having 3 choices for which urn to place the group of 2 balls into and then having 2 choices for which urn to place the other ball. This gives 3(2) = 6.

This gives 1 + 3 + 6 = 10 ways. There is a systematic way to do this, but is not worth our time here. For the curious, please see *www.youtube.com/user/Swartwoodprep*.

36. **B** This is NOT a typo. The answer is C. If you bothered to compute the answer in cm², you would have gotten $100(100^2) = 1,000,000$ cm² = 100 m². However, if you cleverly switched from 100 cm to 1 m from the beginning, you would have gotten $1(1^2) = 1$ m², which is wrong. Why? The problem lies with the fact that the equations base = y and height = y^2 represent different rectangles when different units are used (y, y^2 given one rectangle in cm but a different one in m). Do not let this stress you out—many beginning engineering students (not to mention future dentists) are tripped up by this unit conversion issue. So, why is this problem here? The DAT sometimes has stressful problems (supposedly to keep everyone from getting 30s), but that does not have to stop you from easily topping out (or even getting a 30) if you miss this but keep pushing through the DAT.

37. **C** A direct way is to use average = $\frac{\text{total}}{\text{number}}$.

Then, $30 = \frac{\text{total}}{3} \rightarrow 90 = \text{total \#1}$.

$$70 = \frac{\text{total}}{5} \rightarrow 350 = \text{total}$$

Combined total = 440.

$$\text{average} = \frac{440}{8} = 55$$

38. **A** The answer choices suggest A or B since 5! = 120 seems like the greatest number of ways of arranging 5 things where order matters. But, this assumes that the seats are distinguishable. Since the seats are indistinguishable, we cannot differentiate among seating setups/scenarios in which the people have been rotated around the table in the same way. Pick any particular seating and any particular person, say Rila. For the sake of argument, number the seats 1–5, and let Rila be in seat 1. If everyone's configuration around Rila remains the same, we can move Rila to any of the 4 other seats without changing the seating. This, of course, requires moving everyone else so that they sit the same way around Rila. There are 5 places Rila can be with the same configuration. Since we cannot tell seats 1–5 apart, we cannot distinguish these 5 different arrangements. So, 5!, which assumes that the seats are distinguishable, overcounts 5 times. We must divide by 5 to fix the overcount.

$$\frac{120}{5} = 24$$

39. **B** While this can be solved the usual way, it is faster, perhaps, to notice that:

1. The common denominator is $1(3)(5)(7) = 105$. The equivalent fractions when a common denominator of 105 is used are 105α, $5(7)\alpha$, $3(7)\alpha$, and $3(5)\alpha$.
2. These are exactly the terms in the numerator of the number in column B.
3. But, the denominator is less implying that the fraction on the right is bigger since $\alpha > 1$.

40. **B** The area of the rectangle is $3(6) = 18$.

The area of the triangle can be computed by using the picture below. The smaller triangles have a height of $\sqrt{\frac{8}{3}}$ and bases of 5, 6, and 7. The total area is then

$$\left(\frac{1}{2}\right)\sqrt{\frac{8}{3}}(5) + \left(\frac{1}{2}\right)\sqrt{\frac{8}{3}}(6) + \frac{1}{2}\sqrt{\frac{8}{3}}(7) = \sqrt{216}$$

We can crunch this through the calculator or notice that $18 = \sqrt{18^2} = \sqrt{324}$ is bigger than $\sqrt{216}$.

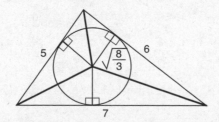

PRACTICE TEST 2

Index